DATE DUE

SEP 27 1994	
OCT 1 0 1994	
OCT 2 1 1994	
NOV - 7 1994	
NOV 2 2 1994	
DEC - 9 1994	
FEB 1 0 1995	
FEB 2 2 1995	
APR 1 7 1995 DEC - 5 1995	
JAN 2 4 1996	
FEB 23 1996	
OCT 2 8 1996	
MAR 2 4 1997	
APR 1 2 1997	
MAR 1 8 2000	
DEC - 8 2000	

BRODART   Cat. No. 23-221

Neurological Aspects of Substance Abuse

Neurological Aspects of Substance Abuse

John C. M. Brust, M.D.

PROFESSOR OF CLINICAL NEUROLOGY, COLUMBIA UNIVERSITY COLLEGE OF PHYSICIANS AND SURGEONS; DIRECTOR, DEPARTMENT OF NEUROLOGY, HARLEM HOSPITAL CENTER, NEW YORK, NEW YORK

Butterworth-Heinemann

Boston London Oxford Singapore Sydney Toronto Wellington

Every effort has been made to ensure that the drug dosage schedules
within this text are accurate and conform to standards accepted at time of
publication. However, as treatment recommendations vary in the light of
continuing research and clinical experience, the reader is advised to verify
drug dosage schedules herein with information found on product information
sheets. This is especially true in cases of new or infrequently used drugs.

Recognizing the importance of preserving what has been written, it is the
policy of Butterworth-Heinemann to have the books it publishes printed on
acid-free paper, and we exert our best efforts to that end.

Library of Congress Cataloging-in-Publication Data

Brust, John C. M. (John Calvin M.), 1936–
    Neurological aspects of substance abuse/John C. M. Brust.
       p.   cm.
    Includes bibliographical references and index.
    ISBN 0-7506-9005-4 (alk. paper):
    1. Psychopharmacology.   2. Substance abuse.   I. Title.
    [DNLM: 1. Substance Abuse.   2. Neurologic Manifestations.
    3. Nervous System—drug effects.   WM270 B912n 1993]
    RM316.B78   1993
    615′.78—dc20
    DNLM/DLC
    for Library of Congress   93-15290
                                                                    CIP

British Library Cataloguing-in-Publication Data

A catalogue record of this book is available from the British Library.

Butterworth-Heinemann
80 Montvale Avenue
Stoneham, MA 02180

10 9 8 7 6 5 4 3 2 1

Printed in the United States of America

For Meridee, Mary, Frederick, and James

Contents

Preface

Reminiscent of "The Sorcerer's Apprentice," we are awash in a deluge of redundant medical texts. Nevertheless, my colleague Dr. Lewis P. Rowland persuaded me that neurologists would welcome a book on drug abuse. If you disagree, blame him. If you agree with the premise but don't like the product, blame me.

The title has been carefully considered, for it is my view that most biomedical aspects of drug abuse are in fact neurological. Accordingly, the text addresses pharmacology and animal studies, overdose and withdrawal, medical and neurological complications, fetal effects, and pharmacotherapy. Historical background and epidemiology are also considered, partly because the subject is often quite entertaining and partly because contradictory and bizarre societal attitudes toward particular substances are better understood in an historical context.

Some of this material has appeared in a chapter on drug dependence I wrote for Joynt's *Clinical Neurology*, and I thank the publishers at Harper & Row for letting me occasionally plagiarize my own sentences without fear of copyright infringement. I also thank Dr. Robert Joynt for inviting me to write that chapter, without which I doubt I would have had the fortitude to proceed with the present text.

Other thanks are due to Nancy Megley, formerly at Butterworth, for early encouragement; Christopher Davis, also formerly at Butterworth, whose cheerful patience remained unflagging as one promised delivery date after another receded into the future; Susan Pioli, currently at Butterworth, who brought the final product to the finish line; Sandra Sands, Janet Rivera, and Jeffrey Green for indispensable assistance with the manuscript; Dr. Edward B. Healton and Ellen Giesow of the Columbia P&S Dean's office at Harlem Hospital Center, for support tangible and intangible; and—even though his suggestion effectively demolished 52 consecutive weekends—Dr. Lewis P. Rowland.

John C. M. Brust, M.D.
New York, New York

Neurological Aspects of Substance Abuse

Chapter 1
Questions and Definitions

Giving up smoking is easy. I've done it hundreds of times.
—Mark Twain

Just say no.   *—Nancy Reagan*

What Do We Mean by *Dependence, Addiction,* and *Abuse*?

In 1964, the World Health Organization (WHO) Expert Committee on Addiction-Producing Drugs recommended that the terms *drug addiction* and *drug habituation* be replaced by *drug dependence,* defined as:

> a state of psychic or physical dependence, or both, on a drug, arising in a person following administration of that drug on a periodic or continuous basis. The characteristics of such a state will vary with the agent involved . . . for example, dependence of morphine type, of barbiturate type, of amphetamine type, etc.[1]

Psychic dependence is " . . . a feeling of satisfaction and a psychic drive that requires periodic or continuous administration of the drug to produce pleasure or avoid discomfort." Physical dependence is " . . . an adaptive state that manifests itself by intense physical disturbances when the administration of the drug is suspended or when its action is affected by administration of a specific antagonist." Psychic dependence thus induces "psychic" symptoms and compulsive drug-seeking behavior. Physical dependence induces "physical" symptoms and objective signs. Psychic and physical dependence can occur independently or together, and only mind-brain dualists need concern themselves over the *voluntary* or *nonorganic* aspects of the former and the *involuntary* or *organic* aspects of the latter.

These definitions were subsequently subjected to a fair amount of tinkering. For example, in 1982, a WHO memorandum suggested replacing *physical dependence* with *neuroadaptive state* and explicitly distinguished dependence from *drug-related disability.*[2]

The American Psychiatric Association's Diagnostic and Statistical Manual (DSM-III-R), moreover, has its own set of criteria for dependence and abuse (Tables 1–1 and 1–2).[3] Nevertheless, the original definitions of physical and psychic dependence have remained in general usage.

Addiction is psychic dependence. An *addict* is someone whose psychic dependence—with or without physical dependence—has made drug procurement a daily preoccupation. Addiction used to be equated with physical dependence; it was believed that prolonged exposure of neurons to a drug led to adaptive responses, which in turn led to craving, which in turn led to drug-seeking. Such a sequence of events would occur whether the drug was self-administered (by an animal or human) or passively administered (by an investigator or nurse). In fact, many patients who receive morphine passively for pain have prominent withdrawal symptoms yet little or no craving for the drug. Conversely, abstinent tobacco smokers often have intense craving without observable physical signs. Conditioning and learning are crucial to the development of addiction[4]—as emphasized by the U.S. Surgeon General, when in 1988 he pronounced tobacco an addictive drug.[5]

The term *drug abuse* is a social judgment. One might be considered a drug abuser for using an illegal substance (e.g., heroin or cocaine), for using a legal substance in amounts that others consider excessive (e.g., ethanol), or for using a legal substance in any amount (e.g., tobacco). Pharmacologists often use the term *abuse liability* to signify a drug's potential for inducing addictive behavior; indeed, that concept is the basis of Drug Enforcement Administration (DEA) drug scheduling under the 1970 Controlled Substances Act (Table 1–3). In clinical

Table 1–1. DSM-III-R Diagnostic Criteria for Psychoactive Substance Dependence

At least 3 of the following:
1. Substance often taken in larger amounts or over a longer period than the person intended
2. Persistent desire or one or more unsuccessful efforts to cut down or control substance use
3. A great deal of time spent in activities necessary to get the substance, taking the substance, or recovering from its effects
4. Frequent intoxication or withdrawal symptoms when expected to fulfill major role obligations at work, school, or home or when substance use is physically hazardous
5. Important social, occupational, or recreational activities given up or reduced because of substance use
6. Continued substance use despite knowledge of having a persistent or recurrent social, psychological, or physical problem that is caused or exacerbated by use of the substance
7. Marked tolerance: need for markedly increased amounts of the substance (i.e., at least a 50% increase) to achieve intoxication or desired effect, or markedly diminished effect with continued use of the same amount

Note: The following items may not apply to cannabis, hallucinogens, or phencyclidine:
8. Characteristic withdrawal symptoms
9. Substance often taken to relieve or avoid withdrawal symptoms

Some symptoms of the disturbance have persisted for at least 1 month or have occurred repeatedly over a longer period of time

Modified from Diagnostic and Statistical Manual of Mental Disorders, Third Edition–Revised. Washington, DC: American Psychiatric Association, 1987, with permission of the publisher.

Table 1–2. DSM-III-R Diagnostic Criteria for Psychoactive Substance Abuse

A maladaptive pattern of psychoactive substance use indicated by at least 1 of the following:
1. Continued use despite knowledge of having a persistent or recurrent social, occupational, psychological, or physical problem that is caused or exacerbated by use of the psychoactive substance
2. Recurrent use in situations in which use is physically hazardous

Some symptoms of the disturbance have persisted for at least 1 month or have occurred repeatedly over a longer period of time

Never met the criteria for Psychoactive Substance Dependence for this substance

Modified from Diagnostic and Statistical Manual of Mental Disorders, Third Edition–Revised. Washington, DC: American Psychiatric Association, 1987, with permission of the publisher.

practice, however, abuse is not the same as addiction. Even one-time use of a drug is abuse if it causes harm to oneself—for example, cocaine—or to others—for example, ethanol. Conversely, although by the above-mentioned definition caffeine is an addicting drug, its legality and lack of perceived harmfulness allow coffee drinkers to pass their days free of social stigma. As we shall see, in the United States neither addiction liability nor physical harm has much bearing on a drug's legal status.

What Is *Tolerance* and What Does It Have to Do with Physical Dependence and Addiction?

Tolerance is " . . . an adaptive state characterized by diminished response to the same quantity of drug or by the fact that a larger dose is required to produce the same degree of pharmacodynamic effect."[1]

There are several kinds of tolerance. Metabolic, dispositional, or pharmacokinetic tolerance results from increased metabolism and decreased availability of the drug at its locus of action. Cellular or pharmacodynamic tolerance, on the other hand, is a reduced response despite unchanging drug concentrations and availability; it signifies an adaptive change in the brain.[6]

Different from pharmacokinetic and pharmacodynamic tolerance are behavioral and environmental tolerance. Behavioral tolerance is a reduced response consequent to a drug's negative effect on reward-seeking or punishment-avoiding behavior.[7] For example, rats intoxicated with ethanol and performing equilibratory tasks develop tolerance to the drug's ataxic effects faster than rats not being tested.[6] Environmental tolerance is the result of a drug being administered in a setting of familiar cues.[8] It could be considered an atypical pavlovian response. Pavlov observed classical conditioning in dogs receiving morphine injections (the unconditioned stimulus); after enough trials, the appearance of the technician (the conditioned stimulus) was sufficient to produce morphine-like effects of salivation, vomiting, and sleep.[9] By contrast, animals receiving morphine "in the context of pre-drug cues" may be *less* sensitive to its analgesic, thermic, locomotor, sedating, and even lethal effects than animals tested in an unfamiliar setting.[8,10] This particular conditioned response—environmental tolerance—seems to result from an *anticipatory compensation*, which attenuates the drug's effect, perhaps by causing environmentally cued changes in drug disposition.[11]

The interrelationships between tolerance, physical dependence, and drug-seeking behavior are complex.[12] In animals, tolerance and physical dependence

Table 1–3. Controlled Substances (Generic Components and Representative Brands), 1992

Schedule I (High Potential for Abuse, No Accepted Medical Use)
Benzymorphine
Dihydromorphine
Heroin
Ketobemidone
Levomoramide
Lysergic acid diethylamide (LSD)
Marijuana
Mescaline
Morphine methylsulfonate
Nicocodeine
Nicomorphine
Peyote
Psilocybin

Schedule II (High Potential for Abuse, Currently Accepted Medical Use)

Generic Components	Representative Brand
Alfentanil HCl	Alfenta
Amobarbital sodium	Amytal Sodium
Amphetamine/dextroamphetamine	Biphetamine
Amphetamine sulfate	Amphetamine Sulfate
Atropine/meperidine	Atropine and Demerol
Cocaine HCl	Cocaine HCl
Codeine	Codeine
Dextroamphetamine sulfate	Dexedrine
Dronabinol	Marinol
Fentanyl citrate	Duragesic
Fentanyl/droperidol	Innovar
Glutethimide	Glutethimide
Hydromorphone HCl	Dilaudid-HP
Hydromorphone/guaifanesin	Dilaudid Cough Syrup
Levorphanol	Levo-Dromoran
Meperidine HCl	Demerol HCl
Meperidine/acetaminophen	Demerol APAP
Meperidine/promethazine	Mepergan
Methadone HCl	Dolophine HCl
Methamphetamine HCl	Desoxyn
Methyphenidate	Ritalin
Morphine sulfate	Infumorph
Opium	Opium
Opium alkaloids	Pantopon
Opium/belladonna	B.&O. Supprettes
Oxycodone HCl	Roxicodone
Oxycodone/acetaminophen	Percocet
Oxycodone/aspirin	Percodan
Oxymorphone HCl	Numorphan HCl
Secobarbital-amobarbital	Tuinal
Secobarbital/phenobarbital/ Butabarbital	Tribarb
Sufentanil citrate	Sufenta

Schedule III (Accepted Medical Use, Lower Potential for Abuse than Schedule I and II Drugs)

Generic Components	Representative Brand
Aspirin/phenacetin/caffeine/codeine	A.P.C. w/Codeine
Acetaminophen/codeine	Phenaphen w/Codeine
Aprobarbital	Alurate
Aspirin/codeine	Empirin w/Codeine
Benzphetamine HCl	Didrex

Table 1–3. *Continued*

Generic Components	Representative Brand
Bismuth/calcium carbonate/opium	Diabismul
Bismuth/kaolin/pectin/paregoric	Biskapec
Butabarbital sodium	Butisol Sodium
Butalbital/caffeine/acetaminophen	Fembutal
Carisoprodol/codeine/aspirin	Soma Compound w/Codeine
Chlorpheniramine/pseudoephedrine/ caffeine/ aspirin/codeine	Vanex
Chlorpheniramine/pseudoephedrine/ hydrocodone	Notuss
Chlorpheniramine/phenylephrine/ hydrocodone/acetaminophen	Hycomine Compound
Chlorpheniramine/phenylephrine/ phenylpropanolamine/hydrocodone	Chemdal HD
Chlorpheniramine/phenylephrine/ codeine/ acetaminophen	Colrex Compound
Chlorpheniramine/phenylephrine/ codeine	Chem-Tuss NE
Chlorpheniramine/phenylephrine/ hydrocodone	Tega-Tussin
Codeine/butalbital/caffeine/aspirin	Florinal w/Codeine
Codeine/butalbital/acetaminophen	G-2
Codeine/salicylamide/acetaminophen	Tega-Code
Codeine/salicylic acid/acetaminophen/caffeine	Codalan
Danazol	Danocrine
Dihydrocodone/aspirin/caffeine	Synalgos-DC
Dovers/atropine/aspirin/phenacetin/caffeine	Kolcaps
Fluoxymesterone	Halotestin
Guaifenesin/codeine	Marcof
Hydrocodone/butalbital/acetaminophen/ caffeine	Anolor DH
Hydrocodone/ammonium chloride/ antihistamines	P-V-Tussin
Hydrocodone/aspirin/acetaminophen/ caffeine	Anodynos-DHC
Hydrocodone/aspirin/caffeine	Damason-P
Hydrocodone/aspirin	Azdone
Hydrocodone/chlorpheniramine	Tussionex
Hydrocodone/guaifenesin	Codiclear DH
Hydrocodone/acetaminophen	Anexsia
Hydrocodone/homatropine	Hycodan
Hydrocodone/phenylpropanolamine	Hycomine
Methandriol dipropionate	Dr-Bolic
Methandrostenolone	Methandrostenolone
Methyltestosterone	Android-10
Nandrolone decanoate	Deca-Durabolin
Nandrolone phenpropionate	Nandrolone phenpropionate
Opium/ipecac/caffeine/aspirin	Aspiro Compound
Oxamdrolone	Oxandrin
Oxymetholone	Anadrol-50
Paregoric	Paregoric
Phendimetrazine tartrate	Appecon
Phenidamine/hydrocodone/guaifenesin	P-V-Tussin Tablets
Phenobarbital/belladonna	Susano
Phenylephrine/hydrocodone	Nalex DH
Phenylephrine/hydrocodone/guaifenesin	Donatussin DC
Phenylephrine/pyrilamine/hydrocodone	Codimal DH
Phenylpropanolamine/hydrocodone/ guaifenesin/salicylamide	Tussanil DH

Table 1–3. *Continued*

Generic Components	Representative Brand
Phenylpropanolamine/phenylephrine/ hydrocodone	Roni-Tuss Green
Phenylpropanolamine/phenylephrine/ hydrocodone/guaifenesin	S-T Forte
Phenylpropanolamine/phenylephrine/ pyrilamine/hydrocodone/guaifenesin	Traminic Expectorant DH
Phenylpropanolamine/phenylephrine/ pyrilamine/pheniramine/ hydrocodone	Rolatuss w/Hydrocodone
Pseudoephedrine/codeine	Nucofed
Pseudoephedrine/hydrocodone	Dutussin
Pseudoephedrine/guaifenesin/ codeine	Nucofed
Pseudoephedrine/hydrocodone/guaifenesin	Hyphed
Secobarbital/phenobarbital/butabarbital	Truxabarb
Stanozolol	Winstrol
Testolactone	Teslac
Testosterone	Testosterone
Testosterone cypionate	Andro-Cyp 100
Testosterone cypionate/estradiol cypionate	Depandrogyn
Testosterone enanthate	Andro L.A. 200
Testosterone enanthate/estradiol valerate	Androgyn L.A.
Testosterone propionate	Testosterone
Thiamylal sodium	Surital
Thiopental sodium	Pentothal

Schedule IV (Lower Potential for Abuse than Schedule III drugs)

Generic Components	Representative Brand
Acetaminophen w/codeine	Acetaminophen w/Codeine
Alprazolam	Xanax
Phenobarbital/hyoscyamine/passiflora/ valerian	Passased
Calcium carbonate/phenobarbital	Anaids
Chloral hydrate	Aquachoral Supprettes
Clorazepate dipotassium	Tranxene SD
Chlordiazepoxide/amitriptyline	Limbitrol 5-12.5
Chlordiazepoxide HCl	Libritabs
Clonazepam	Klonopin
Diazepam	Valium
Diethylpropion HCl	Tenuate
Difenoxin/atropine sulfate	Motofen
Estazolam	Prosom
Ethchlorvynol	Placidyl
Fenfluramine HCl	Pondimin
Flurazepam HCl	Dalmane
Halazepam	Paxipam
Lorazepam	Ativan
Mazindol	Mazanor
Mephobarbital	Mebaral
Meprobamate	Equanil
Meprobamate/aspirin	Equagesic
Meprobamate/benactyzine HCl	Deprol
Methohexital sodium	Brevital Sodium
Midazolam	Versed
Oxazepam	Serax

Table 1–3. *Continued*

Generic Components	Representative Brand
Paraldehyde	Paraldehyde
Pemoline	Cylert
Pentazocine/acetaminophen	Talacen
Pentazocine/aspirin	Talwin Compound
Pentazocine lactate	Talwin Lactate
Pentazocine/naloxone	Talwin NX
Phenobarbital	Luminal Sodium
Phenobarbital/atropine	Phenobarbital and Atropine
Phentermine HCl	Adipex-P
Prazepam	Centrax
Propoxyphene HCl	Darvon
Propoxyphene HCl/acetaminophen	Wygesic
Propoxyphene aspirin/caffeine	Darvon Compound-65
Propoxyphene napsylate	Darvon-N
Propoxyphene napsylate/acetaminophen	Darvocet-N 50
Pseudoephedrine/guaifenesin/codeine	Alamine Expectorant
Quazepam	Doral
Sodium bicarbonate/enzymes/ phenobarbital	Truxaphen
Temazepam	Restoril
Triazolam	Halcion

Schedule V (Lowest Abuse Potential of the Controlled Substances; Includes Over-The-Counter Antitussives and Antidiarrheals)

Generic Components	Representative Brand
Acetaminophen/codeine	Tylenol Elixir w/Codeine
Bismuth/kaolin/pectin/paregoric	Bismuth-Sancl-Opium
Bromodiphenhydramine/codeine	Ambenyl
Brompheniramine/phenylpropanolamine/ codeine	Dimetane-DC
Chlorpheniramine/phenylephrine/codeine/ ammonium chloride/guaifenesin	Efricon
Chlorpheniramine/phenylephrine/ phenylpropanolamine/codeine/ guaifenesin	Chemdal Expectorant
Chlorpheniramine/phenylpropanolamine/ phenylephrine/codeine	T-Koff
Calcium iodide/codeine	Calcidrine
Chlorpheniramine/phenylpropanolamine/ codeine	Decongestant-AT
Chlorpheniramine/pseudoephedrine/ codeine	Novahistine-DH
Chlorpheniramine/phenylephrine/ phenylpropanolamine/ dihydrocodone	Cophene-S
Chlorpheniramine/phenylephrine/codeine	Statuss
Chlorpheniramine/phenylephrine/ hydrocodone	Quendal Expectorant
Chlorpheniramine/phenylephrine/ codeine/potassium iodide	Pediacof
Chlorpheniramine/codeine/guaifenesin	Tussar SF
Codeine/acetaminophen/aspirin/salicylic acid/ caffeine	Codegesic
Codeine/aspirin/acetaminophen	En-Pain
Diphenoxylate HCl w/atropine	Lomotil
Ephedrine/guaifenesin/codeine	Broncholate CS
Guaifenesin/codeine	Scot-Tussin-C

Table 1–3. *Continued*

Generic Components	Representative Brand
Guaifenesin/ammonium chloride/codeine	Cheralin
Homatropine/pectin/paregoric	Dia-Quel
Iodinated glycerol/codeine	Tussi-Organidin
Kaolin/pectin/paregoric	Parepectolin
Kaolin/pectin/paregoric/belladonna	Donnagel-PG
Phenylephrine/pyrilamine/codeine	Codimal PH
Phenylephrine/pheniramine/codeine/ sodium citrate	Tussirex
Phenylpropanolamine/guaifenesin/ codeine	Naldecon-C
Potassium citrate/codeine	Tangecot
Promethazine/codeine	Phenergan w/Codeine
Promethazine/phenylephrine/codeine	Phenergan VC w/Codeine
Pseudoephedrine/dextromethorphan/ guaifenesin/codeine	Ban-Tuss C
Pseudoephedrine/guaifenesin/codeine	Isoclor Expectorant
Pyrilamine/terpin hydrate/codeine	Tricodene
Terpin hydrate/codeine	Terpin Hydrate w/Codeine
Triprolidine/pseudoephedrine/codeine	Actifed w/Codeine

for psychoactive addicting agents tend to develop and persist together, and inhibitors of protein synthesis block both.[13] On the other hand, in humans, marijuana and lysergic acid diethylamide (LSD)–like drugs produce striking tolerance, yet marijuana causes few symptoms of physical dependence, and with hallucinogens withdrawal symptoms do not occur. With opioids, which produce predictable, severe withdrawal symptoms and signs, tolerance is much more marked for psychic and analgesic effects than for smooth muscle actions. Withdrawal from amphetamine and cocaine causes depression, hunger, and intense craving but few objective signs, and although tolerance develops to the euphoric effects of these psychostimulants, there seems to be *reverse tolerance—sensitization,* perhaps comparable to electrophysiologic kindling—to psychosis and abnormal movements. Whether tolerance is required for physical dependence is unclear, and it is possible that an explanation of either phenomenon—in terms of, say, enzyme regulation, receptor change, or functional hypertrophy of alternate pathways—will shed little light on addiction per se.

What Have We Learned from Animal Studies?

There are a variety of animal models for studying addicting drugs.[4,14–17] In drug discrimination studies, animals learn to tell one drug from another (or from saline) for a reward; generalization from one drug to

another implies similar mechanisms of action.[14,18,19] Moreover, many investigators believe that the ability of a drug to act as a discriminative stimulus in animals reflects its subjective rewarding properties in humans—euphorigenic or otherwise. Nearly all drugs that are addicting to humans have discriminative stimulus effects in animals.[4]

Other models more specifically reveal how "reinforcing" or "rewarding" a drug is. In conditioned place preference models, drug and saline injections are paired with different environments, for example, one of two compartments in a cage; an animal's later preference for one or another environment indicates that the drug associated with it was rewarding.[14,20,21]

In other models, drugs are assessed for their ability to lower the threshold for self-stimulation through electrodes implanted in *reward areas*—especially the pathway from the midbrain ventral tegmental area (VTA) through the medial forebrain bundle to the nucleus accumbens (NA).[22]

In self-administration models, animals ingest drugs or self-inject them, either systemically or into various parts of the brain, especially reward areas.[15–17,23–25] In these models, when self-injection of a particular drug increases the rate of responding on subsequent occasions, the animal's response is defined as an operant and delivery of the drug as a reinforcer.[26] Different *schedules of reinforcement* are used, based on whether the reinforcer follows a given number of responses (ratio schedules) or whether it follows a response after a given period of time has elapsed (interval schedules). In ratio schedules, the number of responses required to produce an injection may be constant (fixed ratio), increase over time (progressive ratio), or vary irregularly from injection to injection (variable ratio). With progressive ratio schedules, the response requirement at which responding declines or ceases is called the *breakpoint*.

Drug-seeking behavior has two phases: acquisition and maintenance. Fixed ratio testing measures acquisition: how rapidly an animal learns to self-administer a drug. Progressive ratio testing measures maintenance: how reinforcing a drug continues to be once addiction is established. The *addiction liability* of a drug is usually defined in terms of acquisition. By such criteria, cocaine is more addicting than heroin, for after 5 days of testing, 70% of animals learn to self-administer cocaine, whereas only 30% self-administer heroin. Ethanol is much less addicting than either.[27]

Self-administration studies are complicated by the direct effects of the drugs themselves. For example, increasing rates of cocaine self-administration could be secondary to increased locomotor activity rather than from cocaine's reinforcing properties per se, and decreasing rates of responding might ensue when enough drug has been delivered to be behaviorally disruptive. Such confounding effects vary with the particular schedule of reinforcement selected.

Self-administration studies reveal that animals self-administer most drugs abused by humans, including ethanol, opioids, amphetamine, cocaine, barbiturates, benzodiazepines, phencyclidine, and nicotine. They do not self-administer hallucinogens such as LSD. They do self-administer some drugs not abused by humans, including apomorphine, ketocyclazocine, and procaine. Results with cannabinoids, caffeine, and 3,4-methylenedioxymethamphetamine (MDMA, "ecstasy") have been conflicting.[28]

Striking differences exist in the manner in which animals self-administer "rewarding" drugs. For example, with amphetamine, periodic self-administration tends to alternate with periodic self-imposed abstinence; saline substitution for amphetamine is followed by a few hours of self-administration and then cessation. With morphine, self-administration is done in gradually higher daily doses that prevent both toxicity and signs of withdrawal; with saline substitution, the animal continues to self-administer for weeks.[5,29–31] Perhaps analogously, human parenteral amphetamine abusers tend to "burn out" after a few years; with opioids, physical and psychic dependence can persist for decades.[32,33]

What Is the *Reward Circuit,* and Is It the Anatomic Substrate for All Drug-Seeking Behavior?

As noted, a reinforcer is an event that increases the likelihood of a response. *Reward* is defined similarly, with the added implication of affective pleasure.[34] In 1954, Olds and Milner,[35] studying rats, reported that electrical stimulation of certain parts of the brain, particularly the septal area, was positively reinforcing: animals repeatedly pressed levers to stimulate themselves. Subsequent workers defined a mesocorticolimbic *reward circuit* originating in cells of the midbrain VTA (formerly referred to as A10) and projecting via the medial forebrain bundle to the NA, olfactory tubercle, frontal cortex, amygdala, and septal area. The circuit also includes connections of these regions with the hypothalamus and afferents to the NA from limbic cortex, olfactory cortex, and amygdala. A major NA projection is to the substantia innominata/ventral pallidum (SI/VP), which in turn projects to the pedunculopontine nucleus, the dorsal medial thalamus, and the frontal cortex.[36,37]

The function of this circuit might be "converting emotion into motivated action" by filtering signals from the limbic system that ultimately produce motor acts via extrapyramidal output.[34] Lesions in the system lead to decrease in the locomotor activity ordinarily induced by a novel environment, reduction in the distraction usually associated with irrelevant information, difficulty in certain learning tasks, and perseveration.[34,38,39]

VTA cells of the reward circuit are dopaminergic, and their stimulation in animals produces increased locomotor activity, as does administration of amphetamine, cocaine, morphine, and ethanol, which increase dopamine levels in the NA.[40] Dopamine receptor antagonists—both D1 and D2—reduce self-administration of these drugs in animals.[41,42] Opioids are reinforcing whether injected into the VTA or the NA; VTA actions appear to be dopamine-dependent and NA actions to be dopamine-independent.[34]

The efferent pathway from the NA to the SI/VP is GABAergic.[36] Lesions of the SI/VP not only disrupt self-administration of ethanol, barbiturates, and sedatives (effects of which are largely mediated by GABA receptors), but also decrease self-administration of cocaine and heroin.

That these drugs each affect the reward circuit suggests it is the anatomic and physiologic substrate for drug addiction generally—and maybe also for reward associated with eating, drinking, and sex. Against such a view are the very different effects of different addicting drugs, both acutely and during abstinence. Unitarian views of addiction, however, hold that such effects—especially withdrawal—are secondary. Such a view is supported by several observations. First, human drug-seeking behavior tends to outlast withdrawal symptoms other than craving itself. Second, in rodents, microinjections of opioids into the midbrain periaqueductal gray matter produce physical dependence and withdrawal signs without reinforcement behavior, whereas injections into the VTA produce the opposite.[43] Third, drugs can be reinforcing in animals before physical dependence or withdrawal signs have appeared.

The acquisition of drug abuse or addiction probably depends on a drug's ability to improve mood; in animals, such an effect might be reflected in the increased locomotor activity that follows both the administration of different addicting drugs and the electrical stimulation of the VTA, NA, or medial forebrain bundle.[16,44] Maintenance of addiction, however, may be independent of drug-induced euphoria; human addicts often continue to administer drugs—including ethanol, caffeine, cocaine, heroin, or phencyclidine—in the face of increasing dysphoria.[45]

Some investigators believe that even if avoidance of withdrawal plays a secondary role in establishing addiction, it is nonetheless crucial in maintaining addiction.[36] Others stress the behavioral variables associated with different agents. For example, tobacco addiction most often begins with adolescent peer pressure, and its continuation during adulthood is associated with improved work performance and reduced weight. The sight, smell, and taste of tobacco smoke are also surely relevant, as is the use of a cigarette as a social prop.

How Many Americans Use or Abuse Drugs?

Modern drug abuse prevalence in the United States is crudely estimated by examining data from diverse sources. These include (1) acute medical interventions—for example, reports of hepatitis or acquired immunodeficiency syndrome (AIDS) and statistics from the Drug Abuse Warning Network (DAWN), a federally operated system that monitors emergency rooms, hospital inpatient services, medical examiner offices, and crisis centers; (2) treatment programs, including the National Institute of Drug Abuse's Client Oriented Data Acquisition Process (CODAP); (3) law enforcement agencies; and (4) household, school, and college surveys. Table 1–4 shows life-

Table 1–4. Lifetime Prevalence of Drug Use Among High School Seniors (1989) and U.S. Population Aged 12 and Older (1988)

	Percentage Ever Using	
Substance	Seniors	U.S. Population
Ethanol	90.7	85.0
Tobacco (cigarettes)	65.7	75.1
Marijuana	43.7	33.1
Stimulants	19.1	7.1
Inhalants	18.6	5.7
Cocaine	10.3	10.7
Tranquilizers	7.6	4.8
Hallucinogens	9.9	7.4
Other opioids	8.3	3.5
Sedatives	7.4	3.5
Heroin	1.3	1.0
Any illicit drug	50.9	36.6
Total surveyed	15,200	9,259

Source: Kandel DB. Epidemiological trends and implications for understanding the nature of addiction. In: O'Brien CP, Jaffe JH, eds. Addictive States. Res Publ Assoc Res Nerv Ment Dis 1992; 70:23.

time prevalences of drug use among American high school seniors and the U.S. population aged 12 and older, based on national surveys of schools and households in 1988 and 1989. Table 1–5 shows lifetime prevalence of drug users who during the early 1980s met DSM-III criteria for abuse or dependence disorder. Through the 1980s, use of tobacco, ethanol, and illicit drugs steadily declined—except for cocaine, which peaked in the mid-1980s and then began a downward trend. Daily marijuana use among high school seniors peaked in 1978 at 10.7%; in 1989, it was 2.9%. Although overall use of cocaine declined between 1985 and 1991, however, regular use did not. In 1988, 4% of cocaine users used it

Table 1–5. Life Prevalence of DSM-III Drug Abuse/ Dependence Disorders in Total U.S. Population (1980–1984)

Ethanol	13.8%
Tobacco	36.0%
Marijuana	4.4%
Stimulants	1.7%
Sedatives	1.2%
Opioids	0.7%
Hallucinogens	0.4%
Cocaine	0.2%

Source: Kandel DB. Epidemiological trends and implications for understanding the nature of addiction. In: O'Brien CP, Jaffe JH, eds. Addictive States. Res Publ Assoc Res Nerv Ment Dis 1992; 70:23.

daily compared with 2% in 1985, and 11% used it at least weekly compared with 5%.[46] A 1990 household survey by the National Institute on Drug Abuse (NIDA) found that 662,000 Americans were at least weekly cocaine users, and 1.6 million were at least monthly users; in 1991, those figures had risen to 885,000 and 1.9 million. During the same period, heroin use also rose. What those figures suggest is that although casual drug use—reflecting especially life in suburbia—declined, compulsive drug use—reflecting life in the inner city—did not.[47]

Are Drug Abusers Genetically Prone?

Inbreeding produces strains of rodents with strikingly different responses to particular drugs.[48] For example, there are mice that like to drink ethanol and mice that avoid it. Strains can also be bred that differ in their sensitivity to ethanol-induced ataxia or hypothermia, ethanol tolerance, or ethanol withdrawal seizures. Other strains have different preferences for other agents—including psychostimulants, benzodiazepines, opioids, and nicotine—or different responses to them.[49,50] Such traits are genetically distinct; for example, sensitivity to an effect of ethanol does not predict ethanol liking or disliking.[51,52]

There is a considerable—and controversial—literature on human genetic susceptibility to alcoholism, and there seem to be genetic influences on tobacco addiction (see Chapters 11 and 12). Whether addiction to other drugs—or to drugs in general—is genetically influenced is unknown.

Is There Such a Thing as an *Addictive Personality*?

The answer to this question is easy: no. Animal drug preferences vary between species and strains, but when a highly addictive drug such as cocaine is made available, most animals self-administer it.[53] Similarly, sudden availability of a drug has produced epidemics of human abuse—for example, methamphetamine in Japan in the 1940s and cocaine in the United States in the 1980s. It is of course significant that even when highly reinforcing drugs are plentiful, some animals do not self-administer them, and that among humans who do, most are not compulsive daily users. Drug availability, in other words, does not by itself predict drug addiction. That does not mean, however, that either addicted humans or addicted rats have an *addictive personality*.

Objective psychological testing has repeatedly failed to define a personality profile or psychopathological state specific to drug addiction in general or to abuse of any one substance.[54-67] To be sure, among drug abusers a variety of psychopathologies are overrepresented. Anxiety, emotional immaturity, antisocial personality, or depression can lead to drug use in the first place, and many addicts are self-medicating psychiatric symptoms.[68-75] Some workers report that the majority of drug-abusing or drug-dependent individuals have an additional psychiatric diagnosis.[46] In certain instances—such as depression in cocaine abusers, schizophrenia in phencyclidine abusers, or "apathy" in marijuana users—it is difficult to tell whether psychopathology preceded or followed drug use. Drug abusers tend to be attitudinally and emotionally "different from the average person in society" to the degree that their particular drugs "meet with severe disapproval."[6] Again, such linkage need not imply the existence of an addictive personality, for prior delinquency in itself is conducive to obtaining an illicit drug.[76] As an example, marijuana may or may not serve as a "gateway" drug to more dangerous agents, but if so the reason may simply be that marijuana's illegality brings users in contact with purveyors of cocaine or heroin. Moreover, the prevalence of drug abuse in minority "ghettos" (or, for that matter, in suburban white "ghettos") might reflect reinforcing properties of a drug abuser's lifestyle, offering excitement and risks to those either bored in sterile surroundings or denied normal opportunities for self-fulfillment.

In addition to such operant aspects, drug abuse has pavlovian features. Animals exposed to environmental stimuli previously associated with a drug demonstrate drug-seeking behavior.[77-79] Their human counterparts are successfully detoxified addicts who relapse into drug-seeking on returning to their old neighborhoods.[80] Conversely, patients made physically dependent on morphine while hospitalized usually do not crave the drug on discharge,[81,82] and the great majority of U.S. servicemen addicted to heroin during the Vietnam War did not crave the drug when they returned home.[83]

As already noted, animals exposed to drug-associated surroundings may even display signs of drug intoxication in the absence of drug administration. Their human counterparts are parenteral drug abusers who obtain subjective drug effects after unwittingly self-injecting saline ("needle freaks").

Finally, Siegel[84] suggests that drug "intoxication" is a basic drive in both humans and animals, independent of psychological makeup and no more repressible than eating, drinking, or sex.

How Are Drugs Identified in Body Fluids and Tissues?

A technical discussion of drug detection is beyond the scope of this text. Different testing systems exist for identifying drugs in urine, which is more often analyzed than blood.[85-89] (Testing of hair—which would theoretically detect drug use days to months earlier—is investigational and controversial.[90,91]) Many emergency rooms use thin-layer chromatography, which requires 3 to 4 hours to perform and is insensitive when only small doses of a drug have been taken (especially cocaine and phencyclidine). More sensitive and therefore suitable for screening are immunoassays, which include enzyme immunoassay, radioimmunoassay, fluorescence polarization immunoassay, and latex agglutination inhibition assay. Of these, the qualitative or semiquantitative enzyme immunoassay known as enzyme multiplied immunoassay technique (EMIT) is widely available and inexpensive. With thin-layer chromatography, enzyme immunoassay, radioimmunoassay, and fluorescence polarization immunoassay, positive results for cocaine and marijuana are highly predictive. For amphetamines and opioids, positive results are less specific. Most toxicology laboratories confirm any positive screened sample with gas chromatography/mass spectrometry, which is more expensive, more time-consuming, more sensitive, and more specific. Gas chromatography/mass spectrometry is required for confirmation by the U.S. Armed Forces and by federal regulations for workplace testing. Other confirmatory techniques include high-performance liquid chromatography and gas-liquid chromatography (Table 1–6).[88]

Drug abuse screening has problems in addition to sensitivity and specificity. Persistence of a drug or its metabolite in the urine varies widely among agents and users. For example, urine can be positive for cannabinoids several days after single casual use of marijuana, and in heavy chronic cocaine users, the major metabolite benzoylecgonine is detectable for several weeks. Unless observed, users may substitute "clean" urines (or apple juice) or adulterate urine with water, sodium chloride, vinegar, ammonia, sodium hypochlorite, or soap.[88] "Chain of custody"—the accountability of a specimen from its production to its analysis—must be tightly controlled, and equipment and technique must be continually monitored.[92] These issues are of obvious importance in forensic cases and—along with the problems of invasion of privacy and cost-effectiveness—in the debate over workplace screening.

What About Treatment?

A drug abuser might be treated for overdose, for withdrawal, for medical or neurologic complications, or for addiction itself. Each of these areas is covered in this book, but selectively and, perforce, sometimes superficially. General principles of management in poisoning or overdose are discussed in other texts,[93] and such controversies as whether gastric emptying does more harm than good after ingestion of a poison[94] are outside the bounds of space, time, and my own experience. Similarly, although I address some specific chronic therapies—methadone for heroin abusers, antidepressants for cocaine abusers, disulfiram for alcoholics, nicotine gum for tobacco abusers—readers seeking broad coverage of the treatment of addiction are advised to look elsewhere.[95]

A point worth emphasizing, however, is how artificial unimodal approaches are. For one thing, drug abusers do not usually limit themselves to one agent. A familiar scene is the emergency room patient simultaneously intoxicated with multiple drugs or intoxicated with one agent while withdrawing from another.[96] Heroin addicts frequently become

Table 1–6. Cut-Off Points (in Nanograms per Milliliter) of Different Drugs of Abuse by Different Analytical Techniques

| Drug Group | Immunoassay | | Chromatography | |
	Enzyme Immunoassay	Radioimmunoassay	Thin-Layer Chromatography	Gas Chromatography/ Mass Spectrometry
Cannabinoids	20–100	100	25	1–15
Cocaine	300	300	2000	5
Phencyclidine	75	25	500	5
Dextroamphetamine	300	1000	500	10
Morphine/heroin	300	300	500	5

Source: Schwartz JG, Zollars PR, Okorodudu AO, et al. Accuracy of common drug screen tests. Am J Emerg Med 1991; 9:166.

successfully maintained on methadone and then become alcoholic or addicted to cocaine. Biological, psychological, or socioeconomic approaches to drug abuse are not mutually exclusive, and drug abuse treatment involves (or should involve) them all.[97,98]

What About Prevention?

As with comprehensive treatment, this topic is discussed—when it is discussed at all—*en passant*. American policies on drug abuse prevention are targeted at either supply—crop eradication, border interdiction, and law enforcement—or demand—education and treatment.[99] At the moment, the bulk of money and energy is devoted to the former. To put it gently, I consider such emphasis wrongheaded.

What About *Legalization*?

Although *legalization* is a social, not a medical, issue, the harm a drug does—to a user or to society— has obvious bearing on its legal status. A few points are worth considering in this regard:

1. Nearly every society since recorded history has countenanced the use of one or more mind-altering drugs.
2. Some mind-altering drugs are more harmful than others.
3. Attempts to stamp out abuse of particular drugs by declaring them illegal have been spectacularly unsuccessful.
4. When drugs are freely available, however, more people use them.
5. The two biggest killer drugs in the United States are legal.

For readers who wish to explore this explosive subject free of hypocrisy and cant, I recommend four brief reviews; the authors reach very different conclusions but maintain civil discourse and respect for evidence.[100–103] Such qualities are notably lacking in most political discussions on drug abuse. It is my view that informed participation in the current debate by front-line physicians and other health care workers is overdue but not too late, for—even as the last coca plant is eradicated from the South American continent—the problem is not going to go away.

References

1. Eddy NB, Halbach H, Isbell H, Seevers MH. Drug dependence: its significance and characteristics. Bull WHO 1965; 32:721.

2. Edwards G, Arif A, Hodgson R. Nomenclature and classification of drug and alcohol-related problems: a shortened version of a WHO memorandum. Br J Addict 1982; 77:3.

3. *Diagnostic and Statistical Manual of Mental Disorders, Third Edition-Revised (DSM-III-R)*. Washington, DC: American Psychiatric Association, 1987.

4. Stolerman I: Drugs of abuse: behavioural principles, methods and terms. Trends Pharmacol Sci 1992; 13:170.

5. Department of Health and Human Services. *The Health Consequences of Smoking. A Report of the Surgeon General*. Washington, DC: DHHS Publication No (CDC) 88-8406, US Government Printing Office, 1988.

6. Jaffe JH: Drug addiction and drug abuse. In: Gilman AG, Rall TW, Nies AS, Taylor P, eds. The Pharmacological Basis of Therapeutics, ed 8. New York: Pergamon Press, 1990:522.

7. Dews PB. Behavioral tolerance. In: Krasnegor NA, ed. Behavioral Tolerance: Research and Treatment Implications. Washington, DC: National Institute on Drug Abuse, DHEW Publication No (ADM) 78-551, US Government Printing Office, 1977:18.

8. Siegel S, MacRae J. Environmental specificity of tolerance. Trends Neurosci 1984; 7:140.

9. Pavlov IP. Conditioned Reflexes (Anrep GV, trans). Oxford: Oxford University Press, 1927.

10. Siegel S, Hinson RE, Krank MD, McCully J. Heroin "overdose" death: contribution of drug-associated environmental cues. Science 1982; 216:436.

11. Goudie AJ, Griffiths JW. Environmental specificity of tolerance. Trends Neurosci 1984; 7:310.

12. Dewey WL. Various factors which affect the rate of development of tolerance and physical dependence to abused drugs. In: Sharp CW, ed. *Mechanisms of Tolerance and Dependence*. DHHS, Washington, DC: NIDA Research Monograph 54, 1984:39.

13. Snyder SH. Receptors, neurotransmitters, and drug responses. N Engl J Med 1979; 300:465.

14. Geary N. Cocaine: animal research studies. In: Spitz HI, Rosecan JS, ed. Cocaine Abuse. New Directions in Treatment and Research. New York: Brunner/Mazel, 1987:19.

15. Koob GF, Vaccarino FJ, Amalric M, Serdlow NR. Neural substrates for cocaine and opiate reinforcement. In: Fisher S, Raskin A, Uhlenhuth EH, eds. Cocaine: Clinical and Biobehavioral Aspects. New York: Oxford University Press, 1987:80.

16. Wise RA, Rompre P-P. Brain dopamine and reward. Annu Rev Psychol 1989; 40:191.

17. Singh J, Desiraju T. Differential effects of opioid peptides administered intracerebrally in loci of self-stimulation reward of lateral hypothalamus and ventral tegmental area-substantia nigra. In: Rapaka RS, Dhawan BN, eds. Opioid Peptides: An Update. Washington, DC: NIDA Research Monograph 87, DHHS, 1988:180.

18. Colpaert FC, Janssen PAJ. Factors regulating drug cue sensitivity: limits of discriminability and the role of a

progressively decreasing training dose in cocaine-saline discrimination. Neuropharmacology 1982; 21:1187.

19. Woods JH, Winger GD, France CP. Reinforcing and discriminative stimulus effects of cocaine: analysis of pharmacological mechanisms. In: Fisher S, Raskin A, Uhlehuth EH, eds. Cocaine: Clinical and Biobehavioral Aspects. New York: Oxford University Press, 1987:21.

20. Spyraki C, Fibiger HC, Phillips AG. Cocaine-induced place preference conditioning: lack of effects of neuroleptics and 6-hydroxydopamine lesions. Brain Res 1982; 253:192.

21. Mackey WB, van der Kooy D. Neuroleptics block the positive reinforcing effects of amphetamine but not of morphine as measured by placed conditioning. Pharmacol Biochem Behav 1985; 22:101.

22. Kornetsky C, Bain G. Neuronal basis for hedonic effects of cocaine and opiates. In: Fisher S, Raskin A, Uhlenhuth EH, eds. Cocaine: Clinical and Biobehavioral Aspects. New York: Oxford University Press, 1987:66.

23. Deneau G, Yanigita T, Seevers MH. Self-administration of psychoactive substances by the monkey. Psychopharmacology 1969; 16:30.

24. Johanson CE. Assessment of the dependence potential of cocaine in animals. In: Grabowski J, ed. Cocaine: Pharmacology, Effects, and Treatment of Abuse. Washington, DC: NIDA Research Monograph 50, DHHS, 1984:54.

25. Pettit HO, Ettenberg A, Bloom FL, Koob GF. Destruction of dopamine in nucleus accumbens selectively attenuates cocaine but not heroin self-administration in rats. Psychopharmacology 1984; 84:167.

26. Spealman RD, Goldberg SR. Drug self-administration by laboratory animals: control by schedules of reinforcement. Annu Rev Pharmacol Toxicol 1978; 18:313.

27. Bozarth MA. New perspectives on cocaine addiction: recent findings from animal research. Can J Physiol Pharmacol 1989; 67:1158.

28. Iwamoto E, Martin W. A critique of drug self-administration as a method for predicting abuse potential of drugs. In: Harris LS, ed. Problems of Drug Dependence, 1987. Washington, DC: NIDA Research Monograph 81, DHHS, 1988:457.

29. Johanson CE, Balster RL, Bonese K. Self-administration of psychomotor stimulant drugs: the effects of unlimited access. Pharmacol Biochem Behav 1976; 4:45.

30. Woolverton WL, Balster RL. Reinforcing properties of some local anesthetics in rhesus monkeys. Pharmacol Biochem Behav 1979; 11:661.

31. Downs DA, Harrigan SE, Wiley JN, et al. Continuous stimulant self-administration in rhesus monkeys. Res Commun Psychol Psychiat Behav 1979; 4:39.

32. Kramer JC, Fischman VS, Littlefield DC. Amphetamine abuse: patterns and effects of high doses taken intravenously. JAMA 1967; 201:305.

33. Vaillant G. A 20-year follow-up of New York narcotic addicts. Arch Gen Psychiatry 1973; 29:237.

34. Koob GF. Drugs of abuse: anatomy, pharmacology and function of reward pathways. Trends Pharmacol Sci 1992; 13:177.

35. Olds J, Milner P. Positive reinforcement produced by electrical stimulation of septal area and other regions of rat brain. J Comp Physiol Psychol 1954; 47:419.

36. Koob GF, Bloom FE. Cellular and molecular mechanisms of drug dependence. Science 1988; 242:715.

37. Wise RA, Bozarth MS. Brain reward circuitry: four circuit elements "wired" in apparent series. Brain Res Bull 1984; 12:203.

38. Robbins TW, Everitt BJ. Functional studies of the central catecholamines. Int Rev Neurobiol 1982; 23:303.

39. LeMoal M, Simon H. Mesocorticolimbic dopaminergic network: functional and regulatory roles. Physiol Rev 1991; 71:155.

40. DiChiara G, Imperato A. Opposite effects of mu and kappa opiate agonists on dopamine release in nucleus accumbens and in the dorsal caudate of freely moving rats. J Pharmacol Exp Ther 1988; 244:1067.

41. Nakajima S. Subtypes of dopamine receptors involved in the mechanism of reinforcement. Neurosci Biobehav Rev 1989; 13:123.

42. Woolverton WL, Johnson KM. Neurobiology of cocaine abuse. Trends Pharmacol Sci 1992; 13:193.

43. Wise RA, Bozarth MA. A psychomotor stimulant theory of addiction. Psychol Rev 1987; 94:459.

44. Ward LC, Jones LC. Chronic ingestion of ethanol increases stimulation-induced voluntary activity in the rat. Drug Alcohol Depend 1989; 23:165.

45. Monteiro MG, Schukit MA, Irwin M. Subjective feelings of anxiety in young men after ethanol and diazepam infusions. J Clin Psychiatry 1990; 51:12.

46. Kandel DB. Epidemiological trends and implications for understanding the nature of addiction. In: O'Brien CP, Jaffe JH, eds. *Addictive States*. Res Publ Assoc Res Nerv Ment Dis 1992; 70:23.

47. Massing M. Whatever happened to the "war on drugs"? New York Review of Books, June 11, 1992.

48. Meisch RA, George FR. Influence of genetic factors on drug-reinforced behavior in animals. In: Pickens RW, Svikis DS, eds. Biological Vulnerability to Drug Abuse. Rockville, MD: NIDA Research Monograph 89, DHHS, 1988:9.

49. Goerge FR, Goldberg SR. Genetic approaches to the analysis of addiction processes. Trends Pharmacol Sci 1989; 10:78.

50. Crabbe JC, Belknap JK. Genetic approaches to drug dependence. Trends Pharmacol Sci 1992; 13:212.

51. Cloninger CR. Etiologic factors in substance abuse: an adoption study perspective. In: Pickens RW, Svikis DS, eds. Biological Vulnerability to Drug Abuse. Rockville, MD: NIDA Research Monograph 89, DHHS, 1988:52.

52. Cadoret RJ, Troughton E, O'Gormon TW, Heywood E. An adoption study of genetic and environmental factors in drug abuse. Arch Gen Psychiatry 1986; 43:1131.

53. Dole VP. Addictive behavior. Sci Am 1980; 243:138.

54. Hill HE, Haertzen CA, Davis H. An MMPI factor analysis study of alcoholics, narcotic addicts and criminals. QJ Stud Alcohol 1962; 23:411.

55. Monroe JJ, Ross WF, Berzins J. The decline of the addict as "psychopath": implications for community care. Int J Addict 1971; 6:601.

56. Mott J. The psychological basis of drug dependence: the intellectual and personality characteristics of opiate users. Br J Addict 1972; 67:89.

57. Dole VP. Narcotic addiction, physical dependence, and relapse. N Engl J Med 1972; 286:988.

58. Overall JE. MMPI personality patterns of alcoholics and narcotic addicts. QJ Stud Alcohol 1973; 34:104.

59. Feldstein S, Chesler P, Fink M. Psychological differentiation and the response of opiate addicts to pharmacological treatment. Br J Addict 1973; 68:151.

60. Robins LN, Helzer JE, Davis DH. Narcotic use in southeast Asia and afterward: an interview of 898 Vietnam returners. Arch Gen Psychiatry 1975; 32:955.

61. Craig RJ. Personality characteristics of heroin addicts: review of empirical research 1976–1979. Int J Addict 1982; 17:227.

62. Sutker PB, Moan CE, Goist KC, Allain AN. MMPI subtypes and antisocial behaviors in adolescent alcohol and drug abusers. Drug Alcohol Depend 1984; 13:235.

63. O'Malley PM, Bachman JG, Johnson LD. Period, age, and cohort effects on substance use among American youth, 1976–1982. Am J Public Health 1984; 74:682.

64. O'Mahony P, Smith E. Some personality characteristics of imprisoned heroin addicts. Drug Alcohol Depend 1984; 13:255.

65. Khantzian EJ. The self-medication hypothesis of addictive disorders: focus on heroin and cocaine dependence. Am J Psychiatry 1985; 142:1259.

66. O'Connor L, Berry JW. The drug-of-choice phenomenon: why addicts start using their preferred drug. J Psychoactive Drugs 1990; 22:305.

67. Campbell BK, Stark MJ. Psychopathology and personality characteristics in different forms of substance abuse. Int J Addict 1990; 25:1467.

68. Pope HC. Drug abuse and psychopathology. N Engl J Med 1979; 301:1341.

69. McLellan AT, Woody GE, O'Brien CP. Development of psychiatric illness in drug abusers. Possible role of drug preference. N Engl J Med 1979; 301:1310.

70. Sutker PB, Archer RP, Allain AN. Psychopathology of drug abusers: sex and ethnic considerations. Int J Addict 1980; 15:605.

71. Rounsaville BJ, Novelly RA, Kleber HD. Neuropsychological impairment in opiate addicts: risk factors. Ann NY Acad Sci 1981; 362:79.

72. Weller MP, Ang PC, Zachary A, Latimer-Sayer DT. Substance abuse in schizophrenia. Lancet 1984; 1:573.

73. Marlatt GA, Baer JS, Donovan DM, Kivlahan DR. Addictive behaviors: etiology and treatment. Annu Rev Psychol 1988; 39:223.

74. Butcher JN. Personality factors in drug addiction. In: Pickens RW, Svikis DS, eds. Biological Vulnerability to Drug Abuse. Rockville, MD: NIDA Research Monograph 89, DHHS, 1988:87.

75. Hesselbrock V, Meyer R, Hesselbrock M. Psychopathology and addictive disorders. The specific case of antisocial personality disorder. In: O'Brien CP, Jaffe JH, eds. Addictive States. Res Publ Assoc Res Nerv Ment Dis 1992; 70:179.

76. Robins LN, Murphy GE. Drug use in a normal population of young Negro men. Am J Public Health 1967; 57:1580.

77. Siegel S. Drug anticipation and the treatment of dependence. In: Ray BA, ed. Learning Factors in Substance Abuse. Rockville, MD: NIDA Research Monograph 84, DHHS, 1988:1.

78. Goldberg SR, Woods JH, Schuster CR. Morphine: conditioned increases in self-administration in Rhesus monkeys. Science 1969; 166:1306.

79. Wikler A, Pescor FT, Miller D, Norrell H. Persistent potency of a secondary (conditioned) reinforcer following withdrawal of morphine from physically dependent rats. Psychopharmacologia 1971; 20:103.

80. Wikler A. Interaction of physical dependence and classical and operant conditioning in the genesis of relapse. Res Publ Assoc Res Nerv Ment Dis 1968; 46:280.

81. Dole VP. Narcotic addiction, physical dependence, and relapse. N Engl J Med 1972; 286:988.

82. Foley K. The treatment of cancer pain. N Engl J Med 1985; 313:84.

83. O'Brien CP, Nace EP, Mintz J, et al. Follow-up of Vietnam veterans. 1. Relapse to drug use after Vietnam service. Drug Alcohol Depend 1980; 5:333.

84. Siegel RK. Intoxication. Life in Pursuit of Artificial Paradise. New York: EP Dutton, 1989.

85. Hawks RL, Chiang CN, eds. Urine Testing for Drugs of Abuse. Rockville, MD: NIDA Research Monograph 73, DHHS, 1986.

86. Gold MS, Dackis CA. Role of the laboratory in the evaluation of suspected drug abuse. J Clin Psychiatry 1986; 47(suppl):17.

87. Schwartz RH. Urine testing in the detection of drugs of abuse. Arch Intern Med 1988; 148:2407.

88. Schwartz JG, Zollars PR, Okorodudu AO, et al. Accuracy of common drug screen tests. Am J Emerg Med 1991; 9:166.

89. Weisman RS, Howland MA, Flomenbaum NE. The toxicology laboratory. In: Goldfrank LR, Flomenbaum NE, Lewin NA, et al., eds. Toxicologic Emergencies ed 4. Norwalk, CT: Appleton & Lange, 1990:39.

90. Holden C. Hairy problems for new drug testing method. Science 1990; 249:1099.

91. Nakahara Y, Takahashi K, Shimamine M, Takeda Y. Hair analysis for drug abuse. I. Determination of methamphetamine and amphetamine in hair by stable isotope dilution gas chromatography/mass spectrometry method. J Forensic Sci 1991; 36:70.

92. Wilson JF, Williams J, Walker G, et al. Performance of techniques used to detect drugs of abuse in urine: study based on external quality assessment. Clin Chem 1991; 37:442.

93. Flomenbaum NE, Goldfrank LR, Weisman RS, et al. Management of the poisoned or overdosed patient.

In: Goldfrank LR, Flomenbaum NE, Lewin NA, et al, eds. Toxicologic Emergencies, ed 4. Norwalk, CT: Appleton & Lange, 1990:5.

94. Kulig K. Initial management of ingestions of toxic substances. N Engl J Med 1992; 326:1677.

95. Lowinson JH, Ruiz P, Millman RB, Langrod JG. Substance Abuse: A Comprehensive Textbook, Second Edition. Baltimore, Williams & Wilkins, 1992.

96. Khantzian EJ, McKenna GJ. Acute toxic and withdrawal reactions associated with drug use and abuse. Ann Intern Med 1979; 90:361.

97. McLellan AT, O'Brien CP, Metzger D. How effective is substance abuse treatment—compared to what? In: O'Brien CP, Jaffe JH, eds. Addictive States. Res Publ Assoc Res Nerv Ment Dis 1992; 70:231.

98. Gerstein DR. The effectiveness of drug treatment. In: O'Brien CP, Jaffe JH, eds. Addictive States. Res Publ Assoc Res Nerv Ment Dis 1992; 70:253.

99. Board of Trustees Report. Drug abuse in the United States. Strategies for prevention. JAMA 1991; 265:2102.

100. Nadelmann EA. Drug prohibition in the United States: costs, consequences, and alternatives. Science 1989; 245:939.

101. Goldstein A, Kalant H. Drug policy: striking the right balance. Science 1990; 249:1513.

102. Jarvik ME. The drug dilemma: manipulating the demand. Science 1990; 250:387.

103. Schwartz RH. Legalization of drugs of abuse and the pediatrician. Am J Dis Child 1991; 145:1153.

Chapter 2
Opioids

Thou only givest these gifts to man, and thou hast the
keys of Paradise, O just, subtle, and mighty opium.
—*Thomas De Quincey*

Everything one does in life, even love, occurs in an
express train racing towards death. To smoke opium is to
get out of the train while it is still moving.
—*Jean Cocteau*

Junk is not . . . a means to increased enjoyment of life.
Junk is not a kick. It is a way of life.
—*William Burroughs*

Opium is derived from seed capsules of the poppy, *Papaver somniferum*, indigenous to the Middle East and Southeast Asia. The dried juice (gum opium) contains more than 20 alkaloids, including morphine and codeine.[1] Today there are also commercially available semisynthetic and synthetic opioids, including agonists, antagonists, and mixed agonist-antagonists (Table 2–1).

Pharmacology and Animal Studies

Some investigators use the term *opiate* for morphine-like drugs derived directly or indirectly from opium and *opioid* for drugs with morphine-like actions but quite different chemical structures. To avoid confusion, only opioid is used here, referring to both agonists and antagonists, whether or not they structurally resemble morphine. Similarly misleading is the term *narcotic*, which not only fails to describe why opioids are usually taken (medically or illicitly), but also when used by law enforcement agencies refers to cocaine and marijuana as well.

Some agonist-antagonists (e.g., buprenorphine and nalbuphine) are *partial agonists,* having agonist effects when given alone or in the presence of small doses of strong agonists but antagonizing the effects of large doses. Other agonist-antagonists (e.g., nalorphine and cyclazocine) have agonist effects at low doses but dysphoric psychotomimetic effects at high

doses and antagonize the effects of either low or high doses of pure agonists.[2] Such complex properties have been better understood since the discovery in 1973 of stereospecific opioid receptors in mammalian brain and the subsequent identification of endogenous opioid peptides (endorphins).[3–6]

Exogenous and endogenous opioids have different receptor specificities and anatomic distributions (Tables 2–2 and 2–3).[7–9] Beta-endorphin arises, with adrenocorticotropic hormone (ACTH), from a precursor molecule, proopiomelanocortin. It is at highest concentration in the pars intermedia and pars distalis of the pituitary, the arcuate nucleus of the hypothalamus, the locus coeruleus, limbic areas, and the midbrain and is nearly equipotent at mu and delta receptors.[9] Methionine-enkephalin and leucine-enkephalin, derived from pro-enkephalin, are more widely distributed in the brain and spinal cord. They are especially concentrated in the hypothalamus, the amygdala, and other limbic areas and in brain stem and spinal cord areas involved with pain (e.g., the midbrain, periaqueductal gray matter, the spinal trigeminal nucleus, and laminae I and II or the dorsal horn); enkephalins are also released, with catecholamines, from the adrenal medulla. They are more bound to delta than to mu receptors.[8,9] The dynorphins, derived from pro-dynorphin, contain the leucine-enkephalin amino acid sequence at one end yet have affinity for kappa receptors, in the case of

Table 2–1. Opioids Available in the United States

Agonist
Powdered opium
Tincture of opium (laudanum)
Camphorated tincture of opium (paregoric)
Purified opium alkaloids (Pantopon)
Morphine
Heroin (legally available only for investigational use)
Methadone (Dolophine)
Fentanyl (Sublimaze, and in Innovar)
Sufentanil (Sufenta)
Alfentanil (Alfenta)
Oxymorphone (Numorphan)
Hydromorphone (Dilaudid)
Codeine
Dihydrocodeine (Synalgos)
Oxycodone (in mixtures, e.g., Percodan, Percocet)
Hydrocodone (in mixtures, e.g., Hycodan)
Levorphanol (Levo-Dromoran)
Meperidine (pethidine; Demerol, Pethadol)
Alphaprodine (Nisentil)
Propoxyphene (Darvon, and in Darvocet)
Diphenoxylate (in Lomotil)
Etorphine (for animal use)
Apomorphine

Antagonist
Naloxone (Narcan)
Naltrexone (Trexan)

Mixed Agonist-Antagonist
Pentazocine (Talwin)
Butorphanol (Stadol)
Buprenorphine (Buprenex)
Nalbuphine (Nubain)
Cyclazocine (for investigational use only)
Propiram (for investigational use only)
Profadel (for investigational use only)
Meptazinol (for investigational use only)
Dezocine (for investigational use only)

Table 2–2. Correlation of Opioid Effects with Regional Opioid Receptors

Analgesia	Spinal cord, midbrain peri-aqueductal gray matter, limbic structures
Emotion	Limbic structures, locus coeruleus
Sedation	Midbrain reticular formation, cerebral cortex
Miosis	Midbrain
Hypothermia	Hypothalamic preoptic nucleus
Respiratory depression	Brainstem respiratory centers
Cough suppression	Medulla

Data from references 7–9.

dynorphin A and B to a greater extent than for mu and delta receptors.[8,10] Also widely distributed in the central nervous system (CNS), dynorphins share brain areas with the enkephalins, yet within these areas they often occupy different neuronal groups.

In addition to these well-studied endorphins, the brain contains numerous fragments of propiomelanocortin, pro-enkephalin, and pro-dynorphin, the functional significance of which is uncertain. Even more obscure is the physiologic role in mammalian brain of endogenous morphine, codeine, and 6-acetylmorphine, synthesized in liver (using the same steps as in the opium poppy) and transported across the blood–brain barrier as a presumed *peripheral-to-central hormone.*[11] Finally, a 91-amino acid peptide from the pituitary, beta-lipotropin, also derived from proopiomelanocortin, has a sequence at residues 61 to 65 identical to methionine-enkephalin and at 61 to 91 identical to beta-endorphin, yet beta-lipotropin has no opioid activity itself.[12]

A peptide, Phe-Met-Arg-Phe-NH2 (*FMRF-amide*), originally identified in molluscs, is present in mammalian CNS, where it exerts antiopioid effects. Its physiologic importance is uncertain, but speculation includes a possible role in tolerance and dependence.[13] Rats receiving intrathecal injections of cerebrospinal fluid (CSF) from morphine-tolerant rats develop immediate tolerance to morphine effects, and a FMRF-amide–like peptide precipitates signs of opioid withdrawal.[14]

Mu opioid receptors are widely distributed in the CNS; delta receptors are restricted largely to the forebrain; and kappa receptors are found in limbic and other diencephalic areas, brain stem, and spinal cord (Table 2–4).[15–17] Receptors vary in their affinities for exogenous opioids. For example, the mu receptor has highest affinity for morphine, levorphanol, and fentanyl, and analogs have been developed with selective agonism for mu, delta, and kappa receptors.[9,18] There are also receptor-selective antagonists. Receptors are not functionally specific. For example, mu, delta, and kappa receptors each participate in analgesia, but mu receptors play the major role.[8,19] There are at least two mu receptor subtypes, one (mu-2) affecting pain and respiration equally and the other (mu-1) being more specifically analgesic.[2] Mu-1 receptors bind morphine and the enkephalins with equal affinity; mu-2 receptors bind morphine more avidly than the enkephalins. Mu-1 receptors are antagonized by naloxonazine, which blocks analgesia, prolactin release, acetylcholine turnover, and hypothermia but not respiratory depression, growth hormone release, bradycardia, sedation, inhibition of electrically stimulated guinea

Table 2–3. Receptor Specificities of Natural and Synthetic Opioids

---

Mu
  Beta-endorphin
  Morphine
  Levorphanol
  Fentanyl
  [Met]enkephalyl-Arg-Arg-Val-NH$_2$
  [D-Ala^2-NMePhe^4, Gly-ol]enkephalin (DAGO)
  [Met]enkephalyl-Arg-Arg-Val-Gly-Arg-Pro-Glu-Trp-
    Trp-Met-Asp-Tyr-Gln (BAM 18)
  [Met]enkephalyl-Arg-Phe
  Tyr-D-Arg-Phe-Lys-NH$_2$

Delta
  [Leu]enkephalin
  [Met]enkephalin
  Beta-endorphin
  [D-Ala^2-D-Leu^5]enkephalin (DADLE)
  [D-Pen^2-D-Pen^5]enkephalin (DPDPE)

Kappa
  Dynorphin A (1-17)
  Dynorphin B
  Alpha-neo-beta-neoendorphin
  Dynorphin A (1-18)
  [D-Pro^{18}]dynorphin A (1-11)
  U-69,593
  PD 117302
  Ketocyclazocine
  Pentazocine
  Butorphanol
  Nalbuphine
  Nalorphine

Data from references 7–9.

pig ileum, or dopamine turnover.[20,21]

The relative contributions of mu, delta, and kappa receptors to euphoria are uncertain; all are found in limbic areas including the nucleus accumbens. Morphine is highly mu-specific (more so than any endorphin), and naloxone in doses low enough to be mu-specific blocks heroin-conditioned place preference.[22] Kappa receptors in the CA3 field of the hippocampus contribute to reward seeking; animals self-inject dynorphin A into this area, and stimulation of the hippocampal granule cell layer is rewarding.[7] A number of kappa opioids, including pentazocine, butorphanol, and nalorphine, are self-administered intravenously by rats.[23]

Actions at mu, delta, and kappa receptors are antagonized by naloxone. A fourth receptor type, the sigma receptor, has affinity for mixed agonist-antagonists such as cyclazocine as well as for phencyclidine. Its effects are not blocked by naloxone, and it is currently not classified as an opioid

receptor.[24] Additional opioid receptors or receptor subtypes mediate inhibition of smooth muscle contraction, hypothermia or hyperthermia, and proconvulsant or anticonvulsant effects.[25] Such diversity explains the complex actions of particular opioids. For example, the effects of nalorphine result from competitive antagonism at mu receptors, partial agonism at kappa receptors, and agonism at sigma receptors. Some opioid effects are not understood in terms of any combination of receptors, for example, why morphine produces sedation in some subjects but not others.[2]

The existence of multiple opioid receptor types also helps to explain different abstinence syndromes, for example, of morphine, cyclazocine, and nalbuphine. A partial agonist such as nalbuphine relieves abstinence symptoms in subjects no longer receiving morphine by occupying vacant receptor sites but precipitates abstinence in subjects fully dependent on morphine by replacing a weak agonist for a strong

Table 2–4. Opioid Receptor Distribution

Mu
  Neocortex (especially layers I, III, and IV)
  Caudate and putamen
  Nucleus accumbens
  Thalamus
  Hippocampus
  Amygdala
  Inferior and superior colliculi
  Midbrain periaqueductal gray matter
  Brain stem raphe nuclei
  Nucleus solitarius
  Spinal trigeminal nucleus
  Spinal cord dorsal horn

Delta
  Orbitofrontal olfactory areas
  Neocortex (especially layers II, III, V, and VI)
  Caudate and putamen
  Nucleus accumbens
  Amygdala

Kappa
  Caudate and putamen
  Nucleus accumbens
  Amygdala
  Hippocampus
  Hypothalamus
  Posterior lobe of the pituitary
  Median eminence
  Midbrain periaqueductal gray matter
  Brain stem raphe nuclei
  Spinal trigeminal nucleus
  Spinal cord dorsal horn

Data from reference 15

one. A mixed agonist-antagonist such as cyclazocine precipitates abstinence in subjects dependent on drugs occupying receptor types for which it is a competitive antagonist but does not precipitate abstinence when both it and the drug of dependence are agonists for the same receptors. It and the dependent drug are then cross-tolerant.[2]

Two questions have obvious clinical relevance: First, what are the anatomic substrates of opioid-mediated analgesia, positive reinforcement (euphoria), and physical dependence? Second, are these actions pharmacologically dissociable?

Opioid-related pain control has at least two anatomic and functional components. The first is concerned with pain perception threshold. Beta-endorphin, the enkephalins, and the dynorphins are each present in high concentration in the midbrain periaqueductal gray matter, electrical stimulation of which causes naloxone-reversible analgesia.[26] Analgesia also follows injection of morphine into this area.[27] The periaqueductal gray matter is part of a descending system that ultimately inhibits nociceptive impulses in the dorsal horn of the spinal cord. It probably contributes to analgesia associated with placebo; acupuncture; transcutaneous nerve stimulation; fear; and other stresses such as fighting, sexual arousal, food deprivation, or temperature changes;[19,28,29] each of these analgesic effects is reversible with naloxone.[30-32] The responsible descending pathways are anatomically and pharmacologically complex, with important relays in the nucleus raphe magnus of the medulla and involvement of serotonin, norepinephrine, dopamine, acetylcholine, histamine, somatostatin, thyroid-releasing hormone, neurotensin, and cholecystokinin.[19,28,29,33,34]

The second component of pain control involves psychological response. Morphine-induced analgesia depends as much on relief of the anxiety and tension that accompany pain as on elevation of pain perception threshold; the anatomic basis of this action—presumably limbic—is uncertain. Pain is separable into at least two types. *Phasic* (sudden, sharp) pain is mediated by the lateral spinothalamic tract and relays mainly to the sensory cortex. *Tonic* (persistent) pain is mediated by a more medial system and relays mainly to limbic areas. Opioids appear to affect tonic pain at the limbic rather than the spinal level. Interestingly, although phasic pain shows considerable tolerance to opioid analgesia, tonic pain does not.[35]

Opioid reward has been studied in nondependent animals using place preference, brain stimulation, and self-administration paradigms. Results indicate that opioid positive reinforcement is crucially dependent on the ventral tegmental area (VTA)–nucleus accumbens (NA) *reward circuit*. Microinjections of morphine into the VTA are rewarding, and opioids increase firing of VTA dopaminergic cells,[7] probably by hyperpolarizing local GABA-containing interneurons, with secondary disinhibition.[35a] Opioids injected into the NA are also reinforcing, and this effect, which appears to be secondary to opioid-induced reduction of synaptic transmission,[35b] is independent of VTA dopamine neurons.[36] Neuronal subpopulations that probably participate in opioid reinforcement include dopamine D1 and D2 cells in the VTA and neurons in the NA, frontal cortex, lateral hypothalamus, CA3 hippocampus, medial thalamus, and substantia innominata/ventral pallidum (SI/VP).[7,36-38]

There are no known exogenous or endogenous opioids that are strongly analgesic without producing physical dependence. On the other hand, the mu-1 antagonist naloxonazine reduces morphine analgesia in rats without preventing the development of physical dependence. Such dissociability of analgesia and physical dependence has spurred search for mu-1–selective agonists.

Reward seeking and physical dependence are also dissociable. Rats self-administer morphine directly into the VTA at intervals too long to produce signs of physical dependence,[39] and in place preference and intravenous self-administration models, rats demonstrate heroin seeking for weeks after receiving doses too small to produce physical dependence.[22,40] Conversely, chronic infusion of methionine-enkephalin, beta-endorphin, or morphine into rodent periaqueductal gray matter causes signs of physical dependence following naloxone challenge, but infusion into the VTA does not.[21,39] Animals do not self-administer morphine into the periaqueductal gray matter, and opioids passively injected into the periaqueductal gray matter inhibit rather than facilitate brain stimulation reward.[7] Other investigators, while acknowledging these results, believe there are brain areas that are responsible for both positive and negative reinforcement, even if the latter is manifested in a subtler fashion than frank withdrawal signs (e.g., dysphoria, or, in animals, disruption of motivated operant behavior).[38] The extent to which physical dependence contributes to drug-seeking behavior is a continuing controversy that involves other drugs as well as opioids.

Can there be physical dependence on endogenously released endorphins? Such is suggested by naloxone's ability to precipitate typical opioid withdrawal in physically stressed mice.[41] A child with recurrent apnea and elevated CSF beta-endorphin had signs suggesting opioid withdrawal following treatment with naltrexone.[42]

Is drug-seeking behavior, tolerance, or physical dependence associated with changes in endorphin concentration or in the number or sensitivity of opioid receptors? Although one group reported up-regulation of delta-receptors in rats following either long-term morphine or long-term naltrexone,[43] most studies failed to demonstrate a change in opioid receptor numbers with physical dependence.[44,45] If up-regulation is restricted to particular receptor subtypes, however, it could be difficult to identify.[46] Conditioned place preference for heroin-related cues persists for several weeks in animals no longer receiving the drug and is unaffected by doses of naloxone high enough to block endorphins; this finding suggests that once opioid "addiction" is established, its continued expression in opioid-free subjects is mediated by nonopioid systems.[22] On the other hand, rats receiving chronic morphine do have increased levels of brain encephalinase and decreased levels of pituitary and brain beta-endorphin and enkephalin.[47] Plasma beta-endorphin levels are reduced in heroin-dependent humans and increase during withdrawal.[48] Heroin-dependent humans also have a rise in CSF beta-endorphin during withdrawal; CSF methionine-enkephalin levels rise when acupuncture is additionally given.[49] Heroin users lack a normal circadian rhythm of secretion of the proopiomelanocortin-derived peptides, ACTH, beta-lipotropin, and beta-endorphin.[50] CSF endorphin levels are often abnormally high in humans receiving long-term methadone, and heroin users, in whom levels are quite variable, tend to respond best to methadone maintenance treatment when pretreatment levels are either abnormally low or high.[51,52] Although these reports imply that perturbations of endorphins or their receptors do contribute to symptoms and signs in opioid abusers, they hardly produce a consistent picture.

How do opioids affect other neurotransmitter systems, and could such actions contribute to reinforcement or dependence? In addition to dopamine, investigators have studied serotonin, acetylcholine, adenosine, glutamate, norepinephrine, and cholecystokinin (Table 2–5).[7,45,53–63] As usual, results are conflicting. Particular attention has focused on norepinephrine. Neurons of the locus coeruleus have high concentrations of opioid receptors and fire in response to painful stimuli, an effect blocked by exogenous or endogenous opioids. Locus coeruleus cells also have norepinephrine receptors, and alpha-2-adrenergic agonists such as clonidine decrease cell firing. Naloxone reverses the depressant effect

Table 2–5. Opioid Interactions with Several Neurotransmitter Systems

Serotonin[45]

Serotonin turnover is increased in animals receiving morphine

Serotonin accelerates development of tolerance to morphine

Chemical destruction of serotonergic neurons decreases morphine tolerance and lessens signs of dependence

Acetylcholine[53]

Opioid withdrawal in dependent rats is exacerbated by cholinergic agonists and relieved by antagonists

In nonopioid-dependent dogs, carbachol injected into the midbrain periaqueductal gray matter causes signs indistinguishable from opioid withdrawal

Dopamine[7]

Opioids increase mesolimbic and nigrostriatal dopamine turnover

Dopamine agonists exacerbate opioid withdrawal symptoms, and antagonists decrease them

Neuroleptics in sufficient dosage block heroin self-administration

Adenosine[54,55]

Adenosine and drugs acting at the adenosine A1 receptor suppress, in vitro, naloxone-precipitated withdrawal contractions in opioid-dependent guinea pig ilium and, in vivo, morphine withdrawal signs in mice

Alkylxanthines (theophylline, caffeine), which block adenosine function, antagonize morphine analgesia and precipitate signs suggesting opioid withdrawal

Glutamate[56]

MK-801, which antagonizes N-methyl-D-aspartate receptors, in rats attenuates the development of tolerance to morphine analgesia as well as morphine physical dependence

Norepinephrine[61–63]

Clonidine decreases symptoms of opioid withdrawal and on discontinuation produces similar symptoms itself

Animals self-administer clonidine

Cholecystokinin[57]

The analgesic effect of morphine applied to rat spinal cord is abolished by spinal cord release of the neuropeptide cholecysttokinin. Such *antianalgesia* might play a role in opioid tolerance

of opioids but not of clonidine; piperoxan, an alpha-2-adrenergic antagonist, reverses clonidine inhibition and in nonhuman primates causes behavior resembling opioid abstinence and attributable to noradrenergic hyperactivity. Similar effects follow electrical stimulation of the locus coeruleus and are reversible with either opioids or clonidine.[58] Tolerance develops to suppression of locus coeruleus neurons by exogenous opioids.[59] In humans, clonidine produces analgesia, miosis, sedation, and respiratory depression, and sudden discontinuation causes symptoms resembling opioid withdrawal with increased plasma levels of 3-methoxy-4-hydroxy-phenylglycol (MHPG).[58,60] Clonidine, moreover, decreases abstinence symptoms and elevated MHPG levels following opioid withdrawal in humans.[61] Rats and monkeys self-administer clonidine.[62,63]

Whatever the effects of opioids on dopamine, norepinephrine, or other neurotransmitters, they are indirect and do not explain how opioids ultimately act.[64] Opioid receptor proteins have been purified, revealing molecular weights of 60 kd whether mu, delta, or kappa, and cDNA studies predict amino acid homologies of opioid receptors and the immunoglobulin superfamily, including cell-adhesion molecules, myelin-associated glycoprotein, and platelet-derived growth factor.[65] In 1992 a delta receptor cDNA was cloned and characterized, revealing homology to G-protein-coupled receptors for somatostatin, angiotensin, and interleukin-8.[66,672]

In neuroblastoma–glioma cell cultures possessing opioid receptors, opioids decrease adenyl cyclase levels; tolerance develops to this effect, and opioid withdrawal or addition to the medium of an opioid antagonist causes rebound increase in cyclic adenosine monophosphate (AMP) levels above predrug levels.[67] Opioid inhibition of brain adenylyl cyclase has also been observed.[68] Perhaps related is the observation that sodium ions affect opioid agonists and antagonists differently; the affinity of pure antagonists for opioid receptors is unchanged, that of pure agonists is profoundly decreased, and that of mixed agonist-antagonists is mildly weakened. Sodium may influence receptor interactions with membrane G proteins.[24]

Contrary to expectation, however, cyclic AMP and opioids produced the same effect on neuronal firing. Opioids, through mu, delta, and kappa receptors, reduce neurotransmitter release in many regions of the peripheral nervous system and CNS, and it has been proposed that the mechanism of inhibition is not by affecting cyclic AMP but rather by mobilizing intracellular calcium (via mu and delta agonism) or by modulating voltage-sensitive calcium channels (via kappa agonism). Others describe a dual action of opioids, dependent on concentration and receptor subtype. High concentrations inhibit neurotransmitter release either by increasing potassium conductances or by decreasing calcium conductances, and these effects, blocked by pertussis toxin, are mediated by Gi/Go membrane proteins. Low concentrations stimulate neurotransmitter release by prolonging the calcium component of the presynaptic action potential duration, and this effect, blocked by cholera toxin, is coupled by a Gs-like membrane protein to adenylyl cyclase.[65,69,70]

Historical Background and Epidemiology

The poppy has been harvested for its opioid content for more than 6000 years. Appearing in ancient Assyrian and Egyptian art, it was used for analgesia; whether early use was also for euphoria is unknown.[58,71] Opium was available in Europe by the middle of the 16th century; Paracelsus is said to have formulated laudanum (tincture of opium), and 18th-century physicians recognized its dependence potential.[1,72] By the 19th century, opium was popular in many countries as a euphoriant.[73] In 1839, the British successfully waged the "Opium War" with China to preserve its profitable opium trade, and in Europe during this time, laudanum was readily available; celebrated users include Thomas de Quincey and Samuel Taylor Coleridge. (Such self-styled "opium eaters" were actually "opium drinkers.")

During and after the Civil War, opioid use became widespread in the United States. Morphine was easily obtained with or without a prescription, and opium was present in over-the-counter remedies such as "Dover's Powder," "Godfrey's Cordial," "Darby's Carminative," and "Mrs. Winslow's Soothing Syrup." The invention of the hypodermic needle led to injectable morphine and more rapid and powerful effects than could be achieved with oral preparations. Opium continued to be legally imported, morphine was legally manufactured from it, and opium poppies were legally grown.[74] The number of Americans addicted to opioids by the end of the 19th century is controversial—estimates range from 200,000 to more than 1 million (4% of the population). Most were white, middle-class, middle-aged women taking either opium in patent medicines or injectable morphine.[75] (A possible explanation for female preponderance is that they were not welcome in saloons.) In the 1890s, heroin was introduced as a "nonaddictive" opioid for treating morphine dependence and as an over-the-counter antitussive.[76]

A notable addict of this period was the surgeon, William Halsted, who successfully "cured" a debilitating addiction to cocaine by switching to morphine; maintaining himself on 180 mg daily, he remained professionally productive—and to his colleagues and friends mentally and physically sound—for more than three decades.[77] During this time, it was a common medical practice to try to convert alcoholics to morphine.

The first steps toward opioid prohibition in the United States were racially motivated: Chinese immigrant laborers had brought with them the custom of smoking opium in "dens," and during the 1880s, many localities banned them and restricted the preparations of opium for smoking. The result was a widespread switch to morphine.[74] In 1914, the Harrison Narcotics Act curtailed a physician's right to give opioids to addicts, banned their nonmedical availability, and regulated their manufacture and distribution. Whether the Harrison Act led to a decrease in opioid addiction depends on which figures one accepts for the number of addicts before its passage. In 1918, the number of current American opioid addicts was estimated at 238,000. At least 12,000 received daily morphine from legal dispensing clinics set up by local health departments. In 1924, however, the U.S. Treasury Department closed down these clinics, and thereafter opioid addiction became a crime.[78] (In 1952, the U.S. Supreme Court ruled that imprisonment for merely being an addict represented "cruel and unusual punishment" and was therefore unconstitutional. "Purchase" and "possession" are still punishable, however, making it rather difficult for someone to be addicted to illicit opioids without breaking the law.[74])

During the 1930s, most opioid abusers smoked opium; only 13% injected heroin, and only 17% were black.[79] Following World War II, epidemics of heroin use occurred in black communities, for example, Chicago in the late 1940s, affecting largely nondelinquent adolescents. During the 1950s, heroin-related deaths rose steadily in New York City—from 50 in 1950 to 311 in 1961—with blacks representing more than half. By the mid-1960s, minority use became widespread, especially among unemployed young men who had often been criminally active before they used drugs. In 1972, the number of heroin users in the United States was estimated at more than 600,000, over half of whom were in New York City.[80] A subsequent decline in heroin use was followed by a rise in the 1980s that coincided with increased entry of high-quality heroin into the United States from the Middle East.[81,82] In 1980, 213 deaths from opioid "poisoning" in young men were reported to the Centers for Disease Control (CDC); by 1986, the figure had risen to 619,[83] and similar increases were reported from Europe and Asia.[84-86] In the late 1980s, it was estimated that heroin had been used at least once by more than 2 million Americans—including 1.3% of high school seniors.[87,88] In 1991, a review of data from drug treatment centers, surveys of homeless people, and data from the Federal Bureau of Investigation and the National Institute of Justice estimated the number of Americans addicted to heroin to be between 900,000 and 1 million.[89] (Although American physicians are more likely than their counterparts in the general population to use minor opioids without supervision, they are less likely to abuse heroin or major opioids.[90])

In the early 1970s, when Turkey was reducing its opium crop (estimated at about 80 metric tons in the 1960s), the purity of street heroin averaged about 3% to 5%. A few years later, with opium production in Iran, Afghanistan, and Pakistan estimated at 1600 metric tons, New York City street heroin purity rose as high as 17%.[91] In 1984, 11,000 pounds of heroin were smuggled into the United States, 50% to 75% through New York City.[92] On the West Coast, much heroin has always been imported from Southeast Asia, often of very high purity ("China White");[93] during the 1980s, when the celebrated "Pizza Connection" convictions in New York City destabilized Italian Mafia control of the U.S. heroin trade, the vacuum was filled by Chinese organized crime ("Tongs"), and the amount of American heroin imported from the "Golden Triangle" (the juncture of borders of Thailand, Laos, and Myanmar) rose to more than 50%. New supply sources also flooded the market from South America and West Africa.[94,673] In New York City in 1991, the purity of street heroin was typically 40% to 45%, and the price per milligram had fallen to about 1 dollar.[95,674]

Relevant to attempts by law enforcement agencies to stamp out heroin use by curtailing opium supply abroad is the fact that the amount of heroin imported annually into the United States is derived from less than 2% of world opium production, an amount that would require fewer than 25 square miles of poppy cultivation.[78] Myanmar, Afghanistan, and Pakistan alone produce 20 times as much opium as is needed for the entire U.S. heroin market. The manufacture of heroin is quite simple, and probably less than 15% of what is smuggled into the United States is blocked.[96]

Much of the current American heroin population includes former users who had stopped when the only available material was expensive, scarce, and lowgrade. White-collar workers abuse both parenteral heroin and analgesics prescribed by physicians.[82,97,98] Inner-city users often inject heroin and cocaine together ("speedball"). By the 1990s, in response to falling prices, rising purity, and the threat of acquired immunodeficiency syndrome (AIDS), nonparenteral use—sniffing, snorting, and smoking—became increasingly popular.[99,100]

Often unappreciated is the fact that the majority of heroin users do not take it daily. Most experiment with it for months before obvious dependence develops and repeatedly discontinue use—often for more than a year—after becoming physically dependent.[101–105] Naloxone challenge reveals that up to 45% of applicants to methadone maintenance programs are not physically dependent on opioids.[106,107] In fact, estimates of the prevalence of intermittent or "controlled" heroin users ("chippers," "joy poppers") in the United States have been as high as 4 million.[108]

The relationship between opioid use and crime is complex, yet urban crime rates do rise and fall with heroin retail price.[109–111] The average New York City heroin user engages in almost daily crimes (not including drug trafficking or use), largely thefts, check forgery, and prostitution. Criminal activity frequently precedes heroin use, however,[112] and drug-related violent crime, including homicide, most often involves users and dealers.[80,101]

Acute Effects

Heroin (diacetylmorphine) crosses the blood–brain barrier faster than morphine and is then metabolized to 6-acetylmorphine (which has opioid activity) and morphine. Three milligrams of heroin are equivalent to 10 mg of morphine (Figure 2–1).[1] Experienced users cannot tell heroin from morphine when they are given subcutaneously but are often able to do so when they are given intravenously.[113] It is uncertain if heroin's more rapid effect confers greater dependence liability. (That possibility—along with efficacy, side effects, and potential for street diversion—is relevant to the debate over the comparative merits of heroin and morphine in treating cancer pain.[114] Further complicating the controversy are observations in rats that heroin and 6-acetylmorphine are each more rewarding than morphine[115] and in mice and rats that heroin has direct CNS receptor specificities not shared by morphine.[116])

Illicit heroin—"horse," "crank," "jive," "smack," "junk," "shag," "dope," "shill," "H," "white stuff," "Lady Jane," "boy," "lemonade" (poor-grade heroin), "dynamite" (high-grade heroin)—is usually sold in glassine envelopes ("bags") that contain about 90 mg of white powder, with heroin concentrations ranging from zero to over 90%. (Until the late 1980s, most bags contained 5 to 10 mg heroin.) In New York City five to 40 mg is quinine, originally added in the 1930s for its antimalarial properties and retained because it produces vasodilation, which some users believe enhances the "high," and also, from the dealer's standpoint, because its bitter taste disguises the true content of heroin present.[117] (On the West Coast, quinine is infrequently present in heroin preparations.) The rest of the mixture contains varying quantities of lactose, mannitol, baking soda, procaine, lidocaine, talc, starch, and even on occasion curry powder, Ajax, Vim, or strychnine.[118,119]

Dissolved in unsterile water in a bottle cap or spoon and heated with a match, it is then drawn into an eye dropper or syringe through cotton (purportedly to filter out impurities) and injected either intravenously ("mainlining") or subcutaneously ("skinpopping"). Smokers, "sniffers," or "snorters" are less likely than parenteral users to become compulsive daily users, although some do become severely addicted without ever injecting heroin.[120,121] An additional advantage of nonparenteral use is that overdose is unlikely. (In Europe and India, a growing number of heroin users "chase the dragon": The drug is placed on tinfoil and heated from beneath; the vapor produced is then "chased" and inhaled through a straw or tube.[122] The popularity of this technique seems to have resulted from the ready availability of impure "brown heroin," which is difficult to dissolve for injection.[123,124])

Effects of heroin or morphine include drowsiness, difficulty concentrating, and euphoria, although

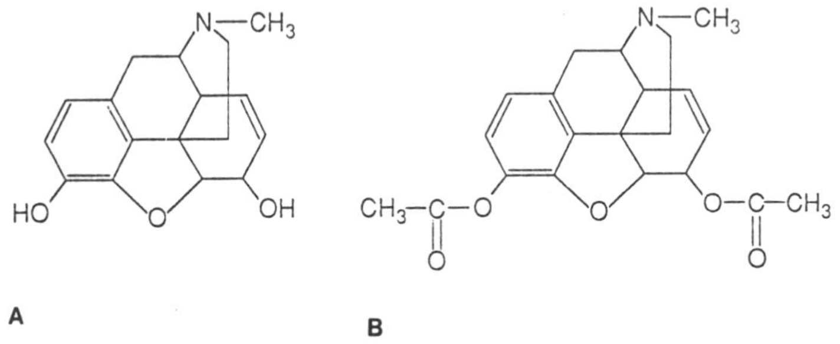

Figure 2–1. Morphine (A) and heroin (B).

A

B

sometimes there is fear or anxiety, especially in non-dependent, pain-free normal subjects (Table 2–6). (Psychotomimetic effects and visual hallucinations can occur after morphine or heroin administration, but are much more often associated with mixed agonist-antagonists such as pentazocine.[125]) Analgesia is more to deep burning pain than to pinprick; both threshold of pain perception and the ability to tolerate pain are increased. Nausea and vomiting occur less often in dependent than naive subjects but can be severe in daily users, who, far from being bothered, refer to the symptoms as "a good sick."[126] Miosis, secondary to stimulation of the autonomic (Edinger-Westphal) nucleus of the oculomotor nerve, may be so marked ("pinpoint") that the light reflex—which opioids do not interrupt—is difficult to discern. Other effects include dryness of the mouth, pruritus, sweating, suppression of the cough reflex, respiratory depression, hypothermia, postural hypotension, constipation (resulting from gastrointestinal hypertonicity and decreased propulsion), reduced gastric acid secretion, biliary tract spasm, and urinary retention. There is electro-encephalographic slowing as in natural sleep, but the time spent in the rapid eye movement (REM) phase is decreased.[127] With high doses, the electroencephalogram may have irritative features, and rarely multifocal myoclonus or seizures occur.[113,128–130] There is increased production of antidiuretic hormone (ADH), prolactin, and calcitonin and reduced secretion of ACTH, luteinizing hormone, and growth hormone.[1,78,131–134] Libido is decreased, although early in the course of dependence potency may be enhanced.[135,136] The insulin response to glucose is reduced, and platelet and coagulation alterations resemble those found in diabetics.[137–139]

Parenteral heroin produces a "rush" ("kick," "thrill," "hit," "flash"), an ecstatic feeling lasting about a minute and often compared to orgasm but usually referred to the abdomen and accompanied by itching and flushing of the skin. The user may then "go on the nod," experiencing a dreamlike, pleasant drowsiness and alternately dozing and suddenly awakening; skeletal muscle tension may be decreased only in the neck and face, so the subject seems asleep on his feet. (A "rosette of cigarette burns on the chest" is an almost pathognomonic sign of "nodding.") Alternatively, there may be "drive," with increased psychomotor activity and garrulous boastfulness ("soap-boxing").

Marked tolerance develops to euphoria, analgesia, and respiratory depression; doses of 500 mg morphine daily have been achieved in only 10 days, and addicts have received 5000 mg morphine without serious consequence. There is less tolerance to smooth muscle effects (e.g., constipation and miosis).[78,140,141] Tolerant users tend to be dysphoric, depressed, hypochondriacal, irritable, and socially withdrawn most of the time except briefly after each injection, and there is greater tolerance to "drive" than to "nodding."[142]

Overdose causes coma with pinpoint but reactive pupils and respiratory depression or apnea. Anoxic brain damage, however, can produce large, unreactive pupils.

Treatment of overdose begins with attention to apnea or shock (Table 2–7). Because opioids depress brain stem carbon dioxide sensitivity, oxygen use should be carefully monitored in patients dependent on hypoxic respiratory drive.[1] Hypotension usually responds quickly to correction of hypoxia and administration of fluids (which, because heroin pulmonary edema may be present, should be given cautiously); vasopressors or plasma expanders are rarely needed.[143]

For patients with respiratory depression, naloxone is given in an initial dose of 2 mg intravenously.[144] If signs are not promptly reversed, boluses of 2 to 4 mg are repeated up to a total dose of 20 mg. High doses may be required for propoxyphene, pentazocine, diphenoxylate, nalbuphine, butorphanol, or buprenorphine overdose, but failure to respond to 20 mg should make one consider alternative diagnoses, superimposed anoxic-ischemic brain damage or additional drugs. Patients who lack adequate veins and are not hypotensive can be given naloxone intramuscularly or subcutaneously. Patients with depressed sensorium but normal respira-

Table 2–6. Acute Effects of Heroin

"Rush"
Euphoria or dysphoria, "drive"
Drowsiness, "nodding"
Analgesia
Nausea and vomiting
Miosis
Dryness of the mouth
Pruritus
Sweating
Suppression of the cough reflex
Respiratory depression
Hypothermia
Postural hypotension
Constipation
Biliary tract spasm
Reduced gastric acid secretion
Urinary retention
Suppression of rapid eye movement sleep

Table 2-7. Treatment of Opioid Overdose

Ventilatory support
If hypotension does not respond promptly to ventilation, IV fluids. (Pressors rarely needed)
Consider prophylactic intubation
If respiratory depression, naloxone, 2 mg IV, IM, or SQ, and then 2 mg to 4 mg repeated as needed up to 20 mg. If no respiratory depression, naloxone, 0.4 mg to 0.8 mg IV, IM, or SQ, and if no response, 2 mg repeated as needed.
Hospitalization and close observation, with additional naloxone as needed
Consider overdose with other drugs, especially cocaine and ethanol

Source: Goldfrank LR, Bresnitz EA. Opioids. In: Goldfrank LR, Flomenbaum NE, Levin NA, et al., eds. Toxicologic Emergencies, ed 4. Norwalk, CT: Appleton & Lange, 1990:433.

tions should initially receive smaller doses to avoid "overshoot" and precipitation of withdrawal signs; 0.4 to 0.8 mg naloxone is given and if there is no response, 2 mg doses are repeated every 2 to 3 minutes. Maximal effect occurs 2 to 3 minutes after intravenous naloxone but only about 15 minutes after intramuscular or subcutaneous administration. In some centers, because of frequent vomiting, routine endotracheal intubation is performed before giving naloxone. Although too much naloxone can precipitate opioid withdrawal symptoms, naloxone is shorter acting than most opioids, and unobserved patients can slip back into coma and apnea. Close observation is required for at least 24 hours with morphine or heroin and for 72 hours with methadone or propoxyphene, and it may be necessary during that time to give naloxone either in 5 mg hourly boluses or by prolonged infusion. (Naloxone infusion can be established at an hourly rate of two-thirds whatever dose reversed respiratory depression; the rate can then be titrated to the reappearance of respiratory depression or the emergence of withdrawal signs.)

A common feature (10% to 15%) of opioid overdose is noncardiogenic pulmonary edema, either present at the outset or appearing during the first 24 hours of hospitalization. It has followed either parenteral or intranasal heroin, and its cause is unclear. Possibilities include anaphylaxis, hypoxia, and vascular damage secondary to street adulterants, especially quinine. Aspiration further complicates the picture. Treatment is with positive pressure ventilation and oxygen, not digitalis, diuretics, or morphine.[1,144]

When heroin is combined with parenteral cocaine or amphetamine, paranoid psychosis can predominate or become unmasked by naloxone.[145] Heroin is also smoked with "crack" cocaine or phencyclidine.[146] Opioids taken with barbiturates or ethanol produce atypical signs including coma unresponsive to naloxone.[147] Conversely, naloxone has reportedly reversed signs of ethanol intoxication, perhaps by inhibiting GABA, and so a response may not be opioid-specific (see Chapter 11).[148]

Dependence and Withdrawal

Accompanying opioid tolerance are psychic and physical dependence and withdrawal symptoms and signs (Table 2-8).[78,149-151] Four to 6 hours after the last heroin dose, drug craving begins. At 8 to 12 hours, irritability and anxiety become marked, and there is weakness, tearing, rhinorrhea, sweating, and yawning, often followed by several hours of restless, tossing sleep from which the addict awakens feeling worse than ever, with achiness, mydriasis, piloerection ("cold turkey"), severe anorexia, nausea, vomiting, abdominal cramps and tenderness, hyperactive bowel sounds, diarrhea, violent yawning, hot flashes, fever, tachycardia, hypertension, and sweating alternating with chills. Pain in the back and limbs accompanies muscle spasms and kicking movements ("kicking the habit"). Erection or ejaculation occur in men and orgasm or menorrhagia in women. The respiratory response to carbon dioxide is exaggerated, with increased respiratory rate. Hypersecretion of bronchial mucous glands

Table 2-8. Symptoms and Signs of Opioid Withdrawal

Drug craving
Irritability, anxiety
Tearing
Rhinorrhea
Sweating
Yawning
Myalgia
Mydriasis
Piloerection
Anorexia, nausea, and vomiting
Diarrhea
Hot flashes
Fever
Tachypnea
Productive coughing
Tachycardia
Hypertension
Abdominal cramps
Muscle spasms
Erection, orgasm

produces clear sputum and rales or rhonchi relieved by coughing. There is increased urinary excretion of epinephrine and 17-hydroxycorticosteroids and often leukocytosis. Dehydration and ketosis can rarely lead to cardiovascular collapse, but in contrast to ethanol or barbiturate abstinence, opioid withdrawal does not cause seizures (except perhaps in newborns), hallucinations, or *delirium tremens* and is hardly ever life-threatening. In fact, the syndrome is often compared to a bad case of "the flu," and its unpleasantness does not fully explain the degree of drug craving. Symptoms peak at 24 to 72 hours with morphine and heroin and usually last 7 to 10 days, but full recovery takes longer—sometimes much longer.

Protracted abstinence is two-phased, with mild behavioral abnormalities and increased pulse, blood pressure, temperature, and carbon dioxide sensitivity lasting several weeks, followed by several months of pulse, blood pressure, temperature, carbon dioxide sensitivity, and pupillary size below predependence levels. During this time, there is increased urinary epinephrine excretion, an elevated cold pressor response, increased response of the autonomic nervous systems to nociceptive stimuli, and continued abnormalities of REM sleep.[150–152]

Protracted abstinence has been observed in animals. Monkeys display signs of acute abstinence for up to several months after withdrawal from morphine, and rats have electroencephalographic abnormalities, "wet-dog" shakes, fever, hypermetabolism, increased water intake, and drug-seeking behavior for up to a year.[153,154] Protracted abstinence may be related to dopamine receptors. Striatal dopamine D2 receptors in rats demonstrated abnormally increased binding during morphine dependence and abnormally decreased binding during protracted abstinence.[155] The degree to which protracted abstinence contributes to persistent drug craving in humans is uncertain but has obvious implications for treatment.

Methadone's action lasts 24 to 36 hours, and there is a similar abstinence syndrome, beginning 8 to 24 hours after the last dose and peaking at 6 days; the most severe symptoms last up to 3 weeks (Figure 2–2). Rifampin, phenytoin, carbamazepine, and barbiturates (but not valproate) accelerate methadone metabolism and precipitate withdrawal symptoms in patients receiving maintenance therapy.[156–158] By unclear mechanisms, metyrapone also precipitates opioid abstinence.[159]

Animal studies suggest that both tolerance and physical dependence can develop after a single opioid dose.[160] The matter is controversial, however; as

Figure 2–2. Methadone.

noted earlier, there are animal models in which widely spaced low doses of opioids produce reward seeking without evidence of tolerance or physical dependence. Human subjects receiving morphine several times daily for 2 weeks develop mild abstinence symptoms when it is stopped. Naloxone precipitates severe abstinence symptoms after only 2 days of morphine and mild symptoms if given within 24 hours of a single dose of morphine or within a week of a single dose of methadone—at a time when acute effects of the opioid are no longer measurable.[161–163] The severity of the abstinence syndrome is dose dependent up to about 500 mg morphine daily.

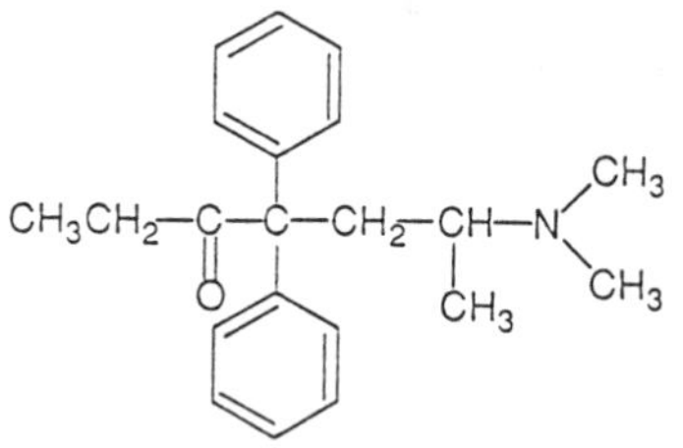

Opioid abstinence symptoms are usually relieved by oral methadone, 20 mg once or twice in the first 24 hours, with subsequent tapering titrated to symptoms.[143] Patients already receiving high doses of methadone as maintenance therapy may require more. About one-fourth of each previous day's dose prevents recurrence. (It is a violation of federal law, however, to give opioids to relieve abstinence symptoms except as "emergency" therapy for inpatients or in federally approved drug-treatment programs.[164]) A British study found that oral heroin also effectively prevented opioid withdrawal symptoms, but frequent doses throughout the day were required, and the mean daily heroin dose (55 mg) was significantly higher than the mean daily methadone dose (36 mg).[165]

The effectiveness of clonidine in suppressing withdrawal symptoms is less certain.[166–168] More sedating and hypotensive than methadone, it carries the theoretical advantage of treatment through nonopioid receptor systems allowing more rapid restoration to baseline status.[58] In contrast to methadone, clonidine suppresses abstinence symptoms without affecting the withdrawal process itself. Its efficacy is probably related to inhibitory action on the locus coeruleus, but additional mechanisms are also possible; in both heroin addicts and controls, clonidine raised plasma beta-endorphin levels. Used in conjunction with methadone, clonidine reduces the time required for detoxification from long-term methadone.[61] In patients detoxified from heroin or methadone, clonidine caused a significant reduction in withdrawal symptoms and signs compared with methadone itself or placebo.[166,169] Comparable success has been claimed with lofexidine, a similar drug.[170] In one study, patients preferred clonidine to placebo even though neither relieved withdrawal symptoms and clonidine produced "substantial impairments in psychomotor performance."[171] In another study, clonidine suppressed objective autonomic signs of morphine withdrawal but not subjective discomfort or craving.[172] Postural hypotension is a common side effect.[173] Clonidine abuse, with psychic dependence, was reported in two patients receiving methadone maintenance treatment.[173a]

The more specific alpha-2-adrenergic agent, guanfacine, in one study relieved autonomic symptoms (e.g., tearing, sweating, hot flashes, orgasm) more than psychological (anxiety), neuromuscular (achiness, tremor), or gastrointestinal (abdominal cramps, diarrhea) symptoms, and craving persisted.[174] In another study, all symptoms except "sleep disturbances" were relieved in over 80% of patients.[175] In a randomized controlled trial, guanfacine was superior to clonidine but inferior to methadone.[173]

Clonidine and naltrexone have been given together to achieve simultaneous opioid withdrawal and initiation of antagonist maintenance.[176,177] Large doses of both agents produced "rapid and comfortable" detoxification in only 4 days.[152,178] (Surprisingly, patients receiving either methadone or heroin had equally short detoxifications.)

Another approach to acute detoxification involves substituting buprenorphine (2 to 8 mg sublingually daily) for heroin or methadone. After a month, it is abruptly stopped, and a high dose (35 mg) of naloxone is given; the resulting abstinence syndrome is usually mild and well tolerated.[152,179] Buprenorphine substitution has also been followed by 1-day detoxification with combined naltrexone and clonidine.[179a]

The dopamine D2 antagonist sulpiride reportedly decreased both objective and subjective symptoms of heroin withdrawal; the effect was attributed to secondary hyperprolactinemia (which inhibits self-administration of heroin in animals) rather than dopamine blockade per se.[180,181]

As might have been predicted from studies with endorphins, acupuncture has relieved abstinence symptoms.[182] In animals, transcutaneous cranial stimulation potentiated analgesia and attenuated opioid abstinence signs.[183]

In newborns of opioid-dependent mothers, withdrawal signs can be severe or even fatal (Table 2–9). Screaming is high-pitched and protracted, diarrhea is explosive, and there is vomiting and poor feeding yet frantic thumb or fist sucking. Myoclonus or seizures can be difficult to tell from severe jitteriness and if they do occur might be secondary to other agents such as barbiturates. Mortality is as high as 90% without treatment, and signs resemble those associated with neonatal hypoglycemia, hypocalcemia, intracranial hemorrhage, meningitis, or sepsis, any of which could coexist.[184–188] Withdrawal signs are especially severe in newborns of mothers taking heroin plus cocaine.[189]

Sudden withdrawal from opioids during pregnancy carries a high risk of premature labor, fetal distress, meconium aspiration, and fetal death.[190,191] Gradual withdrawal with methadone or other agents is impractical when—as it is not unusual—the mother's first appearance at a health care facility is after labor has begun. Even if slow detoxification is accomplished earlier in pregnancy, abstinence through term is unlikely. Methadone maintenance causes its own neonatal withdrawal syndrome—more protracted and, according to some, more severe than that of heroin.[188,192,193] Recommended treatment includes barbiturates, benzodiazepines, phenothiazines, methadone, and paregoric.[185,194] The few empiric data available as well as theoretical considerations of cross-tolerance favor using an opioid; phenobarbital is more useful when there has been prenatal exposure to multiple drugs.[195]

Such infants are often of low birth weight and small for gestational age.[196] The Moro reflex is hyperactive and persists well beyond the usual 20 weeks.[197] Respiratory distress syndrome is common, and there may be an increased frequency of sudden

Table 2–9. Neonatal Opioid Withdrawal

Irritability
Tremor, jitteriness
Increased muscle tone and tendon reflexes
Screaming
Sneezing
Yawning
Tearing
Sweating
Skin pallor or mottling
Fever
Tachypnea and respiratory distress
Tachycardia
Vomiting
Diarrhea
Myoclonus, seizures (?)

infant death.[198] Later in life, there is hyperactivity, disturbed sleep, or impaired cognition.[199,200] Small birth weight and behavioral abnormalities follow intrauterine opioid exposure in animals,[201,202] and both animal and human mothers and offspring have demonstrated chromosomal aberrations.[203–206]

Some of these reports are problematic. Several studies of such children during the first few years of life found no long-term developmental or cognitive sequelae; however, because mothers tend to underreport drug use during pregnancy, differences between users and nonusers could be masked.[207,208] Studies claiming abnormalities have not always addressed the quality of prenatal care, including the use of other drugs, ethanol, or tobacco, or factors such as maternal psychopathology or low intelligence.[196,209–212] A controlled study did show "low average and mildly retarded intellectual performance" in preschool children of mothers taking heroin or methadone during pregnancy, but correlation was with inadequate prenatal care, *prenatal risk score*, and home environment, not with maternal opioid use per se.[213]

Medical and Neurological Complications

Before the AIDS epidemic, the average case fatality rate of heroin addicts in both the United States and Europe was 1% to 2% per year.[214–218] In the late 1960s, heroin-related fatalities were the most common cause of death among New York City men aged 15 to 35.[219] Of these, 40% resulted from violence, especially homicide. Slightly more than half followed overdose or acute adverse reaction to the opioid or an adulterant. Wide variations in the content of street heroin make overdose a continued risk.[85] Subjects dying within 3 hours of injection have higher blood morphine levels than those dying later, and there is strong correlation between the clinical diagnosis of overdose and brain morphine concentrations.[220–222] The frequency of sudden death in a community correlates positively with the amount of heroin in street packages and inversely with prices.[223–225]

Heroin "body packers" swallow or insert in body orifices drug-containing condoms to smuggle or to avoid detection by police.[226,227] Opioid intoxication, intestinal obstruction, and sudden death occur, and attempted endoscopic removal can cause packet rupture. In one case, blood concentration of morphine was 120 mg/L and that of 6-acetylmorphine 184 mg/L.[228] Fatal asphyxiation followed an attempt to swallow a packet of heroin.[229]

In 1985, a striking rise in the number of fatal heroin overdoses in New Mexico was attributed to the availability of Mexican "black tar" heroin, which is difficult to dilute to sublethal levels.[230]

In some patients, coma and death are difficult to explain on the basis of true overdose (Table 2–10). The needle may be found in the vein, implying sudden death. Pulmonary edema is frequently present, and even in the absence of other drugs or anoxic-ischemic brain damage, coma may not respond to naloxone.[223] Death has followed very small amounts of heroin or even oral methadone.[231] Opioids alone can cause pulmonary edema (as noted more than a century ago by Osler);[232] other adulterants damage pulmonary capillaries; and quinine causes cardiac conduction abnormalities, peripheral vasodilation, and ventricular fibrillation. Quinine-related cardiotoxicity has been reported in heroin users.[233,234] Heroin and ethanol are also individually associated with cardiac arrhythmia, and synergism between heroin, ethanol, and quinine could underlie sudden heroin death.[223,225,233,235,236] Hypersensitivity reaction or asthma secondary to histamine release is also possible.[215,223,237] Suggesting an immunologic factor in heroin pulmonary edema is reduction of the C3 component of complement in some patients.[238]

Additional medical complications in heroin users include thrombophlebitis and pulmonary embolism;[239] pulmonary hypertension from talc microemboli;[240] hepatotoxicity;[241] chronic abdominal pain and intestinal pseudo-obstruction;[242] and a syndrome of fever, myalgia, and periarthritis.[243] Heroin nephropathy, probably an immunologic disorder, can cause neurological disease, including uremia, malignant hypertension, hypertensive encephalopathy, and hemorrhagic stroke.[244] Renal damage

Table 2–10. Noninfectious Medical Complications of Heroin Use

"Nonoverdose sudden death"
  Pulmonary edema
  Asthma
  Quinine cardiotoxicity
Thrombophlebitis, pulmonary embolism
Pulmonary hypertension
Hepatotoxicity
Intestinal pseudo-obstruction
Myalgia/periarthritis
Nephropathy
  Immune
  Amyloid
Decreased glucose tolerance
Thrombocytopenia

could also be secondary to amyloidosis or to the immune complex glomerulonephritis of bacterial endocarditis.[245] Altered pulmonary function is common in heroin users, and heroin inhalation has precipitated fatal asthma.[237,246] Heroin users have decreased glucose tolerance.[247] Thrombocytopenia has been associated with antiplatelet antibodies.[248]

Before the AIDS epidemic, infection accounted for about 5% of New York City heroin deaths (Table 2–11). Especially common is infectious hepatitis B. In a survey of New York City parenteral drug abusers, 86% had serologic evidence of hepatitis B infection; none was positive for hepatitis D.[249] Among parenteral drug abusers in the Netherlands, 74% were seropositive for hepatitis C.[250] Of 110 Spanish heroin addicts with acute hepatitis, 63 had hepatitis B and 35 hepatitis C; nearly half of those with hepatitis B also had hepatitis D. All the patients with hepatitis C and 75% of those with hepatitis D developed chronic liver disease.[251] In the early 1980s, an epidemic of hepatitis A in Portland, Oregon, was linked to intravenous drug abuse.[252]

Bacterial infections affect almost any organ and often involve exotic organisms. Skin poppers develop local abscesses, cellulitis, and pyomyositis, and parenteral abusers of any type are at continued risk for sepsis, pneumonia, and a host of direct or blood-borne infections.

Endocarditis is common, affecting in equal frequency the mitral, aortic, and tricuspid valves and

Table 2–11. Non-HIV Infectious Complications of Heroin Abuse

Hepatitis
Skin abscesses, cellulitis
Pyomyositis
Fasciitis
Pneumonia
Sepsis
Infected venous pseudoaneurysm
Enophthalmitis
Chorioretinitis
Episcleritis
Arthritis, including pyogenic sacroiliitis and
  sternocosto-chondritis
Osteomyelitis, including vertebral
Endocarditis
Malaria
Tick-borne relapsing fever
Tetanus
Botulism
Candidiasis, including cardiac and disseminated
Nocardiosis
Mucormycosis
Tuberculosis

most often caused by *Staphylococcus aureus*, which street-purchased antibiotics render resistant to methicillin or oxacillin.[215,218,253–256] The source of the organism appears to be neither the drug itself nor the injection paraphernalia but rather carriage in the nose.[257] Other organisms include *Pseudomonas* (which may be harbored in areas of heart valve fibrosis caused by street heroin additives)[258] and *Candida* (which may necessitate surgical valve replacement)[259] as well as unusual organisms such as *Neisseria subflava* and *Wangiella*.[260,261]

A malaria epidemic among heroin users in California was traced to a Vietnam veteran.[262] Similar cases in Spain were traced to a traveler from Africa.[263]

During a single summer, four heroin users were admitted to the same hospital in Seville, Spain, with tick-borne relapsing fever (*Borrelia*).[264]

Such infections directly or indirectly affect the nervous system. Infectious hepatitis—or its sequela cirrhosis—causes encephalopathy and if clotting is deranged predisposes to traumatic or even spontaneous intracranial hemorrhage.

Vertebral osteomyelitis causes back or neck pain, radiculopathy, and sometimes cord compression.[265–268] Cervical infection is especially common among addicts who inject into the jugular vein.[269] Symptoms frequently precede diagnosis by several weeks. Early in the course, plain cervical radiographs are often normal; computed tomography (CT) is more sensitive. In one series, *S. aureus* was grown in 10 of 14 cases.[269] Others have reported a preponderance of gram-negative organisms, especially *Pseudomonas*.[270–272]

Endocarditis causes intraparenchymal or extraparenchymal abscess of the brain or spinal cord, meningitis, cerebral infarction, diffuse vasculitis, and subarachnoid hemorrhage from rupture of a septic (*mycotic*) aneurysm.[273–276] Subtle or insidiously progressive neurologic or systemic symptoms, such as headache, fever, syncope, hemiparesis, or aphasia, are common with mycotic aneurysms; sudden onset suggesting subarachnoid hemorrhage is less frequent than with saccular aneurysms, and CSF white cell pleocytosis can precede rupture. Although mycotic aneurysms sometimes disappear with antimicrobial therapy, they also persist, enlarge, or burst, arguing for prompt surgical excision once they are identified. At Harlem Hospital and St. Luke's–Roosevelt Hospital in New York City, 28 cerebral mycotic aneurysms were identified in 17 patients; five patients had aneurysmal rupture during or following appropriate antimicrobial therapy, and of 20 aneurysms followed angiographically, 10 became smaller or disappeared, whereas 10 remained unchanged or enlarged, one with fatal rupture (Table 2–12).[277] Mycotic aneurysms in heroin users have occurred on the carotid, subclavian, and pulmonary arteries.[278–280]

Tetanus, usually severe, is especially common in skin poppers with multiple skin abscesses, making it nearly impossible to identify the lesion that harbors *Clostridium tetani*. Quinine, which aggravates anaerobic conditions, further encourages bacillus growth.[281–283] At Harlem Hospital Center, of 34 patients with tetanus seen during a period of 8 years, 30 were heroin users. The case fatality rate was 70% for the drug users and 50% for the nondrug users. Among the drug users, curarization was frequently necessary to control tetanospasms, and even well-controlled patients often had unexplained cardiac arrest (Table 2–13).[281]

Wound botulism with dysphagia, blurred vision, dysphonia, and descending paralysis has occurred in parenteral drug users in several American cities.[284,285]

Heroin users are immunocompromised even in the absence of human immunodeficiency virus (HIV) infection.[286] Endogenous opioids regulate the activation of natural killer (NK) cells and the prolifera-

Table 2–13. Causes of Death in Tetanus Patients at Harlem Hospital Center

Heroin Users	
Inadequately controlled tetanospasms	5
Infection	3
Pulmonary embolism	1
Cardiac arrest	
Secondary to respiratory insufficiency	3
Without apparent cause	9
Nonheroin Users	
Perforated viscus	1
Stroke	1

Source: Brust JCM, Richter RW. Tetanus in the inner city. NY State J Med 1974; 74:1735.

tion of T lymphocytes, and morphine suppresses interferon levels in mice.[287,288] Tuberculosis and fungal infections are therefore frequent in HIV-negative heroin users; reports include devastating cerebral mucormycosis, intravertebral candidiasis, cryptococcal meningitis, nocardial brain abscess, and brain stem chromoblastomycosis.[289–294]

During the 1980s, a rising prevalence of disseminated candidiasis in Europe was associated with the practice of dissolving Iranian "brown heroin" in lemon juice, an excellent culture medium for *Candida albicans*.[295–297] Disseminated candidiasis occurred in a Swiss man who injected buprenorphine tablets dissolved in bottled lemon juice, culture of which grew *C. albicans*.[298] British and Dutch heroin samples were found contaminated with aflatoxin, which could further contribute to immunosuppression.[299]

As of 1992 in the United States nonhomosexual parenteral drug abusers constituted 23% of the 249,000 adults and adolescents with AIDS reported to the CDC (and half of reported women with AIDS). Male homosexual drug abusers constituted another 6%. At that time, the rate of growth of the AIDS epidemic was decreasing among male homosexuals but increasing among parenteral drug abusers.[300,301] In New York City, the majority of AIDS-related deaths occur in parenteral drug abusers. In 1982, 29% of patients in a New York methadone maintenance treatment program had antibodies to HIV; by 1984 the figure was 87%,[302] and 75% of hospitalized parenteral drug abusers had inverted helper-suppressor T lymphocyte ratios.[303] A survey of 242 North Italian heroin users revealed HIV seropositivity in 76%.[304] The prevalence of HIV infection is especially high in communities where needles are shared; in "shooting galleries,"

Table 2–12. Mycotic Aneurysm Behavior in Relation to Antibiotic Therapy

Behavior During Therapy	No. of Aneurysms
Bled before treatment, early excision	4
Bled before treatment, then enlarged during treatment	1
Bled during treatment, then continued to enlarge	1
Bled during treatment, after enlarging	1
Bled during treatment, then early excision	2
Bled following treatment, then early excision	1
Never bled, early excision	1
Never bled, but enlarged or unchanged during or after treatment	7
Never bled, became smaller or disappeared during or after treatment	10
Total	28

Source: Brust JCM, Dickinson PCT, Hughes JEO, Holtzman RHH. The diagnosis and treatment of cerebral mycotic aneurysm. Ann Neurol 1990; 27:238.

drug users rent unsterile equipment previously used by others.[305-307] Such practices contribute to the higher incidence of AIDS among male compared with female drug abusers. Needle sharers have increasingly taken to cleaning their equipment with bleach, and needle exchange programs in Europe and the United States have led to reduced sharing.[308,309] Whether such programs actually slowed the spread of virus is uncertain, and political pressure has limited their expansion in the United States. (In 1991, a New York City judge ruled that AIDS prevention justified the illegal distribution of clean hypodermic needles to drug addicts.[310] The decision reflected American ambivalence over needle distribution programs in particular and drug abuse and AIDS in general.) For a variety of reasons—saturation of high-risk behavior groups, loss of HIV-seropositive drug users from the pool of active drug abusers, entry of HIV-seronegative new drug abusers into the pool, and conscious reduction of risky behavior—in 1987 HIV seroprevalence among parenteral drug abusers in New York City appeared to have stabilized at approximately 60%.[311] Similar stabilization was evident in other cities (e.g., Stockholm, Innsbruck, San Francisco), whereas in some with low prevalence rates (e.g., Los Angeles), the numbers were still rising.

Because AIDS is a sexually transmitted disease and affects heterosexual partners of carriers and because one-third of women entering treatment for opioid abuse engage in prostitution, the disease claims victims lacking the usual risk factors.[312] In the United States, AIDS develops in 13% to 30% of children born to HIV-seropositive mothers, the great majority of whom are either parenteral drug abusers or sexual partners of parenteral drug abusers.[300]

Parenteral drug abusers have the same neurological complications of HIV infection that afflict other risk groups, including CNS opportunistic infections, neoplasms, stroke, peripheral neuropathy, vacuolar myelopathy, and primary HIV encephalopathy (*AIDS-dementia complex*) (Table 2–14). Of special concern is tuberculosis, the prevalence of which had declined steadily in the United States until it rose sharply in the late 1980s. Clinically apparent tuberculosis develops in 10% of HIV-infected patients, and parenteral drug abusers are especially at risk; extrapulmonary tuberculosis—including meningitis, Pott's disease, and CNS tuberculoma or abscess—is encountered far more frequently than in HIV-negative patients with tuberculosis.[313-315] Purified protein derivative (PPD) tuberculin tests are frequently negative in HIV-seropositive parenteral drug abusers, who should be considered positive with

Table 2–14. Major Neurological Complications of HIV Infection

HIV meningitis
Peripheral neuropathy
    Early, Guillain-Barré–like
    Late, sensory, painful
Herpes zoster
Opportunistic CNS infection
    Toxoplasmosis
    Cryptococcal meningitis or granuloma
    Progressive multifocal leukoencephalopathy
    Cytomegalovirus
    Candida, mucor, nocardia, and other fungi
    Herpes simplex
    Tuberculosis (meningitis, Pott's disease, brain
      abscess, or intraparenchymal tuberculoma)
    Syphilis
CNS lymphoma
Stroke (nonbacterial thrombotic endocarditis, cerebral
    vasculitis, intracranial hemorrhage)
Vacuolar myelopathy
HIV encephalopathy (AIDS-dementia complex)

2 mm induration (rather than the usual 5 mm); they should also undergo anergy testing.[316] As if immunosuppression were not enough, in the early 1990s AIDS patients were increasingly infected with tubercle bacilli resistant to conventional antimicrobials.[675] During 1990, tuberculosis was diagnosed in 263 patients at Harlem Hospital Center; 81% were HIV seropositive.

Also of concern is syphilis.[317-324,676] Genital ulcers and promiscuous behavior are added risk factors for HIV infection in drug abusers. Syphilitic meningitis, meningovascular syphilis, and general paresis cause symptoms similar to those of other AIDS-related infections (including HIV encephalopathy); the diagnosis is therefore easy to miss.[317] Moreover, syphilis in HIV-seropositive subjects is reportedly characterized by negative serology (including negative CSF VDRL in the presence of neurosyphilis),[318] an aggressive course,[319] and treatment failures necessitating maintenance therapy.[320] In a study from Miami, 12 of 829 AIDS patients (1.5%) had neurosyphilis; at least 4 were parenteral drug abusers, and 4 had been treated for early syphilis.[321] Of 42 patients from Houston with combined HIV infection and neurosyphilis, 5 had abnormal CSF but were asymptomatic, 9 had meningitic symptoms, 5 of these nine plus 15 others had cranial neuropathies, and 11 had strokes.[322] A recommended alternative to maintenance penicillin in uncomplicated early syphilis is three doses of 2.4×10^6 units of benzathine penicillin; for neurosyphilis, 12 to 24×10^6 units of penicillin daily for 10 days is required.[323]

More than 90% of patients with AIDS have neuropathological abnormalities at autopsy, and up to 92% have neurological symptoms and signs.[314,325–344] The latter high figure is from a prospective study of symptomatic HIV-seropositive patients at Harlem Hospital Center.[344] A retrospective survey of AIDS cases reported to the CDC suggested that parenteral drug abusers are more likely than other risk groups to have cryptococcal meningitis and CNS toxoplasmosis.[345] The Harlem Hospital Center study found no difference between parenteral drug abusers and nondrug-abusing homosexuals in the prevalence of these infections or of such neurological symptoms as dementia, hemiparesis, seizures, ataxia, or peripheral neuropathy.[344] In Baltimore, controlled neuropsychological studies of asymptomatic HIV-seropositive parenteral drug abusers found that they—similar to nondrug-abusing asymptomatic HIV-seropositive homosexuals—had no evidence of significant cognitive impairment.[346]

A Canadian study found that "use of various recreational drugs" did not increase the risk of AIDS developing in men seropositive for HIV,[347] and a Baltimore study found that over an 18-month period CD4 cell counts fell no faster among HIV-seropositive parenteral drug abusers than among other HIV-seropositive groups.[348] A New York City study found no difference in the rate of acceleration to AIDS between HIV-seropositive parenteral drug abusers and non-drug abusers; among drug abusers, however, there was higher pre-AIDS morbidity and mortality, especially from bacterial infection.[348a]

Coinfection with HIV and cytomegalovirus, each presumably from needle sharing, occurred in two intravenous drug abusers. The mononucleosis-like illness that followed perhaps resulted from enhancement of each virus's replication by the other.[349]

Parenteral drug abusers are also subject to infection with either human T cell lymphotropic virus (HTLV)-I or HTLV-II retroviruses.[350–353] HTLV-I is associated with T cell leukemia and myelopathy; HTLV-II is not consistently associated with any disease.[353] In a Veterans Administration study of serum obtained during the 1970s from 585 East Coast methadone maintenance patients, 18% were seropositive for HTLV-II, but none was seropositive for HTLV-I.[354] In a CDC survey of 3217 parenteral drug abusers in 29 American treatment centers, HTLV seroprevalence rates ranged from 0.4% to 18%, with the highest in Los Angeles, New Orleans, and Seattle; 84% of the positive samples were HTLV-II.[353] Similar prevalence and HTLV-II preponderance were reported in northern Italian parenteral drug abusers.[355] None of these surveys described clinically apparent myelopathy, yet myelopathy evidently due to HTLV-I has been reported in parenteral drug abusers from Louisiana, Florida, and Washington, DC.[356–360] From a different vantage, of 25 patients with HTLV-I–associated myelopathy reported to the CDC from 1988 to 1990, three were parenteral drug abusers.[361]

Heroin users are prone to stroke unrelated to liver or kidney disease, endocarditis, or AIDS. A report from Harlem Hospital Center involved six patients aged 25 to 38 years.[362] Four, all normotensive, had cerebral infarcts in association with loss of consciousness after intravenous heroin. In one of these, cerebral angiography was normal. In another, there was stenosis of the internal carotid artery at the siphon and of the early anterior cerebral artery, plus occlusion of the middle cerebral artery; the changes suggested primary vessel disease rather than emboli. Two other active heroin users had occlusive strokes that did not follow overdose or even a recent injection. In one, who was normotensive, cerebral angiography was consistent with widespread small vessel arteritis. Suggesting hypersensitivity, one of the patients had blood eosinophilia, hypergammaglobulinemia, and a positive direct Coombs test, and another had an elevated erythrocyte sedimentation rate and positive latex fixation.

Other reports of occlusive stroke in heroin users include a 19-year-old boy who had taken heroin intravenously for a year, plus intermittent lysergic acid diethylamide (LSD), and developed sudden global aphasia; cerebral angiography suggested diffuse angiitis.[363] A 21-year-old woman devloped hemiparesis 2 weeks after starting daily heroin and 6 hours after an intravenous injection; accompanying symptoms suggested anaphylaxis, with eosinophilia and angiographic changes consistent with cerebral arteritis.[364] Cerebral infarction followed the first heroin injection in several months in a 20-year-old man whose cerebral angiogram showed arterial "beading."[365] A 34-year-old man developed hemiparesis while sniffing heroin; cerebral angiography was normal.[366] Another young man had infarction in the territory of the left anterior choroidal artery after sniffing heroin.[366a] Two Danish patients, aged 30 and 35, awakened from presumed overdose with aphasia and right hemiparesis; cerebral angiography was normal in each.[367] Intracerebral hemorrhage occurred in a young German within minutes of intravenous heroin.[368] A middle-aged woman who had taken daily heroin intranasally for many years had rupture of a cerebellar vascular malformation.[369]

A man using intravenous heroin after 2 years of abstinence developed nalorphine-responsive coma and apnea and then, over several hours, progressive quadriparesis, anarthria, dysphagia, and sensory loss, suggesting a ventral pontine lesion; it was unclear if the cause was vascular.[370]

Heroin could cause stroke by several mechanisms (Table 2–15).[118,371] Hypoventilation causes hypotension and decreased cerebral perfusion, and bilateral globus pallidus infarction is common at heroin-user autopsies. Hemiplegia has appeared on awakening from nalorphine-responsive coma, and overdose has produced dementia, spastic quadriparesis, deafness, seizures, and dystonia. In some cases, an awkward posture of the neck during overdose coma might have kinked the carotid artery and further decreased cerebral perfusion.[367] Delayed postanoxic encephalopathy also occurs.[372]

Refractile particles are observed in the skin of heroin users, and jugular vein injectors sometimes accidentally hit the carotid artery, yet embolization of foreign material to the brain has rarely been documented in heroin users.[373,374] It more often affects parenteral abusers of other drugs.[117,375] In the 1970s, pentazocine (Talwin) and tripelennamine (Pyribenzamine)—"T's and blues"—were widely abused in Chicago and other midwestern cities.[376,377] Crushed oral tablets were suspended in water, passed through cotton or a cigarette filter, and injected intravenously. Cerebral hemorrhages and infarcts resulted.[378] At autopsy, there was often pulmonary arteriolar occlusion by microcrystalline cellulose or particulate magnesium silicate (talc).[379,380] Such microemboli are especially likely to reach the brain when multiple lung emboli have caused pulmonary hypertension and opened functional pulmonary arteriovenous shunts.[118] Lesions consistent with cerebral vasculitis are seen angiographically in T's and blues stroke patients.

Talc microemboli were present at autopsy in the liver, spleen, and brain of a parenteral paregoric abuser.[381] A young man who frequently injected pulverized unfiltered meperidine tablets intravenously had occasional seizures after injection and then impaired memory and visual blurring; there were fundal hemorrhages and arteriolar occlusions, and symptoms improved with abstinence.[382]

Consistent with allergic vasculitis are frequent immunologic abnormalities in heroin users—for example, altered complement, hypergammaglobulinemia (including elevated immunoglobulin M [IgM] independent of IgG and IgA), circulating immune complexes, antibodies to smooth muscle and lymphocyte membranes, and false-positive serology for syphilis.[238,383] Opium, morphine, codeine, and meperidine have caused urticaria, angioneurotic edema, and anaphylaxis.[384] Morphine binding by gamma globulin has been observed in addicts and experimental animals.[385,386]

During heroin withdrawal, platelet alpha-2-adrenoceptors and epinephrine-induced platelet aggregation are increased.[387] Other clotting abnormalities in a heroin user were traced to heparin added to the drug mixture, raising the specter of hemorrhagic strokes should such a practice become popular.[388]

Possibly vascular in origin is heroin myelopathy. Acute paraparesis, sensory loss, and urinary retention usually occur shortly after injection and often follow a period of abstinence.[389–400] Symptoms are sometimes present on awakening from coma. Preserved proprioception in some suggests infarction in the territory of the anterior spinal artery. In one autopsy, there was necrosis "confined almost entirely" to the upper thoracic cord gray matter, and in another there was also involvement of the anterior aspect of the posterior columns and a pyramidal tract in the lower thoracic cord.[396] Possible causes of these lesions, as with heroin cerebral strokes, include "borderzone" cord infarction during a period of coma and hypotension, embolism of foreign material, and direct toxicity or hypersensitivity. Consistent with the latter was a man who, remaining awake, had episodic numbness and weakness of both legs for a few minutes after each injection.[397] An adolescent 11 days after injection developed a rash on his chest and feet and then, following a second injection 6 days later, paraplegia.[399] Cord biopsy in another patient showed vasculitis affecting mainly small arteries and arterioles, with "double refractile fragments" in inflamed tissues.[393] A patient at Harlem Hospital Center developed paraparesis and urinary retention after a friend injected heroin into a vessel over his midthoracic spine; myelography was normal, and it was presumed that the common intercostal origins of the posterior cutaneous and spinal arteries or veins had allowed access of the injected

Table 2–15. Possible Causes of Stroke in Heroin Abusers

Hypertension (nephropathy)
Clotting derangement (liver disease, thrombocytopenia)
Endocarditis (embolic infarction, ruptured mycotic aneurysm)
Overdose, hypoperfusion
Particle embolism
Allergic vasculitis
Toxic vasculitis

Table 2–16. Noninfectious Neurological Complications of Heroin Abuse

Stroke
Myelopathy
Seizures
Peripheral nerve injury
Peripheral neuropathy
Brachial and lumbar plexopathy
Cranial neuropathy
Rhabdomyolysis
Fibrotic myositis
Quinine amblyopia
Lead poisoning
Chloroquine encephalopathy
Spongiform encephalopathy
MPTP parkinsonism

material. In another case, an anterior spinal artery syndrome with quadriplegia followed supraclavicular heroin injection.[401]

A number of other neurological complications affect heroin users (Table 2–16). Peripheral neuropathy includes Guillain-Barré type.[402–404] Peripheral nerves are also damaged by direct injection, by local infection, or by pressure palsies during coma.[405] Bilateral ulnar palsy developed secondary to osteomyelitis affecting the ulnar diaphysis.[406] Two cases of iliopsoas infarction were diagnosed by CT and biopsy; in one, there was also femoral neuropathy.[407] Painful brachial and lumbosacral plexopathies resemble neuralgic amyotrophy, suggesting an immunologic origin.[408–412] Brachial plexopathies have also resulted from septic aneurysm of the subclavian or axillary arteries;[413] angiography should be considered in patients with appropriate symptoms. Persistent vocal cord paralysis has followed repeated jugular vein injections,[414,415] and a young Thai, taking his first heroin dose in several months, awoke with bilateral, severe, permanent sensorineural deafness; the site of pathology was not determined.[416]

Myoglobinuria with renal failure can follow prolonged coma and is likely the result of direct muscle compression. It also follows injection without loss of consciousness, suggesting hypersensitivity;[409,411,417–429] in one instance, recurrent myoglobinuria followed a repeat injection.[425] Rhabdomyolysis has also followed heroin sniffing.[430] In some cases, myocardial involvement with acute ventricular failure has accompanied rhabdomyolysis.[431] A Harlem Hospital Center patient who chronically injected heroin into his deltoids developed fibrotic myositis and abduction contracture of the shoulders.[432] It was unclear if the myopathy was due to nonspecific repeated needle trauma or local toxicity of heroin or an adulterant,[432] but studies of animals receiving systemic morphine suggest chemical toxicity to muscles.[433]

Optic atrophy occurred in a Harlem Hospital Center patient whose heroin mixture provided huge doses of quinine: about 5 g daily. A dealer as well as an addict, he was able to serve as his own control by preparing his heroin without quinine. Vision then improved.[434] A report from Sri Lanka indicated that dyschromatopsia affected 83% of heroin addicts. Quinine was not mentioned, and 40% of patients inhaled the drug.[435]

Abdominal pain and ascending tetraplegia occurred in several Italians who used a batch of unrefined brown heroin contaminated with lead salts.[436] Lead-contaminated heroin caused bilateral brachial plexopathy in another Italian[437] and colic and encephalopathy in a Spaniard.[438]

Adulteration of heroin with chloroquine caused headache, confusion, and visual disturbance in a British user.[439]

Spongiform encephalopathy affected 47 Dutch heroin smokers practicing the technique of "chasing the dragon."[440] Symptoms began with apathy, bradyphrenia, and cerebellar dysarthria and ataxia; some patients then developed spastic hemiparesis or quadriparesis, tremor, chorea, myoclonus, pseudobulbar palsy, fever, blindness, and, in 11 instances, death. CT showed cerebral and cerebellar white matter lucency, and at autopsy there was edema and spongiform white matter degeneration, including the spinal cord. All heroin samples had come from Amsterdam and contained variable amounts of procaine, phenacetin, caffeine, antipyrine, strychnine, quinine, lidocaine, and diethylcarbonate. The disease could not be reproduced in rats or rabbits, and the responsible toxin was not identified. Five similar cases subsequently appeared in Turin, where it was shown that brain stem auditory evoked potentials were frequently prolonged in asymptomatic "dragon chasers."[441,442] Two German "Chinese blowers" developed severe persistent cerebellar signs, and magnetic resonance imaging (MRI) revealed white matter abnormalities.[443] Reversible coma and spasticity developed in a 2-year-old Swiss boy, whose magnetic resonance images revealed cerebral and cerebellar white matter lesions; heroin was present in urine and gastric samples, but route and duration of exposure were unknown.[443a]

In 1979, severe parkinsonism was reported in a young Maryland graduate student who manufactured and self-injected a meperidine analog, 1-methy-4-propionoxy-piperidine (MPPP).[444] He later died of a drug overdose, and at autopsy destruction of the substantia nigra zona compacta was evident; other areas usually involved in Parkinson's disease such as the locus coeruleus and the dorsal motor nucleus of the vagus were spared. Parkinsonism then began appearing in the San Francisco Bay area among users of MPPP sold as "synthetic heroin," and the responsible toxin was identified as a by-product of MPPP synthesis, 1-methy-4-phenyl-1,2,3,6-tetrahydropyridine (MPTP).[445–448] Used commercially as a chemical intermediate, MPTP has also caused parkinsonism in laboratory workers accidentally contaminated by inhalation or skin contact.[449] Bradykinesia and rigidity are severe, with muteness and inability to swallow; one patient could move nothing but his eyes.[445,450] Dementia and autonomic impairment do not occur, however. Appearing within a few days of using the drug, symptoms sometimes progress for a few days after it is stopped.[445] Improvement is then rare, but levodopa/carbidopa and bromocriptine provide relief, often dramatically, and in some instances are probably life-saving.[449,451] Typical side effects of therapy include dyskinesia, on-off phenomenon, and psychiatric symptoms, and attempts after more than a year to wean patients off levodopa/carbidopa have been unsuccessful.[452]

The CSF of affected patients contains elevated protein levels and, as in Parkinson's disease, decreased homovanillic acid levels, but unlike Parkinson's disease, CSF 3-methoxy-4-hydroxyphenyl glycol (MHPG) is normal, implying sparing of norepinephrine systems.[151] In monkeys given MPTP, toxicity is restricted to dopaminergic neurons of the nigrostriatal system.[452–454]

Heroin users exposed to single doses of MPTP have not developed parkinsonian symptoms, but it is feared that the disease might emerge with advancing age and "normal" decreases in dopaminergic activity.[453] Symptoms have been reported in previously asymptomatic patients,[449,452] and positron-emission tomography (PET) (using 18-F-dopa) of asymptomatic drug users exposed to MPTP showed decreased numbers of dopamine-containing neurons.[455]

Parkinsonism caused by MPTP has implications beyond drug abuse. Although species vary greatly in the neurological signs produced by MPTP, with primates most prominently affected, striatal dopamine depletion occurs in every animal studied, including rat, mouse, guinea pig, and frog.[452] MPTP is metabolized to 1-methy-4-phenylpyridinium (MMP+).[456] This reaction and the ability of MPTP to deplete dopamine, destroy neurons, and produce parkinson-ism is blocked by the type B monoamine oxidase (MAO) inhibitors pargyline and deprenyl.[457] MPP+ but not MPTP is selectively taken up by dopaminergic neurons; probably MPTP enters glia (the receptor for it being MAO itself) and is biotransformed there to MPP+, which then enters nigral dopaminergic neurons by way of the dopamine uptake system, binds to neuromelanin, and, by inhibiting mitochondrial oxidation of NADH-linked substrate, destroys the cells.[458–461] The dramatic if serendipitous history of MPTP has raised the possibility that Parkinson's disease itself is caused by an MPTP-like environmental or endogenous toxin and has stimulated new approaches to therapy.[462]

A case-control study at Harlem Hospital Center found that heroin use, both past and current, was a risk factor for new-onset seizures independent of overdose, head injury, infection, stroke, alcohol, or other illicit drugs.[463] In animals, opioids can be convulsant, anticonvulsant, or both and can modify post-ictal phenomena; these effects are variably blocked or not blocked by opioid antagonists. Effects depend on the opioid used, dose, route of administration, seizure type, and opioid receptor subtype.[464–477]

Other Related Agents

MPPP-MPTP and T's and blues demonstrate that when other opioids are more available than heroin, they are abused. The mixed agonist-antagonist pentazocine does not suppress morphine abstinence symptoms and in fact may precipitate them even though it does not antagonize morphine's respiratory depression; it is not liked by heroin addicts.[478] Nonetheless, oral and parenteral abuse do occur independently of T's and blues, and both psychic and physical dependence develops in patients originally taking it for analgesia.[479,480] At low doses, pentazocine causes euphoria, lightheadedness, sedation, impotence, and anhidrosis; higher doses cause headache, nausea, vomiting, blurred vision, diplopia, increased heart rate and blood pressure, urinary retention, respiratory depression, and dysphoric psychotomimetic symptoms including delusions and hallucinations. Seizures occur. In contrast to morphine and heroin, there appears to be a maximally tolerated dose. Withdrawal symptoms are milder than with heroin but include prominent drug-seeking behavior. Treatment of pentazocine withdrawal is with gradually decreasing doses of pentazocine itself.

Pentazocine abusers who inject the drug subcutaneously or intramuscularly develop severe focal skin and muscle fibrosis. Pentazocine injected intramuscularly into all four limbs and the trunk—in one case even the back—has produced symptoms suggesting the stiff man syndrome with hard, tender muscles and disabling contractures. Focal precipitation of acidic pentazocine is probably responsible.[481–483]

T's and blues seem to be a descendent of "blue velvet" (tripelennamine and paregoric) abuse in the 1950s; the combination is believed to avoid both the sedation of the opioid and the occasional stimulation of the antihistamine (although sedation with this agent is actually more common).[377,380,484] In studies with volunteers, tripelennamine in the usual street ratio of 1:2 did increase the euphoric effects of pentazocine.[485] Pentazocine and tripelennamine each cause seizures and psychosis, and in mice the two agents combined are considerably more lethal than either alone.[376,486]

Respiratory insufficiency is common.[487] Staphylococcal infections occur less often in T's and blues users than in heroin users, but *Pseudomonas* infections are more common, perhaps because tripelennamine is inhibitory to the former but not the latter.[488] In 1983, the manufacturer added naloxone to pentazocine tablets. T's and blues abuse then declined but did not disappear—perhaps because naloxone does not block pentazocine's sigma receptor actions and has no effect on tripelennamine.[489,490]

Similar parenteral abuse of the agonist-antagonist butorphanol mixed with diphenhydramine was reported in Mississippi adolescents.[491] Abuse of butorphanol alone—or of the mixed agonist-antagonist nalbuphine—is rare.[1]

Meperidine (Demerol) was originally introduced (like heroin) as a "nonaddicting" analgesic, and its ready availability soon produced a plethora of addicted physicians and nurses.[492] Its action is similar to morphine's despite chemical dissimilarity (Figure 2–3), but it has a shorter duration of action (2 to 4 hours) and is less likely to produce miosis. A toxic metabolite, normeperidine, causes tremor, agitation, confusion, delirium, myoclonus, and seizures.[493–495] (Normeperidine's biologic half-life is greatly prolonged in patients with renal failure, sickle cell disease, and cancer; repetitive doses of meperidine should be avoided in such settings.[144]) The combination of meperidine with MAO inhibitors exacerbates symptoms and can be fatal.[496] An elderly man who took 4000 mg meperidine over 9 days for postoperative pain developed severe parkinsonism that responded to levodopa/carbidopa; symptoms did not recur when treatment was stopped.[497] As with pentazocine, widespread fibrotic myositis com-

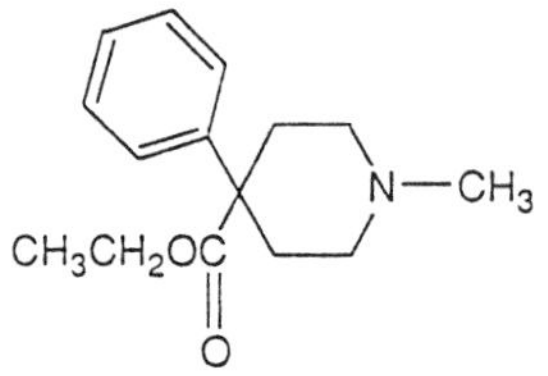

Figure 2–3. Meperidine.

plicates parenteral meperidine abuse.[498] Symptoms of meperidine abstinence usually appear within 3 hours after the last dose, peak at 8 to 12 hours, and decline over 4 to 5 days. There may be intense craving, nervousness, and muscle twitching but often little nausea, vomiting, diarrhea, or mydriasis.[1]

The low abuse potential of propoxyphene (Darvon), an analgesic about as strong as aspirin, is countered by its ready availability, and in 1980 the Food and Drug Administration (FDA), concerned about illicit use, recommended that prescriptions for it not be refillable.[499–502] Abuse may be oral or intravenous.[503] Propoxyphene is often implicated in drug-related deaths, especially in association with ethanol or tranquilizers, but its prevalence as a street drug is less certain.[504–506] Among adolescents arrested for ethanol-related offenses, propoxyphene is often abused but usually along with other drugs.[507] Similarly, propoxyphene or its metabolites were frequently identified at medical examiner autopsies, but when deaths were attributed to drug toxicity, multiple substances (e.g., benzodiazepines, barbiturates, amitriptyline, or ethanol) were present in 89%; although 30% had a history of ethanol or drug abuse, only 1.8% abused propoxyphene alone.[508,509] Propoxyphene abuse seems to occur most often among patients who take it initially for pain and then gradually increase the dose.[502] Intolerable subjective discomfort and craving may be resistant to even very gradual drug withdrawal.[510] Overdose causes delusions, hallucinations, and seizures, and death is often preceded by naloxone-resistant cardiodepression or pulmonary edema.[1,143,505,511–513]

Hydromorphone (Dilaudid) abuse, often parenteral, also spread during the late 1970s.[514] In Washington, DC, during 1987, there was a sharp increase in deaths related to hydromorphone, pills of which were crushed and sold as heroin.[515]

During the same period, New York City, New Jersey, Pennsylvania, and Los Angeles witnessed a rising popularity of glutethimide combined with codeine ("hits," "sets," "loads") or with acetaminophen plus codeine ("4's and doors").[516–518] The euphoric effect of these combinations resembles heroin's but is longer lasting. In 1980–1981 in northeast New Jersey, 236 deaths were attributed to "hits," compared with 126 for heroin and 46 for methadone.[519] In 1985–1987, nine such deaths occurred in Erie, Pennsylvania.[520] The abuse potential of codeine alone is quite low; it partially suppresses morphine withdrawal, and large doses (1200 to 1800 mg daily) produce a mild abstinence syndrome.[521] Upper extremity gangrene followed intra-arterial self-injection of crushed codeine tablets.[522] Reports from Australia describe abuse of codeine linctus, a mixture of codeine phosphate and squill oxymel, a cardiac glycoside; complications include diffuse myopathy with myasthenic features and cardiac atrioventricular dissociation.[523–525]

A woman became addicted to a kaolin and morphine antidiarrheal mixture and developed fatal hypokalemic myocardial necrosis.[526] High doses of the antidiarrheal opioid diphenoxylate produce euphoria and physical dependence, but low aqueous solubility prevents parenteral abuse. Even less likely to be abused is the antidiarrheal opioid loperamide, which is neither euphorigenic nor water soluble.[1]

In 1979, deaths began occurring among Southern California drug users who had thought they were taking high-grade Southeast Asian "China White" heroin but who in fact had been sold alpha-methyl-fentanyl, an analog of fentanyl (Figure 2–4).[527] Used as an anesthetic in major surgery, fentanyl is sometimes abused by health care professionals.[528] Commercially available derivatives include sufentanil, alfentanil, and Innovar (fentanyl plus droperidol, a neuroleptic). Abuse of alpha-methyl-fentanyl spread up the California coast and eastward to Arizona; at the time of its appearance, it was entirely legal, being unclassified as a scheduled drug. It and similar fentanyl analogs are easy and inexpensive to manufacture; chemicals and equipment worth 200 dollars can produce 2 million dollars worth of street drug.[529] More than 1400 potential analogs of fentanyl exist, and at least 10, some of which are thousands of times more potent than heroin, have appeared in the street, accounting for more than 100 overdose deaths.[530] They are usually taken intravenously but are sometimes snorted. Users describe effects different from heroin's: a "fainter rush," longer nod, and more gradual "comedown."[529] By the mid-

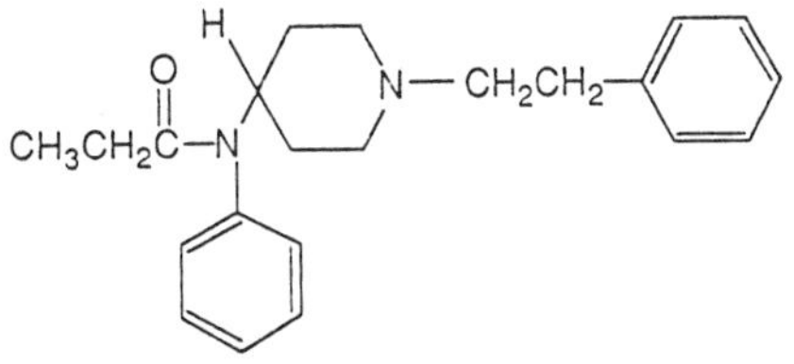

1980s, fentanyl analog "designer drugs" were taken by an estimated 20% of California's 100,000 "heroin" users, especially in suburban areas. Their use then declined sharply in the West, only to emerge in the East.[531–533] During 1988, 16 deaths from methyl-fentanyl were reported from Pittsburgh alone, and during a single weekend in 1991, more than 100 cases of overdose from methyl-fentanyl (nicknamed "Tango and Cash") were treated in New York City, New Jersey, and Connecticut; at least 12 ended fatally.[534]

In the 1950s, lofetamine, a drug that seems to combine opioid and amphetamine-like effects, was widely abused in Japan. In 1989, lofetamine abuse was reported in Italy.[535] Lofetamine may be a partial agonist; it relieves opioid withdrawal, its effects are reversed by naloxone, and pentazocine can be substituted for it.

Long-Term Treatment

The central controversy of whether opioid abuse is a social, a psychological, or a metabolic problem has produced different approaches to treatment.[536] Chronic drug-seeking behavior could be the result of protracted abstinence, consistent with the view that such subjects have a permanent opioid deficiency disease analogous to insulin-dependent diabetes mellitus,[151,537] or it could be more related to environmental psychological conditioning, as exemplified by detoxified patients who relapse into drug craving on returning to their old neighborhoods.[538] A powerful reinforcer might be not only the euphoria or relief of abstinence symptoms following drug intake, but also, as noted in Chapter 1, the risky goal directedness that fills an abuser's days. Many so-called addicts take far too little heroin to cause severe physical dependence and obtain opioid-like euphoria self-injecting saline ("needle freaks").[539] Similarly open to more than one explanation are the tendency of some opioid addicts to "mature out" in middle age,[540] the infrequency with which American soldiers physically dependent on heroin in Vietnam used the drug on returning to the United States,[541] and the rarity with which hospitalized cancer patients physically dependent on opioids experience drug craving after discharge.[35] (In a study of 38 outpatients with chronic noncancer pain who received opioid analgesics orally for several years, only two—both previous drug abusers—developed craving and dose escalation.[543])

Psychological and social factors are considered paramount by advocates of drug-free therapy. Data

Figure 2–4. Fentanyl.

supporting such an approach, however, are either discouraging or difficult to obtain. Relapse occurs in the vast majority of opioid addicts after either voluntary hospitalization or imprisonment (euphemistically called "civil commitment programs").[544–546]

Whatever the role of psychological factors, most workers agree that psychotherapy, although often helpful, has only an ancillary role in the treatment of opioid abuse.[537,547–549] As with drug abusers generally, no *addictive personality* defines opioid users, although a wide variety of psychiatric disturbances are overrepresented among them, especially major depression and antisocial personality.[550–553] Whether a psychiatric illness precedes or follows opioid abuse can be difficult to determine; twin and fostering studies, which have helped to define hereditary subtypes of alcoholism, have not been done with opioid abusers. Compared with relatives of control subjects, relatives of opioid addicts have higher rates of alcoholism, drug abuse, depression, and antisocial personality; however, although relatives of depressed opioid addicts have high rates of depression, anxiety, and antisocial personality, relatives of antisocial addicts do not differ from relatives of controls.[551] Whether these familial clusterings are genetically or environmentally determined is unclear. As would be expected, psychiatric disturbance predicts poor response to therapy of any kind.

Drug-free communities such as Synannon, Daytop, Odyssey House, and Phoenix House reach only a small percentage of abusers and are costly. Data relating to them, although sparse, reveal extremely high relapse rates after patients leave a program.[74,554,555]

Studies of acupuncture in opioid addiction have been either negative or badly designed.[556]

Although chronic opioid use leads to social withdrawal and decreased physical activity, mental performance remains unimpaired. Legalized morphine or heroin, practiced in the United States before restrictive legislation and more recently in Britain, demonstrated that stable daily doses of heroin or morphine are compatible with social productivity.[78,557–559] Heroin must be taken two or three times daily, however, and oral efficacy requires very high doses.[165] It tends to produce lethargy, irritability, and hypochondriasis, and users vary widely in what they consider optimal dosage, leading to frequent illicit supplementation.[559] Although heroin maintenance still has its advocates,[559a] today most British opioid users registered in governmental programs take methadone.[560–563]

Methadone maintenance is based on the premise that opioid abuse is a chronic metabolic disorder and that methadone not only substitutes for a patient's endogenous deficiency, but also "blocks" the effects of other exogenously administered opioids.[564] Cross-tolerant to heroin and morphine, methadone is taken orally in gradually increasing doses, usually up to 80 to 120 mg daily. Although tolerance develops to methadone sedation, euphoria, and analgesia, it does not develop to "blockade." Moreover, methadone is taken up and then slowly released by the liver.[565] Therefore, in contrast to heroin, single daily doses produce high steady-state tissue levels without "cycling between abstinence and narcosis."[564] If someone receiving methadone takes heroin, it may produce paresthesias (caused by histamine release) but not euphoria—at least with heroin doses affordable by most addicts. Methadone itself produces little psychic effect of its own and only minor and acceptable side effects such as constipation, decreased libido, increased sweating, insomnia, and daytime dozing.[565] In contrast to heroin, methadone does not impair NK lymphocyte activity.[566] (Unexplained deaths occurred in several Australians who had recently begun methadone maintenance therapy; all had chronic hepatitis, which possibly caused fatally high methadone tissue levels.[567])

The abstinence rate of Dole and Nyswander's original methadone maintenance pilot study was 98% at 1 year and 60% at 3 years, with striking decreases in arrests and increases in employment or return to school.[568,569] Other programs with less strict entry requirements have had lower retention rates, but they are still severalfold higher (and at considerably less expense) than documented retention rates (and social rehabilitation) of any abstinence program.[570–574]

More than 150,000 Americans have received methadone maintenance therapy, yet it remains a controversial approach.[575–582] Criticisms of methadone maintenance therapy include the objection to keeping someone physically dependent; the observation that some subjects receiving methadone continue to take heroin and may take other illicit drugs (especially cocaine, marijuana, and benzodiazepines) or become ethanol dependent;[583–586] the occurrence among patients of psychic changes, including apathy, daytime "nodding," hypochondriasis, and drug craving as well as impaired male sexual performance;[587] accidental ingestion by children;[588] the fact that methadone does not address socioeconomic or psychological factors;[589] and diversion of methadone into illicit use.[590,591]

These criticisms draw the following rejoinders. First, methadone maintenance is a specific treatment for opioid abuse. Nonopioid abuse, other medical illness, unemployment, or antisocial behavior are separate problems requiring additional supportive services, which governmental regulations hinder.[573–575] (As Jaffe put it, "The best that we can do is get someone to become what they might have been if they had never become a heroin addict."[578]) Addressing the need for comprehensive medical care, an American study—following existing practices in Britain—demonstrated the feasibility of treating selected methadone-maintenance patients in a physician's office, with monthly visits and take-home medication.[592,593] As for other illicit drug use, in reports from New York City and Baltimore cocaine use decreased among heroin addicts when they began methadone maintenance.[594,595] New or continued cocaine use is not unusual, however, especially among depressed patients,[596] and in animal studies methadone increased cocaine conditioned place preference, indicating enhancement of cocaine reinforcement.[596a] Illicit benzodiazepine use—especially diazepam, lorazepam, and alprazolam—is also common among patients receiving methadone, and ethanol abuse is not unusual.[597,598] (Alcoholism in former heroin addicts carries a sad irony; from a medical standpoint, ethanol is a far more harmful drug than heroin.)

Second, heroin abuse among these patients is often, although not always, due to inadequate methadone dosage (i.e., less than 5 mg daily), insufficient to produce the blood concentration of 200 μg/mL necessary for effective blockade.[576,599–601] Low dosage—based, it would appear, on moral posturing rather than medical data[602,603]—leads to dropout and recidivism. Some patients have inadequate blood concentrations even at conventional higher dosage. In a study of 500 patients receiving maintenance methadone, 18 continued to use heroin despite doses of 80 to 100 mg daily; very low serum methadone levels were found, indicating aberrant metabolism and the need for either higher dosage or alternate treatment.[604]

Not only do patients require adequate doses of methadone, but also the great majority must continue maintenance therapy indefinitely.[605,606] As Dole[564] stressed, the treatment is "corrective but not curative," and recidivism among addicts who try to stop or taper methadone is 70% to 80%.[575] Newman[607] suggests that judging methadone maintenance treatment by the number of addicts who relapse when dosage is lowered or terminated is analogous to judging birth control pills by counting the number of pregnancies after treatment is stopped. The goal of methadone maintenance treatment is "rehabilitation, not abstinence."[575] (In 1984, because of budgetary restrictions, California instituted a 2-year limit on methadone maintenance for those unable to pay $200 a month. The result was a predictable fiasco of heroin relapse, with projected savings offset by the cost of incarceration, legal supervision, and medical treatment.[608])

As to diversion for street use, a study of several large American cities found that such methadone is most often taken orally by patients themselves to prevent withdrawal or to detoxify.[609] Of those using methadone illicitly, 95% did so less often than daily. Deaths related to methadone—including accidental ingestion by children and granulomatous disease from intravenous injection of talc-containing tablets—peaked in 1973 and then declined; in 75%, additional drugs were implicated.[610] In 1988, methadone ranked 17th on the Drug Abuse Warning Network, below codeine, Percodan, benzodiazepines, and heroin (which was second).[578] Methadone diversion, however, has led clinics to discontinue take-home medication, requiring daily visits that interfere with vocational rehabilitation.

Additional concern exists over the possible adverse effects of methadone maintenance on children born to treated mothers.[611–613] Withdrawal symptoms are possibly more severe when the mother takes methadone than when she takes heroin.[188,614] Such symptoms can persist for several months, and affected infants have impaired fetal respiratory movements, are small, and may be prone to sudden infant death and later impaired perceptual-motor performance.[198,611,615,616] In one study, infants of mothers who conceived while taking heroin and were then treated with methadone had smaller birth weight, length, and head circumference than nondrug controls; at 9 months of age, weight and length had caught up to control levels, but at 2 years, head circumference remained smaller than that of controls even though psychomotor development appeared normal.[617] In another study, infants of mothers maintained on methadone had lower weight and smaller head circumference at birth but by 6 months of age were no different developmentally from drug-free controls.[618] Another study found no difference in withdrawal symptoms between heroin-exposed and methadone-exposed infants and no neonatal complications other than withdrawal in methadone-exposed infants.[619] Factors other than in utero opioid exposure could of course be responsible for neonatal or development abnormalities.[209,213,620] Birth weight was significantly lower, however, in methadone-treated monkeys compared with controls.[621]

Opioid delta receptors are not well developed in fetal brains; a potential alternative to methadone during pregnancy would therefore be a delta agonist. The validity of such an approach remains to be demonstrated.[43]

The AIDS epidemic has lent a new urgency to the controversy over methadone-maintenance therapy.[622] In New York City in 1990, fewer than 10% of heroin addicts enrolled in methadone maintenance programs before 1980 were HIV seropositive compared with 60% enrolled after 1987.[582] Similar figures have been reported from other American cities and from Europe.[623–626] Not only does methadone maintenance reduce parenteral drug abuse, but also the setting provides opportunities for counseling and other AIDS risk reduction.[627]

A young man developed choreic movements of the arms, torso, and muscles of speech after 2 years of maintenance methadone; chorea disappeared when treatment was discontinued.[628] A 71-year-old man developed bilateral ballism during methadone withdrawal.[629]

A potential alternative to methadone is the related agonist methadyl acetate (levo-alpha-acetylmethadol [LAAM]), which suppresses opioid withdrawal for 72 hours and does not suppress plasma testosterone levels.[630,631] Trials comparing LAAM with methadone, however, found higher dropout rates in the LAAM group.[632]

Another possible maintenance treatment is high-dose propoxyphene napsylate. In animals, the napsylate preparation is less toxic than the hydrochloride; it is also less water soluble, discouraging parenteral abuse. The drug must be given in divided daily doses, however.[633–635]

Anecdotal suggestions that propranolol prevented heroin-induced euphoria, precipitated withdrawal symptoms, and decreased craving after withdrawal were not confirmed by a controlled study.[636]

In contrast to those who favor maintenance therapy, proponents of opioid antagonist treatment view opioid abuse as "a chronic relapsing, frequently temporary self-limited condition," with drug-taking behavior related to psychological reinforcement.[637] Cyclazocine, a combined agonist-antagonist, is taken orally twice daily. Low doses produce effects similar to low doses of morphine. At higher doses, there is sedation with a tendency to fall asleep but awaken quickly feeling nervous and restless; some subjects have racing thoughts, dysphoric delusions, unpleasant hallucinations, and respiratory depression.[638] As with other agonist-antagonists, there is an atypical withdrawal syndrome, beginning with lightheadedness, fainting spells, or a sensation compared with "electric shocks in the head," followed by tachycardia, mydriasis, tearing, rhinorrhea, yawning, anorexia, diarrhea, chills, fever, and sometimes myoclonic jerks but, in contrast to pentazocine, no drug craving. Trials with cyclazocine have failed to demonstrate therapeutic efficacy.[639]

Naloxone, a pure antagonist, has weak oral efficacy and short duration of action. Naltrexone, another pure antagonist, is orally effective and blocks heroin's effects for more than 24 hours.[640] It has been recommended for intermittent use in highly motivated patients who are otherwise drug free and receiving appropriate supportive therapy.[637] In follow-up studies of patients receiving naltrexone, dropout rates have been high; long-term opioid abstinence seems to require at least 3 months of continuous naltrexone.[641,642] These disappointing results may be a consequence of dysphoria secondary to blockade of endorphins.[643] Such an effect would not only limit the efficacy of any antagonist treatment, but could even aggravate the problem.[564]

Buprenorphine, a combined agonist-antagonist, has reportedly been effective without causing the unacceptable side effects of cyclazocine.[644,645] In a randomized, double-blind trial buprenorphine 8 mg daily was as effective as methadone 60 mg daily in reducing illicit opioid use over 25 weeks; both regimens were superior to methadone 20 mg daily.[646] In studies involving heroin-cocaine "speedballers," combined treatment with buprenorphine and naltrexone was more effective than methadone in reducing abuse of either drug; cocaine produced euphoria in patients receiving methadone and dysphoria in those receiving buprenorphine.[647] In another study of speedball addicts, daily buprenorphine, 4 or 8 mg sublingually, completely blocked the subjective effects of 10 mg intravenous morphine and reduced craving for heroin. Effects on cocaine craving varied, however, and some subjects reported enhancement of the subjective effects of intravenous cocaine.[648]

In monkeys buprenorphine suppressed self-administration of both cocaine and the opioid alfentanil, but much higher doses were required to suppress cocaine reinforcement.[649] Others have also observed buprenorphine suppression of cocaine self-administration in monkeys,[650] but a possible interpretation is that the rate of self-administration decreases because buprenorphine and cocaine are *additively* rewarding.[651] In monkeys, morphine also decreases the rate of cocaine self-administration,[652] and in rats, cocaine and buprenorphine are synergistic in producing conditioned place preference and in raising extracellular dopamine levels in the nucleus accumbens.[651] In rats, buprenorphine lowered threshold for brain self-stimulation reward.[653] In baboons, buprenorphine is mildly reinforcing, maintaining moderate levels of self-injection in some animals and none in others.[654] In monkeys, buprenorphine is reinforcing but, similar to methadone, less so than heroin.[655] Its dependence liability in humans has been described as "minimal,"[656] and it produces mild abstinence symptoms.[657] More severe withdrawal has been observed, however, and buprenorphine abuse has been reported in several countries.[658-670] A man who took a single dose of buprenorphine for pain developed auditory hallucinations and attempted suicide.[671]

References

1. Jaffe JH, Martin WR. Opioid analgesics and antagonists. In: Gilman AG, Goodman LS, Nies AS, Taylor P, eds. The Pharmacological Basis of Therapeutics, ed 8. New York: Pergamon Press, 1990:491.
2. Martin WR. Pharmacology of opioids. Pharmacol Rev 1984; 35:283.
3. Pert CB, Snyder SH. Opiate receptor demonstration in nervous tissue. Science 1973; 179:1011.
4. Simon EJ, Hiller JM, Edelman I. Stereospecific binding of the potent narcotic analgesic 3H-etorphine to rat brain homogenate. Proc Natl Acad Sci USA 1973; 70:1947.
5. Terenius L. Stereospecific interaction between narcotic analgesics and a synaptic plasma membrane fraction of rat cerebral cortex. Acta Pharmacol Toxicol 1973; 32:317.
6. Hughes J, Smith TW, Kosterlitz HW, et al. Identification of two related pentapeptides from the brain with potent opiate agonist activity. Nature 1975; 258:577.
7. Wise RA. Opiate reward: sites and substrates. Neurosci Biobehav Rev 1989; 13:129.
8. Zukin RS, Zukin SR. The case for multiple opiate receptors. Trends Neurosci 1984; 7:160.
9. Kosterlitz AW, Corbett AD, Paterson SJ. Opioid receptors and ligands. In: Harris LS, ed. Problems of Drug Dependence 1989. Rockville, MD: NIDA Research Monograph 95, DHHS, 1990:159.
10. Smith AP, Lee NM. Pharmacology of dynorphin. Annu Rev Pharmacol Toxicol 1988; 28:123.
11. Weitz CJ, Lowney LI, Faull KF, et al. 6-acetyl morphine: a natural product present in mammalian brain. Proc Natl Acad Sci USA 1988; 85:5335.
12. Cox, BM, Goldstein A, Li CH. Opioid activity of a peptide, beta-lipotropin (61–91) derived from beta-lipotropin. Proc Natl Acad of Sci USA 1976; 73:1821.
13. Raffa RB. The actions of FMRF-NH2 and FMRF-NH2 related peptides on mammals. In: Harris L, ed. Problems of Drug Dependence 1990. Rockville, MD: NIDA Research Monograph 105, DHHS, 1991:243.
14. Malin DH, Lake JR, Fowler DE, et al. FMRF-NH2-like mammalian peptide precipitates opiate withdrawal syndrome in the rat. Peptides 1990; 11:277.
15. Mansour A, Khachaturian H, Lewis ME, et al. Anatomy of CNS opioid receptors. Trends Neurosci 1988; 11:308.
16. Fujimoto JM, Arts KS. Intracerebroventricular (ICV) clonidine produces an antialgesic effect through spinal dynorphin A (1-17) mediation. In: Harris LS, ed. Problems of Drug Dependence 1989. Rockville, MD: NIDA Research Monograph 95, DHHS, 1990:306.
17. Faden AL. Opioid and nonopioid mechanisms may contribute to dynorphin's pathophysiological actions in spinal cord injury. Ann Neurol 1990; 27:67.
18. Porreca F, Mosberg HI, Omnaas JR, et al. Supraspinal and spinal potency of selective opioid agonists in the mouse writhing test. J Pharmacol Exp Ther 1987; 240:890.
19. Levine J. Pain and analgesia: the outlook for more rational treatment. Ann Intern Med 1984; 100:269.
20. Adler MW, Geller EB. The opioid system and temperature regulation. Annu Rev Pharmacol Toxicol 1988; 28:429.
21. Ling GSF, MacLeod JM, Lee S, et al. Separation of morphine analgesia from physical dependence. Science 1984; 226:462.
22. Hand TL, Stinus L, LeMoal M. Differential mechanisms in the aquisition and expression of heroin-induced place preference. Psychopharmacology 1989; 98:61.
23. Iwamoto ET. Characterization of dynorphin A (1-17)-induced place preferences in rats. In: Harris LS, ed. Problems in Drug Dependence 1989. Rockville, MD: NIDA Research Monograph 95, DHHS, 1990:308.
24. Snyder SH. Drugs and neurotransmitter receptors in the brain. Science 1984; 224:22.
25. Traynor J. Subtypes of the k-opioid receptor: fact or fiction? Trends Pharmacol Sci 1989; 10:52.
26. Akil H, Mayer JC, Liebeskind CR. Antagonism of stimulation-produced analgesia by naloxone, a narcotic antagonist. Science 1976; 191:961.
27. Pert A, Yaksh T. Site of morphine induced analgesia in the primate brain: relation to pain pathways. Brain Res 1974; 80:135.
28. Basbaum AI, Fields HL. Endogenous pain control systems: brainstem spinal pathways and endorphin circuitry. Annu Rev Neurosci 1984; 7:309.
29. Terman GW, Shavit Y, Lewis JW, et al. Intrinsic mechanisms of pain inhibition: activation by stress. Science 1984; 226:1270.
30. Faneslow MS. What is conditioned fear? Trends Neurosci 1984; 7:460.
31. Fields HL, Levine JD. Placebo analgesia—a role for endorphins? Trends Neurosci 1984; 7:271.
32. Gracely RH, Dubner R, Wolskee PJ, Deeter WR. Placebo and naloxone can alter post-surgical pain by separate mechanisms. Nature 1983; 306:264.
33. Hayman JS, Vaught JL, Raffa RB, Porreca F. Can supraspinal delta-opioid receptors mediate antinociception? Trends Pharmacol Sci 1988; 9:134.
34. Watkins LR, Johannesson JN, Kinscheck IB, Mayer DJ. The neurochemical basis of footshock analgesia:

the role of spinal cord serotonin and norepinephrine. Brain Res 1984; 290:107.

35. Melzack R. The tragedy of needless pain. Sci Am 1990; 262:27.

35a. Johnson SW, North RA. Opioids excite dopamine neurons by hyperpolarization of local interneurons. J Neurosci 1992; 12:483.

35b. Yuan XR, Madamba S, Siggins GR. Opioid peptides reduce synaptic transmission in the nucleus accumbens. Neurosci Lett 1992; 134, 223.

36. Steward J, Vezina P. A comparison of the effects of intra-accumbens injections of amphetamine and morphine on reinstatement of heroin intravenous self-administration behavior. Brain Res 1988; 457:287.

37. Hakan RL, Callaway C, Henriksen SJ. Electrophysiological analysis of the neural circuitry underlying opiate effects in the nucleus accumbens septi. Neurosci Lett 1989; 101:163.

38. Koob GF, Stinus L, LeMoal M, Bloom FE. Opponent process theory of motivation: neurobiological evidence from studies of opiate dependence. Neurosci Biobehav Rev 1989; 13:135.

39. Bozarth MA, Wise RA. Anatomically distinct opiate receptor fields mediate reward and physical dependence. Science 1984; 224:514.

40. Dai S, Corrigall WA, Coen K-M, Kalant H. Heroin self-administration by rats: influence of dose and physical dependence. Pharmacol Biochem Behav 1989; 32:1009.

41. Christie MJ, Chester GB. Physical dependence on physiologically released endogenous opiates. Life Sci 1982; 30:1173.

42. Myer EC, Morris DL, Brase DA, et al. Naltrexone therapy of apnea in children with elevated cerebrospinal fluid beta-endorphin. Ann Neurol 1990; 27:75.

43. Rothman RB, Long JB, Bykov V, et al. Site-directed affinity ligands as tools to study the phenomenology and mechanisms of morphine-induced upregulation of opioid receptors. In: Harris LS, ed. Problems in Drug Dependence 1989. Rockville, MD: NIDA Research Monograph 95, DHHS, 1990:1928.

44. Koob CF, Bloom FE. Cellular and molecular mechanisms of drug dependence. Science 1988; 242:715.

45. Redmond DE, Krystal JH. Multiple mechanisms of withdrawal from opioid drugs. Annu Rev Neurosci 1984; 7:443.

46. Rothman RB, Yang H-Y-T, Long JB. Upregulation of rat brain opioid receptors by the chronic administration of morphine: possible evidence for an anti-opiate model of tolerance and dependence. In: Harris L, ed. Problems of Drug Dependence 1990. Rockville, MD: NIDA Research Monograph, DHHS, 1991:264.

47. Sweep CG, Weigant VM, DeVry J, Van Ree JM. Beta-endorphin in brain limbic structures as a neurochemical correlate of psychic dependence on drugs. Life Sci 1989; 44:1133.

48. O'Brien CP, Terenius LY, Nyberg F, et al. Endogenous opioids in cerebrospinal fluid opioid-dependent humans. Biol Psychiatry 1988; 24:649.

49. Clement-Jones V, McLaughlin L, Lowry PJ, et al. Acupuncture in heroin addicts: changes in met-enkephalin and endorphin in blood and cerebrospinal fluid. Lancet 1979; 2:380.

50. Facchinetti F, Volpe A, Nappi G, et al. Impairment of adrenergic-induced proopiomelanocortin-related peptide release in heroin addicts. Acta Endocrinol 1985; 108:1.

51. Holmstrand J, Gunne LM, Wahlstrom A, Terenius L. CSF endorphins in heroin addicts during methadone maintenance and during withdrawal. Pharmacopsychiatry 1981; 14:126.

52. O'Brien CP, Terenius L, Wahlstrom A, et al. Endorphin levels in opioid-dependent human subjects: longitudinal study. Ann NY Acad of Sci 1982; 398:377.

53. Sharpe LG, Pickworth WB. Morphine abstinence syndrome: cholinergic mechanisms in the ventral periaqueductal gray of the dog. In: Harris LS, ed. Problems of Drug Dependence 1983. Washington, DC: NIDA Research Monograph 49, DHHS, 1984:143.

54. Collier HOJ, Tucker JF. Novel form of drug-dependence—on adenosine in guinea pig ileum. Nature 1983; 302:618.

55. Tucker JF, Plant NT, van Uexkull A, Collier HOJ. Inhibition by adenosine analogs of opiate withdrawal effects. In: Harris LS, ed. Problems of Drug Dependence 1983. Washington, DC: NIDA Research Monograph 49, DHHS, 1984:85.

56. Trujillo KA, Akil H. Inhibition of morphine tolerance and dependence by the NMDA receptor antagonist MK-801. Science 1991; 251:85.

57. Wiertelak EP, Maier SF, Watkins LR. Cholecystokinin antianalgesia: safety cues abolish morphine analgesia. Science 1992; 256:830.

58. Gold MS, Rea WS. The role of endorphins in opiate addiction, opiate withdrawal, and recovery. Psychiat Clin North Am 1983; 6:489.

59. Aghajanian GK. Tolerance of locus coeruleus neurones to morphine and suppression of withdrawal response by clonidine. Nature 1978; 276:186.

60. Bailey RR. Clondine (Catapres) overshoot. NZ Med J 1975; 81:268.

61. Gold MS, Redmond DE, Kleber HD. Clonidine blocks acute opiate-withdrawal symptoms. Lancet 1978; 2:599.

62. Shearman G, Hynes M, Fielding S, Lal H. Clonidine self-administration in the rat: a comparison with fentanyl self-administration. Pharmacologist 1977; 19:171.

63. Woolverton WL, Wessinger WD, Balster RL. Reinforcing properties of clonidine in rhesus monkeys. Psychopharmacology 1982; 77:17.

64. Haynes L. Opioid receptors and signal transduction. Trends Pharmacol Sci 1988; 9:390.

65. Loh HH, Smith AP. Molecular characterization of opioid receptors. Annu Rev Pharmacol Toxicol 1990; 30:123.

66. Evans CJ, Keith DR, Morrison H, et al. Cloning of a delta opioid receptor by functional expression. Science 1992; 258:1952.

67. Sharma SK, Bhatia M, Ralhan R. Mechanism of development of tolerance and dependence in neuroblastoma X glioma hybrid cells and mice. In: Rapake RS, Dhawan BN, ed. Opioid Peptides: An Update. Washington, DC: NIDA Research Monograph 87, DHHS, 1988:157.

68. Klee WA, Milligan G, Simonds WF, Tocque B. The role of adenylcyclase in opiate tolerance and dependence. In: Sharp CW, ed. Mechanisms of Tolerance and Dependence. Washington, DC: NIDA Research Monograph 54, DHHS, 1984:109.

69. Werz MA, Macdonald RL. Opioid peptides with differential affinity for mu and delta receptors decrease sensory neuron calcium-dependent action potentials. J Pharmacol Exp Ther 1983; 227:394.

70. Crain SM, Shen KF. Opioids can evoke direct receptor-mediated excitatory effects on sensory neurons. Trends Pharmacol Sci 1990; 11:77.

71. Emboden W. Narcotic Plants. New York: MacMillan, 1979:26.

72. Paulshock BZ. William Heberden and opium—some relief to all. N Engl J Med 1983; 308:53.

73. Haller JS. Heroin addiction; insights from Alexis de Tocqueville. NY State J Med 1986; 86:121.

74. Brecher EM. Licit and Illicit Drugs. Boston: Little, Brown, 1972.

75. Musto D. Opium, cocaine, and marijuana in Amerian history. Sci Am 1991; 265:40.

76. Higby GJ. Heroin and medical reasoning: the power of analogy. NY State J Med 1986; 86:137.

77. Penfield W. Halsted of Johns Hopkins. The man and his problem as described in the secret records of William Osler. JAMA 1969; 210:2214.

78. Blaine JD, Bozetti LP, Ohlson KE. The narcotic analgesics: the opiates. In: Drug Use in America: Problem in Perspective. The Technical Papers of the Second Report of the National Commission on Marijuana and Drug Abuse. Washington, DC: US Government Printing Office, 1973:60.

79. Hughes PH, Barker NW, Crawford GA, Jaffe JH. The natural history of a heroin epidemic. Am J Public Health 1972; 62:995.

80. Stimmel B. The socioeconomics of heroin dependency. N Engl J Med 1972; 287:1275.

81. Dogoloff LI, Devine CM. International patterns of drug abuse and control. Ann NY Acad of Sci 1981; 363:16.

82. Raab S. Flood of heroin and cocaine changing patterns of drug use in New York. NY Times, May 29, 1984.

83. Leads from the MMWR. Unintentional poisoning mortality—United States, 1980–1986. JAMA 1989; 261:1870.

84. Jannsen W, Trubner K, Puschel K. Death caused by drug addiction: a review of the experiences in Hamburg and the situation in the Federal Republic of Germany in comparison with the literature. Forens Sci Int 1989; 43:223.

85. Steentoft A, Kaa E, Worm K. Fatal intoxications in the age group 15–34 years in Denmark in 1984 and in 1985. A forensic study with special reference to drug addicts. Z Rechtsmed 1989; 103:93.

86. Gossop M. The detoxification of high dose heroin addicts in Pakistan. Drug Alcohol Depend 1989; 24:143.

87. Kreek MJ. Opiate-ethanol interactions: implications for the biological basis and treatment of combined addictive diseases. In: Harris LS, ed. Problems of Drug Dependence 1987. Washington, DC: NIDA Research Monograph 81, US Government Printing Office, 1988:428.

88. Kandel, DB. Epidemiological trends and implications for understanding the nature of addiction. In: O'Brien CP, Jaffe JH, eds. Addictive States. Res Publ Assoc Res Nerv Ment Dis 1992; 70:23.

89. Halloway M. Treatment for addiction. Sci Am 1991; 265:94.

90. Hughes PH, Brandenburg N, Baldwin DC, et al. Prevalence of substance use among U.S. physicians. JAMA 1992; 267:2333.

91. Maitland L, Nossiter BD. U.S. tries new tack in drug fight as global supply and use mount. NY Times, January 30, 1983.

92. Raab S. Strategies differ in the war on drugs. NY Times, May 22, 1984.

93. Smith DE. West Coast and East Coast drug abuse patterns, 1979–80. Ann NY Acad of Sci 1981; 363:22.

94. Massing M. Whatever happened to the "war on drugs"? New York Review of Books, June 11, 1992.

95. Treaster JB. A more potent heroin makes a comeback in a new, needleless form. NY Times, April 28, 1991.

96. Skolnick JH. The limits of narcotics law enforcement. J Psychoact Drugs 1984; 16:119.

97. Longmark M, Olesen J. Drug abuse in migraine patients. Pain 1984; 19:81.

98. McNairy SL, Maruta T, Ivnik RJ, et al. Prescription medication dependence and neuropsychologic function. Pain 1984; 18:169.

99. Treaster JB. Heroin use rising as crack use wanes, report says. NY Times, June 18, 1991.

100. Treaster JB. Cocaine users adding heroin and a plague to their menus. NY Times, July 21, 1990.

101. Nicholi AM. The non-therapeutic use of psychoactive drugs. A modern epidemic. N Engl J Med 1983; 308:925.

102. Newman RG. The need to redefine "addiction." N Engl J Med 1983; 308:1096.

103. Robertson JR. Drug users in contact with general practice. BMJ 1984; 290:34.

104. Vaillant GE. The natural history of narcotic drug addiction. Semin Psychiatry 1970; 2:486.

105. Robertson JR, Bucknall AB, Skidmore CA, et al. Remission and relapse in heroin users and implications for management: treatment control or risk reduction. Int J Addict 1989; 24:229.

106. Blachy PH. Naloxone for diagnosis in methadone programs. JAMA 1973; 244:334.

107. Glaser FB. Psychologic vs pharmacologic heroin dependence. N Engl J Med 1974; 290:231.

108. Harding G. Patterns of heroin use: what do we know? Br J Addict 1988; 83:1247.
109. DuPont RL, Greene MH. The dynamics of a heroin addiction epidemic. Science 1973; 181:716.
110. Musto DF. The American Disease: Origins of Narcotic Control. New Haven, CT: Yale University Press, 1973.
111. Nurco DN, Ball JC, Shaffer JW, Hanton TE. The criminality of narcotic addicts. J Nerv Ment Dis 1985; 173:94.
112. Shaffer JW, Nurco DN, Ball JC, et al. The relationship of preaddiction characteristics to the types and amounts of crime committed by narcotic addicts. Int J Addict 1987; 22:153.
113. Martin WR, Fraser HF. A comparative study of physiological and subjective effects of heroin and morphine administered intravenously in postaddicts. J Pharmacol Exp Ther 1961; 133:388.
114. Levine MN, Sackett DL, Bush H. Heroin vs morphine for cancer pain? Arch Intern Med 1986; 146:353.
115. Hubner CB, Kornetsky C. Heroin, 6-acetylmorphine and morphine effects on threshold for rewarding and aversive brain stimulation. J Pharmacol Exp Ther 1992; 260:562.
116. Rady JJ, Roerig SC, Fujimoto JM. Heroin acts on different opioid receptors than morphine in Swiss Webster and ICR mice to produce antinociception. J Pharmacol Exp Ther 1991; 256:448.
117. Sapira JD. The narcotic addict as a medical patient. Am J Med 1968; 45:555.
118. Caplan LR, Hier DB, Banks G. Stroke and drug abuse. Stroke 1982; 13:869.
119. Eskes D, Brown JK. Heroin-caffeine-strychnine mixtures—where and why? Bull Narc 1975; 27:67.
120. French JF, Stafford J. AIDS and intranasal heroin. Lancet 1989; 1:1082.
121. Casriel C, Rockwell R, Stepherson B. Heroin sniffers: between two worlds. J Psychoactive Drugs 1988; 20:437.
122. Gossop M, Griffiths P, Strang J. Chasing the dragon: characteristics of heroin chasers. Br J Addict 1988; 83:1159.
123. Madden S. Chasing the dragon and syringe-exchange programs. Br J Addict 1989; 84:697.
124. Strang J, Gossop M, Griffiths P, Farrel M. The technology of dragon chasing. Br J Addict 1989; 84:699.
125. Foley KM. Opioids. In: Brust JCM, ed. Neurologic Complications of Drug and Alcohol Abuse. Neurol Clin 1993, in press.
126. Fraser HF, Isbell H. Comparative effects of 290 mg morphine sulfate in non-addicts and former morphine addicts. J Pharmacol Exp Ther 1952; 105:498.
127. Kay DC, Eisenstein RB, Jasinski DR. Morphine effects on human REM state, waking time, and NREM sleep. Psychopharmacologia 1969; 14:404.
128. Frenk H, Liban A, Balamuth R, Urca G. Opiate and non-opiate aspects of morphine induced seizures. Brain Res 1982; 253:253.

129. Volavka J, Zaks A, Roubicek J, Fink M. Electroencephalographic effects of diacetylmorphine (heroine) and naloxone in man. Neuropharmacology 1970; 9:587.
130. Larpin R, Vincent A, Perret C. Morbidite et mortalite hospitalieres de l'intoxicaiton aigue par les opices. Presse Med 1990; 19:1403.
131. McCann SM, Lumpkin MD, Mizunuma H, et al. Peptidergic and dopaminergic control of prolactin release. Trends Neurosci 1984; 7:127.
132. Tagliero F, Capra F, Dorizzi R, et al. High serum calcitonin levels in heroin addicts. J Endocrinol Invest 1984; 7:331.
133. Vescovi PP, Girasole G, Caccavari R, et al. Metyrapone effects on beta-endorphin, ACTH, and cortisol levels after chronic opiate receptor stimulation in man. Neuropeptides 1990; 15:129.
134. Genazzami AR, Petraglia F. Opioid control of luteinizing hormone secretion in humans. J Steroid Biochem 1989; 33:751.
135. Buffum JC. Pharmacosexuality update: heroin and sexual function. J Psychoact Drugs 1983; 15:317.
136. Mendelson JH, Mello NK. Hormones and psychosexual development in young men following chronic heroin use. Neurobehav Toxicol Teratol 1982; 4:441.
137. Ceriello A, Dello Russo P, Curcio F, et al. Depressed antithrombin III biological activity in opiate addicts. J Clin Pathol 1984; 37:1040.
138. Giugliano D. Morphine, opioid peptides, and pancreatic islet function. Diab Care 1984; 7:92.
139. Passariello N, Gugliano I, Ceriello A, et al. Increased platelet aggregation in opiate addicts. Blood 1982; 60:276.
140. Higgins ST, Stitzer ML, McCaul ME, et al. Pupillary response to methadone challenge in heroin users. Clin Pharmacol Ther 1985; 37:460.
141. Jaffe JH. Drug addiction and drug abuse. In: Gilman AG, Goodman LS, Nies AS, Taylor D, eds. The Pharmacological Basis of Therapeutics, ed 8. New York: Pergamon Press, 1990:522.
142. Haertzen CA, Hooks NT. Changes in personality and subjective experience associated with the chronic administration and withdrawal of opiates. J Nerv Ment Dis 1969; 148:606.
143. Khantzian EJ, McKenna GJ. Acute toxic and withdrawal reactions associated with drug use and abuse. Ann Intern Med 1979; 90:361.
144. Goldfrank LR, Bresnitz EA. Opioids. In: Goldfrank LR, Flomenbaum NE, Levin NA, et al, eds. Toxicologic Emergencies, ed 4. Norwalk, CT: Appleton & Lange, 1990:433.
145. Choudry N, Doe J. Inadvertent abuse of amphetamines in street heroin. Lancet 1986; 2:817.
146. Kramer TH, Fine J, Bahari B, Ottomanelli G. Chasing the dragon: the smoking of heroin and cocaine. J Subst Abuse Treatment 1990; 7:65.
147. Kreek MJ. Opioid interaction with alcohol. Adv Alcohol Subst Abuse 1984; 3:35.

148. Sorensen SC, Mattison K. Naloxone as an antagonist in severe alcohol intoxication. Lancet 1978; 2:688.
149. Himmelsbach CK. The morphine abstinence syndrome, its nature and treatment. Ann Intern Med 1941; 15:829.
150. Martin WR, Jasinski DR. Physiological parameters of morphine dependence in man: tolerance, early abstinence, protracted abstinence. J Psychiat Res 1967; 7:9.
151. Jasinski DR. Opiate withdrawal syndrome: acute and protracted aspects. Ann NY Acad Sci 1981; 362:183.
152. Kosten TR. Current pharmacotherapies for opioid dependence. Psychopharmacol Bull 1990; 26:69.
153. Nash P, Colasanti B, Khazan N. Long-term effects of morphine on the electroencephalogram and behavior of the rat. Psychopharmacologia 1973; 29:271.
154. Goldberg SR, Schuster CR. Nalorphine: increased sensitivity of monkeys formerly dependent on morphine. Science 1969; 166:1548.
155. Carlson KR, Cooper DO. Morphine dependence and protracted abstinence. Regional alternations in CNS radioligand binding. Pharmacol Biochem Behav 1985; 23:1059.
156. Liu SJ, Wang RI. Case report of barbiturate-induced enhancement of methadone metabolism and withdrawal syndrome. Am J Psychiatry 1984; 141:1287.
157. Tong TG, Pond SM, Kreek MJ, et al. Phenytoin-induced methadone withdrawal. Ann Intern Med 1981; 94:349.
158. Saxon AJ, Whittaker S, Hawkes CS. Valproic acid, unlike other anticonvulsants, has no effect on methadone metabolism: two cases. J Clin Psychiatry 1989; 50:228.
159. Kennedy JA, Harman N, Sbriglio R, et al. Metyrapone-induced withdrawal symptoms. Br J Addict 1990; 85:1133.
160. Cochin J, Kornetsky C. Development and loss of tolerance to morphine in rat after single and multiple injections. J Pharmacol Exp Ther 1964; 145:1.
161. Wright C, Bigelow GE, Stitzer ML. Acute physical dependence in man: repeated naloxone-precipitated withdrawal after a single dose of methadone. In: Harris LS, ed. Problems of Drug Dependence 1989. Rockville, MD: NIDA Research Monograph 95, DHHS, 1990:395.
162. Bickel WK, Stitzer ML, Liebson IA, Bigelow GE. Acute physical dependence in man: effects of naloxone after brief morphine exposure. J Pharmacol Exp Ther 1988; 244:126.
163. Heishman SJ, Stitzer ML, Bigelow GE, Liebson IA. Acute opioid physical dependence: naloxone dose effects after brief morphine exposure. J Pharmacol Exp Ther 1989; 248:127.
164. FDA Regulations Governing Methadone. In: Federal Register, Vol XXXVII, Section 130.44, 1972.
165. Ghodse AH, Creighton FJ, Bhat AV. Comparison of oral preparations of heroin and methadone to stabilize opiate misusers as inpatients. BMJ 1990; 300:719.
166. Gold MS, Pottash AC, Sweeney DR, Kleber HD. Opiate withdrawal using clonidine: a safe, effective, and rapid non-opiate treatment. JAMA 1980; 243:343.
167. Hoder EL, Leckman JF, Ehrenkrantz R, et al. Clonidine in neonatal narcotic-abstinence syndrome. N Engl J Med 1981; 305:1284.
168. Johnson DA, Bohan ME. Propoxyphene withdrawal with clonidine. Am J Psychiatry 1983; 140:1217.
169. Cami J, DeTorres S, San L, et al. Efficacy of clonidine and of methadone in the rapid detoxification of patients dependent on heroin. Clin Pharmacol Ther 1985; 38:336.
170. Gold MS, Pottash AC, Annitto WJ, et al. Lofexidine: a clonidine analogue effective in opiate withdrawal. Lancet 1981; 1:992.
171. Preston KL, Bigelow GE, Liebson IA. Self-administration of clonidine and oxazepam by methadone detoxification patients, In: Harris LS, ed. Problems of Drug Dependence 1983. Washington, DC: NIDA Research Monograph 49, DHHS, 1984:192.
172. Jasinski DR, Johnson RE, Kocher TR. Clonidine in morphine withdrawal. Arch Gen Psychiatry 1985; 42:1063.
173. San L, Cami J, Peri JM, et al. Efficacy of clonidine, guanfacine, and methadone in the rapid detoxification of heroin addicts: a controlled clinical trial. Br J Addict 1990; 85:141.
173a. Lauzon P. Two cases of clonidine abuse/dependence in methadone-maintained patients. J Subst Abuse Treat 1992; 9:125.
174. Schubert H, Fleischhacker WW, Meise V, Theohar C. Preliminary results of guanfacine treatment of acute opiate withdrawal. Am J Psychiatry 1984; 141:1271.
175. Soler-Insa PA, Bedate-Villar J, Theohar C, Yotis A. Treatment of heroin withdrawal with guanfacine: an open clinical investigation. Can J Psychiatry 1987; 32:679.
176. Kleber HD, Topazian M, Gaspari J, et al. Clonidine and naltrexone in the outpatient treatment of heroin withdrawal. Am J Drug Alcohol Abuse 1987; 13:1.
177. Brewer C, Rezae H, Bailey C. Opioid withdrawal and naltrexone induction in 48–72 hours with minimal dropout, using a modification of the naltrexone-clonidine technique. Br J Psychiatry 1988; 153:340.
178. Vining E, Kosten TR, Kleber HD. Clinical utility of rapid clonidine naltrexone detoxification for opioid abusers. Br J Addict 1988; 83:567.
179. Kosten TR, Kleber HD. Buprenorphine detoxification from opioid dependence. A pilot study. Life Sci 1988; 42:635.
179a. Stine SM, Kosten TR. Use of drug combinations in treatment of opioid withdrawal. J Clin Psychopharmacol 1992; 12:203.
180. Drago F, Scapagnini U. Effects of endogenous hyperprolactinemia on opiate-induced behavioral changes in rats. Brain Res 1985; 336:215.

181. Patti F, Drago F, Marano P, et al. Effects of sulpiride on chronic abstinence syndrome in addicted patients. Clin Neuropharmacol 1986; 9:469.

182. Newmeyer JA, Johnson G, Klot S. Acupuncture as a detoxification modality. J Psychoact Drugs 1984; 16:241.

183. Auriacombe M, Tignol J, LeMoal M, Stinus L. Transcutaneous electrical stimulation with Limoge current potentiates morphine analgesia and attenuates opiate abstinence syndrome. Biol Psychiatry 1990; 28:650.

184. Glass L, Rajegowda BK, Kahn EJ, Floyd MV. Effect of heroin withdrawal on respiratory rate and acid-base status in the newborn. N Engl J Med 1972; 286:746.

185. Kahn EJ, Newman LL, Polk G. The course of the heroin withdrawal syndrome in newborn infants treated with phenobarital or chlorpromazine. J Pediatr 1969; 75:495.

186. Kandell SR, Gartner LM. Late presentation of drug withdrawal symptoms in newborns. Am J Dis Child 1974; 127:58.

187. Klenka HM. Babies born in a district general hospital to mothers taking heroin. BMJ 1986; 293:745.

188. Zelson C, Lee SJ, Casalino M. Neonatal narcotic addiction: comparative effects of maternal intake of heroin and methadone. N Engl J Med 1973; 289:1216.

189. Fulroth R, Phillips B, Durand DJ. Perinatal outcome of infants exposed to cocaine and/or heroin in utero. Am J Dis Child 1989; 143:905.

190. Rementeria JL, Nunag NN. Narcotic withdrawal in pregnancy: stillbirth incidence with a case report. Am J Obstet Gynecol 1973; 116:1152.

191. Thomas CS, Osborn M. Inhaling heroin during pregnancy. BMJ 1988; 296:1672.

192. Herszlinger RA, Kandell SR, Vaughan HG. Neonatal seizures associated with narcotic withdrawal. J Pediatr 1977; 91:638.

193. Rosen TS, Johnson HL. Children of methadone maintained mothers: follow-up to 18 months of age. J Pediatr 1982; 101:192.

194. Pacifico P, Nardelli E, Pantarotto MF. Neonatal heroin withdrawal syndrome: evaluation of different pharmacological treatments. Pharmacol Res 1989; 21:63.

195. Finnegan LP, Michael H, Leifer B, Desai S. An evaluation of neonatal abstinence treatment modalities. In: Harris LS, ed. Problems of Drug Dependence 1983. Washington, DC: NIDA Research Monograph 49, DHHS, 1984:282.

196. Finnegan LP. The effects of narcotics and alcohol on pregnancy and the newborn. Ann NY Acad Sci 1981; 362:136.

197. Chasnoff IJ, Burns WJ. The Moro reaction: a scoring system for narcotic withdrawal. Dev Med Child Neurol 1984; 26:484.

198. Peterson DR. SIDS in infants of drug-dependent mothers. J Pediatr 1980; 96:734.

199. Wilson GS, Desmond MM, Verniaud WM. Early development of infants of heroin-addicted mothers. Am J Dis Child 1973; 126:457.

200. Kletter R, Jeremy RJ, Rumsey C, et al. Developmental decline in infants born to HIV-infected intravenous drug-using mothers. In: Harris LS, ed. Problems of Drug Dependence 1989. Rockville, MD: NIDA Research Monograph 95, DHHS, 1990:409.

201. Kirby MC. Effects of morphine on spontaneous activity of 18-day rat fetus. Dev Neurosci 1979; 2:238.

202. Taeusch HW, Carson SH, Wang NS, Avery ME. Heroin induction of lung maturation and growth retardation in fetus rabbits. J Pediatr 1972; 82:869.

203. Piatti E, Rizzi R, Chiesara E. Genotoxicity of heroin and cannabinoids in humans. Pharmacol Res 1989; 21:59.

204. Fischman HK, Roizin L, Moralishvili E, et al. Clastogenic effects of heroin in pregnant monkeys and their offspring. Mut Res 1983; 118:77.

205. Amarose AP, Norusis MJ. Cytogenetics of methadone managed and heroin addicted pregnant women and their newborn infants. Am J Obstet Gynecol 1976; 124:635.

206. Shafer DA, Falek A, Donahoe RM, Madden JJ. Biogenetic effects of opiates. Int J Addict 1990–91; 25:1.

207. Maynard EC. Material abuse of cocaine and heroin. Am J Dis Child 1990; 144:520.

208. Hingson R, Zuckerman B, Amaro H, et al. Maternal marijuana use and neonatal outcome: uncertainty posed by self-reports. Am J Public Health 1986; 76:667.

209. Kaltenbach K, Finnegan LP. Developmental outcome of children born to methadone maintained women: a review of longitudinal studies. Neurobehav Toxicol Teratol 1984; 6:271.

210. Marcus J, Hans SL, Jeremy RJ. A longitudinal study of offspring born to methadone-maintained women. III. Effects of multiple risk factors on development at 4, 8, and 12 months. Am J Drug Alcohol Abuse 1984; 10:195.

211. Oats JN, Beischer NA, Breheny JE, Pepperell RJ. The outcome of pregnancies complicated by narcotic drug addiction. Aust NZ J Obstet Gynaecol 1984; 24:14.

212. Strauss ME, Reynolds KS. Psychological characteristics and development of narcotic-addicted infants. Drug Alcohol Depend 1983; 12:381.

213. Lifeschitz MH, Wilson GS, Smith EO, Desmond MM. Factors affecting head growth and intellectual function in children of drug addicts. Pediatrics 1985; 75:269.

214. Barr HL, Antes D, Oldenberg DJ, Rosen A. Mortality of treated alcoholics and drug addicts: the benefits of abstinence. J Stud Alcohol 1984; 45:440.

215. Cherubin CE. The medical sequelae of narcotic addiction. Ann Intern Med 1967; 67:23.

216. Ghodse AH, Sheehan M, Taylor C, Edwards G. Deaths of drug addicts in the United Kingdom, 1967–1981. BMJ 1985; 290:425.

217. Haastrop S, Jepson PW. Seven year follow-up of 300 young drug abusers. Acta Psychiatr Scand 1984; 70:503.

218. Louria DB, Hensle T, Rose J. The major medical complications of heroin addiction. Ann Intern Med 1967; 67:1.

219. Richter RW. Drug abuse. In: Rowland LP, ed. Merritt's Textbook of Neurology, ed 8. Philadelphia: Lea & Febiger, 1989:909.

220. Garriott JC, Sturner WQ. Morphine concentration and survival in acute heroin fatalities. N Engl J Med 1973; 289:1276.

221. Pare EM, Montforte JR, Thibert RJ. Morphine concentrations in brain tissue from heroin associated deaths. J Anal Toxicol 1984; 8:213.

222. Steentoft A, Worm K, Christensen H. Morphine concentrations in autopsy material from fatal cases after intake of morphine and/or heroin. J Forens Sci Soc 1988; 28:87.

223. Ruttenber AJ, Luke JL. Heroin-related deaths: new epidemiologic insight. Science 1984; 226:14.

224. Centers for Disease Control. Heroin-related deaths—District of Columbia, 1980–1982. MMWR 1983; 32:321.

225. Ruttenber AJ, Kalter HD, Santinga P. The role of ethanol abuse in the etiology of heroin-related death. J Forens Sci 1990; 35:891.

226. Introna F, Smialek JE. The "mini-packer syndrome." Fatal injection of drug containers in Baltimore, Maryland. Am J Forens Med Pathol 1989; 10:21.

227. Stewart A, Heaton ND, Hognin B. Body packing—a case report and review of the literature. Postgrad Med J 1990; 66:659.

228. Joynt BP, Mikhael NZ. Sudden death of a heroin body packer. J Anal Toxicol 1985; 9:238.

229. Simpson LR. Sudden death while attempting to conceal drugs; laryngeal obstruction by a package of heroin. J Forens Sci 1976; 21:378.

230. Sperry K. An epidemic of intravenous narcoticism deaths associated with the resurgence of black tar heroin. J Forens Sci 1988; 33:1156.

231. Monforte JR. Some observations concerning blood morphine concentrations in narcotic addicts. J Forens Sci 1977; 22:718.

232. Osler W. Oedema of left lung—morphia poisoning. Montreal Gen Hosp Rep 1880; 1:291.

233. Levine LH, Hiroch CS, White LW. Quinine cardiotoxicity: a mechanism for sudden death in narcotic addicts. J Forens Sci 1973; 18:167.

234. Lupovich P, Pilewski R, Sapira JD, Juselius R. Cardiotoxicity of quinine as adulterant in drugs. JAMA 1970; 212:1216.

235. Labi M. Paroxysmal atrial fibrillation in heroin intoxication. Ann Intern Med 1969; 71:951.

236. Lipaki J, Stimmel B, Donoso E. The effect of heroin and multiple drug abuse on the electrocardiogram. Am Heart J 1973; 86:663.

237. Hughes S, Calverley PM. Heroin inhalation and asthma. BMJ 1988; 297:1511.

238. Becker C. Medical complications of drug abuse. Adv Intern Med 1979; 24:183.

239. Kurtin P, Wagner J. Deep vein thrombosis in intravenous drug abusers presenting as a systemeic illness. Am J Med Sci 1984; 287:44.

240. Magnan A, Ottomani A, Garbe L, et al. Detresse espiratoire chez une heroinomane seropositive pour le virus de l'immunodeficience humaine. Ann Fr Anesth Reanim 1991; 10:74.

241. deAraujo MS, Gerard F, Chossegros P, et al. Vascular hepatotoxicity related to heroin addiction. Virchows Arch [A] 1990; 417:497.

242. Sandgren JE, McPhee MS, Greenberger NJ. Narcotic bowel syndrome treatment with clonidine. Ann Intern Med 1984; 101:331.

243. Pastan RS, Silverman SL, Goldenberg DL. A musculoskeletal syndrome in intravenous heroin users. Association with brown heroin. Ann Intern Med 1977; 87:22.

244. Cunningham EE, Brentjens JR, Zielezny MA, et al. Heroin nephropathy: a clinicopathologic and epidemiologic study. Am J Med 1980; 47:58.

245. Dubrow A, Mittman N, Ghali V, Flamenbaun W. The changing spectrum of heroin-associated nephropathy. Am J Kidney Dis 1985; 5:36.

246. Overland ES, Nolan AJ, Hopewell PC. Alteration of pulmonary function in intravenous drug abusers: prevalence, severity, and characterization of gas exchange abnormalities. Am J Med 1980; 68:231.

247. Giugliano D, Quatraro A, Ceriello A, D'Onofrio F. Endogenous opiates, heroin addiction, and non-insulin dependent diabetes. Lancet 1985; 2:769.

248. Savona S, Nardi MA, Lennette ET, Karpatkin S. Thrombocytopenic purpura in narcotic addicts. Ann Intern Med 1985; 102:737.

249. Brown LS, Kreek MJ, Trepo C, et al. Human immunodeficiency virus and viral hepatitis seroepidemiology in New York City intravenous drug abusers (IVDAs). In: Harris LS, ed. Problems of Drug Dependence 1989. Rockville, MD: NIDA Research Monograph 95, DHHS, 1990:443.

250. van den Hoek JA, van Haastrecht HJ, Goudsmit J, et al. Prevalence, incidence, and risk factors of hepatitis C virus infection among drug users in Amsterdam. J Infect Dis 1990; 162:823.

251. Gimeno V, Escudero A, Gonzales R, et al. Hepatitis agunda en heroinomanos: estudio etiologico y evolutivo de 110 casos. Rev Clin Esp 1989; 184:360.

252. Shade CP, Komorwska D. Continuing outbreak of hepatitis A, linked with intravenous drug abuse in Multnomah County. Public Health Rep 1988; 105:452.

253. Richter RW, Pearson J, Bruun B, et al. Neurological complications of addiction to heroin. Bull NY Acad Med 1973; 49:3.

254. Gattell JM, Miro JM, Para C, Garcia-San Miguel J. Infective endocarditis in drug addicts. Lancet 1984; 1:228.

255. Hubbell G, Cheitlin MD, Rapaport E. Presentation, management, and follow-up of infective endocarditis in drug addicts. Am Heart J 1981; 138:85.

256. Novick DM, Ness GL. Abuse of antibiotics by abusers of parenteral heroin or cocaine. South Med J 1984; 77:302.

257. Tuazon CU, Sheagren JN. Staphylococcal endocarditis in parenteral drug abusers: source of the organism. Ann Intern Med 1975; 82:788.

258. Reyes MP, Palutke WA, Wylin RF, et al. Pseudomonas endocarditis in the Detroit Medical Center, 1969–1972. Medicine 1973; 52:173.

259. Harris PD, Yeoh CB, Breault J, et al. Fungal endocarditis secondary to drug addiction. Recent concepts in diagnosis and therapy. J Thorac Cardiovasc Surg 1972; 6:980.

260. Pollack S, Magtader A, Lange M. Neisseria subflava endocarditis. Case report and review of the literature. Am J Med 1984; 76:752.

261. Vartian CV, Shlaes DM, Padhye AA, Ajello L. Wangiella dermatitides endocarditis in an intravenous drug user. Am J Med 1985; 78:703.

262. Bick RL, Anhalt JE. Malaria transmission among narcotic addicts: a report of 10 cases and review of the literature. Calif Med 1971; 115:56.

263. Gonzalez-Garcia JJ, Arnalich F, Pena JM, et al. An outbreak of *Plasmodium vivax* malaria among heroin users in Spain. Trans R Soc Trop Med Hyg 1986; 80:549.

264. Lopez-Cortes L, Lozamo deLeon F, Gomez-Mateos JM, et al. Tick-borne relapsing fever in intravenous drug abusers. J Infect Dis 1989; 159:804.

265. Koppel BS, Tuchman AJ, Mangiardi JR, et al. Epidural spinal infection in intravenous drug abusers. Arch Neurol 1988; 45:1331

266. Jabbari B, Pierce JF. Spinal cord compression due to Pseudomonas in a heroin addict. Neurology 1977; 27:1034.

267. Kaplan SS. Pseudomonas disc space infection in an occasional heroin user. Ariz Med 1974; 31:916.

268. Messer HD, Litvinoff J. Pyogenic cervical osteomyelitis. Arch Neurol 1976; 33:571.

269. Endress C, Guyot DR, Fata J, Salciccioli G. Cervical osteomyelitis due to IV heroin use: radiologic findings in 14 patients. Am J Roentgenol 1990; 155:133.

270. Lewis R, Gorback S, Alter P. Spinal Pseudomonas chondroosteomyelitis in heroin users. N Engl J Med 1972; 286:1330.

271. Wiesseman GJ, Wood VE, Kroll LL. Pseudomonas vertebral osteomyelitis in heroin addicts: report of five cases. J Bone Joint Surg 1973; 55A:1416.

272. Smith MA, Trowers NRH, Klein RS. Cervical osteomyelitis caused by *Pseudomonas cepecia* in an intravenous drug abuser. J Clin Microbiol 1985; 21:445.

273. Amine AB. Neurosurgical complications of heroin addiction: brain abscess and mycotic aneurysm. Surg Neurol 1977; 7:385.

274. Gilroy J, Andaya L, Thomas VJ. Intracranial mycotic aneurysms and subacute endocarditis in heroin addiction. Neurology 1973; 23:1193.

275. Greenman RL, Arcey SM, Gutterman DA, Zweig RM. Twice-daily intramuscular ceforanide therapy of *Staphylococcus aureus* endocarditis in parenteral drug abusers. Antimicrob Agents Chemother 1984; 25:16.

276. Jaffe RB. Cardiac and vascular involvement in drug abuse. Semin Roentgenol 1983; 18:207.

277. Brust JCM, Dickinson PCT, Hughes JEO, Holtzman RHH. The diagnosis and treatment cerebral mycotic aneurysm. Ann Neurol 1990; 27:238.

278. Ho K, Rassekh Z. Mycotic aneurysm of the right subclavian artery. A complication of heroin addiction. Chest 1978; 74:116.

279. Ledgerwood AM, Lucas CE. Mycotic aneurysm of the carotid artery. Arch Surg 1974; 109:496.

280. Navarro C, Dickinson PCT, Kondlapoedi P, Hagstrom JW. Mycotic aneurysm of the pulmonary arteries in intravenous drug addicts. Report of three cases and review of the literature. Am J Med 1984; 76:1124.

281. Brust JCM, Richter RW. Tetanus in the inner city. NY State J Med 1974; 74:1735.

282. Heurich AE, Brust JCM, Richter RW. Management of urban tetanus. Med Clin North Am 1973; 57:1373.

283. Redmond J, Stritch M, Blaney P. Severe tetanus in a narcotic addict. Ir Med J 1984; 77:325.

284. MacDonald KL, Rutherford GW, Friedman SM, et al. Botulism and botulism-like illness in chronic drug abusers. Ann Intern Med 1985; 102:616.

285. Elston HR, Wang M, Loo LK. Arm abscesses caused by *Clostridium botulinum*. J Clin Microbiol 1991; 29:2678.

286. Weber RJ, Band LC, de Costa B, et al. Neural control of immune function: opioids, opioid receptors and immunosuppression. In: Harris L, ed. Problems of Drug Dependence 1990. Rockville, MD: NIDA Research Monograph 105, DHHS, 1991:96.

287. Chang K-J. Opioid peptides have actions on the immune system. Trends Neurosci 1984; 7:234.

288. Novick DM, Ochshorn M, Ghali V, et al. Natural killer cell activity and lymphocyte subsets in parenteral heroin abusers and long-term methadone maintenance patients. J Pharmacol Exp Ther 1989; 250:606

289. Chmel H, Grieco MH. Cerebral mucomycosis and renal aspergillosis in heroin addicts without endocarditis. Am J Med Sci 1973; 266:225.

290. Hershewe GL, Davis LE, Bicknell JM. Primary cerebellar brain abscess from nocardiosis in a heroin addict. Neurology 1988; 38:1655.

291. Kasantikul V, Shuangshoti S, Taecholarn C. Primary phycomycosis of the brain in heroin addicts. Surg Neurol 1987; 28:468.

292. Morrow R, Wong B, Finkelstein WE, et al. Aspergillosis of the cerebral ventricles in a heroin abuser. Case report and review of the literature. Arch Intern Med 1983; 143:161.

293. Pierce PF, Soloman SL, Kaufman L, et al. Zygomycetes brain abscesses in narcotic addicts with serological diagnosis. JAMA 1982; 248:2881.

294. Kasantikul V, Shuangshoti S, Sampatanukul P. Primary chromoblastomycosis of the medulla oblon-

gata: complication of heroin addiction. Surg Neurol 1988; 29:319.

295. Etienne M, Nemery A, Darcis JM, et al. Disseminated candidiasis in heroin addicts. Report of two cases and review of the literature. Acta Clin Belg 1986; 41:18.

296. Hay RJ. Systemic candidiasis in heroin addicts. BMJ 1986; 292:1096.

297. Rowe IF, Wright ED, Higgens CS, Burnie JP. Intravertebral infection due to *Candida albicans* in an intravenous heroin abuser. Ann Rheum Dis 1988; 47:522.

298. Scheidegger C, Frei R. Disseminated candidiasis in a drug addict not using heroin. J Infect Dis 1989; 159:1007.

299. Hendrickse RG, Maxwell SM, Young R. Aflatoxins and heroin. BMJ 1989; 299:492.

300. Anderson RM, May RM. Understanding the AIDS epidemic. Sci Am 1992; 267:58.

301. Centers for Disease Control. HIV/AIDS Surveillance. Year End Edition. Atlanta, GA: DHHS, 1992.

302. Spira TJ, DesJarlais DC, Marmor M, et al. Prevalence of antibody to lymphadenopathy-associated virus among drug-detoxification patients in New York. N Eng J Med 1984; 311:467.

303. Layon J, Idris A, Warzyunski M, et al. Altered T-lymphocyte subsets in hospitalized intravenous drug abusers. Arch Intern Med 1984; 144:1376.

304. Mandelli C, Cesana M, Ferroni P, et al. HBV, HDV, and HIV infections in 242 drug addicts: two-year follow-up. Eur J Epidemiol 1988; 4:318.

305. Magura S, Grossman JI, Lipton DS, et al. Determinants of needle sharing among intravenous drug users. Am J Public Health 1989; 79:459.

306. Schoenbaum EE, Hartel D, Selwyn PA, et al. Risk factors for human immunodeficiency virus infection in intravenous drug users. N Engl J Med 1989; 321:874.

307. Schrager L, Friedland G, Feiner C, Kahl P. Demographic characteristics, drug use, and sexual behavior of IV drug users with AIDS in Bronx, New York. Public Health Rep 1991; 106:78.

308. Saxon A, Calsyn DA, Whittaker S, Freeman G. Needle obtainment and cleaning habits of addicts. In: Harris LS, ed. Problems of Drug Dependence 1989. Rockville, MD: NIDA Research Monograph 95, DHHS, 1990:418.

309. Ingold FR, Ingold S. The effects of the liberalization of syringe sales on the behavior of intravenous drug users in France. Bull Narc 1989; 41:67.

310. Sullivan R. Needle-exchangers had right to break law, Judge rules. NY Times, June 26, 1991.

311. DesJarlais DC, Friedman SR, Novick DM, et al. HIV-1 infection among intravenous drug users in Manhattan, New York City, from 1977 through 1987. JAMA 1989; 261:1008.

312. Brookmeyer R. Reconstruction and future trends of the AIDS epidemic in the United States. Science 1991; 253:37.

313. Bishburg E, Sunderam G, Reichman LB, Kapila R. Central nervous system tuberculosis with the acquired immunodeficiency syndrome and its related complex. Ann Intern Med 1986; 105:210

314. Mallolas J, Gatell JM, Rovira M, et al. Vertebral arch tuberculosis in two human immunodeficiency virus-seropositive heroin addicts. Arch Intern Med 1988; 148:125.

315. Barnes PF, Bloch AB, Davidson PT, Snider DE. Tuberculosis in patients with human immunodeficiency virus infection. N Engl J Med 1991; 324:1644.

316. Graham NMH, Nelson KE, Solomon L, et al. Prevalence of tuberculin positivity and skin test anergy in HIV-1-seropositive and seronegative intravenous drug users. JAMA 1992; 267:369.

317. Lukehart SA, Hook EW, Baker-Zander SA, et al. Invasion of the central nervous system by T pallidum: implications for diagnosis and treatment. Ann Intern Med 1988; 109:855.

318. Feraru ER, Aronow HA, Lipton RB. Neurosyphilis in AIDS patients: initial CSF VDRL may be negative. Neurology 1990; 49:541.

319. Johns DR, Tierney M, Felsenstein D. Alteration in the natural history of neurosyphilis by concurrent infection with the human immunodeficiency virus. N Engl J Med 1987; 316:1569.

320. Berry CD, Hooten TM, Collier AC, Lukehart SA. Neurologic relapse after benzathine penicillin therapy for secondary syphilis in a patient with HIV infection. N Engl J Med 1987; 316:1587.

321. Katz DA, Berger JR. Neurosyphilis in acquired immunodeficiency syndrome. Arch Neurol 1989; 46:895.

322. Musher DM, Hammill RJ, Baughn RE. The effect of human immunodeficiency virus infection on the course of syphilis and the response to treatment. Ann Intern Med 1990; 113:872.

323. Musher DM. Syphilis, neurosyphilis, penicillin, and AIDS. J Infect Dis 1991; 163:1201.

324. Berger JR. Neurosyphilis in human immunodeficiency virus type 1-seropositive individuals. Arch Neurol 1991; 48:700.

325. Anders KH, Guerra WF, Tomiyasu U, et al. The neuropathology of AIDS. UCLA experience and review. Am J Pathol 1986; 124:537.

326. Anders K, Verity MA, Concilla PA, Vinters HV. Acquired immune deficiency syndrome (AIDS): neuropathologic studies. J Neuropathol Exp Neurol 1984; 43:315.

327. Berger JR, Moskowitz L, Fischl M, Kelly RE. Neurologic disease as the presenting manifestation of acquired immunodeficiency syndrome. South Med J 1987; 80:683.

328. Britton CB. HIV infection. In: Brust JCM, ed. Neurologic complications of drug and alcohol abuse. Neurol Clin 1993, in press.

329. Ho DD, Bredesen DE, Vinters HV, Daar ES. The acquired immunodeficiency syndrome (AIDS) dementia complex. Ann Intern Med 1989; 111:400.

330. Porter SB, Sande MA. Toxoplasmosis of the central nervous system in the acquired immunodeficiency syndrome. N Engl J Med 1992; 327:1643.

331. Koppel BS, Wormser GP, Tuchman AJ, et al. Central nervous system involvement in patients with acquired

immune deficiency syndrome. Acta Neurol Scand 1985; 71:337.

332. Kovacs JA, Kovacs AA, Polis M, et al. Cryptococcosis in the acquired immunodeficiency syndrome. Ann Intern Med 1985; 103:553.

333. Levy RM, Bredesen DE, Rosenblum ML. Neurological manifestations of the acquired immunodeficiency syndrome (AIDS): experiences at UCSF and review of the literature. J Neurosurg 1985; 62:475

334. Levy RM, Pons VG, Rosenblum ML. Intracerebral mass lesions in the acquired immunodeficiency syndrome (AIDS). N Engl J Med 1983; 309:1454.

335. Levy RM, Pons VG, Rosenblum ML. Central nervous system mass lesions in the acquired immunodeficiency syndrome. J Neurosurg 1984; 61:9.

336. McArthur JC. Neurologic manifestations of AIDS. Medicine 1987; 66:407.

337. Moskowitz LB, Hensley GT, Chan JC, et al. The neuropathology of acquired immune deficiency syndrome. Arch Pathol Lab Med 1984; 108:867.

338. Niedt GW, Scinella RA. Acquired immunodeficiency syndrome. Clinicopathologic study of 56 autopsies. Arch Pathol Lab Med 1985; 109:727.

339. Petito CK. Review of central nervous system pathology in human immunodeficiency virus infection. Ann Neurol 1988; 23(suppl):554.

340. Rosenberg S, Lopes MBS, Tsanaclis AM. Neuropathology of acquired immunodeficiency syndrome (AIDS). Analysis of 22 Brazilian cases. J Neurol Sci 1986; 76:187.

341. Snider WD, Simpson DM, Aronyk KE, Nielsen SL. Primary lymphoma of the nervous system associated with acquired immune deficiency syndrome. N Engl J Med 1983; 308:45.

342. Snider WD, Simpson DM, Nielsen S, et al. Neurological complications of acquired immune deficiency syndrome: analysis of 50 patients. Ann Neurol 1983; 14:403.

343. Wong B, Gold JWM, Brown AE, et al. Central nervous system toxoplasmosis in homosexual men and parenteral drug abusers. Ann Intern Med 1984; 100:36.

344. Malouf R, Dobkin J, Jacquette G, Brust JCM. Neurologic complications of HIV infection in parenteral drug abusers. Arch Neurol 1990; 47:1002.

345. Levy RM, Janssen RS, Bush TJ, Rosenbaum ML. Neuroepidemiology of acquired immunodeficiency syndrome. AIDS 1988; 1:31.

346. Concha M, Selnes OA, Munoz A, et al. Factors associated with neuropsychological performance in a cohort of intravenous drug users (IVDUs) infected with HIV-1. Neurology 1992; 42(suppl 3):192.

347. Coates RA, Farewell VT, Raboud J, et al. Co-factors of progression to acquired immunodeficiency syndrome in a cohort of male sexual contacts of men with human immodeficiency virus disease. Am J Epidemiol 1990; 132:717.

348. Margolick JB, Munoz A, Vlahov D, et al. Changes in T-lymphocyte subsets in intravenous drug users with HIV-1 infection. JAMA 1992; 267:1631.

348a.Selwyn PA, Alcabes P, Hartel D, et al. Clinical manifestations and predictors of disease progression in drug users with human immunodeficiency virus infection. N Engl J Med 1992; 327:1697.

349. Bonetti A, Weber R, Vogt MW, et al. Co-infection with human immunodeficiency virus type 1 (HIV-1) and cytomegalovirus in two intravenous drug users. Ann Intern Med 1989; 111:293.

350. Lee H, Swanson P, Shorty VS, et al. High rate of HTLV-II infection in seropositive IV drug abusers in New Orleans. Science 1989; 244:471.

351. Robert-Guroff M, Weiss SH, Giron JA. Prevalence of antibodies to HTLV-I, II, and III in intravenous drug abusers from an AIDS epidemic region. JAMA 1986; 255:3133.

352. Gradilone A, Zani M, Barillari G, et al. HTLV-I and HIV infection in drug addicts in Italy. Lancet 1986; 2:753.

353. Khabbaz RF, Onorato IM, Cannon RO, et al. Seroprevalence of HTLV-I and HTLV-II among intravenous drug users and persons in clinics for sexually transmitted diseases. N Engl J Med 1992; 326:375.

354. Bigger RJ, Buskell-Bales Z, Yakshe PN, et al. Antibody to human retroviruses among drug users in three east coast American cities, 1972–1976. J Infect Dis 1991; 163:57.

355. Zanetti AR, Galli C. Seroprevalence of HTLV-I and HTLV-II. N Engl J Med 1992; 326:1783.

356. Parry GJ, Erlemeier S, Malamut R, Garcia C. HTLV-I-associated myelopathy (HAM) in native Louisiana drug abusers. Neurology 1990; 40(suppl):239.

357. Honig LS, Lipka JJ, Young KK, et al. HTLV-I-associated myelopathy in a Californian: diagnosis by reactivity to a viral recombinant antigen. Neurology 1991; 41:448.

358. McKendall RR, Oas J, Lairmore MD. HTLV-I-associated myelopathy endemic in Texas-born residents and isolation of virus from CSF cells. Neurology 1991; 41:831.

359. Berger JR, Svenningsson A, Raffanti S, Resnick L. Tropical spastic paraparesis-like illness occurring in a patient dually infected with HIV-1 and HTLV-II. Neurology 1991; 41:85.

360. Berger JR, Svenningsson A, McCarthy M, et al. The role of HTLV in HIV-I neurologic disease. Neurology 1991; 41:197.

361. Janssen RS, Kaplan JE, Khabbaz RF, et al. HTLV-I-associated myelopathy/tropical spastic paraparesis in the United States. Neurology 1991; 41:1355.

362. Brust JCM, Richter RW. Stroke associated with addiction to heroin. J Neurol Neurosurg Psychiatry 1976; 39:194.

363. Lignelli GJ, Buchheit WA. Angiitis in drug abusers. N Engl J Med 1971; 284:112.

364. Woods BT, Strewler GJ. Hemiparesis occurring six hours after intravenous heroin injection. Neurology 1972; 22:863.

365. King J, Richards M, Tress B. Cerebral arteritis associated with heroin abuse. Med J Aust 1978; 2:444.

366. Herskowitz A, Gross E. Cerebral infarction associated with heroin sniffing. South Med J 1973; 66: 778.

366a. Bartolomei F, Nicoli F, Swaider L, et al. Accident vasculaire cerebral ischemique apres prise nasale d'heroine. Une nouvelle observation. Presse Med 1992; 21:983.

367. Jensen R, Olsen TS, Winther BB. Severe non-occlusive ischemic stroke in young heroin addicts. Acta Neurol Scand 1990; 81:354.

368. Knoblauch AL, Buchholz M, Koller MG, Kistler H. Hemiplegie nach Injektion von Heroin. Schweiz Med Wochenschr 1983; 113:402.

369. Sloan MA, Kittner SJ, Rigamonti D, Price TR. Occurrence of stroke associated with use/abuse of drugs. Neurology 1991; 41:1358.

370. Hall JH, Karp HR. Acute progressive ventral pontine disease in heroin abuse. Neurology 1973; 23:6.

371. Brust JCM. Stroke and substance abuse. In: Barnett HJM, Mohr JP, Stein BM, Yatsu FM, eds. Stroke: Pathophysiology, Diagnosis, and Management. New York: Churchill-Livingstone, 1992:875.

372. Protass LM. Delayed post-anoxic encephalopathy after heroin use. Ann Intern Med 1971; 74:738.

373. Hirsch CS. Dermatopathology of narcotic addiction. Hum Pathol 1972; 3:37.

374. Ostor A. The medical complications of narcotic addiction. Med J Aust 1977; 1:497.

375. Atlee W. Talc and cornstarch emboli in eyes of drug abusers. JAMA 1972; 219:49.

376. Lahmeyer HW, Steingold RG. Pentazocine and tripelennamine: a drug abuse epidemic? Int J Addict 1980; 15:1219.

377. Wadley C, Stillie GD. Pentazocine (Talwin) and tripelennamine (Pyribenzamine): a new drug combination or just a revival. Int J Addict 1980; 15:1285.

378. Caplan LR, Thomas C, Banks G. Central nervous system complications of addiction to "T's and Blues." Neurology 1982; 32:623.

379. Houck RJ, Bailey G, Daroca P, et al. Pentazocine abuse. Chest 1980; 77:227.

380. Szwed JJ. Pulmonary angiothrombosis caused by "blue velvet" addiction. Ann Intern Med 1970; 73:771.

381. Butz WC. Disseminated magnesium and silicate associated with paregoric addiction. J Forens Sci 1970; 15:581.

382. Lee J, Sapira JD. Retinal and cerebral microembolization of talc in a drug abuser. Am J Med Sci 1973; 265:75.

383. Ortona L, Laghi V, Cauda R. Immune function in heroin addicts. N Engl J Med 1979; 300:45.

384. Shaikh WA. Allergy to heroin. Allergy 1990; 45:555.

385. Ryan JJ, Parker CW, Williams RL. Gamma-globulin binding of morphine in heroin addicts. J Lab Clin Med 1972; 80:155.

386. Baranek JT. Morphine binding by serum globulins from morphine-treated rabbits. Fed Proc 1974; 33:474.

387. Garcia-Sevilla JA, Ugedo L, Ulibarri I, Guitierrez M. Platelet alpha-2 adrenoceptors in heroin addicts during withdrawal and after treatment with clonidine. Eur J Pharmacol 1985; 114:365.

388. Maqbool Z, Billett HH. Unwitting heparin abuse in a drug addict. Ann Intern Med 1982; 96:790.

389. Ell JJ, Unley D, Silver JR. Acute myelopathy in association with heroin addiction. J Neurol Neurosurg Psychiatry 1981; 44:448.

390. Goodhart LC, Loizou LA, Anderson M. Heroin myelopathy. J Neurol Neurosurg Psychiatry 1982; 45:562.

391. Grassa C, Montanari E, Scaglioni A, et al. Acute heroin myelopathy—case report. Ital J Neurol Sci 1984; 5:63.

392. Guidotti M, Passerini D, Brambilla M, Landi G. Heroin myelopathy. A case report. Ital J Neurol Sci 1985; 6:99.

393. Judice DJ, LeBlanc HJ, McGarry PA. Spinal cord vasculitis presenting as spinal cord tumor in a heroin addict. J Neurosurg 1978; 48:131.

394. Krause GS. Brown-Sequard syndrome following heroin injection. Ann Emerg Med 1983; 12:581.

395. Lee MC, Randa DC, Gold LH. Transverse myelopathy following the use of heroin. Minn Med 1976; 59:82.

396. Pearson J, Richter RW, Baden MM, et al. Transverse myelopathy as an illustration of the neurologic and neuropathologic features of heroin addiction. Hum Pathol 1972; 3:109.

397. Richter RW, Rosenberg RN. Transverse myelitis associated with heroin addiction. JAMA 1968; 206:1255.

398. Rodriguez E, Smokvina M, Sokolow J, Grynbaum BB. Encephalopathy and paraplegia occurring with the use of heroin. NY State J Med 1971; 71:2879.

399. Schein PS, Yessayun L, Mayman CI. Acute transverse myelitis associated with intravenous opium. Neurology 1971; 21:101.

400. Thompson WR, Waldman MB. Cervical myelopathy following heroin administration. J Med Soc NJ 1970; 67:223.

401. Fleishon H, Mandel S, Arenas A. Anterior spinal artery syndrome after cervical injection of heroin. Arch Neurol 1982; 39:739.

402. Smith WR, Wilson AF. Guillain-Barré syndrome in a heroin addict. JAMA 1975; 231:1367.

403. Ammueilaph R, Boongird P, Leechawengwongs M, Vejjajiva A. Heroin neuropathy. Lancet 1973; 1:1517.

404. Loizou LA, Boddie HG. Polyradiculoneuropathy associated with heroin abuse. J Neurol Neurosurg Psychiatry 1978; 41:855.

405. Ritland D, Butterfield W. Extremity complications of drug abuse. Am J Surg 1973; 126:639.

406. Colavita N, Orazi C, LaVecchia G, et al. An unusual kind of muscular and skeletal involvement in a heroin addict. Arch Orthop Trauma Surg 1984; 103:140.

407. Kaku DA, So YT. Acute femoral neuropathy and iliopsoas infarction in intravenous drug abusers. Neurology 1990; 40:1317.

408. Challenor YB, Richter RW, Bruun B, Pearson J. Non-traumatic plexitis and heroin addiction. JAMA 1973; 225:958.

409. Herdmann J, Benecke R, Meyer BU, Freund HJ. Erfolgreiche Kortikeidbehandlung einer lumbosakralen Plexusneuropathie bei Heroinabusus. Klinik, Electrophysiologie, Therapie und Verlauf. Nervenarzt 1988; 59:683.

410. Stamboulis E, Psimaris A, Malliara-Loulakaki S. Brachial and lumbar plexitis as a reaction to heroin. Drug Alcohol Depend 1988; 22:205.

411. Hecker E, Friedli WG. Plexusiasionen, Rhabdomyolysis, und Heroin. Schweiz Med Wochenschr 1988; 118:1982.

412. Delcker A, Dux R, Diener HC. Akute Plexuslasionen bei Heroinabhangigkeit. Nervenarzt 1992; 63:240.

413. Miller CM, Sangiulo P, Schanzer H, et al. Infected false aneurysms of the subclavian artery: a complication in drug addicts. J Vasc Surg 1984; 1:684.

414. Raz S, Ramanathan V. Injection injuries of the recurrent laryngeal nerve. Laryngoscope 1984; 94:197.

415. Hillstrom RP, Cohn AM, McCarroll KA. Vocal cord paralysis resulting from neck injections in the intravenous drug use population. Laryngoscope 1990; 100:503.

416. Polpathapee S, Tuchinda P, Chiwapong S. Sensorineural hearing loss in a heroin addict. J Med Assoc Thai 1984; 67:57.

417. Aeschlimann, Mall T, Sandoz P, Probst A. Course and complications of rhabdomyolysis following heroin poisoning. Schweiz Med Wochenschr 1984; 114:1236.

418. Nolte KB, McDonough ET. Rhabdomyolysis and heroin abuse. Am J Forensic Med Pathol 1991; 12:273.

419. deGans J, Stan J, Van Winjungaarden GK. Rhabdomyolysis and neurological lesions after intravenous heroin abuse. J Neurol Neurosurg Psychiatry 1985; 48:1057.

420. Fames M, Radu EW, Harder F. Rabdomyolyse und Kompartment-syndrome bei Heroinabusus. Helv Chir Acta 1984; 50:745.

421. Gibb WR, Shaw IC. Myoglobinuria due to heroin abuse. J R Soc Med 1985; 78:862.

422. Kathrein H, Kirchmair W, Koning P, Diettrich P. Rhabdomyolyse mit akuten Nierenversagen nach Heroinintoxikation. Dtsch Med Wochenschr 1983; 108:464.

423. Owen CA, Mubarak SJ, Hargens AR, et al. Intramuscular pressures with limb compression. N Engl J Med 1979; 300:1169.

424. Penn AS, Rowland LP, Fraser DW. Drugs, coma, and myoglobinuria. Arch Neurol 1972; 26:336.

425. Richter RW, Challenor YB, Pearson J, et al. Acute myoglobinuria associated with heroin addiction. JAMA 1971; 216:1172.

426. Schreiber SN, Liebowitz MR, Bernstein LH. Limb compression and renal impairment (crush syndrome) following narcotic and sedative overdose. J Bone Joint Surg 1972; 54A:1683.

427. Schwartzfarb L, Singh G, Marcus D. Heroin-associated rhabdomyolysis with cardiac involvement. Arch Intern Med 1977; 137:1255.

428. Chan YF, Wong PK, Chow TC. Acute myoglobinuria as a fatal complication of heroin addiction. Am J Forens Med Pathol 1990; 11:160.

429. Claros-Gonzolez I, Banos-Gallardo M, Forascepi-Roza R, Arguelles-Torana M. Rabdomiolisis atraumatica y fracaso renal agudo secundario a sobredosis de heroina. Rev Clin Esp 1988; 182:338.

430. Aunane D, Teboul JF, Richard C, Auzepy P. Severe rhabdomyolysis related to heroin sniffing. Intens Care Med 1990; 16:410.

431. Scherrer P, Delaloye-Bischof A, Turini G, Perret C. Participation myocardique a la rhabdomyolyse non traumatique apres surdosage aux opiaces. Schweiz Med Wochenschr 1985; 115:1116.

432. Chen SS, Chien CH, Yu HS: Syndrome of deltoid and/or gluteal fibrotic contracture: an injection myopathy. Acta Neurol Scand 1988; 78:167.

433. Pena J, Aranda C, Luque E, Vaamonde R. Heroin-induced myopathy in rat skeletal muscle. Acta Neuropathol 1990; 80:72.

434. Brust JCM, Richter RW. Quinine amblyopia related to heroin addiction. Ann Intern Med 1971; 74:84.

435. Dias PLR. Dyschromatopsia in heroin addicts. Br J Addict 1990; 85:241.

436. Dalessandro-Gandolfo L, Macci A, Biolcati G, et al. Inconsueta modalita d'intossicazione da piombo. Presentazione di un caso. Recenti Prog Med 1989; 80:140.

437. Antonini G, Palmieri G, Spagnoli G, Millefiorini M. Lead brachial neuropathy in heroin addiction. A case report. Clin Neurol Neurosurg 1989; 91:167.

438. Parras F, Patier JL, Ezpeteta C. Lead-contaminated heroin as a source of inorganic-lead intoxication. N Engl J Med 1987; 316:755.

439. O'Gorman P, Patel S, Notcutt S, Wicking J. Adulteration of "street" heroin with chloroquine. Lancet 1987; 1:746.

440. Wolters ECH, Van Winjungaarden GK, Stam FC, et al. Leukoencephalopathy after inhaling "heroin pyrolysate." Lancet 1982; 2:1233.

441. Schiffer D, Brignolio F, Giordena MT, et al. Spongiform encephalopathy in addicts inhaling pre-heated heroin. Clin Neuropathol 1985; 4:174.

442. Bianco C, Cocito D, Benna P, et al. Brain-stem auditory evoked potential alterations in heroin addicts. J Neurol 1985; 232:262.

443. Hungerbuhler H, Waespe W. Leukoencephalopathie nach Inhalation von Heroin-Pyrolysat. Schweiz Med Wochenschr 1990; 120:1801.

443a. Roulet Perez E, Maeder P, Rivier L, et al. Toxic leukencephalopathy after heroin ingestion in a 2½-year old child. Lancet 1992; 340:729.

444. Davis GC, Williams AC, Markey SP, et al. Chronic parkinsonism secondary to intravenous injection of meperidine analogues. Psychiatry Res 1979; 1:249.

445. Langston JW, Ballard P, Tetrud JW, Irwin I. Chronic parkinsonism in humans due to a product of meperidine-analog synthesis. Science 1983; 219: 9789.
446. Leads from the MMWR. Street drug contaminant causing parkinsonism. JAMA 1984; 252:331.
447. Stern Y. MPTP-induced parkinsonism. Prog Neurobiol 1990; 34:107.
448. Wright JM, Wall RA, Perry TL, Paty DW. Chronic parkinsonism secondary to intranasal administration of a product of meperidine-analogue synthesis. N Engl J Med 1984; 310:325.
449. Langston JW, Ballard PA. Parkinson's disease in a chemist working with 1-methyl-4-phenyl-1,2,5,6 tetrahydropyridine. N Engl J Med 1983; 309:310.
450. Ballard PA, Tetrud JW, Langston JW. Permanent human parkinsonism due to 1-methyl-4-phenyl-1,2,3,6-tedrahydropyridine (MPTP): seven cases. Neurology 1985; 35:949.
451. Langston JW, Ballard P. Parkinsonism induced by 1-methyl-4-phenyl-1,2,3,6-tetrahydropyridine (MPTP): implications for treatment and the pathogenesis of Parkinson's disease. Can J Neurol Sci 1984; 11: 160.
452. Langston JW. MPTP and Parkinson's disease. Trends Neurosci 1985; 8:79.
453. Burns RS, LeWitt PA, Ebert MH, et al. The clinical syndrome of striatal dopamine deficiency. Parkinsonism induced by 1-methyl-4-phenyl-1,2,3,6-tetrahydropyridine (MPTP). N Engl J Med 1985; 312: 1418.
454. Langston JW, Forno LS, Rebert CS, Irwin I. Selective nigral toxicity after systemic administration of 1-methyl-4-phenyl-1,2,5,6-tetrahydropyridine (MPTP) in the squirrel monkey. Brain Res 1984; 292: 390.
455. Calne DB, Langston JW, Stoessl AJ, et al. Positron emission tomography after MPTP. Observations relating to the cause of Parkinson's disease. Nature 1986; 317:246.
456. Markey SP, Johannessen JN, Chiveh CC, et al. Intraneuronal generation of a pyridinium metabolite may cause drug-induced parkinsonism. Nature 1984; 311:464.
457. Heikkila RE, Manzino L, Cabbat FS, Duvoisin RC. Protection against the dopaminergic neurotoxicity of 1-methyl-4-phenyl-1,2,5,6-tetrahydropyridine by monoamine oxidase inhibitors. Nature 1984; 311: 467.
458. Kindt MV, Nicklas WJ, Sonsalla PK, Heikkila RE. Mitochondria and the neurotoxicity of MPTP. Trends Pharmacol Sci 1986; 7:473.
459. Snyder SH. MPTP: a neurotoxin relevant to the patholophysiology of Parkinson's disease. Neurology 1986; 36:250.
460. Kindt MV, Heikkila RE, Nicklas WJ. Mitochondrial and metabolic toxicity of 1-methyl-4-phenyl-1,2,3,6-tetrahydropyridine. J Pharmacol Exp Ther 1987; 242:858.
461. Weingarten HL. 1-methyl-4-phenyl-1,2,3,6-tetrahydropyridine (MPTP): one designer drug and serendipity. J Forens Sci 1988; 33:588.
462. The Parkinson Study Group. Effects of tocopheral and deprenyl on the progression of disability in early Parkinson's disease. N Engl J Med 1993; 328:176.
463. Ng SKC, Brust JCM, Hauser WA, Susser M. Illicit drug use and the risk of new onset seizures: contrasting effects of heroin, marijuana, and cocaine. Am J Epidemiol 1990; 40:1017.
464. Albertson TE, Joy RM, Stark LF. Modification of kindled amygdaloid seizures by opiate agonists and antagonists. J Pharmacol Exp Ther 1984; 228:620.
465. Bohaus DW, Rigsbee LC, McNamara JO. Intranigral dynorphin 1-13 suppressed kindled seizures by a naloxone-sensitive mechanism. Brain Res 1987; 405:358.
466. Chugani HT, Ackermann RF, Chugani DC, Engel J. Opioid-induced epileptogenic phenomena: anatomical, behavioral, and electroencephalographic features. Ann Neurol 1984; 15:361.
467. Dua AK, Pinsky C, LaBella FS. Mu- and delta-opioid receptor mediated epileptoid responses in morphine-dependent and nondependent rats. Electroencephalogr Clin Neurophysiol 1985; 61:569.
468. Foote F, Gale K. Morphine potentiates seizures induced by GABA antagonists and attenuates seizures induced by electroshock in the rat. Eur J Pharmacol 1983; 95:259.
469. Foote F, Gale K. Proconvulsant effect of morphine on seizures induced by pentylenetetrazol in the rat. Eur J Pharmacol 1984; 105:179.
470. Frenk H. Pro- and anticonvulsant actions of morphine and the endogenous opioids: involvement and interactions of multiple opiate and non-opiate systems. Brain Res 1983; 287:197.
471. Frey HH. Interactions between morphine-like analgesics and anticonvulsant drugs. Pharmacol Toxicol 1987; 60:210.
472. Garant DS, Gale K. Infusion of opiates into substantia nigra protects against maximal electroschock seizures in rats. J Pharmacol Exp Ther 1985; 234:45.
473. Ikonomidou-Turski C, Cavalheiro EA, Turski WA, et al. Convulsant action of morphine, [D-Ala2,-D-Leu5] enkephalin and naloxone in the rat amygdala: electroencephalographic, morphological, and behavioral sequelae. Neuroscience 1987; 20:671.
474. Tortella FC. Endogenous opioid peptides and epilepsy: quieting the seizing brain? Trends Pharmacol Sci 1988; 9:366.
475. Tortella FC, Robles L, Holaday JW. U50,488, a highly selective kappa opioid: anticonvulsant profile in rats. J Pharmacol Exp Ther 1986; 237:49.
476. Tortella FC, Robles L, Mosberg HI. Evidence for mu opioid receptor mediation of enkephalin-induced electroencephalographic seizures. J Pharmacol Exp Ther 1987; 240:571.
477. Walker GE, Yaksh TL. Studies on the effects of intrathecally injected DADL and morphine on nocicep-

tive thresholds and electroencephalographic activity: a thalamic delta receptor syndrome. Brain Res 1986; 383:1.

478. Schuster CR, Smith BB, Jaffe JH. Drug abuse in heroin users: an experimental study of self-administration of methadone, codeine, and pentazocine. Arch Gen Psychiatry 1971; 24:359.

479. Lewis JR. Misprescribing analgesics. JAMA 1974; 228:1155.

480. Sandoval RG, Wang RIH. Tolerance and dependence on pentazocine. N Engl J Med 1969; 280:1391.

481. Choucair AK, Ziter FA. Pentazocine abuse masquerading as familial myopathy. Neurology 1984; 34:524.

482. Schlicher JE, Zuchlke RL, Lynch PJ. Local changes at the site of pentazocine injection. Arch Dermatol 1971; 104:90.

483. Steiner JC, Winkelman AC, deJesus PV. Pentazocine-induced myopathy. Arch Neurol 1973; 28:408.

484. Shannon HF, Su TP. Effects of the combination of tripelennamine and pentazocine at the behavioral and molecular levels. Pharmacol Biochem Behav 1982; 17:789.

485. Jasinski DR, Boren JJ, Henningfield JE, et al. Progress report from the NIDA Addiction Research Center, Baltimore, MD. In: Harris LS, ed. Problems of Drug Dependence 1983. Washington, DC: NIDA Research Monograph 49, DHHS, 1984:69.

486. Waller DP, Katz NL, Morris RW. Potentiation of lethality in mice by combinations of pentazocine and tripelennamine. Clin Toxicol 1980; 16:17.

487. Itkonen J, Schnoll S, Daghestani A, Glassroth J. Accelerated development of pulmonary complications due to illicit intravenous use of pentazocine and triplennamine. Am J Med 1984; 76:617.

488. Botsford KB, Weinstein RA, Nathan CR, Kabins SA. Selective survival in pentazocine and triplennamine of *Pseudomonas aeruginosa* serotype Oii from drug addicts. J Infect Dis 1985; 151:209.

489. Baum C, Hsu JP, Nelson RC. The impact of the addition of naloxone on the use and abuse of pentazocine. Public Health Rep 1987; 102:426.

490. Reed DA, Schnoll SH. Abuse of pentazocine-naloxone combination. JAMA 1986; 256:2562.

491. Smith SG, Davis WM. Nonmedical use of butorphanol and diphenhydramine. JAMA 1984; 252:1010.

492. Rasor RW, Orecraft HJ. Addiction to meperidine (Demerol) hydrochloride. JAMA 1955; 157:654.

493. Hershey LA. Meperidine and central neurotoxicity. Ann Intern Med 1983; 98:548.

494. Hochman MS. Meperidine-associated myoclonus and seizures in long-term hemodialysis patients. Ann Neurol 1983; 14:593.

495. Kaiko RF, Foley KM, Grabinski PY, et al. Central nervous system excitatory effects of meperidine in cancer patients. Ann Neurol 1983; 13:180.

496. Meyer D, Halfin V. Toxicity secondary to meperidine in patients on monoamine oxidase inhibitors: a case report and critical review. J Clin Psychopharmacol 1981; 1:319.

497. Lieberman AN, Goldstein M. Reversible parkinsonism related to meperidine. N Engl J Med 1985; 312:509.

498. Aberfeld DC, Bienenstock H, Shapiro MS, et al. Diffuse myopathy related to meperidine addiction in a mother and daughter. Arch Neurol 1968; 19:384.

499. Collins GB, Kiefer KS. Propoxyphene dependence. Postgrad Med J 1981; 70:57.

500. Lader M. Abuse of weak opioid analgesics. Hum Toxicol 1984; 3(suppl):229S.

501. Physicians asked to write "no refill" on propoxyphene Rxes. FDA Drug Bull 1980; 10:11.

502. Wall R, Linford SMJ, Akhter M. Addiction to Ditalgesic (dextropropoxyphene). BMJ 1980; 1:1213.

503. Chambers CD, Taylor WJR. Patterns of propoxyphene abuse. Int J Clin Pharmacol 1971; 4:240.

504. Chard P. Darvon dependence: three case studies. Chem Depend 1980; 4:65.

505. Finkle BS. Self-poisoning with dextropropoxyphene and dextropropoxyphene compounds; the USA experience. Hum Toxicol 1984; 3(suppl):115S.

506. Hooper HE, Santo Y. Use of propoxyphene (Darvon) by adolescents admitted to drug programs. Contemp Drug Prob 1980; 9:357.

507. Schuckit MA, Morrisey ER. Propoxyphene and phencyclidine (PCP) use in adolescents. J Clin Psychiatry 1978; 39:7.

508. Finkle BS, Caplan YH, Garriott JC, et al. Propoxyphene in postmortem toxicology, 1976–1978. J Forens Sci 1981; 26:739.

509. Litman RE, Diller J, Nelson F. Deaths related to propoxyphene or codeine or both. J Forens Sci 1983; 28:128.

510. D'Adadie NB, Lenton JD. Propoxyphene dependence: problems in management. South Med J 1984; 77:229.

511. Young RJ. Dextropropoxyphene overdosage. Pharmacological considerations and clinical management. Drugs 1983; 26:70.

512. Amsterdam EA, Rendig SV, Henderson L, Mason DT. Depression of myocardial contractile function by propoxyphene and norpropoxyphene. J Cardiovasc Pharmacol 1981; 3:129.

513. Henry JA, Cassidy SL. Membrane stabilizing activity: a major cause of fatal poisoning. Lancet 1986; 1:1414.

514. McBride DC, McCoy CB, Rivers JE, Lincoln LA. Dilaudid use: trends and characteristics of users. Chem Depend 1980; 4:85.

515. Leads from the MMWR. Dilaudid-related deaths— District of Columbia, 1987. JAMA 1988; 260:903.

516. Feuer E, French J. Descriptive epidemiology of mortality in New Jersey due to combinations of codeine and glutethimide. Am J Epidemiol 1984; 119:202.

517. Shamoian CA. Codeine and glutethimide: euphoretic, addicting combination. NY State J Med 1975; 75:97.

518. Sramek JJ, Khajawall A. "Loads." N Engl J Med 1981; 305:231.

519. Feuer E, French J. Death related to narcotics overdose in New Jersey. J Med Soc NJ 1984; 81:291.

520. Bender FH, Cooper JV, Dreyfus R. Fatalities associated with an acute overdose of glutethimide (Doriden) and codeine. Vet Hum Toxicol 1988; 30:322.

521. Murray RM. Minor analgesic abuse: the slow recognition of a public health problem. Br J Addict 1980; 75:9.

522. Goldberg I, Bahar A, Yosipovitch Z. Gangrene of the upper extremity following intra-arterial injection of drugs. A case report and review of the literature. Clin Orthop 1984; 188:223.

523. Curry KH, Stanhope JM. Codeine linctus and myopathy. Med J Aust 1984; 140:247.

524. Kilpatrick C, Braund W, Burns R. Myopathy with myasthenic features possibly induced by codeine linctus. Med J Aust 1982; 2:410.

525. Seow SS. Abuse of APF Linctus codeine and cardiac glycoside toxicity. Med J Aust 1984; 140:54.

526. Barragry JM, Morris DV. Fatal dependence on kaolin and morphine mixture. Postgrad Med J 1980; 56:180.

527. Ayres WA, Starsiak MJ, Sokolay P. The bogus drug: 3-ethyl and alpha-methyl fentanyl sold as "China White." J Psychoact Drugs 1981; 13:91.

528. Silsby HD, Kruzich DJ, Hawkins MR. Fentanyl citrate abuse among health care professionals. Milit Med 1984; 149:227.

529. LaBarbera M, Wolfe T. Characteristics, attitudes, and implications of fentanyl use based on reports from self-identified fentanyl users. J Psychoact Drugs 1983; 15:293.

530. Carroll FL, Boldt KG, Huang PT, et al. Synthesis of fentanyl analogs. In: Harris LS, ed. Problems of Drug Dependence 1989. Rockville, MD: NIDA Research Monograph 95, DHHS, 1990:497.

531. Henderson GL. Designer drugs: past history and future prospects. J Forens Sci 1988; 33:569.

532. Martin M, Hecker J, Clark R, et al. China White epidemic: an eastern United States emergency department experience. Ann Emerg Med 1991; 20:158.

533. Hibbs J, Perper J, Winek CL. An outbreak of designer drug-related deaths in Pennsylvania. JAMA 1991; 265:1011.

534. Nieves E. Toxic heroin has killed 12, officials say. NY Times, February 4, 1991.

535. Mannelli P, Janiri L, DeMarinis M, Tempesta E. Lofetamine: new abuse of an old drug: clinical evaluation of opioid activity. Drug Alcohol Depend 1989; 24:95.

536. Meyer RE. What treatments for the heroin addict? JAMA 1986; 256:511.

537. Dole VP. Addictive behavior. Sci Am 1980; 243:18.

538. Wikler A. Dynamics of drug dependence. Implications of a conditioning theory for research and treatment. Arch Gen Psychiatry 1973; 28:611.

539. Levine DG. Needle freaks. Compulsive self-injection by drug abusers. Am J Psychiatry 1974; 131:297.

540. Musto DF, Ramos MR. Notes on American medical history. A follow-up study of the New Haven morphine maintenance clinic of 1920. N Engl J Med 1981; 304:1071.

541. O'Brien CP, Nace EP, Mintz J, et al. Follow-up of Vietnam veterans. 1. Relapse to drug use after Vietnam service. Drug Alcohol Depend 1980; 5:333.

542. Foley KM. The treatment of cancer pain. N Engl J Med 1985; 313:84.

543. Portenoy RK, Foley KM. Chronic use of opioid analgesics in non-malignant pain: report of 38 cases. Pain 1986; 25:171.

544. Baganz PC, Maddux JF. Employment status of narcotic addicts one year after hospital discharge. Public Health Rep 1965; 80:615.

545. Vaillant G. A 20-year follow-up of New York narcotic addicts. Arch Gen Psychiatry 1973; 29:237.

546. Kramer JC, Bass RA. Institutionalization patterns among civilly committed addicts. JAMA 1969; 208:2297.

547. Kosten TR, Rounsaville BJ, Kleber HD. A 2.5 year follow-up of depression, life crises, and treatment effects on abstinence among opioid addicts. Arch Gen Psychiatry 1986; 43:733.

548. Rounsaville BJ, Kleber HD. Psychotherapy/counseling for opiate addicts: strategies for use in different treatment settings. Int J Addict 1985; 20:869.

549. Woody GE, McLellan AT, Luborsky L, et al. Severity of psychiatric symptoms as a predictor of benefits from psychotherapy: the Veterans Administration-Penn Study. Am J Psychiatry 1984; 141:1172.

550. Anglin MD, Weisman CP, Fisher DG. The MMPI profiles of narcotics addicts. I. A review of the literature. Int J Addict 1989; 24:867.

551. Rounsaville BJ, Kosten TR, Weissman MM, et al. Psychiatric disorders in relatives of probands with opiate addiction. Arch Gen Psychiatry 1991; 48:33.

552. Khantzian EJ, Treece C. DSM-III psychiatric diagnosis of narcotic addicts: recent findings. Arch Gen Psychiatry 1985; 42:1067.

553. Rounsaville BJ, Weissman MM, Kleber HD, Wilber CH. Heterogeneity of psychiatric diagnosis in treated opiate addicts. Arch Gen Psychiatry 1982; 39:161.

554. Bale RN, Zarcone VP, Van Stone WW, et al. Three therapeutic communities. A prospective controlled study of narcotic addiction treatment: process and two-year follow-up results. Arch Gen Psychiatry 1984; 41:185.

555. DeLeon G, Schwartz S. Therapeutic communities: what are the retention rates? Am J Drug Alcohol Abuse 1984; 10:267.

556. Ter-Riet G, Kleijnen J, Knipschild P. A meta-analysis of studies into the effect of acupuncture on addiction. Br J Gen Pract 1990; 40:379.

557. Koran LM. Heroin maintenance for heroin addicts: issues and evidence. N Engl J Med 1973; 288:654.

558. Pillard RC. Shall we allow heroin maintenance? N Engl J Med 1973; 288:682.

559. Hawks D. The proposal to make heroin available legally to intravenous drug abusers. Med J Aust 1988; 149:455.

559a.Parry A. Taking heroin maintenance seriously: the politics of tolerance. Lancet 1992; 339:350.

560. Burr A. A British view of prescribing pharmaceutical heroin to opiate addicts: a critique of the "heroin solution" with special reference to the Piccadilly and Kensington Market drug scenes in London. Int J Addict 1986; 21:83.

561. Connell PH, Mitcheson M. Necessary safeguards when prescribing opioid drugs to addicts: experience of drug dependence clinics in London. BMJ 1984; 288:767.

562. Bayer R. Heroin maintenance: an historical perspective on the exhaustion of liberal narcotics reform. J Psyched Drugs 1976; 8:157.

563. Ghodse H. Drugs and Addictive Behavior: A Guide to Treatment. Boston: Blackwell Scientific, 1989.

564. Dole VP. Implications of methadone maintenance for theories of narcotic addiction. JAMA 1988; 260:3025.

565. Kreek MJ. Medical safety and side effects of methadone in tolerant individuals. JAMA 1973; 223:665.

566. Novick DM, Ochshorn M, Ghali V, et al. Natural killer cell activity and lymphocyte subsets in parenteral heroin abusers and long-term methadone maintenance patients. J Pharmacol Exp Ther 1989; 250:606.

567. Drummer OH, Syrjanen M, Opeskin K, Cordner S. Deaths of heroin addicts starting on a methadone maintenance program. Lancet 1990; 1:108.

568. Dole VP, Robinson JW, Orraca J, et al. Methadone treatment of randomly selected criminal addicts. N Engl J Med 1969; 280:1372.

569. Dole VP, Nyswander ME. Methadone maintenance treatment: a ten-year perspective. JAMA 1976; 235:2117.

570. Bass UF, Brown BS, Barry S. Methadone maintenance and methadone detoxification: a comparison of retention rates and client characteristics. Int J Addict 1975; 8:889.

571. Bourne PG. Methadone. Benefits and Shortcomings. Washington, DC: Drug Abuse Council (Publication MS-12), 1975.

572. Newman RG, Whitehill WB. Double blind comparison of methadone and placebo maintenance treatments of narcotic addicts in Hong Kong. Lancet 1979; 2:485.

573. Zinberg N. The crisis in methadone maintenance. N Engl J Med 1977; 296:1000.

574. Gerstein DR, Lewin LS. Treating drug problems. N Engl J Med 1990; 323:844.

575. Zweben JE. Methadone maintenance in the treatment of opioid dependence. A current perspective. West J Med 1990; 152:588.

576. Dole VP, Nyswander ME, DesJarlais D, Joseph H. Performance-based rating of methadone maintenance programs. N Engl J Med 1982; 306:169.

577. Kreek MJ. Rationale for maintenance pharmacotherapy of opiate dependence. In: O'Brien CP, Jaffe JH, eds. Addictive States. Res Publ Assoc Res Nerv Ment Dis 1992; 70:205.

578. Kirn TF. Methadone maintenance treatment remains controversial after 23 years of experience. JAMA 1988; 260:2970.

579. Arif A, Westermeyer J. Methadone Maintenance in the Management of Opioid Dependence: An International Review. New York: Praeger, 1990.

580. Liappas JA, Jenner FA, Viente B. Literature on methadone maintenance clinics. Int J Addict 1988; 23:927.

581. Hubbard RL, Marsden ME, Rachal JV, et al. Drug Abuse Treatment: A National Study of Effectiveness. Chapel Hill, NC: University of North Carolina Press, 1989.

582. Newman RE. Advocacy for methadone treatment. Ann Intern Med 1990; 113:819.

583. Smith DE, Landry MJ. Benzodiazepine dependency discontinuation: focus on the chemical dependency detoxification setting and benzodiazepine-polydrug abuse. J Psychiat Res 1990; 24(suppl 2):145.

584. Kolar AF, Brown BS, Weddington WW, Ball JC. A treatment crisis: cocaine use by clients in methadone maintenance programs. J Subst Abuse Treatment 1990; 7:101.

585. Saxon AJ, Calsyn DA, Blaes PA, et al. Marijuana use by methadone maintenance patients. In: Harris L, ed. Problems of Drug Dependence 1990. Rockville, MD: NIDA Research Monograph 105, DHHS, 1991:306.

586. Lehman WE, Barrett ME, Simpson DD. Alcohol use by heroin addicts 12 years after drug abuse treatment. J Stud Alcohol 1990; 51:233.

587. Cicero TJ, Bell RD, Wiest WG, et al. Function of the male sex organs in heroin and methadone users. N Engl J Med 1975; 292:882.

588. Aronow R, Paul SD, Woolley PV. Childhood poisoning: an unfortunate consequence of methadone availability. JAMA 1972; 219:321.

589. Jonas S. Methadone maintenance programs. N Engl J Med 1982; 306:1493.

590. Stephens RC, Weppner RC. Legal and illegal use of methadone: one year later. Am J Psychiatry 1973; 130:1391.

591. Weppner RS, Stephens RC, Conrad HT. Methadone: some aspects of its legal and illegal use. Am J Psychiatry 1972; 129:451.

592. Novick DM, Pascarelli EF, Joseph H, et al. Methadone maintenance patients in general medical practice. A preliminary report. JAMA 1988; 259:3299.

593. Wesson DR. Revival of medical maintenance in the treatment of heroin dependence. JAMA 1988; 259:3314.

594. Hanbury R, Sturiano V, Cohen M, et al. Cocaine use in persons on methadone maintenance. Adv Alcohol Subst Abuse 1986; 6:97.

595. Nurco DN, Kinlock TW, Hanlon TE, Ball JC. Non-narcotic drug use over an addiction career—a study of heroin addicts in Baltimore and New York City. Compr Psychiatry 1988; 29:450.

596. Batki SL, Sorensen JL, Gibson DR, Maude-Griffin P. HIV-infected IV drug users in methadone treatment: outcome and psychological correlates—a prelimi-

nary report. In: Harris LS, ed. Problems of Drug Dependence 1989. Rockville, MD: NIDA Research Monograph 95, DHHS, 1990:405.

596a. Bilsky EJ, Montegut MJ, Delong CL, et al. Opioidergic modulation of cocaine conditioned place preference. Life Sci 1992; 50:85.

597. Iguchi MY, Griffiths RR, Bickel WK, et al. Relative abuse liability of benzodiazepines in methadone maintained population in three cities. In: Harris LS, ed. Problems in Drug Dependence 1989. Rockville, MD: NIDA Research Monograph 95, DHHS, 1990:364.

598. Anglin MD, Almog IJ, Fisher DG, Peters KR. Alcohol use by heroin addicts: evidence for an inverse relationship. A study of methadone maintenance and drug-free treatment samples. Am J Drug Alcohol Abuse 1989; 15:191.

599. Bell J, Bowron P, Lewis J, Batey R. Serum levels of methadone in maintenance clients who persist in illicit drug use. Br J Addict 1990; 85:1599.

600. Bell J, Seres V, Bowron P, et al. The use of serum methadone levels in patients receiving methadone maintenance. Clin Pharmacol Ther 1988; 43:623.

601. Caplehorn JR, Bell J. Methadone dosage and retention of patients in maintenance treatment. Med J Aust 1991; 154:195.

602. D'Aunno T, Vaughn TE. Variations in methadone treatment practices. Results from a national study. JAMA 1992; 267:253.

603. Cooper JR. Ineffective use of psychoactive drugs. Methadone treatment is no exception. JAMA 1992; 267:281.

604. Tennant FS. Inadequate plasma concentrations in some high dose methadone patients. Am J Psychiatry 1987; 144:1349.

605. Cushman P. Detoxification after methadone maintenance treatment. Ann NY Acad Sci 1981; 262: 217.

606. DesJarlais DC, Joseph H, Dole VP. Long-term outcomes after termination from methadone maintenance treatment. Ann NY Acad Sci 1981; 262:231.

607. Newman RG. Methadone treatment: defining and evaluating success. N Engl J Med 1987; 317:447.

608. Murphy S, Rosenbaum M. Money for methadone II: unintended consequences of limited-duration methadone maintenance. J Psychoact Drugs 1988; 20:397.

609. Inciardi JA. Methadone Diversion: Experiences and Issues. Washington, DC: DHEW Publication No (ADM) 78-488, US Government Printing Office, 1977.

610. Sieniewitz DJ, Nidecker AC. Conglomerate pulmonary disease: a form of talcosis in intravenous methadone abusers. Am J Roentgenol 1980; 135:697.

611. Chasnoff IJ, Hatcher R, Burns WJ. Early growth patterns of methadone-addicted infants. Am J Dis Child 1980; 134:1049.

612. Chasnoff IJ, Hatcher R, Burns WJ. Polydrug and methadone-addicted newborns: a continuum of impairment? Pediatrics 1982; 70:210.

613. Rosen TS, Honson HL. Children of methadone-maintained mothers: follow-up to 18 months of age. J Pediatr 1982; 101:192.

614. Mass U, Kattner E, Weighart-Jesse B, et al. Infrequent neonatal opiate withdrawal following maternal methadone detoxification during pregnancy. J Perinat Med 1990; 18:111.

615. Richardson BS, O'Grady JP, Olsen GD. Fetal breathing movements and the response to carbon dioxide in patients on methadone maintenance. Am J Obstet Gynecol 1984; 150:400.

616. Davis DD, Templer DI. Neurobehavioral functioning in children exposed to narcotics in utero. Addict Behav 1988; 13:275.

617. Chasnoff IJ, Burns KA, Burns WJ, Schnoll SH. Prenatal drug exposure: effects on neonatal and infant growth and development. Neurobehav Toxicol Teratol 1986; 8:357.

618. Kaltenbach K, Finnegan LP. Perinatal and development outcome of infants exposed to methadone in utero. In: Harris LS, ed. Problems of Drug Dependence 1986. Rockville, MD: NIDA Research Monograph 76, DHHS, 1987:276.

619. Stimmel B, Goldberg J, Reisman A, et al. Fetal outcome in narcotic-dependent women: the importance of the type of maternal narcotic used. Am J Drug Alcohol Abuse 1982–1983; 9:383.

620. Edelin KC, Gurganious L, Golar K, et al. Methadone maintenance in pregnancy: consequences to care and outcome. Obstet Gynecol 1988; 71; 399.

621. Hein PR, Schatorje J, Frencken HJ. The effect of chronic methadone treatment on intra-uterine growth of the cynomolgus monkey (Macaca fasciularis). Eur J Obstet Gynecol Reprod Biol 1988; 27:81.

622. Cooper JR. Methadone treatment and the acquired immunodeficiency syndrome. JAMA 1989; 262: 1664.

623. Dole VP. Methadone treatment and the acquired immunodeficiency syndrome epidemic. JAMA 1989; 262:1681.

624. Novick DM, Joseph H, Croxson TS, et al. Absence of antibody to human immunodeficiency virus in long-term, socially rehabilitated methadone maintenance patients. Arch Intern Med 1990; 150:97.

625. Bourne PG. AIDS and drug use. An international perspective. J Psychoact Drugs 1988; 20:153.

626. Serraino D, Franceschi S. Methadone maintenance programs and AIDS. Lancet 1989; 2:1522.

627. Magura S, Grossman JI, Lipton S, et al. Correlates of participation in AIDS education and HIV antibody testing by methadone patients. Public Health Rep 1989; 104:231.

628. Wasserman S, Yahr MD. Choreic movements induced by the use of methadone. Arch Neurol 1980; 37:727.

629. Palmer W-R, Haferkame G. Involuntary movements associated with methadone. Arch Neurol 1981; 38:737.

630. Ling W, Dorus W, Hargreaves WA, et al. Alternative induction and crossover schedules for methadyl acetate. Arch Gen Psychiatry 1984; 41:193.

631. Mendelson JH, Ellingboe J, Judson B, Goldstein A. Plasma testosterone and luteinizing hormone levels during levo-alpha-acetylmethadol maintenance and withdrawal. Clin Pharmacol Ther 1984; 36:239.

632. Ling W, Charuvastra VC, Kain SC, Kleet CJ. Methadyl acetate and methadone as maintenance treatment for heroin addicts. Arch Gen Psychiatry 1976; 33:709.

633. Woody GE, McLellan AT, O'Brien CP. Lack of toxicity of high dose propoxyphene napsylate when used for treatment of addiction. Clin Toxicol 1980; 16:473.

634. Tennant FS, Rawson RA. Outpatient treatment of prescription opioid dependence: comparison of two methods. Arch Intern Med 1982; 142:1845.

635. Wang RIH, Kochar C, Hasegawa AT, Roh BL. Propoxyphene napsylate compared to methadone for opiate dependence. Psychopharmacology 1981; 75:355.

636. Resnick RB, Kestenbaum RS, Schwartz LK, Smith A. Evaluation of propranolol in opiate dependence. Arch Gen Psychiatry 1976; 33:993.

637. Schecter A. The role of narcotic antagonists in the rehabilitation of opiate addicts: a review of naltrexone. Am J Drug Alcohol Abuse 1980; 7:1.

638. Freedman AM, Fink M, Sharoff R, Zaks A. Clinical studies of cyclazocine in the treatment of narcotic addiction. Am J Psychiatry 1968; 124:1499.

639. Goldstein MJ. Cyclazocine in the treatment of opiate addiction: a review with recommendations. Int J Addict 1980; 15:939.

640. Gonzalez JP, Brogden RN. Naltrexone: a review of its pharmacodynamic and pharmacokinetic properties and therapeutic efficacy in the management of opioid dependence. Drugs 1988; 35:192.

641. Crabtree BL. Review of naltrexone, a long-acting opiate antagonist. Clin Pharm 1984; 3:273.

642. Kosten TR, Kleber HD. Strategies to improve compliance with narcotic antagonists. Am J Drug Alcohol Abuse 1984; 10:249.

643. Crowley TJ, Wagner JE, Zebe G, et al. Naltrexone-induced dysphoria in former opioid addicts. Am J Psychiatry 1985; 142:1081.

644. Resnick RB, Galanter M, Pycha C, et al. Buprenorphine: an alternative to methadone for heroin dependence treatment. Psychopharmacol Bull 1992; 28:109.

645. Fudala PJ, Jaffe JH, Dax EM, Johnson RE. Use of buprenorphine in the treatment of opiate addiction. II. Physiologic and behavioral effects of daily and alternate-day administration and abrupt withdrawal. Clin Pharmacol Ther 1990; 47:525.

646. Johnson RE, Jaffe JH, Fudala PJ. A controlled trial of buprenorphine treatment for opioid dependence. JAMA 1991; 267:2750.

647. Kosten TR, Kleber HD, Morgan CH. Treatment of cocaine abuse using buprenorphine. Biol Psychiatry 1989; 26:637.

648. Mendelson JH, Mello NK, Teoh SK, et al. Buprenorphine treatment for concurrent heroin and cocaine dependence: Phase I study. In: Harris L, ed. Problems of Drug Dependence 1990. DHHS, Rockville, MD: NIDA Research Monograph 105, 1991:196.

649. Winger G, Skjoldager P, Woods JH. Effects of buprenorphine and other opioid agonists and antagonists on alfentanil- and cocaine-reinforced responding in rhesus monkeys. J Pharmacol Exp Ther 1992; 261:311.

650. Mello NK, Mendelson JH, Bree MP, Lukas SE. Buprenorphine suppresses cocaine self-administration by rhesus monkeys. Science 1989; 245:859.

651. Brown EE, Finlay JM, Wong JTF, et al. Behavioral and neurochemical interactions between cocaine and buprenorphine: implications for the pharmacotherapy of cocaine abuse. J Pharmacol Exp Ther 1991; 256:119.

652. Stretch R. Discrete-trial control of cocaine self-injection behavior in squirrel monkeys: effects of morphine, naloxone, and chlorpromazine. Can J Physiol Pharmacol 1977; 55:778.

653. Hubner CB, Kornetsky C. The reinforcing properties of the mixed agonist-antagonist buprenorphine as assessed by brain-stimulation reward. Pharmacol Biochem Behav 1988; 30:195.

654. Lukas SE, Brady JV, Griffiths RR. Comparison of opioid self-injection and disruption of scheudule-controlled performance in the baboon. J Pharmacol Exp Ther 1986; 238:924.

655. Mello NK, Lukas SE, Bree MP, Mendelson JH. Progressive ratio performance maintained by buprenorphine, heroin and methadone in macaque monkeys. Drug Alcohol Depend 1988; 21:81.

656. Mello NK, Mendelson JH, Kuehnle JC. Buprenorphine effects on human heroin self-administration: an operant analysis. J Pharmacol Exp Ther 1982; 223:30.

657. Johnson RE, Cone EJ, Henningfield JE, Fudala PJ. Use of buprenorphine in the treatment of opiate addiction. I. Physiologic and behavioral effects during a rapid dose induction. Clin Phamacol Ther 1989; 46:335.

658. Harper I. Temgesic abuse. N Z Med J 1983; 96:777.

659. O'Conner JJ, Moloney E, Travers R, Campbell A. Buprenorphine abuse among opiate addicts. Br J Addict 1988; 83:1085.

660. Quigley AJ, Bredemeyer DE, Seow SS. A case of buprenorphine abuse. Med J Aust 1984; 140:425.

661. Rainey HB. Abuse of buprenorphine. N Z Med J 1986; 99:72.

662. Richert S, Strauss A, von Arnim T, et al. Drug dependence of buprenorphine. MMWR 1983; 125:1195.

663. Robertson JR, Bucknall ABV. Burprenorphine: dangerous drug or over-looked therapy. BMJ 1986; 292:1465.

664. San Molina L, Porta-Serra M. Addiction to buprenorphine. Rev Clin Esp 1987; 181:288.

665. Strang J. Abuse of buprenorphine. Lancet 1985; 2:725.

666. Wodak AD. Buprenorphine: new wonder drug or new hazard? Med J Aust 1984; 140:389.

667. Lewis JW. Buprenorphine. Drug Alcohol Depend 1985; 14:362.
668. Chowdhury AN, Chowdhury S. Buprenorphine abuse: report from India. Br J Addict 1990; 85:1349.
669. San L, Tremoleda J, Olle JM, et al. Prevalencia del consumo de buprenorphina en heroinomanos en tratamiento. Med Clin 1989; 93:645.
670. San L, Cami J, Fernandez T, et al. Assessment and management of opioid withdrawal symptoms in buprenorphine-dependent subjects. Br J Addict 1992; 87:55.
671. Paraskevaides EC. Near fatal auditory hallucinations after buprenorphine. BMJ 1988; 296:214.
672. Kieffer BL, Befort K, Gaveriaux-Ruff, Hirth CG. The delta opioid receptor: isolation of a cDNA by expression cloning and pharmacological characterization. Proc Natl Acad Sci USA 1992; 89:12048.
673. Golden T. Violently, drug traffic in Mexico rebounds. N.Y. Times, March 8, 1993.
674. Cowell A. Heroin pouring through porous European borders. N. Y. Times, February 5, 1993.
675. Frieden TR, Sterling T, Pablos-Mendez A, et al. The emergence of drug-resistant tuberculosis in New York City. N Engl J Med 1993; 328:521.
676. Katz DA, Berger JR, Duncan RC: Neurosyphilis. A comparative study of the effects of infection with human immunodeficiency virus. Arch Neurol 1993; 50:243.

Chapter 3

Amphetamine and Other Psychostimulants

I love coffee! I love tea!
I love the Java jive, and it loves me!   —*The Ink Spots*

Who put the Benzedrine in Mrs. Murphy's Ovaltine?
                    —*Harry "The Hipster" Gibson*

Speed kills.   —*DEA slogan*

This chapter discusses drugs that are taken for psychostimulation, especially amphetamine and related indirect bioamine agonists[1,2] but also other substances with different pharmacological properties. (Cocaine, because in the 1980s it became a major American preoccupation, is considered separately in Chapter 4.) Amphetamine-like drugs are used for narcolepsy and attention deficit disorder. It has long been believed that their anorectic effects wear off in a matter of weeks, yet a 1992 study found that weight loss was sustained as long as the drugs were taken.[3] They are rarely of value in depressive disorders. Although their manufacture decreased following regulatory legislation in the 1960s and 1970s,[4] amphetamine-like psychostimulants are still produced in huge quantities, both legally and illegally (Table 3–1, Figure 3–1).

Pharmacology and Animal Studies

Amphetamine is both a central stimulant and a peripheral sympathomimetic. In animals, it raises systolic and diastolic blood pressure. Low doses reflexly slow the heart rate; higher doses cause tachycardia or cardiac arrhythmia. Stimulation of the medullary respiratory center increases the rate and depth of respiration, and excitatory actions on the brain stem, diencephalon, and cerebrum produce increased locomotor activity, sleeplessness, and increased body temperature.[2,5] Higher or repeated doses cause stereotypic motor behavior (exploration, nose poking,

head bobbing) and then tremor, dyskinesias, or catalepsy. Seizures are less frequent than with cocaine; in fact, amphetamine raises the threshold for electroshock seizures. Also in contrast to cocaine, amphetamine increases the cerebral metabolic rate for oxygen ($CMRO_2$).[6] As a central nervous system (CNS) stimulant, the d-isomer of amphetamine (dextroamphetamine) is four times more potent than the 1-isomer. Methamphetamine is more potent than either.[7]

Amphetamine produces appetite suppression and weight loss by inhibiting the lateral hypothalamic feeding center. By unclear mechanisms, it potentiates the analgesic effects of opioids, and it is itself weakly analgesic.[8]

Similar to cocaine, amphetamine enhances an animal's rate of self-stimulation through electrodes implanted in the medial forebrain bundle, and rats or monkeys self-inject the drug itself either systemically or directly into the nucleus accumbens (NA) or medial prefrontal cortex.[9] Preferring amphetamine to food or water, animals eventually develop fatal seizures and hyperthermia.[10] (Perhaps relevant to human psychostimulant abuse, animals with preexisting pronounced locomotor responses to novel stimuli are more likely to self-administer amphetamine compulsively.[11]) Animals also self-administer methamphetamine, methylphenidate, phentermine, diethylpropion, phenmetrazine, phendimetrazine, benzphetamine, methylenedioxyamphetamine (MDA), methylenedioxymethamphetamine (MDMA), and, to a lesser degree, ephedrine, clotermine, and

Table 3–1. Amphetamine and Related Agents

Amphetamine (Benzedrine)
Dextroamphetamine (Dexedrine)
Amphetamine and dextroamphetamine (Biphetamine)
Methamphetamine (Methedrine; Desoxyn; Fetamin)
Ephedrine
Pseudoephedrine
Methylphenidate (Ritalin)
Pemoline (Cylert)
Phenmetrazine (Preludin; Prelu-2)
Diethylpropion (Tenuate; Tepanil)
Benzphetamine (Didrex)
Fenfluramine (Pondimin)
Phendimetrazine (Plegine; Bontril)
Phentermine (Ionamin; Wilpo; Adipex-P; Fastin)
Mazindol (Sanorex; Mazanor)
Phenylpropanolamine (Propadrine; Propagest; and in decongestants and diet pills)
Propylhexedrine (Benzedrex nasal inhaler)
Naphzoline (Privine nasal solution; Naphcon ophthalmic solution)
Tetrahydrozoline (Tyzine nasal solution; Visine ophthalmic solution)
Oxymetazoline (Afrin nasal solution; Ococlear ophthalmic solution)
Xylometazoline (Otrivin nasal solution)
Phenoxazoline (nasal solutions)

chlorphentermine. They do not self-administer fenfluramine, methoxyamphetamine, 2,5-dimethoxy-4-methylamphetamine (DOM), or dimethoxyethylamphetamine (DOET).[12]

The psychostimulants enhance the synaptic activity of biogenic amines: norepinephrine, dopamine, and serotonin.[13] Peripheral cardiovascular effects depend on norepinephrine, which probably also contributes to alerting, anorexia, and locomotor stimulation. Stereotypy and dyskinesias are related to neostriatal dopamine. Reinforcement (self-administration) seems to depend on dopaminergic neurons in the mesencephalic ventral tegmental area (VTA) projecting to the NA and medial prefrontal cortex.[14] Dopamine-depleting lesions of either the VTA or the NA disrupt self-administration of amphetamine by animals. Lesions of the norepinephrine system (locus coeruleus) do not. Dopamine antagonists increase response rates for intravenous self-administration of amphetamine (presumably a compensatory response). Norepinephrine antagonists have no effect.[9,15]

The role of serotonin in the effects of psychostimulants differs among agents. It is reasonable to speculate that serotonin contributes to amphetamine-induced psychosis and hallucinations. Self-administration of amphetamine by rats, is reduced by pretreatment with L-tryptophan (a serotonin precursor) or fluoxetine (a serotonin reuptake blocker) and enhanced by dihydroxytryptamine (which selectively destroys serotonergic neurons).[16] Serotonin probably contributes little to the subjective effects of amphetamine in humans. With MDA and MDMA, its contribution is greater, and with those agents not self-administered by animals (e.g., DOM) it plays a

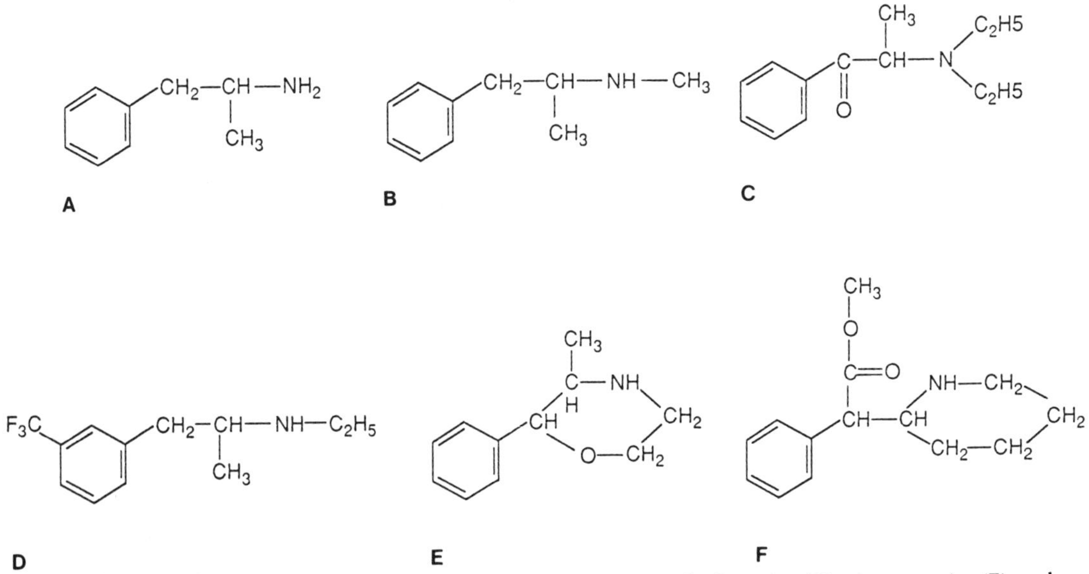

Figure 3–1. Amphetamine (A), methamphetamine (B), diethylpropion (C), fenfluramine (D), phenmetrazine (E), and methylphenidate (F).

dominant role. (In humans, such drugs produce lysergic acid diethylamide (LSD)–like effects; see Chapter 7.)

The psychostimulants have been subdivided into two pharmacologically distinct groups, based on whether the increased locomotor activity and stereotypies produced in animals are blocked by reserpine.[17] The *nonamphetamine class* of stimulants (methylphenidate, pipradrol, nomifensine, mazindol, cocaine) are inhibited by pretreatment with reserpine, which depletes nerve endings of catecholamines in the granular (storage) pool. The *amphetamine class* of stimulants (amphetamine, methamphetamine, phenmetrazine, pemoline) are not inhibited by reserpine. By contrast, alpha-methyltyrosine (AMT), which blocks catecholamine synthesis, inhibits the amphetamine class of stimulants but not the nonamphetamine class. Similarly, amphetamine-induced release of dopamine into cat lateral ventricle is enhanced by reserpine and inhibited by AMT; methylphenidate release of dopamine is inhibited by reserpine but not by AMT. Amphetamine's mechanism of action thus depends on the cytoplasmic, newly synthesized, rapidly metabolized pool of dopamine. Methylphenidate's mechanism of action depends on the granular storage pool. Both mechanisms appear to involve the presynaptic *dopamine uptake transporter*, which carries dopamine in either direction across presynaptic nerve endings. Amphetamine potentiates release of dopamine from these terminals. Once it has entered nerve terminals, amphetamine inhibits storage of dopamine by the granular pool and degradation of dopamine by monoamine oxidase, thereby increasing levels of dopamine in the cytoplasmic pool. Binding to the transporter, dopamine is then carried out into the synaptic cleft.[7] By contrast, methylphenidate (and cocaine) block reuptake of dopamine from the synaptic cleft back into the nerve ending.[18] This blockade then makes the granular storage pool of dopamine available for release, accounting for the ability of reserpine and the inability of AMT to block methylphenidate's action.[17] Additionally, by occupying the reuptake carrier, nonamphetamine-class stimulants in reserpinized mice block the locomotor effects of amphetamine-class stimulants.[19]

With both classes of psychostimulants, there is tolerance to the anorectic, cardiovascular, hyperthermic, and lethal effects but sensitization (*reverse tolerance*) to dyskinesias.[20,21] Such sensitization to systemic amphetamine can be induced by injecting amphetamine directly into mesencephalic dopamine neurons (VTA and substantia nigra) but not into their terminal areas (NA and striatum).[22] Possible

mechanisms of action of sensitization include down-regulation of dopamine inhibitory autoreceptors,[23] decreased neurotransmitter release in response to stimulation of dopaminergic neurons,[22] change in the functional state of dopamine terminals or their postsynaptic neurons,[24] and long-term accumulation of amphetamine metabolites in the brain.[25]

In monkeys, chronic amphetamine administration damages brain dopaminergic nerve terminals, with lasting depletion of brain dopamine.[26] In rats, methamphetamine similarly affects both dopamine and serotonergic nerves.[27] Methylphenidate displays no such toxicity to either neurotransmitter system. It would appear that the cytoplasmic, newly synthesized transmitter pool is required for amphetamine and methamphetamine neurotoxicity, which is blocked by inhibition of dopamine synthesis.[13,28,29] The mechanism of damage is unknown. Possibilities include a toxic metabolite such as 6-hydroxydopamine, formed as a result of amphetamine inhibition of monoamine oxidase.[21,30] Excitatory neurotransmitters (glutamate or aspartate) could also play a role; in mice, the N-methyl-D-aspartate (NMDA) receptor blockers MK-801 and phencyclidine protect against methamphetamine neurotoxicity.[31] A possible consequence of amphetamine toxicity is persistence of behavioral tolerance to the drug long after administration is stopped.[21] Rats so treated appear behaviorally normal, but of course subtle cognitive changes, testable in humans, would be difficult to detect in rodents.[29]

Historical Background and Epidemiology

In the 1920s, the search for an oral antiasthmatic led to the discovery of ephedrine in the ma huang plant (*Ephedra vulgaris*), which had been used for that purpose in China for centuries. In 1932, the synthetic ephedrine analog, amphetamine, was introduced and sold in over-the-counter form in Benzedrine inhalers; 250 mg of the drug was contained in a cotton plug. The ability of amphetamine to ward off sleep and elevate mood was quickly recognized, and users learned either to extract drug from the plug or to ingest it whole.[7,32,33] By the late 1930s, warnings appeared in medical journals of amphetamine's abuse liability.[34] During the Second World War, amphetamine was provided to soldiers of both sides and in Japan to the civilian population as well. (The most famous wartime amphetamine addict was Adolf Hitler, who, after his assassination attempt, took daily cocaine as well.[35]) Following the war, Japanese pharmaceutical companies continued to promote the drug, leading to an epidemic of amphet-amine abuse in which 5% of all Japanese aged 16 to 25 became physically dependent.[32] The epidemic subsided following passage of stringent control laws.

During the 1950s, drug companies tried to de-velop amphetamine analogs with selective effects, ei-ther stimulation without appetite suppression (e.g., methylphenidate) or appetite suppression without stimulation (e.g., phenmetrazine, diethylpropion, or phendimetrazine). Among the latter group, selective action proved less than claimed. In Sweden during the 1950s, amphetamine was regulated but phen-metrazine was not, and an epidemic of phenmetra-zine abuse led to removal of the drug from the market.[36] (Another amphetamine analog, fenflu-ramine, does suppress appetite without CNS stimu-lation and perhaps for that reason has never been very popular among the obese.)

Attempts to temper amphetamine stimulation by combining it with a sedative were also fruitless. Dur-ing the 1950s in Britain, a mixture of amphetamine and amobarbital (Drinamyl, "purple hearts") was widely abused.

In the United States, amphetamine was available in over-the-counter form until 1954, and with or without a prescription, its popularity has continued among students and truck drivers who want to stay alert, athletes who seek increased endurance, and dieters who actually use it for mood elevation, often in conjunction with sedatives or ethanol.[37–40] Acute intoxication has been an ongoing accompani-ment.[41–43] Oral amphetamines are also common illicit street drugs ("uppers," "ups," "bennies," "dexies," "pep pills," "jelly beans").

Amphetamine began to be used intravenously by American servicemen in Korea and Japan during the early 1950s. Presaging the current "speedball," it was often combined with heroin. The practice was then taken up in the San Francisco Bay area, where, in addition, intravenous amphetamine was prescribed illegally by physicians to "treat" heroin addicts. By the 1960s, intravenous abuse of amphet-amine and methamphetamine ("speed," "crank") was a well-publicized problem in the United States, resulting in removal of Desoxyn ampules from the market and restriction of Methedrine ampules to hospitals.[44] In 1965, the Federal Drug Abuse Con-trol Amendments further restricted manufacture and distribution of amphetamines, and supply shifted to illicit manufacture ("speed labs"). Although seem-ingly overshadowed by the cocaine epidemic of the 1980s, abuse of amphetamine and methamphet-amine has remained a major drug problem in the United States and other countries. Most street amphetamine is manufactured by legitimate labora-tories and taken orally (although most people who think they are taking illicit amphetamine are actually taking "lookalike pills"—see later). By contrast, most street methamphetamine is manu-factured in illegal "garage laboratories" and taken intravenously.[45]

In 1982, an estimated 13 million Americans had used amphetamine or methamphetamine without medical supervision, including over one-third of high school seniors.[46] In a 1988 survey of 1152 parenteral drug abusers in a Stockholm prison, 958 had used amphetamine, compared with only 194 who had used heroin.[47] During the late 1980s, American methamphetamine abuse increased fur-ther, especially on the West Coast. Injected, snorted, or drunk in beverages, methamphetamine also began appearing in a crystalline smokable form ("ice," "crystal"), comparable to smokable alkaloidal cocaine ("crack").[7] Amphetamine is frequently com-bined with ephedrine, phenylpropanolamine, co-caine, heroin ("speedball"), ethanol, or sedatives. In 1987, 2900 urine toxicology profiles were performed at the University of California Medical Center in San Diego, and 290 (10%) were positive for amphet-amine or methamphetamine, a prevalence compara-ble to cocaine's.[48] Twelve percent of positive urine tests were from neonates. By 1989, in Hawaii "ice" had replaced "crack" as the illicit drug of choice.[49]

Acute Effects

In human novices, 10 to 30 mg oral dextroamphet-amine produces alertness, euphoria, increased motor activity, improved coordination, and greater physical endurance, but the feeling of well-being can lead to overconfidence and impaired judgment.[50] Some sub-jects are initially drowsy, becoming hyperalert only after 1 or 2 hours.[51] Some experience agitation, dys-phoria, confusion, headache, palpitations, and fa-tigue. Systolic blood pressure is raised, often with reflex bradycardia, and there is mild pupillary dilation.[52] Sleep is reduced as well as the percent-age of time spent in the rapid eye movement (REM) phase, and there is a shift toward higher frequencies in the resting electroencephalogram.[2]

Intravenous amphetamine produces a brief "flash" or "rush," a sharp awakening that may be compared to an electric shock or orgasm but is qual-itatively different from an opioid "rush." Because the transit time from lung to brain is shorter than from antecubital vein to brain, the rush is even more rapid and powerful following inhalation of "ice."

With either route of administration, there is a lingering euphoria. Amphetamine's biological half-life is about 8 hours, and methamphetamine's is about 12 hours; powerful psychic effects can therefore last several hours (compared with 30 to 90 minutes for cocaine).[53] With repeated use, moreover, drug accumulation occurs. Amphetamine delays genital orgasm and heightens it when it occurs.[54]

Tolerance to these effects develops rapidly. Although 100 mg amphetamine can be fatal to a novice, addicts have taken thousands of milligrams daily. Intravenous users of amphetamines ("speed freaks") often take the drug in a familiar pattern.[55] After a period of oral use, injections begin. There then develops a "run": several days of intravenous injections every 2 or 3 hours in increasing dosage up to 100 to 300 mg per injection, during which time the subject is continuously awake. Toxic symptoms appear: tremor, bruxism, dystonia, choreoathetosis, picking and excoriations, sweating, thirst, difficulty with micturition, and sometimes cardiac arrhythmia. Anorexia leads to marked weight loss when "runs" occur successively. Suspiciousness and rapid mood changes occur as well as preoccupation with one's thoughts and a sense of profundity. Stereotyped repetitive behavior might consist of taking apart and trying to put together mechanical objects or stringing beads for hours. Paranoia eventually develops in nearly all chronic abusers, and frank psychosis is common. Hallucinations are auditory, visual, olfactory, or haptic (the feeling of bugs or vermin crawling over and under the skin). The emergence of dyskinesias and psychosis during chronic amphetamine use is a good example of drug sensitization (reverse tolerance), all the more striking when it occurs while tolerance is developing to "rush," euphoria, anorexia, hyperthermia, cardiovascular effects, and lethality. A contributor to tolerance may be anorexia, which causes ketosis and increases amphetamine excretion. More important, however, is cellular responsiveness (pharmacodynamic tolerance), not tissue levels of drug (pharmacokinetic tolerance). Dyskinesias usually resolve within a few days of stopping amphetamine but can last weeks, months, or even years.[56]

In subjects tolerant to cardiovascular effects, amphetamine may be overlooked as the cause of schizophrenic symptoms,[2] although the extent to which psychotic symptoms actually resemble schizophrenia is disputed.[57–59] Amphetamine produces positive schizophrenic symptoms (e.g., paranoia, hallucinations) but in contrast to phencyclidine does not produce negative symptoms (e.g., emotional withdrawal, motor retardation) or a formal thought disorder.[60] Paranoia sometimes leads to violence, including suicide and homicide. Subjects carry weapons and attack strangers who fit into their persecutory delusions.[58] Psychosis may emerge gradually over months or occur during a single "run." Amphetamine can precipitate psychotic symptoms in known schizophrenics, and premorbid psychopathology is common in chronic abusers, but psychosis also occurs in apparently normal subjects, and it is unusual for psychotic symptoms to persist after the drug is stopped.[59] Moreover, some schizophrenic patients receiving amphetamines have had symptomatic improvement.[59–61] In one report, schizophrenic patients already receiving haloperidol became more active and had improved performance on the Wisconsin Card Sorting Test after receiving amphetamine; the authors proposed that the combined treatment selectively enhanced cortical dopaminergic activity.[62]

Acute overdose of amphetamine or methamphetamine causes excitement, confusion, headache, chest pain, hypertension, tachycardia, flushing, profuse sweating, and mydriasis, progressing to delirium, hallucinations, hyperpnea, cardiac arrhythmia, hyperpyrexia (sometimes over 109°F), seizures, shock, coma, and death.[63–67] Small children display head banging, mutilation of digits by biting, and violent purposeless movements.[64] Myoglobinuria occurs, and shock has resulted from loss of intravascular volume into necrotic muscle. Some subjects have acute pyrogenic reactions following previously tolerated doses.[68] Disseminated intravascular coagulation may be secondary to hyperthermia, and death may be from heat stroke itself. At autopsy, diffuse cerebral edema and petechiae are found.[43,63] Dogs and rabbits given lethal doses of amphetamines had severe hyperpyrexia and, at autopsy, subendocardial and epicardial hemorrhage, myocardial fiber necrosis, and neuronal degeneration in the cerebral cortex and cerebellum.[69,70] Curare prevented the fever and the fatal course, suggesting that muscle hyperactivity was critical.[71] Fever may have contributed to similar pathological findings in the brains of cats receiving chronic methamphetamine, although in that study neuronal catecholamine depletion was considered the primary cause.[72]

Seizures are less frequent among amphetamine users than cocaine users. In a report from San Francisco General Hospital of 49 recreational drug-induced seizures, 11 occurred in users of amphetamine, either alone (8) or with cocaine, phencyclidine, or heroin. Seizures occurred in both first-time and chronic users, were independent of route of administration (intravenous, intranasal, or oral), and were not always associated with other signs of overdose.[73]

The usual fatal dose of amphetamine for a nontolerant adult is 20 to 25 mg/kg and for children 5 mg/kg, but idiosyncratic reactions sometimes follow low doses. Treatment of overdose usually begins with reducing excitement and protecting against injury.[74] Because psychostimulant poisoning is infrequently lethal, physical restraints and sedation should be used only as necessary. One should try to maintain verbal contact with the patient in a quiet, lighted room. If sedation is necessary, it should be instituted cautiously. Barbiturates can aggravate delirium, potentiate postexcitatory depression, and, if amphetamine has been taken with a sedative, precipitate stupor or coma. Neuroleptics also have drawbacks, especially if the diagnosis is uncertain or amphetamine has been taken with another drug. They can precipitate seizures in cocaine intoxication, aggravate delirium in anticholinergic intoxication, contribute to myoglobinuria in phencyclidine intoxication, and produce hypotension in any setting. Chlorpromazine effectively reversed delirium and self-injury in a series of small children poisoned by amphetamine, methamphetamine, or phenmetrazine.[64] Others recommend haloperidol on the grounds that chlorpromazine prolongs the half-life of amphetamine.[75] The current sedative of choice in most emergency rooms, however, is intravenous diazepam.[74]

Cardiorespiratory support is provided as needed. If seizures occur, they are treated conventionally with diazepam and phenytoin. For severe hypertension, beta blockers carry the risk of unopposed alpha-adrenergic activity and aggravation of blood pressure. Alteratives include selective beta-1 agents (e.g., labetalol), alpha blockers (e.g., phenoxybenzamine or phentolamine), or direct vasodilators (e.g., nitroprusside). Forced diuresis and acidification of urine enhance drug excretion, but acidification is given only in the absence of metabolic acidosis and myoglobinuria.[76] For severe refractory cases, peritoneal dialysis or hemodialysis can be instituted.[64]

Dependence and Withdrawal

Amphetamines produce psychic and probably physical dependence, and there are often only a few months between first exposure and chronic use.[54] Withdrawal from prolonged use is followed by depression, fatigue, and increased appetite and sleep, including time spent in the REM phase.[77] Following a "run," the subject, because of tenseness, paranoia, or exhaustion, stops taking the drug and falls asleep for usually 12 to 18 hours ("crashing"). Sometimes sedatives are taken to induce sleep, but usually drowsiness occurs within a few hours of the last "fix" and cannot be resisted without taking more stimulant. Longer "runs" are followed by more prolonged sleep, sometimes lasting several days. Psychotic symptoms are usually absent on awakening, but there is hunger (often ravenous), lethargy, and depression. Injections are then resumed, and a new "run" begins.

Withdrawal symptoms are not life-threatening, but depression, sometimes suicidal, can last for weeks, requiring hospitalization and treatment with tricyclic antidepressants. Drug craving can persist for months. In contrast to opioid addicts, amphetamine abusers tend to "burn out" after a few years.[54,78]

Medical and Neurological Complications

Parenteral psychostimulant use leads to many of the same medical sequelae that beset parenteral abusers of other drugs. Infections often involve unusual organisms and affect the nervous system.[79,80] There is also, of course, a risk for human immunodeficiency virus (HIV) infection. In Stockholm, where amphetamine is the most prevalent parenteral drug of abuse, 5.9% of users were HIV-seropositive.[55]

A 19-year-old boy developed pneumomediastinum while snorting amphetamine.[81]

Myocardial infarction is less often associated with amphetamine than with cocaine. It has occurred in young, otherwise healthy men taking amphetamine alone or with heroin[82,83] and has followed snorting of methamphetamine.[84] Acute cardiomyopathy with normal coronary angiography has followed intravenous amphetamine use,[85] and congestive cardiomyopathy has followed chronic oral amphetamine use.[86]

A frequent complication of amphetamine abuse is stroke, both occlusive and hemorrhagic. More than 30 patients, ages 16 to 60 years, have been reported with intracranial hemorrhage after amphetamine use.[87–114] Routes of administration have been oral, intravenous, or nasal. Most patients were chronic users, but in five stroke followed first exposure. Dosage was usually unknown but in one case was less than 80 mg. Except for one instance each of diethylpropion and pseudoephedrine, all took amphetamine or methamphetamine; seven also took methylphenidate, LSD, DOM, cocaine, heroin, or barbiturates. Symptoms usually began with severe headache within minutes of drug use. Blood pressure was elevated in more than half, with diastolic pressure as high as 120 mm Hg. Computed tomography (CT) has shown intracerebral hemorrhage (often lobar), intraventricular hemorrhage, subarachnoid hemorrhage, or no abnormality. Cerebral angiography in 12 patients showed irregular narrowing ("beading") of distal cerebral vessels, consistent with vasculitis, which was found at autopsy in three patients. In one case, a cerebral vascular malformation was identified at both angiography and CT.

High fever and disturbed clotting were not noted in any of these patients. Some of the hemorrhages appeared to be secondary to acute hypertension, some to vasculitis, and some to a combination of the two, but in others neither feature was apparent. Moreover, acute hypertension could have been either causal or a transient result of the stroke, and fleeting blood pressure elevations could have been missed.

Amphetamine-induced cerebral vasculitis has caused occlusive as well as hemorrhagic stroke and appears to be of more than one type. Necrotizing angiitis occurred in 14 Los Angeles abusers of multiple drugs, including amphetamine, methamphetamine, barbiturates, chlordiazepoxide, diazepam, marijuana, hydroxyzine, LSD, heroin, meperidine, mescaline, oxycodone, oxymorphone, DOM, and strychnine.[115] All but two patients used methamphetamine, and one used it exclusively. Five patients were asymptomatic, and in others there were a variety of systemic symptoms and signs, including skin rash, anemia, hypertension, arthralgia, pneumonitis, renal failure, and peripheral neuropathy. One, with "*progressive encephalopathy,*" at autopsy had vasculitis affecting pontine arterioles. Another, with "*mental obtundation,*" had brain vasculitis with cerebral and brain stem infarcts and cerebellar hemorrhage. Vessel changes affected only muscular arteries and arterioles and were considered typical for polyarteritis nodosa, although unassociated with Australia antigen.[116,117]

Such brain lesions have been observed pathologically in other polydrug abusers.[101,118] Sometimes, however, cerebral arteritis has been presumed on the basis of cerebral angiography, and the relation to amphetamine has not always been obvious.[93–95,99,100,106,118] Widespread angiographic beading of cerebral arteries, with multiple occlusion of arterioles, was reported in 19 young drug abusers (mostly intravenous methamphetamine) admitted for coma or stroke.[119] Ischemic stroke has followed intranasal inhalation of methamphetamine, with intervals from last use to stroke ranging from 12 hours to 2 weeks. Angiographically occluded or "beaded" vessels have

included the extracranial and supraclinoid internal carotid, distal middle cerebral, lenticulostriate, and thalamoperforating arteries.[120,121]

Monkeys given intravenous methamphetamine underwent serial angiograms.[122] Some showed beaded small cerebral vessels at 10 minutes with a return to normal at 24 hours. In others, both small and large vessels were affected, and the changes persisted or progressed over a 2-week period. Clinically there was hypertension and behavioral change. At autopsy, some animals had subarachnoid hemorrhage with brain petechiae, infarcts, microaneurysms, and perivascular white cell cuffing. More severe vasculitic changes occurred in a later study of monkeys receiving intravenous methamphetamine three times weekly for up to a year.[123] In rats given intravenous methamphetamine, electron microscopy revealed endothelial cell changes in vessels too small (under 100 μ) to be seen angiographically. Angiographic and histologic changes have also occurred in monkeys and rats receiving intravenous methylphenidate.[123]

These lesions differ from those of polyarteritis nodosa, in which elastic arteries, capillaries, and veins are spared. It is unclear if they are the result of hypersensitivity or direct toxicity or if subarachnoid hemorrhage itself contributes.

In an adolescent amphetamine abuser with mononeuritis multiplex, sural nerve biopsy showed apparent hypersensitivity angiitis of medium and small arteries, arterioles, venules, and veins; there were no CNS symptoms.[124] Amphetamine-induced angiitis has also caused renal failure.[125]

Tourette's syndrome has been exacerbated and precipitated by amphetamine, methylphenidate, and pemoline, sometimes clearing with discontinuation of the drug but sometimes persisting.[126–128] Also occasionally persistent are the bruxism and choreiform movements that develop with chronic amphetamine use.[56]

Two methamphetamine users from Oregon developed lead poisoning. One had hallucinations, constipation, hepatic tenderness, and jaundice initially misdiagnosed as infectious hepatitis; the other had weakness, malaise, headache, abdominal pain, myalgia, chills, sweating, and weight loss. Lead acetate had been used in the illicit manufacture of the drug.[129]

Whether amphetamine causes permanent psychiatric or cognitive disturbance is uncertain. Users often report decreased memory or poor concentration after achieving abstinence, and there are anecdotal reports of lasting psychosis or dementia.[54,59,78] Formal studies of cognitive performance in chronic amphetamine abusers have been methodologically flawed.[129a]

Obstetric and Pediatric Aspects

The literature on amphetamine use during pregnancy is scanty compared with that dealing with cocaine. At the Presbyterian Hospital in New York, amphetamine metabolites were detected in 13% of more than 500 women admitted for delivery (compared with 10% for cocaine). The screens did not distinguish between metabolites of amphetamine and other drugs such as cold remedies. Medical histories predicted none of the amphetamine-positive samples.[130]

Newborns of methamphetamine-using mothers have had abnormal sleep patterns, poor feeding, tremor, and hypertonia as well as higher than expected rates of prematurity, intrauterine growth retardation, and smaller head circumference.[131,132] An anecdotal report described dysgenesis of the corpus callosum following in utero exposure to amphetamine and septo-optic dysplasia following in utero exposure to the amphetamine-like agent phenylpropanolamine.[133] In another study, echoencephalographic abnormalities were found in 9 of 24 neonates exposed to methamphetamine, including white matter cavities (1), white matter densities (3), intraventricular hemorrhage (4), subarachnoid hemorrhage (4), subependymal hemorrhage (3), and ventricular enlargement (2).[134] As with cocaine and other substances, the effects of amphetamine use per se are difficult to separate from those of inadequate prenatal care, including use of other drugs, ethanol, and tobacco.[135] In animal studies, maternal amphetamine administration led to reduced brain norepinephrine levels in newborn mice and impaired performance on some behavioral tests.[136] There are no long-term follow-up studies of the effects of fetal amphetamine exposure in humans.

Amphetamine use at 36 weeks gestation precipitated eclampsia with seizures in a 19-year-old gravida 3, para 2 who had not had eclampsia or preeclampsia before.[137]

Other Related Agents

Federal restrictions on amphetamine do not apply to phenylpropanolamine, a similar but less potent drug found, sometimes combined with ephedrine or caf-

Table 3–2. "Cold" or Allergy Medications Containing Phenylpropanolamine

Alka-Seltzer Plus Cold Medicine
Allerest
Bayer Children's Cold Tablets
Children's CoTylenol
Comtrex
Contac
Coricidin-D
Coryban-D
Deconex
Dehist
Dimetapp
Duadacin
Four-Way Cold Tablets
Histabid Duracap
Naldecon Pediatric Syrup
Noraminic
Oraminic
Ornade
Sinarest
Sine-off Sinus Medicine
Sinubid
Spect-T Decongestant Lozenges
St Joseph's Cold Tablets for Children
Sucrets Cold Decongestant
Triaminic

feine, in over-the-counter diet pills (e.g., Dex-a-diet, Dexatrim, Anorexin, Maxi-slim) and decongestants (Table 3–2).[138] Although the Food and Drug Administration (FDA) has restricted combinations of phenylpropanolamine, ephedrine, and caffeine,[139] an estimated 5 billion doses of phenylpropanolamine are used annually in the United States.[140] Animal studies suggest that the addiction liability of phenylpropanolamine is low—it is not self-administered by pigeons or monkeys[141]—and studies with human volunteers reveal little stimulant or euphoric properties at therapeutic doses.[142] (In one such study, very high doses of phenylpropanolamine produced "arousal" and "vigor" but in contrast to amphetamine did not cause euphoria.[143]) Nonetheless, phenylpropanolamine, alone or combined with ephedrine or caffeine, is a well-known illicit street drug, often misrepresented as amphetamine ("look-alike pills," "pseudospeed," "pea shooters").[45] Phenylpropanolamine is also sold by mail order as a "legal stimulant."[144] (Legally manufactured stimulants, in compliance with FDA regulations, contain only one drug.[45])

A narrow margin of safety exists between recommended and toxic doses of phenylpropanolamine, and in a study of normal volunteers, there was considerable variability between subjects in phenyl-propanolamine's pressor effects.[145] Complications of phenylpropanolamine include acute hypertension and severe headache;[146–150] intractable nausea and vomiting;[151] cardiac arrhythmia;[152–154] hallucinations, paranoia, and homicidal behavior;[154–156] and seizures.[147,156–158] Hemorrhagic stroke, intracerebral and subarachnoid, has followed recommended as well as excessive dosage.[151,159–171] Of those with intracerebral hemorrhage, several have had multiple simultaneous lesions, suggesting diffuse vessel abnormalities, and vasculitis has been both implied angiographically and demonstrated pathologically. A young woman, 3 weeks postpartum, had an intracerebral hemorrhage following a single dose of Dexatrim, Extra Strength; leptomeningeal and brain biopsy demonstrated necrotizing vasculitis of small arteries and veins with infiltration of polymorphonuclear leukocytes.[165] Phenylpropanolamine with caffeine, from a commercial diet preparation, caused subarachnoid hemorrhage in rats receiving it parenterally in several times the recommended dose.[138]

Ephedrine and pseudoephedrine are also present in over-the-counter decongestants and bronchodilators. Ephedrine's margin of safety is as low as phenylpropanolamine's; pseudoephedrine's is greater, but both agents have caused anxiety, headache, tachyarrhythmia, and hypertensive crisis.[144,163,171–173] The abuse potential of these drugs is low, but dependence occurs.[174] Ephedrine is also taken by athletes to enhance performance.[40] Psychosis has been reported in abusers of ephedrine or pseudoephedrine either alone or in combination with other agents (e.g., Actifed, containing pseudoephedrine and triprolidine.)[175–177] In Britain, over-the-counter Do-Do tablets containing ephedrine, caffeine, and theophylline, are a popular form of stimulant abuse.[177] A young man who had previously used "speed" and LSD had a subarachnoid hemorrhage within an hour of ingesting pills that turned out to be ephedrine; cerebral angiography, initially normal, a week later showed beading and branch occlusions, and biopsy of normal-appearing skin revealed deposits of immunoglobulin M (IgM) and the C3 component of complement in dermal vessels, suggesting circulating immune complexes.[178] Intracranial hemorrhage has also followed pseudoephedrine use.[179]

A number of other amphetamine-like drugs are promoted mainly as diet pills, and they vary in their abuse potential (which in turn correlates loosely with their Drug Enforcement Administration [DEA] scheduling). Phenmetrazine, which is self-administered by animals and causes psycho-stimulation and euphoria in humans, is widely

abused.[142,180,181] So is phentermine, inadvertent arterial injection of which has caused subclavian and carotid mycotic aneurysms.[182] Phentermine was also implicated in two young women with occlusive stroke, one of whom also took phendimetrazine and oral contraceptives and showed angiographic changes consistent with vertebrobasilar angitis.[182a] Less often abused is diethylpropion and then usually orally.[183,184] Paranoid psychosis with auditory and visual hallucinations has affected diethylpropion users.[185] The anorectic benzphetamine is also self-administered by animals and produces amphetamine-like effects in humans, but abuse seems to be rare.[142] The anorectic mazindol (which does not structurally resemble amphetamine) is self-administered by monkeys,[181] yet in humans it not only fails to produce euphoria, but also in one study was dysphoric.[142,143] (The rarity of mazindol abuse shows that animal studies do not always predict human dependence liability.) Also more often dysphoric than euphoric is fenfluramine, which is not self-administered by animals;[2] nonetheless, fenfluramine abuse—taken in large oral doses for its psychic effects—was reported among young South Africans.[186]

Intravenous abuse of crushed methylphenidate tablets ("poor man's cocaine") has been reported throughout the United States. Classified as a Schedule II drug, methylphenidate is often prescribed by unwary physicians in drug-seeking scams. Of 22 methylphenidate abusers in Baltimore, 9 had children who were taking methylphenidate for "hyperactivity."[187] In Seattle, methylphenidate abuse was especially common among patients receiving methadone maintenance therapy.[188] Water-insoluble constituents of the tablets lead to a high incidence of pulmonary complications, including chest pain, wheezing, hemoptysis, abnormal pulmonary function tests, and eventually fibrosis or even fatal pulmonary hypertension.[187,189] Deep neck abscesses in methylphenidate abusers are also attributed to foreign body reaction to tablet fillers followed by superinfection.[190] Other users have developed a syndrome of fever, myalgia, arthralgia, and eosinophilia.[191] Methylphenidate neuropsychiatric toxicity is similar to that of other psychostimulants. Acutely syncope is common, and dyskinesias and psychosis develop during the course of a binge.[192–194] Seizures, appearing as a late complication, suggest the "kindling" pattern seen with cocaine.

Cerebrovascular complications have also been reported. Right hemiplegia in a young woman followed attempted injection into the left jugular vein of crushed methylphenidate tablets; 2 weeks later, left hemiplegia followed a similar right injection.[195] Talc microemboli have been seen in the fundi of intravenous methylphenidate abusers, sometimes with retinal and vitreous hemorrhages and neovascularization; in one such patient, who had not had a clinical stroke, talc and cornstarch emboli were also present in brain and lung.[196,197] Infarction of the medulla followed intravenous methylphenidate in a young woman; at autopsy, there were talc deposits in small vessels around the infarct.[198] A 12-year-old boy taking methylphenidate orally in prescribed dosage for attention deficit disorder developed hemiparesis and aphasia; angiography revealed occlusion of the anterior cerebral artery and a branch of the middle cerebral artery, plus vessel irregularities suggestive of arteritis.[199]

Pemoline, used to treat attention deficit disorder, is considered to have much less addiction liability than methylphenidate, but it has been abused. Choreoathetosis severe enough to cause myoglobinuria followed ingestion of more than 1000 mg pemoline within 24 hours in a middle-aged man without other signs of toxicity.[200]

Propylhexedrine and 1-desoxyephedrine replaced amphetamine in Benzedrex inhalers, and complications of oral or parenteral abuse have included psychosis, myocardial infarction, cardiomyopathy, pulmonary hypertension, and sudden death.[33,201–204] An adolescent who had previously used cocaine and amphetamine developed headache, nausea, numbness of hands and feet, precordial chest pain, and palpitations after intravenously injecting epinephrine from a bronchodilator inhaler.[205] Cerebral infarction and retinal artery branch occlusion were reported in chronic intranasal abusers of sprays and drops containing phenoxazoline or oxymetazoline.[206,207]

Khat (*Catha edulis*) is a shrub indigenous to East Africa and the Arabian peninsula; its leaves contain cathinone, a compound similar to amphetamine.[208,209] Animals self-administer cathinone at rates higher than amphetamine but lower than cocaine.[210] Cathinone's duration of action is shorter than amphetamine's, and tolerance develops more rapidly to its anorectic effects. Today several million people in East Africa (especially Ethiopia and Kenya) and the southwest Arabian peninsula (especially Yemen) chew khat leaves for their stimulating properties.[209] Users include participants in social "khat sessions," where the goal is euphoria and loquacity, and farmers and manual laborers, who use the drug to reduce hunger and fatigue. Khat's toxic psychic effects are limited by its bulkiness and by the slow absorption and rapid metabolism of the psy-

choactive cathinone, but aggressive behavior, hallucinatory psychosis, and fatal hyperthermia have occurred.[211,212] Similarly, although withdrawal symptoms are usually mild, severe depression, suicide, and homicide have followed abstinence. Bilateral optic atrophy with central scotomas were reported in several khat users, in one of whom electroretinography suggested retinal toxicity in addition to optic neuropathy.[213,214] Although prohibited in a number of African and Arabian countries, khat use increased in that part of the world during the 1980s. Moreover, although the leaves lose their effect within a few days of harvesting, air travel and creative gardening have allowed khat chewing to spread beyond its originally indigenous areas.[215] Psychosis has been reported in users in Italy, Britain, and the United States.[212,216–219]

In the 1960s 3,4-methylenedioxyamphetamine (MDA) became a popular street drug, and it was soon evident that it was a different kind of agent than either amphetamine or the so-called hallucinogenic amphetamines such as mescaline or dimethoxymethylamphetamine (DOM).[220,221] At low doses, MDA produces decreased anxiety and a sense of self-awareness, with a desire to talk with other people (the "love drug").[222] As the dose is increased, the drug becomes hallucinogenic and then psychostimulatory.[223] MDA abuse continues in the United States, but in the 1980s its popularity was exceeded by a similar drug, 3,4-methylenedioxymethamphetamine (MDMA, Figure 3–2). Developed in 1914 as an appetite suppressant, MDMA for many years was legally available and occasionally used in psychiatric treatment for its ability to create a pleasant state of introspection and facilitate communication.[224] By the 1980s, it was widely abused, especially on college campuses, and in 1985, the DEA made it a Schedule I controlled substance.[225]

Animals trained to discriminate MDA generalize to MDMA and vice versa but not to amphetamine or typical hallucinogens.[220] Animals self-administer MDA and MDMA but not hallucinogens.[226,227] MDMA-induced locomotor stimulation in animals is blocked by the serotonin antagonist methysergide; the mechanism may be disinhibition of dopaminergic neurons from serotonergic modulation. This and

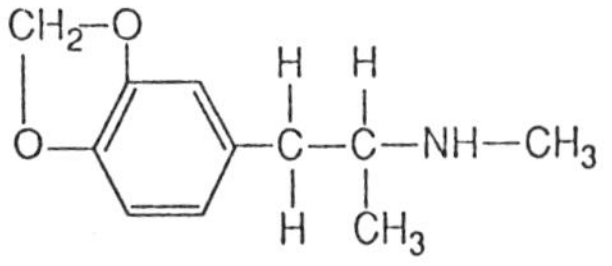

Figure 3–2. 3,4-methylendioxymethamphetamine (MDMA).

other evidence suggests that MDA and MDMA act predominantly as serotonin agonists with only weak dopaminergic activity.[9,228-230]

MDMA is known as "Ecstasy" (and also as "Adam," "XTC," "M&M," "the Yuppie Drug," "Essence," "Clarity," "Venus," "Zen," and "Doctor"); a similar drug, 3,4-methylenedioxyethyamphetamine (MDEA), is known as "Eve."[231-233] Available as powders or pills, they are usually taken orally in group sessions; typically 100 mg is followed by supplemental doses of 40 mg, up to several hundred milligrams over 30 to 120 minutes. Infrequently MDMA is taken intranasally or parenterally; compulsive use rarely if ever occurs. Desired effects include "enhanced communication, empathy, or understanding;" euphoria or ecstasy; and "transcendental or religious experiences."[231,234] Perceptual changes include vivid color enhancement, illusions, and hallucinations (visual, tactile, auditory, olfactory, or gustatory); visual hallucinations are either formed or unformed, and polyopia has been reported. Undesirable side effects include anxiety, tremor, muscle tightness, jaw clenching, diaphoresis, profuse salivation, blurred vision, ataxia, tachycardia, hypertension, and nausea. Mydriasis and horizontal or vertical nystagmus are seen.[235] Effects usually disappear within 24 hours, but users have reported jaw tightness, blurred vision, fatigue, nausea, anxiety, depression, or insomnia lasting days or even weeks, and "flashbacks" have occurred.[236] Tolerance may develop more rapidly to MDMA's desirable effects than to its undesirable effects.[237]

As with amphetamine, overdose with MDA, MDMA, or MDEA causes hyperthermia, hypertensive crisis, tachyarrhythmia, panic, paranoia, psychosis, delirium, disseminated intravascular coagulation, rhabdomyolysis, seizures, coma, and death.[235-240]

In contrast to amphetamine, which damages dopaminergic nerve terminals, and methamphetamine, which damages both dopaminergic and serotonergic nerve terminals, MDMA and MDA (and, less potently, MDEA) selectively destroy serotonin nerve terminals in rat and primate brain.[241,242] In monkeys, this effect requires only two to three times the usual human dose. As with amphetamine, the mechanism of neurotoxicity is unclear, but it is prevented if serotonin uptake blockers such as fluoxetine are administered within 12 hours of MDMA administration.[243] It is also prevented by combined pretreatment with parachlorophenylalanine and reserpine, which deplete both releasable and storage serotonin.[244] The damage, moreover, is partially reversible—a year later serotonin uptake sites have returned to control levels, yet the content of serotonin

in these areas remains lower than normal.[245] The significance of these findings to human users is unknown, but evidence for persistently altered CNS serotonin function was provided in a study of MDMA users in whom the normal prolactin response to L-tryptophan was absent 20 to 180 days after last use.[246] Neurotoxicity similar to that of MDMA has been produced in animals with the anorectic fenfluramine.[247]

Similar to psychostimulant drugs, monoamine oxidase inhibitors increase the availability of biogenic amines at synapses, and so it is not surprising that some users experience amphetamine-like effects: euphoria and a sense of increased energy. Tranylcypromine (Parnate) abuse, with craving and dose escalation, was reported in three patients who received the drug for treatment of depression associated with amphetamine abuse.[248] Taking tranylcypromine, they developed progressive irritability, violent outbursts, and paranoia. Interestingly, none had complications when ingesting tyramine-containing cheese or wine. Other reports describe psychological dependence on tranylcypromine or phenylzine, with withdrawal depression, irritability, and "shivering."[249-252] One woman who abused tranylcypromine developed status epilepticus on abrupt discontinuation.[253] Other monoamine oxidase inhibitor users have reportedly had delirium, hallucinations, and paranoid psychosis following withdrawal.[254] It can be difficult telling symptoms of antidepressant withdrawal from the symptoms that led to taking antidepressants in the first place.

Oral abuse of the tricyclic antidepressant amitriptyline (Elavil) is well recognized, although whether it is taken for its effects on biogenic amines or for its anticholinergic properties is uncertain.[255] Amitriptyline has sedative effects, and its abuse is largely limited to abusers of other drugs. In a survey of 346 patients enrolled in a New York City methadone maintenance treatment program, 86 (25%) admitted to taking amitriptyline for its euphoric properties.[256] Overdose resembles atropine poisoning (see Chapter 10), and abrupt cessation has precipitated panic, headache, myalgia, nausea, vomiting, diarrhea, sweating, tremor, and palpitations—symptoms considered to be withdrawal phenomena and not simply reappearance of predrug anxiety or depression.[254-258]

The antidepressant nomifensine blocks synaptic reuptake of norepinephrine but has only slight dopamine-releasing effects. In normal humans, it "enhances drive" without producing euphoria.[259] Abuse of nomifensine, with dosage escalation, was reported in a woman who had previously abused sedatives.[260]

Yohimbine, derived from the bark of *Corynanthe yohimbi* in West and Central Africa, has been touted (probably incorrectly) as an aphrodisiac for more than a century. In the United States, it can be purchased without prescription from mail-order companies. An alpha-2-adrenergic receptor antagonist, yohimbine produces nervousness, palpitations, hot and cold flashes, tremor, piloerection, and systolic hypertension. It precipitates panic attacks in patients suffering from panic disorders and in fact is considered the best current pharmacological model of anxiety.[261,262] At high doses, it also causes a dissociative mental state and hallucinations. As a street drug, it is known as "yo-yo."[263]

For thousands of years, ginseng root preparations have been used as all-purpose tonics in the Orient. The plant—genus *Panax*, that is, panacea—also grows in the United States, and between 5 and 6 million Americans use ginseng. Preparations include roots, capsules, tablets, teas, extracts, cigarettes, chewing gum, and candy; routes of administration include oral, intranasal, smoking, and intravenous.[264] The desired effects are stimulation and euphoria, but the pharmacological mechanisms are uncertain; ginseng contains a variety of glycosides and steroidal saponins. Chronic users experience nervousness, insomnia, diarrhea, tachycardia, and hypertension, and abrupt withdrawal has precipitated weakness, tremor, and hypotension.[264,265]

In East Africa, India, Southeast Asia, Indonesia, and the Philippines, 200 million people chew betel made from the nut of the palm, *Areca catechu;* the preparation also contains quicklime and leaves from nutmeg or other local psychoactive plants. Active ingredients from the palm nut include arecoline and arecaidine. The effect is psychostimulation, often with ataxia and tremor, followed the next day by fatigue, apathy, and headache. Addiction occurs, with ability to work dependent on the drug. High doses cause toxic psychosis and auditory hallucinations. Betal stains the teeth red and increases the risk of oral cancer.[266]

An unusual substance abuse has been studied in Malaysia and Thailand. Leaves of the kratour tree (*Mitragyna speciosa*) are chewed as an opium substitute, with a mild opioid-like withdrawal syndrome, yet acute effects are both stimulating and calming, comparable to chewing coca leaves and smoking opium simultaneously. The active agent is an indole, mitragynine.[267,268]

A large number of herbal preparations are sold in the United States as capsules, teas, and cigarettes, many for their euphoriant and stimulating effects. Some contain such well-defined ingredients as ephedrine, nutmeg, or yohimbine; others produce their effects by unclear mechanisms (Table 3–3).[265,269]

Caffeine

The most widely used psychoactive drug in the world is caffeine (Figure 3–3). Tea, prepared from leaves of the bush *Thea sinensis*, originated in China probably thousands of years ago and today is consumed by more than half the world's population. Coffee, made from the fruit of *Coffea arabica*, first appeared in Ethiopia more than 1000 years ago and today is the major source of caffeine in the United States; coffee is drunk in 98% of American households, and 30% of adult Americans drink three to five cups a day. Other sources of caffeine include cola-flavored drinks (containing extracts of the nut of *Cola acuminata*), cocoa and chocolate (from seeds of *Theobroma cacao* and containing theobromine plus small amounts of caffeine), and both prescription and over-the-counter medications (Table 3–4).[270,271] (As

Table 3–3. Herbal Preparations Sold as Stimulants in the United States

Herb	Source	Active Ingredients	Use
Cinnamon	*Cinnamon camphora*	Unknown. Contains tannins and oils	Bark smoked, often with marijuana
Hydrangea	*Hydrangea paniculata*	Hydrangin glycoside, saponin, cyanogenic glycoside	Smoke (marijuana substitute)
Damiana	*Turnera diffusa aphrodisiaca*	Unknown. Contains volatile oils, resins, tannins, and "damianin"	Liquid, pill, smoke (marijuana substitute)
Passion flower	*Passiflora caerulea*	Harmine alkaloids, cyanogenic glycosides	Capsules, tea, smoke (marijuana substitute)
Prickly poppy	*Argemona mexicana*	Isoquinolone alkaloids, prolopine, berberine	Smoke seeds

Source: Lewin NA, Howland MA, Goldfrank LR. Herbal preparations. In: Goldfrank LR, Flomenbaum NE, Levin NA, et al., eds. Toxicologic Emergencies, ed 4. Norwalk, CT: Appleton & Lange, 1990:587.

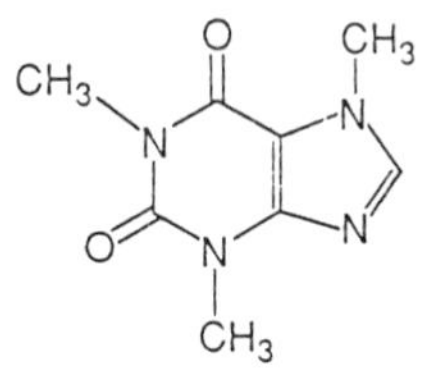

Figure 3–3. Caffeine.

already noted, the FDA has banned over-the-counter diet pills containing both phenylpropanolamine and caffeine.)

Similar to theophylline and theobromine, caffeine is a methylxanthine. Its actions include inhibition of cyclic nucleotide phosphodiesterases and adenosine; the latter action probably accounts for most of its pharmacological effects.[272] Adenosine receptors, which are of two major types, are ubiquitous throughout the body and are believed to regulate oxygen availability and utilization. Among many actions, adenosine dilates cerebral blood vessels and decreases neuronal firing rates in the CNS. Adenylyl

cyclase is inhibited by A-1 receptors and stimulated by A-2 receptors. At concentrations within the therapeutic range, caffeine antagonizes both actions. Whether it does so by binding to adenosine receptors is disputed.[270,273]

In animals, caffeine stimulates locomotor activity.[274] In drug discrimination studies, low doses generalize not only to other methylxanthines, but also to amphetamine, methylphenidate, and cocaine; high doses generalize only to other methylxanthines.[275] Self-administration studies have been inconsistent. Both primates and rats show wide individual differences, and many animals develop preference for caffeine only after forced exposure, suggesting that physical dependence potentiates reinforcement. Caffeine maintains self-administration much less reliably than amphetamine or cocaine.[276]

Tolerance develops to caffeine-stimulated locomotor activity, without cross-tolerance to nonmethylxanthine psychostimulants. By contrast, tolerance to caffeine's rate-decreasing effects on food-reinforced operant responding generalizes both to

Table 3–4. Caffeine Concentrations in Beverages and Pharmaceuticals

Product	Caffeine Concentration
Beverage and Food (mg/100 mL)	
Coffee	
Brewed	40–120 (usual cup: about 85 mg)
Decaffeinated	1–3
Tea	13–60 (usual cup: about 50 mg)
Cola drinks	10–15
Cocoa	4–10
Milk chocolate	20
Prescription Medication (mg/tablet)	
Cafergot	100
Darvon compound	32
Synalgos	30
Fiorinal	40
Migral	50
Migraine	100
Over-the-counter Preparation (mg/tablet)	
Anacin	32
Midol	32
Excedrin	65
Cope, Easy Mens	32
Many cold preparations	40
Dristan	16.2
Prolamine	140
Spantrol	150
Vanquish	33
No-Doz	100

Modified from Lewin NA, Goldfrank LR, Melinek M, Weisman RS. Caffeine. In: Goldfrank LR, Flomenbaum NE, Lewin NA, et al., eds. Toxicologic Emergencies, ed 4. Norwalk, CT: Appleton & Lange, 1990:607, with permission of the publisher.)

methylxanthine and to nonmethylxanthine psycho-stimulants.[274]

In humans, caffeine reduces drowsiness and fatigue and improves the flow of thought. Heart rate and blood pressure increase moderately, gastric acid and pepsin secretion is stimulated, and there is diuresis. The oils of coffee cause diarrhea; the tannins of tea cause constipation. Higher doses of caffeine cause nervousness, anxiety, tremor, insomnia, tachycardia, and ventricular premature contractions. Caffeine seems to be an example of a drug that produces craving independent of euphoria or otherwise pleasant effects; in some individuals, consumption continues in the face of increasing dysphoria.[276]

Toxic doses of caffeine cause agitation, dry mouth, dysesthesias, myalgia, "restless legs," tinnitus, ocular dyskinesias, scotomas, nausea, vomiting, and cardiac arrhythmia.[270,277–280] Panic attacks have been induced and schizophrenic symptoms exacerbated. Very high doses of caffeine cause delirium, seizures, and coma. Fatalities are rare but have been reported in both children and adults.[281–288] The lethal dose in adults has usually been 5 to 10 g, but serious toxicity can follow ingestion of only 1 g. Treatment includes induced vomiting if the patient is seen early; activated charcoal; catharsis; and respiratory, cardiac, and blood pressure support. Resin hemoperfusion has been used, and antacids and ranitidine are given for gastritis. Benzodiazepines can be used for sedation and, with phenytoin or phenobarbital, for seizures.

Peak serum levels of caffeine occur after 30 to 60 minutes, and its half-life is 3 to 7 hours.[270] Metabolites include theophylline and theobromine. Both tolerance and physical dependence develop to caffeine. Withdrawal symptoms include headache, yawning, drowsiness, irritability, difficulty concentrating, depression, diarrhea, and nausea.[270,289] In a double-blind, placebo-controlled study, such symptoms occurred even after low to moderate caffeine intake—mean 235 mg daily, equivalent to 2.5 cups of coffee.[290] Headache can be severe, and symptoms are sometimes called flu-like. Neonatal caffeine withdrawal causes irritability, jitteriness, and vomiting.[291]

Abuse of caffeine-containing "legal stimulants," with dosage escalation to more than 1 g daily, has been reported in abusers of other drugs and in alcoholics.[288,292] A middle-aged woman began using No Doz and Vivarin during periods of cocaine unavailability.[292] Death resulted from coffee enemas in a health food faddist.[286]

Although an association of caffeine and cardiovascular disease has been reported,[293] the weight of evidence is against caffeine carrying risk for myocardial infarction, peripheral vascular disease, hypertension, or stroke.[270,294,295] Coffee raises serum levels of both high-density and low-density lipoprotein cholesterol; the effect seems to be independent of caffeine.[296] In rodents, caffeine reduces ischemic damage, perhaps by up-regulating adenosine receptors.[297–299]

An alleged association of caffeine with pancreatic or renal cancer was refuted by subsequent studies. Huge doses of caffeine have been teratogenic in mammals, but the amounts consumed in beverages or medications do not appear to increase the risk for fetal malformations or low birth weight.[281] Caffeine increases the risk of osteoporosis in the elderly.[300]

References

1. Foltin RW, Fischman MW. Assessment of abuse liability of stimulant drugs in humans: a methodological survey. Drug Alcohol Dep 1991; 28:3.
2. Hoffman BB, Lefkowitz RJ. Catecholamines and sympathomimetic drugs. In: Gilman AG, Rall TW, Nies AS, Taylor P, eds. The Pharmacological Basis of Therapeutics, ed 8. New York: Pergamon Press, 1990:187.
3. Weintraub M. Long-term weight control study: conclusions. Clin Pharmacol Ther 1992; 51:642.
4. Treffert DA, Johanson D. Restricting amphetamines. JAMA 1981; 245:1336.
5. Hill H, Horita A. Inhibition of amphetamine hyperthermia by blockade of dopamine receptors in rabbits. J Pharm Pharmacol 1971; 23:715.
6. Berntman L, Carlsson C, Hagerdal M, Siesjo BK. Excessive increase in oxygen uptake and blood flow in the brain during amphetamine intoxication. Acta Physiol Scand 1976; 97:264.
7. Cho AK. Ice: a new dosage form of an old drug. Science 1990; 249:631.
8. Forrest WH, Brown BW, Brown CR. Dextroamphetamine with morphine for the treatment of postoperative pain. N Engl J Med 1977; 296:712.
9. Gold LH, Geyer MA, Koob GF. Neurochemical mechanisms involved in behavioral effects of amphetamines and related designer drugs. In: Asghar K, DeSouza E, eds. Pharmacology and Toxicology of Amphetamine and Related Designer Drugs. Rockville, MD: NIDA Research Monograph 94, DHHS, 1989: 146.
10. Pickens R, Harris WC. Self-administration of d-amphetamine by rats. Psychopharmacologia 1968; 12:158.
11. Piazza PV, Deminiere J-M, LeMoal M, Simon H. Factors that predict individual vulnerability to amphetamine self-administration. Science 1989; 245:1511.
12. Sannerud CA, Brady JV, Griffiths RR. Self-injection in baboons of amphetamines and related designer drugs. In: Asghar K, DeSouza E, eds. Pharmacology and

Toxicology of Amphetamine and Related Designer Drugs. Rockville, MD: NIDA Research Monograph 94, DHHS, 1989:30.

13. Seiden LS, Kleven MS. Methamphetamine and related drugs: toxicity and resulting behavioral changes in response to pharmacological probes. In: Asghar K, DeSouza E, eds. Pharmacology and Toxicology of Amphetamine and Related Designer Drugs. Rockville, MD: NIDA Research Monograph 94, DHHS, 1989:146.

14. Moghaddam B, Bunney BS. Differential effect of cocaine on extracellular dopamine levels in rat medial prefrontal cortex and nucleus accumbens: comparison to amphetamine. Synapse 1989; 4:156.

15. Lyness WH, Friedle NM, Moore KE. Increased self-administration of d-amphetamine after destruction of 5-hydroxydopamine neurons. Pharmacol Biochem Behav 1980; 12:937.

16. Leccese AP, Lyness WH. The effects of putative 5-hydroxytryptamine receptor active agents on d-amphetamine median forebrain bundle lesions. Brain Res 1984; 303:153.

17. McMillen BA. CNS stimulants: two distinct mechanisms of action for amphetamine-like drugs. Trends Pharmacol Sci 1983; 4:429.

18. Madras BK, Fahey MA, Bergman J, et al. Effects of cocaine and related drugs in non-human primates. 1. [3-H]Cocaine binding sites in caudate-putamen. J Pharmacol Exp Ther 1989; 251:131.

19. Heikkila RE. Differential effects of several dopamine uptake inhibitors and releasing agents on locomotor activity in normal and in reserpinized mice. Life Sci 1981; 28:1967.

20. Rebec GV, Lee EH. Tolerance to amphetamine-induced inhibition of neuronal activity in the central amygdaloid nucleus. Pharmacol Biochem Behav 1983; 19:219.

21. Jaffe JH. Drug addiction and drug abuse. In: Gilman AG, Rall TW, Nies AS, Taylor P, eds. The Pharmacological Basis of Therapeutics, ed 8. New York: Pergamon Press, 1990:522.

22. Kalivas PW, Weber B. Amphetamine injection into the ventral mesencephalon sensitizes rats to peripheral amphetamine and cocaine. J Pharmacol Exp Ther 1988; 245:485.

23. Robinson TE, Becker JB. Enduring changes in brain and behavior produced by chronic amphetamine administration. A review and evaluation of animal models of amphetamine psychosis. Brain Res Rev 1986; 11:157.

24. Barnett JV, Segal DS, Kuczenski R. Repeated amphetamine pre-treatment alters the responsiveness of striatal dopamine-stimulated adenylate cyclase to amphetamine-induced desensitization. J Pharmacol Exp Ther 1987; 242:40.

25. Dougan D, Wade D, Duffield P. How metabolites may augment some psychostimulant actions of amphetamine. Trends Pharmacol Sci 1987; 8:277.

26. Ellinwood EH, Kilbey MM. Fundamental mechanisms underlying altered behavior following chronic administration of psychomotor stimulants. Biol Psychiatry 1980; 15:749.

27. Ricaurte GA, Seiden LS, Schuster CR. Further evidence that amphetamines produce long-lasting dopamine neurochemical deficits by destroying dopamine nerve fibers. Brain Res 1984; 303:359.

28. Gibb JW, Stone DM, Johnson M, Hanson GR. Role of dopamine in the neurotoxicity induced by amphetamines and related designer drugs. In: Asghar K, DeSouza E, eds. Pharmacology and Toxicology of Amphetamine and Related Designer Drugs. Rockville, MD: NIDA Research Monograph 94, DHHS, 1989:161.

29. Fuller RW. Recommendations for future research on amphetamines and related designer drugs. In: Asghar K, DeSouza E, eds. Pharmacology and Toxicology of Amphetamine and Related Designer Drugs. Rockville, MD: NIDA Research Monograph 94, DHHS, 1989:341.

30. Gawin FH, Ellinwood EH. Cocaine and other stimulants. Actions, abuse, treatment. N Engl J Med 1988; 318:1173.

31. Sonsalla PK, Nicklas WJ, Heikkila RE. Role for excitatory amino acids in methamphetamine-induced nigrostriatal toxicity. Science 1989; 243:398.

32. Snyder SH. Drugs and the Brain. New York: Scientific American Library, 1986.

33. Anderson RJ, Reed WG, Hillis LD, et al. History, epidemiology, and medical complications of nasal inhaler abuse. J Toxicol Clin Toxicol 1982; 19:95.

34. Munroe RR, Drell HJ. Use of stimulants obtained from inhalers. JAMA 1937; 135:909.

35. Post JM. Drunk with power. Alcohol and drug abuse among the leadership elite. Washington Post National Weekly Edition, Feb 5, 1990:39.

36. Cohen S. Stimulant abuse in Sweden. In: Drug Dependence, No 2, National Clearinghouse for Mental Health Information. Bethesda, MD: National Institute of Mental Health, 1969:30.

37. Brecher EM. Licit and Illicit Drugs. Boston: Little, Brown, 1972:267.

38. Kalant OJ. The Amphetamines: Toxicity and Addiction, ed 2. Springfield, IL: Charles C. Thomas, 1973.

39. Scarpino V, Arrigo A, Benzi G, et al. Evaluation and prevalence of "doping" among Italian athletes. Lancet 1990; 336:1048.

40. Catlin DH, Hatton CK. Use and abuse of anabolic and other drugs for athletic enhancement. Adv Intern Med 1991; 36:399.

41. Smith LC. Collapse with death following the use of amphetamine sulfate. JAMA 1939; 113:1022.

42. Norman J, Shea JT. Acute hallucinosis as a complication of addiction to amphetamine sulfate. N Engl J Med 1945; 233:270.

43. Harvey JK, Todd CW, Howard JH. Fatality associated with Benzedrine ingestion. A case report. Delaware State M J 1949; 21:111.

44. Grinspoon L, Hedblom P. The Speed Culture: Amphetamine Use and Abuse in America. Cambridge, MA: Harvard University Press, 1975.

45. Lake CR, Quirk RS. CNS stimulants and the look-alike drugs. Psychiat Clin North Am 1984; 7:689.

46. Nicholi AM. The nontherapeutic use of psychoactive drugs. N Engl J Med 1984; 16:241.

47. Kall KI, Olin RG. HIV status and changes in risk behavior among intravenous drug users in Stockholm 1987–1988. AIDS 1990; 4:153.

48. Bailey DN. Amphetamine detection during toxicology screening of a university medical center patient population. Clin Toxicol 1987; 25:399.

49. Jackson JG. Hazards of smokable methamphetamine. N Engl J Med 1989; 321:907.

50. Weiss B, Laties VG. Enhancement of human performance by caffeine and the amphetamines. Pharmacol Rev 1962; 14:1.

51. Tecce JJ, Cole JO. Amphetamine effects in man: paradoxical drowsiness and lowered electrical brain activity (CNV). Science 1974; 185:451.

52. Martin WR, Sloan JW, Sapira JD, Jasinski DR. Physiologic, subjective, and behavioral effects of amphetamine, methamphetamine, ephedrine, phenmetrazine, and methylphendiate in man. Clin Pharmacol Ther 1971; 12:245.

53. Cook CE, Jeffcoat AR, Perez-Reyes M, et al. Plasma levels of methamphetamine after smoking methamphetamine hydrochloride. In: Harris L, ed. Problems of Drug Dependence, 1990. Rockville, MD: NIDA Research Monograph 105, DHHS, 1991:578.

54. Kramer JC, Fischman VS, Littlefield DC. Amphetamine abuse: patterns and effects of high doses taken intravenously. JAMA 1967; 201:305.

55. Cox C, Smart RG. The nature and extent of speed use in North America. Can Med Assoc J 1970; 102:724.

56. Lundh H, Tunving K. An extrapyramidal choreiform syndrome caused by amphetamine addiction. J Neurol Neurosurg Psychiatry 1981; 44:728.

57. Connell HP. Amphetamine Psychosis. London: Chapman and Hall Ltd, 1958.

58. Bell DS. Comparison of amphetamine psychosis and schizophrenia. Br J Psychiatry 1965; 111:701.

59. Angrist B, van Kammen DP. CNS stimulants as tools in the study of schizophrenia. Trends Neurosci 1984; 7:388.

60. Javitt DC, Zukin SR. Recent advances in the phencyclidine model of schizophrenia. Am J Psychiatry 1991; 148:1301.

61. van Kammen D, Bunney WE, Docherty JP, et al. D-amphetamine-induced heterogeneous changes in psychotic behavior in schizophrenia. Am J Psychiatry 1982; 139:991.

62. Goldberg TE, Bigelow LB, Weinberger DR, et al. Cognitive and behavioral effects of the coadministration of dextroamphetamine and haloperidol in schizophrenia. Am J Psychiatry 1991; 178:78.

63. Zalis EG, Parmley LF. Fatal amphetamine poisoning. Arch Intern Med 1963; 112:822.

64. Espelin DE, Done AK. Amphetamine poisoning. N Engl J Med 1968; 278:1361.

65. Edison GR. Amphetamines. A dangerous illusion. Ann Intern Med 1971; 74:605.

66. Cohen S. Amphetamine abuse. JAMA 1975; 231:414.

67. Kojima T, Une I, Yashiki M, et al. A fatal methamphetamine poisoning associated with hyperpyrexia. Forens Sci Int 1984; 24:87.

68. Kendrick WC, Hull AR, Knochel JP. Rhabdomyolysis and shock after intravenous amphetamine administration. Ann Intern Med 1977; 86:381.

69. Kasirsky G, Zaidi IH, Tansy MF. LD50 and pathologic effects of acute and chronic administration of methamphetamine HCl in rabbits. Res Commun Chem Pathol Pharmacol 1972; 3:215.

70. Zalis EG, Lundberg GD, Knutson RA. The pathophysiology of acute amphetamine poisoning with pathologic correlation. J Pharmacol Exp Ther 1967; 158:115.

71. Zalis EG, Kaplan G, Lundberg GD, Knutson RA. Acute lethality of the amphetamines in dogs and its antagonism with curare. Proc Soc Exp Biol Med 1965; 18:557.

72. Duarte Escalante O, Ellinwood EH. Central nervous system cytopathological changes in cats with chronic methedrine intoxication. Brain Res 1970; 21:151.

73. Alldredge BK, Lowenstein DH, Simon RP. Seizures associated with recreational drug abuse. Neurology 1989; 39:1037.

74. Goldfrank LR, Kirstein RH. Amphetamines. In: Goldfrank LR, Flomenbaum NE, Lewin NA, et al., eds. Toxicologic Emergencies, ed 4. Norwalk, CT: Appleton & Lange, 1990:509.

75. Lemberger L, Witt EP, David J, Kopin IJ. The effects of haloperidol and chlorpromazine on amphetamine metabolism and amphetamine stereotype behavior in rat. J Pharmacol Exp Ther 1970; 174:428.

76. Khantzian EJ, McKenna GJ. Acute toxic and withdrawal reactions associated with drug use and abuse. Ann Intern Med 1979; 90:361.

77. Oswald I, Thacore VR. Amphetamine and phenmetrazine addiction. Physiological abnormalities in the abstinence syndrome. BMJ 1963; 2:427.

78. Angrist BM, Gershon D. Psychotic sequelae of amphetamine use. In: Shader R, ed. Psychiatric Complications of Medical Drugs. New York: Raven Press, 1972:175.

79. Kantor HL, Emsellem HA, Hogg JE, Simon GL. *Candida albicans* meningitis in a parenteral drug abuser. South Med J 1984; 77:404.

80. Brooks GF, O'Donoghue JM, Rissing JP, et al. *Eikenella corrodens*, a recently recognized pathogen: infections in medical-surgical patients and in association with methylphenidate abuse. Medicine 1974; 53:325.

81. Seaman ME. Barotrauma related to inhalational drug abuse. J Emerg Med 1990; 8:141.

82. Carson P, Oldroyd K, Phadke K. Myocardial infarction due to amphetamine. BMJ 1987; 294:1525.

83. Packe GE, Garton MJ, Jennings K. Acute myocardial infarction caused by intravenous amphetamine abuse. Br Heart J 1990; 64:23.

84. Furst SR, Fallon SP, Reznik GN, Shah PK. Myocardial infarction after inhalation of methamphetamine. N Engl J Med 1990; 323:1147.

85. Call TD, Hartneck J, Dickinson WA, et al. Acute cardiomyopathy secondary to intravenous amphetamine abuse. Ann Intern Med 1982; 97:559.

86. Smith HJ, Roche AHG, Jagusch MF, Hersdon PB. Cardiomyopathy associated with amphetamine administration. Am Heart J 1976; 91:792.

87. Poteliakhoff A, Roughton BC. Two cases of amphetamine poisoning. BMJ 1956; 1:26.

88. Lloyd JTA, Walker DRH. Death after combined dexamphetamine and phenylzine. BMJ 1965; 2:168.

89. Coroner's report: Amphetamine overdose kills boy. Pharmaceut J 1967: 198:172.

90. Kane FJ, Keeler MH, Reifler CB. Neurological crisis following methamphetamine. JAMA 1969; 210:556.

91. Goodman SJ, Becker DP. Intracranial hemorrhage associated with amphetamine abuse. JAMA 1970; 212:480.

92. Weiss SR, Raskind R, Morganstern NL, et al. Intracerebral and subarachnoid hemorrhage following use of methamphetamine ("speed"). Int Surg 1970; 53:123.

93. Margolis MT, Newton TH. Methamphetamine ("speed") arteritis. Neuroradiology 1971; 2:179.

94. Tibbetts JC, Hinck VC. Conservative management of a hematoma in the fourth ventricle. Surg Neurol 1973; 1:253.

95. Chynn KY. Acute subarachnoid hemorrhage. JAMA 1973; 233:55.

96. Hall CD, Blanton DE, Scatliff JH, Morris CE. Speed kills: fatality from the self administration of methamphetamine intravenously. South Med J 1973; 66:650.

97. Yatsu FM, Wesson DR, Smith DE. Amphetamine abuse. In: Richter RW, ed. Medical Aspects of Drug Abuse. Hagerstown, MD: Harper & Row, 1975:50.

98. Olsen ER. Intracranial hemorrhage and amphetamine usage. Angiology 1977; 28:464.

99. Yarnell PR. "Speed" headache and hematoma. Headache 1977; 17:69.

100. Edwards K. Hemorrhagic complications of cerebral arteritis. Arch Neurol 1977; 34:549.

101. Kessler JT, Jortner BS, Adapon BD. Cerebral vasculitis in a drug abuser. J Clin Psychiatry 1978; 39:559.

102. LoVerme S. Complications of amphetamine abuse. In: Culebras A, ed. Clini-Pearls, Vol 2, No 8. Syracuse, NY: Creative Medical Publications, 1979:5.

103. Delaney P, Estes M. Intracranial hemorrhage with amphetamine abuse. Neurology 1980; 30:1125.

104. Gericke OL. Suicide by ingestion of amphetamine sulfate. JAMA 1980; 128:1125.

105. D'Souza T, Shraberg D. Intracranial hemorrhage associated with amphetamine use. Neurology 1981; 31:922.

106. Cahill DW, Knipp H, Mosser J. Intracranial hemorrhage with amphetamine abuse. Neurology 1981; 31:1058.

107. Shukla D. Intracranial hemorrhage associated with amphetamine use. Neurology 1982; 32:917.

108. Harrington H, Heller HA, Dawson D, et al. Intracerebral hemorrhage and oral amphetamine. Arch Neurol 1983; 40:503.

109. Yu YJ, Cooper DR, Wallenstein DE, Block B. Cerebral angiitis and intracerebral hemorrhage associated with methamphetamine abuse. J Neurosurg 1983; 58:109.

110. Lukes SA. Intracerebral hemorrhage from an arteriovenous malformation after amphetamine injection. Arch Neurol 1983; 40:60.

111. Matick H, Anderson D, Brumlik J. Cerebral vasculitis associated with oral amphetamine overdose. Arch Neurol 1983; 40:253.

112. Salanova V, Taubner R. Intracerebral hemorrhage and vasculitis secondary to amphetamine use. Postgrad Med J 1984; 60:429.

113. Imanse J, Vanneste J. Intraventricular hemorrhage following amphetamine abuse. Neurology 1990; 40:1318.

114. Delaney P. Intracranial hemorrhage associated with amphetamine use. Neurology 1981; 31:923.

115. Citron BP, Halpern M, McCarron M, et al. Necrotizing angiitis associated with drug abuse. N Engl J Med 1970; 283:1003.

116. Citron BP, Peters RL. Angiitis in drug abusers. N Engl J Med 1971; 284:112.

117. Gocke DJ, Christian CL. Angiitis in drug abusers. N Engl J Med 1971; 284:112.

118. Bostwick DG. Amphetamine induced cerebral vasculitis. Hum Pathol 1981; 12:1031.

119. Rumbaugh CL, Bergeron RT, Fang HCH, McCormick R. Cerebral angiographic changes in the drug abuse patient. Radiology 1971; 101:335.

120. Rothrock JF, Rubenstein R, Lyden PD. Ischemic stroke associated with methamphetamine inhalation. Neurology 1988; 38:589.

121. Sachdeva K, Woodward KG. Caudal thalamic infarction following intranasal methamphetamine use. Neurology 1989; 39:305.

122. Rumbaugh CL, Bergeron T, Scanlon RL, et al. Cerebral vascular changes secondary to amphetamine abuse in the experimental animal. Radiology 1971; 101:345.

123. Rumbaugh CL, Fang HCH, Higgins RE, et al. Cerebral microvascular injury in experimental drug abuse. Invest Radiol 1976; 11:282.

124. Stafford CR, Bogdanoff BM, Green L, Spector HB. Mononeuropathy multiplex as a complication of amphetamine angiitis. Neurology 1975; 25:570.

125. Rifkin SI. Amphetamine-induced angiitis leading to renal failure. South Med J 1977; 70:108.

126. Golden GS. Gilles de la Tourette's syndrome following amphetamine administration. Dev Med Child Neurol 1976; 16:76.

127. Pollack MA, Cohen NL, Friedhoff AJ. Gilles de la Tourette's syndrome: familial occurrence and precipitation by methylphenidate therapy. Arch Neurol 1977; 34:630.

128. Bonthala CM, West A. Pemoline induced chorea and Gilles de la Tourette's syndrome. Br J Psychiatry 1983; 143:300.

129. Allcott JV, Barnhart RA, Mooney LA. Acute lead poisoning in two users of illicit methamphetamine. JAMA 1987; 258:510.

129a. Weinrieb RM, O'Brien CP. Persistent cognitive deficits attributed to substance abuse. In: Brust JCM, ed.: Neurologic Complications of Drug and Alcohol Abuse. Neurol Clin 1993, in press.

130. Matera C, Warren WB, Moomjy M, et al. Prevalence of use of cocaine and other substances in an obstetrics population. Am J Obstet Gynecol 1990; 163:797.

131. Oro AS, Dixon SD. Perinatal cocaine and methamphetamine exposure: maternal and neonatal correlates. J Pediatr 1987; 11:571.

132. Eriksson M, Larsson G, Zetterstrom R. Amphetamine addiction and pregnancy. Acta Obstet Gynecol Scand 1981; 60:253.

133. Dominguez R, Vila-Coro AA, Slopis JM, Bohan TP. Brain and ocular abnormalities in infants with in utero exposure to cocaine and other street drugs. Am J Dis Child 1991; 145:688.

134. Dixon SD, Bejar R. Electroencephalographic findings in neonates associated with maternal cocaine and methamphetamine use: incidence and clinical correlates. J Pediatr 1989; 115:770.

135. Kandall SR. Perinatal effects of cocaine and amphetamine use during pregnancy. Bull NY Acad Med 1991; 67:240.

136. Middaugh LD. Prenatal amphetamine effects on behavior: possible mediation by brain monoamines. Ann NY Acad Sci 1989; 562:308.

137. Elliott RH, Rees GB. Amphetamine ingestion presenting as eclampsia. Can J Anaesth 1990; 37:130.

138. Mueller SM, Ertel PJ. Subarachnoid hemorrhage associated with over-the-counter diet medications. Stroke 1983; 14:16.

139. FDA announces new drug status of OTC combination products containing caffeine, phenylpropanolamine, and ephedrine. Natl Assoc Boards of Pharmacy 1982; IA 4:3.

140. Lasagna L. Phenylpropanolamine: A Review. New York: John Wiley & Sons, 1988.

141. Woolverton WL, Johanson CE, de la Garza R, et al. Behavorial and neurochemical evaluation of phenylpropanolamine. J Pharmacol Exp Ther 1986; 237:926.

142. Chait LD, Uhlenhuth EH, Johanson CE. Reinforcing and subjective effects of several anorectics in normal human volunteers. J Pharmacol Exp Ther 1987; 242:777.

143. Chait LD, Uhlenhuth EH, Johanson CE. The discriminative stimulus and subjective effects of phenylpropanolamine, mazindol, and d-amphetamine in humans. Pharmacol Biochem Behav 1986; 24:1665.

144. Pentel P. Toxicity of over-the-counter stimulants. JAMA 1984; 252:1898.

145. O'Connell MB, Pentel PR, Zimmerman CL. Individual variability in the blood pressure response to intravenous phenylpropanolamine: a pharmacokinetic and pharmacodynamic investigation. Clin Pharmacol Ther 1989; 45:252.

146. Bernstein E, Diskant B. Phenylpropanolamine, a potentially hazardous drug. Ann Emerg Med 1982; 11:315.

147. Bale JF, Fountain MT, Shaddy R. Phenylpropanolamine associated CNS complications in children and adolescents. Am J Dis Child 1984; 138:683.

148. Waggoner WC. Phenylpropanolamine overdosage. Lancet 1983; 2:1503.

149. Mueller SM. Neurologic complications of phenylpropanolamine use. Neurology 1983; 33:650.

150. Hyams JS, Leichtner AM, Breiner RG, et al. Pseudopheochromocytoma and cardiac arrest associated with phenylpropanolamine. JAMA 1985; 253:1609.

151. LeCoz P, Woimant F, Rougemont D, et al. Angiopathies cerebrales benigues et phenylpropanolamine. Rev Neurol 1988; 144:295.

152. Peterson RB, Vasquez LA. Phenylpropanolamine-induced arrhythmias. JAMA 1973; 233:324.

153. Woo OF, Benowitz NL, Baily FW, et al. Atrioventricular conduction block caused by phenylpropanolamine. JAMA 1985; 253:2646.

154. Norvenius G, Widerlov E, Lonnerholm G. Phenylpropanolamine and mental disturbances. Lancet 1979; 2:1367.

155. Schaffer CB, Pauli MW. Psychotic reaction caused by proprietary oral diet agents. Am J Psychiatry 1980; 137:1256.

156. Cornelius JR, Soloff PH, Reynolds CF. Paranoia, homicidal behavior and seizures associated with phenylpropanolamine. Am J Psychiatry 1984; 141:120.

157. Mueller SM, Solow EB. Seizures associated with a new combination "pick-me-up" pill. Ann Neurol 1982; 11:322.

158. Howrie DL, Wokfson JM. Phenylpropanolamine-induced seizure. J Pediatr 1983; 102:143.

159. King J. Hypertension and cerebral hemorrhage from Trimolets ingestion. Med J Aust 1979; 2:258.

160. Lovejoy FH. Stroke and phenylpropanolamine. Pediatr Alert 1981; 12:45.

161. Mueller SM, Muller J, Asdell SM. Cerebral hemorrhage associated with phenylpropanolamine in combination with caffeine. Stroke 1984; 15:119.

162. Mesnard B, Ginn DR. Excessive phenylpropanolamine ingestion followed by subarachnoid hemorrhage. South Med J 1984; 77:939.

163. Stoessl AJ, Young GB, Feasby TE. Intracerebral hemorrhage and angiographic beading following ingestion of catecholaminergics. Stroke 1985; 16:734.

164. Kikta DG, Devereaux MW, Chandar K. Intracranial hemorrhages due to phenylpropanolamine. Stroke 1985; 16:510.

165. Fallis RJ, Fisher M. Cerebral vasculitis and hemorrhage associated with phenylpropanolamine. Neurology 1985; 35:405.

166. Kizer KW. Intracranial hemorrhage associated with overdose of decongestant containing phenylpropanolamine. Am J Emerg Med 1986; 2:180.

167. Kase CS, Foster TE, Reed JE, et al. Intracerebral hemorrhage and phenylpropanolamine use. Neurology 1987; 37:399.

168. Maertens P, Lum G, Williams JP, et al. Intracerebral hemorrhage and cerebral angiopathic changes in a suicidal phenylpropanolamine poisoning. South Med J 1987; 80:584.

169. Glick R, Hoying J, Cerullo L, Perlman S. Phenylpropanolamine: an over-the-counter drug causing central nervous system vasculitis and intracerebral hemorrhage. Neurosurgery 1987; 20:969.

170. Forman HP, Levin S, Stewart B, et al. Cerebral vasculitis and hemorrhage in an adolescent taking diet pills containing phenylpropanolamine: case report and review of literature. Pediatrics 1989; 83:737.

171. Sloan MA, Kittner SJ, Rigamonti D, Price TR. Occurrence of stroke associated with use/abuse of drugs. Neurology 1991; 41:1358.

172. Garcia-Albea E. Subarachnoid hemorrhage and nasal vasoconstrictor abuse. J Neurol Neurosurg Psychiatry 1983; 46:875.

173. Mariani PJ. Pseudoephedrine-induced hypertensive emergency: treatment with labetalol. Am J Emerg Med 1986; 4:141.

174. Pugh CR, Howie SM. Dependence on pseudoephedrine. Br J Psychiatry 1986; 149:789.

175. Lambert MT. Paranoid psychosis after abuse of proprietary cold remedies. Br J Psychiatry 1987; 151:548.

176. Whitehorse M, Duncan JM. Ephedrine psychosis rediscovered. Br J Psychiatry 1987; 150:258.

177. Loosmore S, Armstrong D. Do-Do abuse. Br J Psychiatry 1990; 157:278.

178. Wooten MR, Khangure MS, Murphy MJ. Intracerebral hemorrhage and vasculitis related to ephedrine abuse. Ann Neurol 1983; 13:337.

179. Loizou LA, Hamilton JG, Tsementzis SA. Intracranial hemorrhage in association with pseudoephedrine overdose. J Neurol Neurosurg Psychiatry 1982; 45:471.

180. Mellar J, Hollister LE. Phenmetrazine: an obselete problem drug. Clin Pharmacol Ther 1982; 32:671.

181. Corwin RL, Woolverton WL, Schuster CR, Johanson CE. Anorectics: effects on food intake and self-administration in rhesus monkeys. Alcohol Drug Res 1987; 7:351.

182. Hamer R, Phelp D. Inadvertent intra-arterial injection of phentermine. A complication of drug abuse. Ann Emerg Med 1981; 10:148.

182a. Kokkinos J, Levine SR. Possible association of ischemic stroke with phentermine. Stroke 1993; 24:310.

183. Caplan J. Habituation to diethylpropion (Tenuate). Can Med Assoc J 1963; 88:943.

184. Cohen S. Diethylpropion (Tenuate): an infrequently abused anorectic. Psychosomatics 1977; 18:28.

185. Carney MWP. Diethylpropion and psychosis. Clin Neuropharmacol 1988; 11:183.

186. Levin A. The non-medical use of fenfluramine by drug-dependent young South Africans. Postgrad Med J 1975; 51:186.

187. Parran TV, Jasinski DR. Intravenous methylphenidate abuse. Arch Intern Med 1991; 151:781.

188. Raskind M, Bradford T. Methylphenidate (Ritalin) abuse and methadone maintenance. Dis Nerv Syst 1975; 36:9.

189. Lewman LV. Fatal pulmonary hypertension from intravenous injection of methylphenidate (Ritalin) tablets. Hum Pathol 1972; 3:67.

190. Zemplenyi J, Colman MF. Deep neck abscesses secondary to methylphenidate (Ritalin) abuse. Head Neck Surg 1984; 6:858.

191. Wolf J, Fein A, Fehrenbacher L. Eosinophilic syndrome with methylphenidate abuse. Ann Intern Med 1978; 89:224.

192. Spensley J, Rockwell DA. Psychosis during methylphenidate abuse. N Engl J Med 1972; 286:880.

193. Hahn HH, Schweid AI, Beaty HN. Complications of injecting dissolved methylphenidate tablets. Arch Intern Med 1969; 123:656.

194. Extein I. Methylphenidate-induced choreoathetosis. Am J Psychiatry 1978; 135:252.

195. Chillar RK, Jackson AL. Reversible hemiplegia after presumed intracarotid injection of Ritalin. N Engl J Med 1981; 304:1305.

196. Atlee W. Talc and cornstarch emboli in eyes of drug abusers. JAMA 1972; 219:49.

197. Tse DT, Ober RR. Talc retinopathy. Am J Ophthalmol 1980; 90:624.

198. Mizutami T, Lewis R, Gonatas N. Medial medullary syndrome in a drug abuser. Arch Neurol 1980; 37:425.

199. Trugman JM. Cerebral arteritis and oral methylphenidate. Lancet 1988; 1:584.

200. Briscoe JG, Curry SC, Gerkin RD, Ruiz RR. Pemoline-induced choreoathetosis and rhabdomyolysis. Med Toxicol 1988; 3:72.

201. McIntyre D. Psychosis due to nasal decongestant abuse. Br J Psychiatry 1976; 112:93.

202. White L, DiMiao VJM. Intravenous propylhexedrine and sudden death. N Engl J Med 1977; 297:1071.

203. Anderson R, Garza H, Garriott JC, DiMaio V. Intravenous propylhexedrine (Benzedrex) abuse and sudden death. Am J Med 1979; 67:15.

204. Croft CH, Firth BG, Hillis LP. Propylhexedrine-induced left ventricular dysfunction. Ann Intern Med 1982; 97:560.

205. Hall AH, Kulig KW, Rumack BH. Intravenous epinephrine abuse. Am J Emerg Med 1987; 5:64.

206. Margaral LE, Sandborn GE, Donoso LA, Gander JR. Branch retinal artery occlusion after excessive use of nasal spray. Ann Ophthalmol 1985; 17:500.

207. Montalban J, Ibanez L, Rodriguez C, et al. Cerebral infarction after excessive use of nasal decongestants. J Neurol Neurosurg Psychiatry 1989; 52:541.

208. Brenneisen R, Fisch HU, Koelbing U, et al. Amphetamine-like effects in humans of the khat alkaloid cathinone. Br J Clin Pharmacol 1990; 30:825.

209. Kalix P. Pharmacological properties of the stimulant khat. Pharmacol Ther 1990; 48:397.

210. Yanagita T. Intravenous self-administration of cathinone and of 2-amino-(2,5-dimethyl-4-methyl)-phenyl-

propane in rhesus monkeys. Drug Alcohol Depend 1986; 17:135.

211. Pantelis C, Hindler C, Taylor J. Use and abuse of khat: distribution, pharmacology, side effects and description of psychosis attributed to khat chewing. Psychol Med 1989; 19:657.

212. Kalix P. Amphetamine psychosis due to khat leaves. Lancet 1984; 1:46.

213. Baird DA. A case of optic neuritis in a khat addict. East Afr Med J 1952; 29:325.

214. Roper JP. The presumed neurotoxic effects of Catha edulis—an exotic plant now available in the United Kingdom. Br J Ophthalmol 1986; 70:779.

215. Browne DL. Qat use in New York City. In: Harris L, ed. Problems of Drug Dependence, 1990. Rockville, MD: NIDA Research Monograph 105, DHHS, 1991:464.

216. Giannini AJ, Castelanni S. A manic-like psychosis due to khat (Catha elulis). J Toxicol Clin Toxicol 1982; 19:455.

217. Gough SP, Cookson IB. Khat-induced schizophreniform psychosis in UK. Lancet 1984; 1:455.

218. Mayberry J, Morgan G, Perkin E. Khat-induced schizophreniform psychosis in UK. Lancet 1984; 1:455.

219. Nencini P, Grassi M, Botan A, et al. Khat chewing spread to the Somali community in Rome. Drug Alcohol Depend 1989; 23:255.

220. Nichols DE, Oberlender R. Structure-activity relationships of MDMA-like substances. In: Asghar K, DeSouza E, eds. Pharmacology and Toxicology of Amphetamine and Related Drugs. Rockville, MD: NIDA Research Monograph 94, DHHS, 1989:1.

221. Jackson B, Reed A. Another abusable amphetamine. JAMA 1970; 211:830.

222. Weil A. The love drug. J Psychoact Drugs 1976; 8:335.

223. Climko RP, Roehrich H, Sweeney DR, Al-Rari J. Ecstasy: a review of MDMA and MDA. Int J Psychiatr Med 1986; 16:359.

224. Grinspoon L, Bakalar JB. Can drugs be used to enhance the psychotherapeutic process? Am J Psychother 1986; 15:393.

225. Peroutka SJ. Incidence of recreational use of 3,4-methylenedimethoxymethamphetamine (MDMA, "Ecstasy") on an undergraduate campus. N Engl J Med 1987; 317:1542.

226. Beardsley PM, Balster RL, Harris LS. Self-administration of methylenedioxymethamphetamine (MDMA) by Rhesus monkeys. Drug Alcohol Depend 1986; 18:149.

227. Lamb RJ, Griffiths RR. Self-injection of d,1-3,4-methylenedioxymethamphetamine (MDMA) in the baboon. Psychopharmacology 1987; 91:268.

228. Gold LH, Koob GF, Geyer MA. Stimulant and hallucinogenic behavioral profiles of 3,4-methylenedioxymethamphetamine (MDMA) and N-ethyl-3,4-methylenedioxyamphetamine (MDEA) in rats. J Pharmacol Exp Ther 1988; 247:547.

229. Stone D, Stahl D, Hanson G, Gibb J. The effects of 3,4-methylenedioxymethamphetamine and 3,4- methylenedioxyamphetamine (MDA) on monoaminergic systems in the rat brain. Eur J Pharmacol 1986; 128:41.

230. Oberlender R, Nichols DE. (+)-N-Methyl-1-(1,3-benzodioxol-5-yl)-2-butanamine as a discriminative stimulus in studies of 3,4-methylenedioxymethamphetamine-like behavioral activity. J Pharmacol Exp Ther 1990; 255:1098.

231. Siegel RK. MDMA. Nonmedical use and intoxication. J Psychoact Drugs 1986; 18:349.

232. Bost RO. 3,4-methylenedioxymethamphetamine (MDMA) and other amphetamine derivatives. J Forens Sci 1988; 33:576.

233. Boja JW, Schechter MD. Behavioral effects of N-ethyl-3,4-methylenedioxyamphetamine (MDEA; "Eve"). Pharmacol Biochem Behav 1987; 28:153.

234. Peroutka SJ, Newman H, Harris H. Subjective effects of 3,4-methylenedioxymethamphetamine in recreational users. Neuropsychopharmacology 1988; 1:273.

235. Brown C, Osterloh J. Multiple severe complications from recreational ingestion of MDMA ("Ecstasy"). JAMA 1987; 258:780.

236. Hayner GN, McKinney H. MDMA. The dark side of ecstasy. J Psychoact Drugs 1986; 18:341.

237. Dowling GP, McDonough ET, Bost RO. "Eve" and "Ecstasy"—Garden of Eden or serpent? A report of five deaths associated with the use of MDEA and MDMA. JAMA 1987; 257:1615.

238. Suarez RV, Riemorsma R. "Ecstasy" and sudden cardiac death. Am J Forens Med Pathol 1988; 9:339.

239. Whitaker-Azmitia PM, Aronson TA. "Ecstasy" (MDMA)-induced panic. Am J Psychiatry 1989; 146:119.

240. Simpson DL, Rumack BH. Methylenedioxyamphetamine. Clinical description of overdose, death, and review of pharmacology. Arch Intern Med 1981; 141:1507.

241. Battaglia G, Yeh SY, O'Hearn E, et al. 3,4-methylenedioxymethamphetamine and 3,4-methylenedioxyamphetamine destroy serotonin terminals in rat brain: quantification of neurodegeneration by measurement of [^{3}H]paroxetine-labelled serotonin uptake sites. J Pharmacol Exp Ther 1987; 242:911.

242. Ricuarte GA, Forno LS, Wilson MA, et al. 3,4-methylenedioxymethamphetamine selectively damages central serotonergic neurons in nonhuman primates. JAMA 1988; 260:51.

243. Schmidt CJ. Neurotoxicity of the psychedelic amphetamine, methylenedioxymethamphetamine. J Pharmacol Exp Ther 1986; 240:1.

244. Molliver ME, Mamounas LA, Wilson MA. Effects of neurotoxic amphetamines on serotonergic neurons: immunocytochemical studies. In: Asghar K, DeSouza E, eds. Pharmacology and Toxicology of Amphetamine and Related Drugs. Rockville, MD: NIDA Research Monograph 94, DHHS, 1989:270.

245. DeSouza EB, Battaglia G. Effects of MDMA and MDA on brain serotonin neurons: evidence from neurochemical and autoradiographic studies. In: Asghar K, DeSouza E, eds. Pharmacology and Toxicology of Amphetamine and Related Drugs. Rockville, MD: NIDA Research Monograph 94, DHHS, 1989:196.

246. Price LH, Ricaurte GA, Krystal JH, Heninger GR. Neuroendocrine and mood responses to intravenous L-tryptophan in 3,4-methylenedioxymethamphetamine (MDMA) users. Arch Gen Psychiatry 1989; 46:20.

247. Kleven MS, Schuster CR, Seiden LS. The effect of depletion of brain serotonin by repeated fenfluramine on neurochemical and anorectic effects of acute fenfluramine. J Pharmacol Exp Ther 1988; 246:1.

248. Shopsin B, Kline NS. Monoamine oxidase inhibitors: potential for drug abuse. Biol Psychiatr 1976; 11:451.

249. Ben-Arie O, George GCW. A case of tranylcypromine (Parnate) addiction. Br J Psychiatry 1979; 135:273.

250. Griffin N, Draper RJ, Webb MGT. Addiction to tranylcypromine. BMJ 1981; 283:346.

251. Pitt B. Withdrawal symptoms after stopping phenelzine? BMJ 1974; 2:332.

252. LeGassicke J, Ashcrof GW, Eccelston D, et al. The clinical state, sleep, and amine metabolism of a tranylcypromine (Parnate) addict. Br J Psychiatry 1965; 111:357.

253. Vartzopoulos D, Krull F. Dependence on monoamine oxidase inhibitors in high dose. Br J Psychiatry 1991; 158:856.

254. Dilsaver SC. Heterocyclic antidepressant, monoamine oxidase inhibitor and neuroleptic withdrawal phenomena. Prog Neuropsychopharmacol Biol Psychiatry 1990; 14:137.

255. Cohen MJ, Hanbury R, Stimmel B. Abuse of amitriptyline. JAMA 1978; 240:1372.

256. Cantor R. Methadone maintenance and amitriptyline. JAMA 1979; 241:2378.

257. Bialos D, Giller E, Jatlow P, et al. Recurrence of depression after long-term amitriptyline treatment. Am J Psychiatry 1982; 139:325.

258. Charney DS, Heninger GR, Sternberg DE, Landis H. Abrupt discontinuation of tricyclic antidepressant drugs—evidence for noradrenergic hyperactivity. Br J Psychiatry 1982; 141:377.

259. Siegfried K, Taeuber K. Pharmacodynamics of nomifensine: a review of studies in healthy subjects. J Clin Psychiatry 1984; 45:33.

260. Boning J, Fuchs G. Nomifensine and psychological dependence—a case report. Pharmacopsychiatry 1986; 19:386.

261. Charney DS, Heninger GR, Breier A. Noradrenergic function on panic anxiety. Effects of yohimbine in healthy subjects and patients with agoraphobia and panic disorder. Arch Gen Psychiatry 1984; 41:751.

262. Lader M, Bruce M. States of anxiety and their induction by drugs. Br J Clin Pharmacol 1986; 22:251.

263. Linden CH, Vellman WP, Rumrack B. Yohimbine: a new street drug. Ann Emerg Med 1985; 14:1002.

264. Siegel RK. Ginseng abuse syndrome. Problems with the panacea. JAMA 1979; 241:1614.

265. Lewin NA, Howland MA, Goldfrank LR. Herbal preparations. In: Goldfrank LR, Flomenbaum NE, Lewin NA, et al., eds. Toxicologic Emergencies, ed. 4. Norwalk, CT: Appleton & Lange, 1990:587.

266. Cawte J. Psychoactive substances of the South Seas: betal, kava and pituri. Aust NZ J Psychiatry 1985; 19:83.

267. Suwanlert S. A study of Kratom eaters in Thailand. Bull Narc 1975; 27:21.

268. Jansen KLR, Prast CJ. Psychoactive properties of mitragynine (Kratom). J Psychoact Drugs 1988; 20:455.

269. Siegel RK. Herbal intoxication. Psychoactive effects from herbal cigarettes, tea, and capsules. JAMA 1976; 236:473.

270. Rall TW. Drugs used in the treatment of asthma. In: Gilman AG, Rall TW, Nies AS, Taylor P, eds. The Pharmacological Basis of Therapeutics, ed 8. New York: Pergamon Press, 1990:618.

271. Lewin NA, Goldfrank LR, Melinek M, Weisman RS. Caffeine. In: Goldfrank LR, Flomenbaum NE, Lewin NA, et al, eds, Toxicologic Emergencies. ed 4. Norwalk, CT: Appleton & Lange, 1990:607.

272. Williams M, Jarvis MF. Adenosine antagonists as potential therapeutic agents. Pharmacol Biochem Behav 1988; 29:433.

273. Katz JL, Prada JA, Goldberg SR. Effects of adenosine analogs alone and in combination with caffeine in the squirrel monkey. Pharmacol Biochem Behav 1988; 29:429.

274. Holtzman SG, Finn IB. Tolerance to behavioral effects of caffeine in rats. Pharmacol Biochem Behav 1988; 29:411.

275. Mumford GK, Holtzman SG. Quantitative differences in the discriminative stimulus effects of low and high doses of caffeine in the rat. J Pharmacol Exp Ther 1991; 258:857.

276. Griffiths RR, Woodson PP. Reinforcing properties of caffeine: studies in humans and laboratory animals. Pharmacol Biochem Behav 1988; 29:419.

277. Myers MG. Effects of caffeine on blood pressure. Arch Intern Med 1988; 148:115.

278. Myers MG. Caffeine and cardiac arrhythmias. Chest 1988; 94:4.

279. Lutz EG. Restless legs, anxiety, and caffeinism. J Clin Psychiatry 1978; 39:693.

280. Charney DS, Heninger GR, Jatlow PI. Increased anxiogenic effects of caffeine in panic disorders. Arch Gen Psychiatry 1985; 42:233

281. Curatolo PW, Robertson D. The health consequences of caffeine. Ann Intern Med 1983; 98:641.

282. DiMaio VJM, Garriott JC. Lethal caffeine poisoning in a child. Forens Sci Int 1974; 3:275.

283. Turner JE, Cravey RH. A fatal ingestion of caffeine. Clin Toxicol 1977; 10:341.

284. Sullivan JL. Caffeine poisoning in an infant. J Pediatr 1977; 90:1022.

285. Banner W, Czajka PA. Acute caffeine overdose in a neonate. Am J Dis Child 1980; 134:495.

286. Eisele JW, Reay DT. Deaths related to coffee enemas. JAMA 1980; 244:1608.
287. Zimmerman PM, Pulliam J, Schwengels J, MacDonald SE. Caffeine intoxication. A near fatality. Ann Emerg Med 1985; 14:1227.
288. Garriott JC, Simmons LM, Poklis A, Mackell MA. Five cases of fatal overdose from caffeine-containing "look-alike" drugs. J Anal Toxicol 1985; 9:141.
289. Hughes JR, Higgins ST, Bickel WK, et al. Caffeine self-administration, withdrawal, and adverse effects among coffee drinkers. Arch Gen Psychiatry 1991; 48:611.
290. Silverman K, Evans SM, Strain EC, Griffiths RR. Withdrawal syndrome after the double-blind cessation of caffeine consumption. N Engl J Med 1992; 327:1110.
291. McGowan JD, Altman RE, Kanto WP. Neonatal withdrawal symptoms after chronic maternal ingestion of caffeine. South Med J 1988; 81:1092.
292. Russ NW, Sturgis ET, Malcolm RJ, Williams L. Abuse of caffeine in substance abusers. J Clin Psychiatry 1988; 49:457.
293. LaCroix AZ, Mead LA, Liang K-Y, et al. Coffee consumption and the incidence of coronary heart disease. N Engl J Med 1986; 315:977.
294. Dawber TR, Kannel WB, Gordon T. Coffee and cardiovascular disease. Observations from the Framingham Study. N Engl J Med 1974; 291:871.
295. Grobbee DE, Rimm EB, Giovannucci E, et al. Coffee, caffeine, and cardiovascular disease in men. N Engl J Med 1990; 323:1026.
296. Fried RE, Levine DM, Kwiterovich PO, et al. The effect of filtered-coffee consumption on plasma lipid levels. Results of a randomized clinical trial. JAMA 1992; 267:811.
297. Rudolphi KA, Keil M, Fastbom J, Fredholm BB. Ischaemic damage in gerbil hippocampus is reduced following upregulation of adenosine (A1) receptors by caffeine treatment. Neurosci Lett 1989; 103:275.
298. Li H, Bruederlin B, Buchan AM. Chronic caffeine protects hippocampal CA_1 cells from severe forebrain ischemia. Stroke 1991; 22:132.
299. Sutherland GR, Peeling J, Lesiuk HJ, et al. The effects of caffeine on ischemic neuronal injury as determined by magnetic resonance imaging and histopathology. Neuroscience 1991; 42:171.
300. Kiel DP, Felson DT, Hannan MT. Caffeine and the risk of hip fracture: the Framingham Study. Am J Epidemiol 1990; 132:675.

Chapter 4
Cocaine

If you are forward you will see who is the stronger,
a gentle little girl who doesn't eat enough or a big wild
man who has cocaine in his body.
—*Sigmund Freud to his fiancée Martha Bernays*

I would rather live ten years with coca than one million
centuries without coca.
—*Italian neurologist Paolo Mantegazza, 1859*

If coke is a lady, crack is a bitch.
—*Anonymous West Coast user*

Cocaine, the only naturally occurring local anesthetic, is also a central nervous system (CNS) stimulant (Figure 4–1). Pharmacologically it is similar to amphetamine and related psychostimulants (see Chapter 3). In the 1980s, cocaine became the most feared illicit drug in the United States. It thereby merits its own chapter.

Pharmacology and Animal Studies

In animals, cocaine produces an alerting response with increased exploration, locomotion, grooming, and rearing.[1,2] Repeated administration leads to stereotypic movements (*sensitization, reverse tolerance*) and seizures at previously subthreshold doses (*kindling*).[3,4] The basis of sensitization is unclear. It does not occur in animals prevented from moving or with continuous steady drug levels, and it can last months or years in animals or humans.[5] According to one hypothesis, sensitization results from decreased tonic inhibition of dopamine neurons in the midbrain ventral tegmental area (VTA) by dopamine D-2 autoreceptors and gamma-aminobutyric acid (GABA) receptors.[6,7] Cocaine's local anesthetic properties may contribute to seizures; similar kindling occurs with other local anesthetics that do not produce locomotor or stereotypic effects.[8,9] Excitatory amino acid neurotransmitters probably play an additional role in cocaine-induced seizures, which in mice were prevented by the N-methyl-D-aspartate (NMDA) receptor antagonists MK-801 and phencyclidine.[10] In rats, MK-801 prevented both seizures and stereotypy; haloperidol prevented stereotypy but not seizures.[11]

In contrast to these effects, other actions of cocaine in animals and humans—including cardiovascular effects and reward seeking—show tolerance, although not consistently.[2,12]

Cocaine is highly reinforcing in every species tested, using place preference, self-stimulation, and self-administration designs.[2] As with amphetamine, animals self-inject cocaine even when they receive electric shocks and in preference to food and water until they die.[2,13–15] In one experiment, rats self-administering heroin established a stable pattern of use with gradually increasing intake and preserved grooming, body weight, and general health; by contrast, rats self-administering cocaine did so erratically and excessively and tended to cease grooming, to lose weight, and to deteriorate in general health. After 30 days, mortality was 36% for the heroin animals and 90% for the cocaine animals.[16] Others have shown—with obvious relevance to human patterns of use—that when access in animals is limited to a few hours daily, stable regular patterns of self-injection ensue, but when access is unlimited, such stability disappears and the drug is taken erratically, excessively, and fatally.[17]

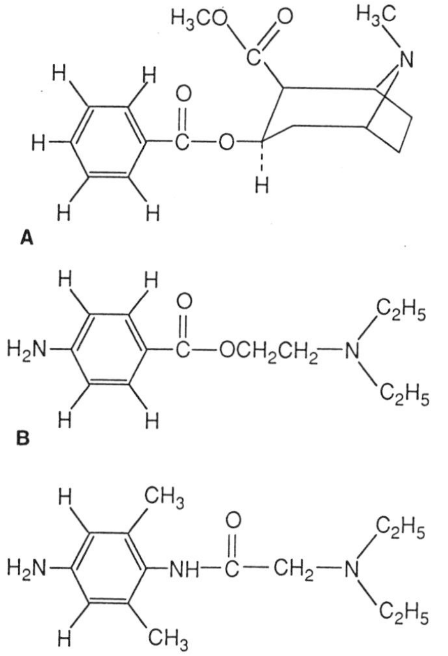

Figure 4–1. Cocaine (A), procaine (B), and lidocaine (C).

Self-administration studies of this type carry the confounding factor of direct cocaine effects, which produce increased responding independent of reinforcement. The dose-response curve of cocaine self-administration, moreover, is often an inverted U: At high doses, direct cocaine effects *reduce* response rates.[2] The problem of separating cocaine's direct stimulant effects from reinforcement per se can be circumvented by measuring the break point in progressive ratio schedules rather than the rate of responding.[18] In one such study, monkeys responded up to 12,800 times for each 0.48 mg/kg dose of cocaine.[19]

Cocaine's principal synaptic action is to block reuptake of dopamine, norepinephrine, and serotonin, acting through cocaine-binding sites on bioamine uptake transporters.[20–22] (Complementary DNAs for the cocaine-sensitive dopamine and norepinephrine transporters have been cloned and, interestingly, have homology to the GABA transporter.[23–25]) In addition, cocaine (like methylphenidate but unlike amphetamine) releases dopamine from granular storage vesicles.[26]

Several lines of evidence support the contention that dopamine in the nigrostriatal system mediates cocaine-induced stereotypy and that dopamine in the mesocorticolimbic reward system mediates cocaine euphoria and reinforcement. First, in discriminative stimulus (DS) studies, animals that have learned to discriminate cocaine from saline to obtain a reward generalize to other stimulants that share its dopaminergic effects (amphetamine, methamphetamine, diethylpropion, phenmetrazine, phentermine, cathinone, and methylphenidate) but not to stimulants that do not (fenfluramine, strychnine).[27,28] Partial substitution occurs with the direct dopamine agonists bromocriptine, amantadine, and piribedil,[2] and both the dopamine D-2 antagonists haloperidol and pimozide and the dopamine D-1 antagonist SCH23390 partially block cocaine DS.[28–30] Alpha-adrenergic and beta-adrenergic receptor blockers and acetylcholine and serotonin receptor blockers do not affect cocaine DS.[28] Consistent with cocaine's greater pharmacological resemblance to methylphenidate than to amphetamine (see Chapter 3), reserpine, which depletes dopamine from granular storage vesicles, blocks cocaine DS but not amphetamine DS,[2] and conversely alpha-methyltyrosine (AMT), which depletes newly formed dopamine, blocks amphetamine DS but not cocaine DS.[28] Some DS studies suggest that dopamine alone cannot account for all of cocaine's effects. Type B but not type A monoamine oxidase inhibitors substitute for cocaine DS, implying a role for beta-phenylethylamine.[31] In one study, procaine but not lidocaine partially substituted for cocaine,[32] whereas in another study, lidocaine partially substituted.[33]

Second are self-administration studies. Rats self-inject the dopamine D-2 receptor agonists apomorphine and piribedil,[34,35] and monkeys self-administer these agents but not the D-1 agonist SKF38393 or the noradrenergic uptake blocker nisoxetine.[36,37] Dogs do not self-administer the noradrenergic agonist methoxamine.[38] The potencies of cocaine and related drugs in self-administration studies correlate with their potencies in inhibiting the binding of [H-3]-mazindol to dopamine transport sites in rat striatum[39] and with extracellular release of dopamine in the nucleus accumbens (NA).[40] Dopamine receptor blockers (chlorpromazine, perphenazine, sulpiride, alpha-flupenthixol) alter cocaine self-administration by animals;[2] alpha-adrenergic and beta-adrenergic blockers do not.[37]

Third are lesion studies. 6-Hydroxydopamine lesions in the NA of rats decrease self-administration of cocaine but not of food or water and do not affect the descending limb of the dose-response curve (which reflects direct rate-decreasing effects of cocaine).[41] Lesions in the ventral pallidum (to which the NA projects) and the VTA (which projects to the NA) also disrupt cocaine self-administration.[42,43]

Fourth are studies involving intracranial self-administration. These have demonstrated maximal cocaine effects after injection into the prefrontal cortex (to which the VTA also projects).[44] Local injection of the dopamine antagonist sulpiride blocks such effects;[44] blockers of alpha-noradrenergic and beta-noradrenergic and cholinergic receptors do not.[45] It has been suggested that the prefrontal cortex initiates cocaine effects, whereas the NA maintains them.[2]

Fifth, cocaine acutely reduces the threshold current that maintains electrical self-stimulation of these reward areas in animals.[46]

Sixth, in rats low doses of cocaine selectively increased regional cerebral blood flow in the amygdala, ventral pallidum, olfactory tubercle, and medial prefrontal cortex, and higher doses increased blood flow in the nucleus accumbens.[46a]

Finally, studies in monkeys show close correspondence between the ability of different drugs to block dopamine reuptake, to displace radiolabeled cocaine from caudate-putamen binding sites, and to produce cocaine-like behavioral effects.[22,47]

Cocaine's rewarding properties involve both D-1 and D-2 dopamine receptors, but the relative importance of each is uncertain. Also involved are other neurotransmitter systems, including adrenergic (alpha-2-adrenoceptors) and serotonergic ($5-HT_{1A}$). L-dopa/carbidopa activates dopamine and noradrenergic systems but is not serotonergic, and it is not self-administered by animals or abused by humans. Purely serotonergic agonists or antagonists similarly lack rewarding properties. It has been proposed that serotonergic or other inputs to dopaminergic reward pathways augment the effects of dopamine reuptake blockade, contributing to euphoria.[48]

Opioids are also probably involved in cocaine's rewarding effects. Similar to cocaine, opioids increase extracellular dopamine levels in the NA,[50] and in rats, naloxone or naltrexone attenuates cocaine's effects on intracranial self-stimulation,[51] self-administration of low (but not high) doses of cocaine,[52] cocaine-induced locomotor activity, and place preference conditioning.[53] Postsynaptic opioid mu-receptors in the NA are down-regulated by dopamine denervation and up-regulated by chronic cocaine administration.[54,55] In mice, cocaine greatly enhances morphine analgesia,[56] and in rats, cocaine blocks the development of tolerance to morphine analgesia.[57]

Like methylphenidate (but unlike amphetamine), cocaine does not cause morphologic damage to dopamine nerve terminals.[26] However, cocaine does deplete dopamine in rat frontal cortex and hypothalamus and reduces tyrosine hydroxylase in rat striatum.[58,59] Some investigators attribute these reductions to supersensitivity of dopamine D-2 inhibitory autoreceptors.[60] In chronic cocaine abusers, increased prolactin and decreased homovanillic acid levels reflect decreased dopaminergic activity, and in animals, chronic cocaine administration eventually raises the threshold for intracranial electrical self-stimulation, consistent with dopaminergic down-regulation. Dopamine receptors are supersensitive in animals chronically receiving cocaine, and if inhibitory dopamine autoreceptors are more supersensitive than postsynaptic dopamine receptors, the net effect would be decreased dopaminergic neurotransmission.[49] (A potential paradox should be noted here: *Decreased* dopamine autoreceptor inhibition has been invoked to explain sensitization to cocaine effects.) Reduced serotonergic activity has also been observed in animals chronically receiving cocaine.[1] At a more basic level, cocaine, acting through dopamine D-1 receptors, increases the C-fos proto-oncogene, implying altered synaptic activity through effects on the cell nucleus.[61]

In contrast to amphetamine, cocaine depresses cerebral oxygen metabolism and decreases the amplitude of the P300 component of an auditory evoked response.[62] Perhaps related to its local anesthetic actions, cocaine is more likely than amphetamine to cause seizures after a single dose, yet in some settings it has anticonvulsant properties, and it produces electrical changes in the amygdala more resembling those caused by lysergic acid diethylamide (LSD) than by amphetamine.[62–64]

Following any route of administration, the plasma half-life of cocaine is about 40 to 60 minutes; it is detectable in urine for up to 36 hours.[65] Cocaine is metabolized by liver and plasma cholinesterases mainly to benzoylecgonine and ecgonine methyl ester, with smaller amounts of ecgonine, norcocaine, and other hydroxylated products.[66] Benzoylecgonine is itself a potent CNS stimulant and persists in the brain long after cocaine has disappeared.[67] It is usually detectable in plasma for 2 to 3 days but in heavy users has been identified after 3 weeks.[68] Fetuses, infants, elderly men, pregnant women, and patients with liver disease have low plasma cholinesterase levels and are sensitive to low doses of cocaine, as are those with congenital cholinesterase deficiency.[69]

Benzoylecgonine can be detected in hair after blood and urine tests have become negative. The procedure is time-consuming and costly, however.[70,71]

Historical Background and Epidemiology

Cocaine is obtained from the South American shrub, *Erythroxylon coca*, leaves of which have been chewed by South American Indians for many centuries.[2,72] (In an imaginative study, hair was analyzed from eight Chilean mummies dating between 2000 and 1500 BC; all were positive for benzoylecgonine.[73]) The Incas considered the coca plant a gift of the Sun God, and its use was restricted to priests and the ruling class. Following the conquest of the Incas by the Spanish in the 16th century, coca use was at first banned as idolatrous but later encouraged when it was recognized that Inca slaves worked harder when it was available. Then, as today, the leaves were chewed with lime or ash to increase the release of cocaine.

Perhaps because the plant decayed on passage from South America and was difficult to grow in the European climate, coca did not become popular in Europe until after the isolation of cocaine by Niemann in 1855. Vin Mariani, a coca wine developed by Angelo Mariani, became enormously popular in Europe and the United States; enthusiasts included President William McKinley, Thomas Edison, and the Czar of Russia, and Mariani received a medal of appreciation from the Pope. In 1886, John Pemberton of Georgia introduced Coca Cola, originally an elixir containing both cocaine and caffeine and promoted as a headache remedy and stimulant.[74] Alcohol was removed in 1888 and cocaine in 1906 (the year the Pure Food and Drug Act was passed).

In 1884, Sigmund Freud published "Ueber Coca," in which he referred to cocaine as "a far more potent and far less harmful stimulant than alcohol."[75] In this and later papers, Freud recommended cocaine as a stimulant and aphrodisiac and for treatment of digestive disorders, cachexia, asthma, and addiction to ethanol and morphine. It was Freud's colleague Karl Koller, however, who successfully developed cocaine as a local anesthetic, which quickly became recognized as its only legitimate medical use.[76] (It was as an anesthetic that cocaine came to the attention of the ophthalmologist A. Conan Doyle; Sherlock Holmes was a celebrated recreational user.) In the meantime, Freud had treated his friend Ernst Fleishl's morphine addiction with cocaine, only to convert Fleishl into a cocaine addict.[77] (In a reversed approach, the surgeon William Halsted treated his own cocaine addiction with morphine and became a morphine addict.[78]) As early as 1886, the Viennese chemist Erlenmeyer had labeled cocaine "the third scourge of humanity," along with ethanol

and morphine.[76] In 1914, the Harrison Narcotic Act banned the use of cocaine in proprietary medicines and strictly regulated its importation, manufacture, and medical use.

From the 1920s to the 1960s, recreational use of cocaine in the United States was largely restricted to jazz musicians, actors, and the "cultural avant garde."[72] Its cost limited spread and made it a status drug for the affluent. In the early 1970s, there began a steady rise in the prevalence of cocaine use that continued over the next two decades.[79] The number of Americans who had tried cocaine at least once rose from 5.4 million in 1974 to 21.6 million in 1982, including up to 20% of high school seniors and 28% of those aged 18 to 25.[80,81] It was estimated that if the cocaine industry were included in American corporate listings, it would, with at least 27 billion dollars annual gross income, rank seventh, between Gulf Oil and the Ford Motor Company.[82]

The appearance in 1985 of commercially manufactured alkaloidal cocaine ("crack") led to acceleration of the epidemic and with it lawlessness and violence in American cities reminiscent of Prohibition in the 1920s. By 1988, in the United States there were 5000 new cocaine users daily, 6 million people were regular users, and nearly 1 million were "compulsive users."[83]

Estimates of cocaine-related fatality have been based on figures from the Center for Disease Control's National Center for Health Statistics (NCHS), which monitors death certificates, and the Drug Abuse Warning Network (DAWN), which surveys hospital emergency rooms and medical examiners' and coroners' offices. During the 6-year period 1983 to 1988, NCHS reported that cocaine-related deaths increased fivefold, from 218 to 1179, with a total of 3466. During the same period, DAWN reported a sixfold increase in deaths, from 314 to 1952, with a total of 6057. Seventy-nine percent of NCHS deaths and 69% of DAWN deaths were attributed to poisoning; the rest were ascribed to injury or disease.[84] A review of forensic cases from Arizona, Utah, Virginia, New York City, Michigan, and San Diego implied even higher mortality rates than these federal estimates would indicate;[85-91] for example, of 151 cocaine intoxication deaths reported by the New York City Medical Examiner during 1986, only 7 were identified by NCHS.[88]

In 1986, one-third of male homicides in Manhattan were drug related.[92] In New York City in 1987, more than 40% of all felony indictments were for drug law violations, and a 1988 study by the National Institute of Justice in 10 large American cities revealed that one-half to three-quarters of all arrestees were taking illicit drugs (excluding marijuana).[93,94] During 1989 in Atlanta, Georgia, 40% of 224 homicide victims tested had cocaine metabolites in their blood.[95] In Memphis, 46 of 84 cocaine-related deaths were homicides, and cocaine metabolites were present in 17% of all homicide victims.[96]

Violence is related to drug abuse in three different ways.[97] *Pharmacological violence* refers to violent behavior induced by the drugs themselves. *Economic compulsive violence* refers to violent crime committed to obtain drugs. *Systemic violence* refers to violence intrinsic to the lifestyles and business methods of drug traffickers. Although most ethanol-related violence is pharmacological in origin, cocaine-related violence is overwhelmingly of the systemic type.[98]

From 1984 to 1987, one-fourth of New York City drivers aged 16 to 45 who died in automobile accidents had cocaine or a metabolite in blood or urine.[99]

Increased cocaine consumption in the United States occurred despite enormous expenditures that were mainly targeted at crop eradication in South America, interdiction at United States borders, and local law enforcement. During 1990, federal expenditures for the "War on Drugs" amounted to nearly $10 billion, of which nearly $4 billion were for criminal justice activities and more than $2 billion were for drug interdiction programs.[100] (A high point of the latter effort was the military kidnapping and extradition on drug trafficking charges of the Chief of State of Panama—an event apparently without historical precedent.)

Approximately 2.5 million square miles of South American land are potentially cultivatable for coca; approximately 700 square miles are currently being used for that purpose.[94] By the 1990s, as military pressure was increasing against distribution centers in Medellin, Colombia, and cultivation areas in Peru and Bolivia, distribution shifted to the Colombian city of Cali, and both cultivation and distribution spread to other South American countries, including Venezuela, Brazil, Ecuador, Uruguay, and Suriname.[101] (*Erythroxylon coca* also grows abundantly in Mexico, the West Indies, and Indonesia.[102]) As for interdiction, cocaine is easy to smuggle (in contrast to bulky marijuana), and huge profits provide big incentives. In 1991, 1 kg of cocaine purchased for $1200 in Colombia sold wholesale in the United States for approximately $20,000; after conversion to "crack," its retail value (at about $5.00 per vial) was roughly three times that amount.[103]

Despite the evident futility of eradication, interdiction, and jailing of "drug kingpins," casual use of cocaine, estimated by the National Household Survey, and high school use, estimated by the High School Senior Survey, peaked during the mid-1980s[104,105] The decline was likely related to growing middle class awareness of cocaine's addictive liability and lethal effects (e.g., the death of the athlete Len Bias). In other words, the major factor was reduced demand—the result of education and changing attitudes, including the predictable decline of a fad—rather than reduced supply.[106] Indeed, although federal appropriations for drug control were targeted at interdiction, cocaine continued to be plentiful and cheap throughout the "War on Drugs," and compulsive use, especially within inner cities—the poor, the homeless, high school dropouts, and arrestees—did not decline at all.[105,107,108] In 1991, the number of Americans who used cocaine at least weekly was estimated at 1.75 to 1.9 million—a 29% increase from the year before—and during the early 1990s cocaine-related emergency room visits reported to DAWN rose steadily—30% in 1991 and 12% in the first three months of 1992.[104,105,108a] (In 1991 a survey of 23 American medical schools revealed that 2.8% of senior medical students had used cocaine during the previous 30 days.[109])

Preparation and Methods of Use

Cocaine is effective orally, and its absorption by South American natives who chew coca leaves is probably from swallowed saliva as well as across oral mucous membranes. Harvested leaves are soaked in alkali; kerosene and sulfuric acid (and sometimes potassium permanganate) are then added, producing semisolid "coca-paste," which contains alkaloidal ("free-base") cocaine, plus impurities. Coca-paste ("bazooka") is widely smoked in South America, and, less commonly, in Panama, the Caribbean, the Netherlands, and the United States.[110] Further refining produces cocaine hydrochloride, which is then adulterated with inactive substances such as mannitol, boric acid, lactose, dextrose, sucrose, inositol, talc, flour, or corn starch, and active substances such as procaine, lidocaine, benzocaine, ephedrine, amphetamine, phenylpropanolamine, caffeine, or strychnine.[67,111] Street preparations ("snow," "flake," "coke," "girl," "lady," "dama blanca," "blow," "jam," "happy trails," "rock," "nose candy," "leaf," "gold," "dust") sell by the gram, with purity ranging from 7% to 100%.[67]

When cocaine is inhaled nasally (snorting), users usually lay out a "line" of powder (20 to 50 mg) and sniff it through a straw.[112] It can also be taken parenterally, usually intravenously; more than 80% of New York City heroin users concomitantly inject cocaine ("speedball").[113] Because cocaine hydrochloride is destroyed at very high temperatures, smoking requires conversion back to "free base," which before the emergence of "crack" was made from cocaine hydrochloride using commercially available extraction kits. To make "free-base," cocaine hydrochloride is dissolved in water and converted to the alkaloidal form by adding a strong base such as ammonium hydroxide. The alkaloid is extracted with an organic solvent such as petroleum ether, and the free base is then crystallized. In the process, most adulterants are left behind.[114] The preparation of crack is even simpler: Adding baking soda or sodium bicarbonate to cocaine hydrochloride in heated water precipitates alkaloidal cocaine, which is then dried by evaporation into a cake-like solid. In this process, adulterants are more likely to be co-precipitated. (The basis of the term *crack* is disputed. One version is that the small "rocks" sold are "cracked" off larger pieces. Another is that when smoked in a pipe, it makes a crackling sound.) Usually 50 to 120 mg of free base or "crack" is inhaled per "hit," sometimes repeated every few minutes in binges (resembling amphetamine "runs") lasting 30 minutes to 96 hours. Sometimes single binges last days, separated by a few days of abstinence. During binges, all thoughts are focused on the drug; food, sleep, family, and even survival become secondary.[49] Tolerance leads to higher doses, and 3000 mg have been taken in a single "hit."[67]

Intranasal snorting of 96 mg cocaine hydrochloride produced peak plasma levels of 150 to 200 ng/mL. Intravenous injection of 32 mg cocaine produced peak levels of 300 ng/mL. Chronic smoking of alkaloidal cocaine produced plasma levels of 800 to 900 ng/mL 3 hours after smoking.[115]

Cocaine has also been taken rectally, sublingually, vaginally, and intraurethrally, and sudden death has followed such routes of administration.[116–118] Seizures and death have even followed topical application of TAC (tetracaine, adrenaline, cocaine) solution to wounds or mucous membranes.[119] The slow rise in tissue levels achieved by oral cocaine probably explains its unpopularity, even though levels are eventually as high as by other routes.[120]

A special form of administration is "body packing," in which smuggled cocaine is swallowed or inserted rectally in packets wrapped with latex, and "body stuffing," in which packaged cocaine is more hurriedly swallowed to avoid detection. Rupture of packets in the gastrointestinal tract of smugglers ("mules") has caused severe toxicity, sometimes fatal, and bowel obstruction has required surgery.[121]

Acute Effects

Injected or smoked cocaine produces, similar to amphetamine, a brief "rush," peaking at one-half to 2 minutes and followed by euphoria, excitement, garrulousness, and a sense of increased mental and physical powers.[49,122] Experienced users are often unable to tell the drugs apart except that cocaine's effects are shorter lived, lasting usually 20 to 40 minutes.[123,124] (The rapid transit time from lung to brain—5 to 10 seconds—means cocaine smoking can produce an even more intense "rush" than intravenous use.[125]) Snorted cocaine produces qualitatively similar stimulation for up to 90 minutes without the initial "rush," peaking at about 30 minutes and lasting about 1 hour.[122] (Snorted cocaine limits its own absorption by causing vasoconstriction of the nasal mucosa.) As with amphetamine, a cocaine user's sense of increased mental power is not borne out with objective testing.[123]

Low doses of cocaine slow the heart rate (because of vagal stimulation); higher doses cause symptoms and signs of sympathetic overactivity: tachycardia, tachypnea, and hypertension. (In dogs, the hypertensive response to cocaine is reduced by pretreatment with the ganglionic blocker hexamethonium, suggesting that cocaine increases sympathetic activity through CNS actions.[126]) In rats, cocaine's pressor effects depend on alpha-1-adrenergic vasoconstriction and are two-phased, with a centrally mediated initial peak response and a peripherally-mediated sustained but more modest response.[126a,126b] Skin pallor is secondary to vasoconstriction. Other symptoms of mild to moderate overdose are most often cardiopulmonary, psychiatric, or neurological and can occur alone or together (Table 4–1). Of 233 visits to Grady Memorial Hospital in Atlanta for "cocaine-related medical problems," the most common symptoms were chest pain (40%) (most often considered nonischemic), shortness of breath (22%), palpitations (21%), anxiety (22%), dizziness (13%), and headache (12%). Only 10% of patients required admission.[127]

More severe symptoms can be life-threatening, and some, including psychiatric and neurological, show sensitization (reverse tolerance) with repeated cocaine use.[128–132] Patients may be agitated, combative, paranoid, depressed, lethargic, or comatose.

Table 4–1. Acute Toxic Effects of Cocaine

Cardiopulmonary
  Chest pain
  Shortness of breath
  Palpitations
  Diaphoresis
  Pulmonary edema
  Cardiac arrhythmia
  Myocardial infarction
  Cardiac arrest

Psychiatric
  Anxiety
  Insomnia
  Paranoia
  Agitation, violence
  Depression, suicide
  Hallucinations
  Psychosis

Neurological
  Dizziness, syncope
  Vertigo
  Paresthesias
  Headache
  Tremor
  Stereotypy
  Bruxism
  Chorea
  Dystonia
  Myoclonus
  Seizures
  Lethargy
  Coma
  Ischemic or hemorrhagic stroke

Other
  Throat tightness
  Blurred vision (mydriasis)
  Nasal congestion
  Nausea, vomiting
  Abdominal pain
  Weakness
  Fever
  Chills
  Myalgia
  Back pain
  Rhabdomyolysis

Modified from Brody SL, Slovis CM, Wrenn KD. Cocaine-related medical problems: Consecutive series of 233 patients. Am J Med 1990; 88:325, with permission of the publisher.

There may be hyperreflexia, tremor, stereotypic movements, dystonia, chorea, myoclonus, or seizures. Metabolic acidosis can be marked, and cardiac arrhythmia or pulmonary edema can precede cardiac arrest. In the Atlanta series, the heart rate ranged from 34 to 168/minute, the systolic blood pressure from 70 to 240 mm Hg, and the respiratory rate from 6 to 50/minute.[127] Fever can be high enough to suggest heat stroke, and rhabdomyolysis causes renal failure.[133–141] Disseminated intravascular coagulation has occurred.[142]

Migraine-like headaches, sometimes accompanied by hemiparesis or vertigo, are especially common during cocaine binges, whether snorting, smoking, or parenterally injecting.[143,144] They are often promptly relieved by additional cocaine, perhaps attributable to blockade of serotonin reuptake.[145] Dependency developed in a patient who began using cocaine as a treatment for migraine.[146]

In volunteers, 4-hour infusions of cocaine induced suspiciousness,[147] and chronic users are increasingly likely to develop pathological behavior.[148] At first there is irritability, hyperactivity, impaired interpersonal relations, and disturbed eating and sleeping. Symptoms then progress to anxiety, stereotypic compulsive behavior, confusion, paranoia, and frank psychosis. Hallucinations are visual ("snow lights"), auditory, gustatory, olfactory, or tactile ("cocaine bugs," the sensation of insects crawling beneath the skin).[1,2,60] Psychosis occurs regardless of predrug personality. During an epidemic of freebase use in the Bahamas, paranoia and bizarre violent behavior in some patients lasted several weeks.[149] Similar protracted psychopathology accompanied an epidemic of coca paste smoking in Peru.[150] A patient receiving repeated topical anesthesia containing 3 mL of 10% cocaine developed psychosis that lasted 60 hours.[151]

Seizures occur immediately or within a few hours of cocaine administration with or without other signs of toxicity.[152–159,159a] Single major motor seizures are most common, but focal seizures occur, and status epilepticus is sometimes refractory to anticonvulsant therapy. Among 32 cases of cocaine-related seizures seen at San Francisco General Hospital, routes of administration included intranasal, intravenous, smoking, and oral, and seizures occurred from 10 minutes to "under 24 hours" after use.[158] Nine patients used additional drugs, including marijuana, amphetamine, phencyclidine, and methylphenidate, and LSD. Of 474 patients seen at Hennepin County Medical Center in Minneapolis for acute cocaine intoxication, 44 (9.3%) had seizures within 90 minutes of cocaine use.[159] In 32, seizures were new onset, and of these the great majority were induced by either intravenous or "crack" cocaine. In 12, seizures occurred in patients who had had previous seizures unrelated to cocaine, and among these patients intranasal use was more common than intravenous or "crack" cocaine. In both groups, 40% of seizures followed first-time cocaine use.

In a subsequent report from Minneapolis, seizures occurred in 98 (10%) of 945 patients admitted for cocaine intoxication, with striking sex differences: 18.4% of women but only 6.2% of men had seizures. Patients with single generalized seizures (the most common type) all had normal cranial CT scans and electroencephalography. Patients with new onset focal seizures had evidence of cerebral infarction or hemorrhage. Four patients with status epilepticus had ingested massive (2 to 8gm) doses of cocaine, were resistant to treatment, and had considerable morbidity and mortality.[159b]

The prevalence of seizures among cocaine-intoxicated patients is higher in the Minneapolis series than in others. At Bronx Municipal Hospital in New York, only 4 of 283 (1.4%) hospitalized cocaine users had seizures,[155] and at San Francisco General Hospital, seizures occurred in 29 of 1275 (2.3%) cocaine users.[153] Phone surveys of users detect much higher seizure prevalences.[160] A large survey of adolescent drug abusers in Virginia found that seizures occurred in none of the intranasal cocaine users, in 1% of "experimental" crack smokers, and in 9% of heavy crack smokers.[161] In a case-control series of new onset seizures from Harlem Hospital Center, cocaine use was not identified as a risk factor; the reasons for this surprising finding are probably that only incident (new onset) seizures were included and the study was conducted before the advent of "crack."[162] In fact, the Harlem Hospital study would have excluded most of the patients reported from Minneapolis.

A young woman who smoked "crack" over 3 days developed bizarre behavior that turned out to be complex partial status epilepticus, a diagnosis easy to overlook in patients with other reasons for behavioral abnormality.[163]

Relevant to the observation that seizures sometimes occur several hours or more after use of cocaine are studies in rats that demonstrate epileptogenicity of the cocaine metabolite benzoylecgonine. In contrast to cocaine-induced seizures, those associated with benzoylecgonine had longer latencies and less often resulted in death.[163a]

Acute dystonia and chorea following cocaine use have lasted minutes to a few days and in some instances have emerged during early abstinence.[164-167] Cocaine reportedly exacerbated symptoms in a patient with idiopathic dystonia and in another with neuroleptic-induced tardive dystonia.[167a] Haloperidol has precipitated acute dystonia in heavy cocaine users,[168] and patients with Tourette's syndrome, well controlled with haloperidol, have developed severe tics and vocalizations after using cocaine intranasally.[169-171] Tics have also followed cocaine use in previously asymptomatic patients.[170] Diffuse myoclonus and opsoclonus followed cocaine snorting in a young woman, clearing over 4 weeks.[172]

Rhabdomyolysis can occur without other symptoms or signs of toxicity and has been attributed to muscle ischemia.[133] In one case, it recurred with repeated cocaine use.[141] Elevated serum creatine kinase and even myoglobinuria can occur in the absence of any muscle symptoms.[173-176] Combined muscle and skin infarction has also been reported.[177]

The lethal dose of cocaine in human novices is about 500 to 800 mg but is quite variable and can follow any route of administration.[123,178] As much as 14 g alkaloidal cocaine has been smoked daily without serious complications, yet death has followed intravenous injection of only 20 mg. In rats, the lethal dose ranges from 35 to 100 mg/kg and in dogs from 16.5 to 24.4 mg/kg. Postmortem blood levels in human overdose have ranged from 1 to 25 μg/ml.[179] A young man who died after swallowing a bag of cocaine to avoid arrest had a blood level of 212 mg/L.[180] Sudden death may be from ventricular fibrillation or, rarely, anaphylactic response to impurities.[128,131] Patients with blood levels much lower than those associated with true overdose have suddenly died following delirium and extreme hyperthermia resembling the neuroleptic malignant syndrome.[181,182] (A patient with a rectal temperature of 114°F survived.[183]) Such patients tend to have dystonic movements rather than muscular rigidity.[184] In some fatalities, autopsy has revealed pulmonary edema and ascites, perhaps neurogenic in origin.[185]

Other drugs could play a role in cocaine-related fatalities, and psychosis predisposes to violence, accidental death, and suicide.[186-190] Of 925 persons dying in New York City with cocaine in their bodies, death was attributed to cocaine overdose in 4% and to combined cocaine and heroin overdose in 12%; 38% were attributed to homicide, 7% to suicide, and 8% to accidents.[88] It is estimated that 60% to 80% of cocaine users consume ethanol at the same time.[191] Users have taken cocaine with organophosphates—creating their own pseudocholinesterase deficiency to prolong the drug's half-life.[102] Cocaine toxicity is also enhanced by concomitant use of monoamine oxidase inhibitors, cyclic antidepressants, phenylpropanolamine, alpha-methyldopa, and reserpine.[102]

Treatment of Overdose

Treatment of cocaine overdose depends on symptoms and signs and may require sedation, bicarbonate for acidosis, artificial ventilation, oxygen, blood pressure support, antihypertensives, cardiac monitoring, or antiarrhythmia drugs.[152] Urinary acidification accelerates excretion but is contraindicated if myoglobinuria is present.[128] Hyperthermia can be treated with an ice water bath and a fan, plus sedation.[122]

The choice of specific medications is controversial, for animal studies are conflicting and human studies anecdotal. In rats, dogs, swine, and primates, diazepam and other sedatives prevent seizures and death.[192–195] Neuroleptics, which would theoretically have antidopaminergic, antiadrenergic, sedative, and antihyperthermic effects, are less obviously helpful. In cocaine-intoxicated primates, chlorpromazine unexpectedly raised rather than lowered the seizure threshold.[195] In dogs, all animals developed seizures, yet chlorpromazine prevented mortality.[196] In rats, haloperidol, a dopamine D-2 antagonist, had no effect on cocaine lethality, and the D-1 antagonist SCH23390 was effective only if given before the cocaine.[197] In swine, haloperidol did not prevent cocaine-induced seizures.[194] In human volunteers, domperidone, a D-2 antagonist, did not prevent cocaine-induced hypertension, tachycardia, or elevated catecholamine levels in subjects at rest and with exercise actually aggravated these responses, a finding of obvious relevance to agitated patients.[198]

In mice, propranolol reduced pulmonary edema and ascites and improved survival.[185] Reports on the use of propranolol in humans have been conflicting, however; in some cases, nonselective beta blockade seems to have left alpha stimulation unopposed, causing a further increase in blood pressure.[62,199] Such an effect might be preventable by using combined beta and alpha blockade (e.g., labetolol) or selective beta-1 blockade (e.g., metoprolol).[128,200–202] Case reports claiming efficacy of labetolol, however, are countered by animal studies showing no benefit,[194,203] and seven cocaine-intoxicated patients had no benefit from the short-acting beta-blocker esmolol, with side effects—exacerbation of hypertension, hypotension, and lethargy and vomiting— developing in three.[204] On the basis of such reports, vasodilators such as nitroprusside or alpha-adrenergic blockers such as phentolamine have been recommended for cocaine-induced hypertensive crisis.[122]

Animal studies with calcium channel blockers have also been conflicting. In one report, nitrendipine suppressed cardiac arrhythmias and seizures and increased survival in cocaine-intoxicated rats.[205] In another study, pretreatment of rats with diltiazem, nifedipine, or verapamil potentiated seizures and death.[206] (In that study, both calcium channel blockers and cocaine were given intraperitoneally, raising the possibility that local vasodilation increased cocaine absorption.)

In mice acute cocaine lethality was reduced by the opioid partial agonist buprenorphine but not by the pure antagonists naloxone or naltrexone, suggesting that buprenorphine might be useful in cases of combined heroin-cocaine ("speedball") toxicity.[206a] Other reportedly beneficial agents are pancuronium (which prevented fatalities in dogs without affecting cardiovascular signs)[192,196] and tricyclic antidepressants (which, despite aggravation of some effects, decreased cocaine's cardiac actions in rats).[207] Lidocaine exacerbated seizures and death in cocaine-intoxicated rats.[208]

On the basis of such studies, Goldfrank and Hoffman[122] recommend that cocaine-intoxicated patients receive oxygen and sedation with a benzodiazepine (Table 4–2). Hypertension is treated with nitroprusside or phentolamine (or if the patient is pregnant hydralazine). Myocardial ischemia is treated with nitrates and calcium channel blockers or combined alpha-adrenergic and beta-adrenergic blockade. Calcium channel blockers or combined alpha-adrenergic and beta-adrenergic blockade are appropriate for patients with atrial tachyarrhythmia; combined alpha-adrenergic and beta-adrenergic blockade, lidocaine, or sodium bicarbonate is appropriate for those with ventricular tachyarrhythmia.

Recovery from cocaine overdose is usually within a few hours unless there is hypoxic-ischemic brain damage.[128]

Table 4–2. Treatment of Cocaine Overdose

Sedation with benzodiazepine
Oxygen
Bicarbonate for acidosis
Anticonvulsants (diazepam, phenobarbital, or phenytoin)
Antihypertensives (nitroprusside, phentolamine, or hydralazine)
Artificial ventilation
Blood pressure support
Cardiac monitoring
    For atrial arrhythmia: cooling if febrile, calcium channel blockers or combined alpha- and beta-adrenergic blockade
    For ventricular arrhythmia: combined alpha- and beta-adrenergic blockade, sodium bicarbonate, lidocaine
Urinary acidification (unless already acidosis or rhabdomyolysis)
For hyperthermia: ice water bath, fan, sedation

Modified from Goldfrank LR, Hoffman RS. The cardiovascular effects of cocaine. Ann Emerg Med 1991; 20:165, with permission of the publisher.

When other drugs are taken with cocaine, they confuse the clinical picture and complicate treatment.[112,209] Ethanol reportedly enhances cocaine toxicity, perhaps because in the presence of ethanol cocaine is metabolized to cocaethylene, which binds to the dopamine transporter and blocks dopamine reuptake as avidly as cocaine itself.[191,210] Cocaine is often injected with heroin, and heroin-cocaine mixtures are smoked.[112] Volunteers receiving intravenous cocaine and morphine combinations had cardiovascular effects similar to those caused by cocaine alone and subjective effects reflecting the particular "highs" of each drug.[210a] Methadone maintenance patients frequently use cocaine,[211] which both acutely and chronically reduces the severity of naloxone-precipitated opioid withdrawal.[212] Parenteral cocaine users and crack smokers often take sedatives to induce sleep.[67] Crack cocaine is also often smoked with marijuana ("grimmie"), tobacco ("caviar" or "cavies"), or phencyclidine ("whack" or "spacebase").[114]

Dependence and Withdrawal

The "high" of snorted or intravenous cocaine usually lasts less than an hour and is followed by fatigue and depression. Effects of intramuscular or subcutaneous injection are longer lasting, whereas those of smoking are more intense but shorter.[67] In volunteers, 4-hour cocaine infusions maintained the drug euphoric "high" but not the initial "rush"; haloperidol pretreatment did not affect the cocaine "rush" but partially attenuated the euphoric "high."[213]

As with amphetamine, there seems to be tolerance for subjective and cardiovascular effects, including lethality, and reverse tolerance or sensitization for psychosis, stereotypic movements, and seizures.[123,214] In one study, a single intranasal 96-mg dose produced acute tolerance to heart rate and subjective effects.[215] Another study found tolerance to heart rate but not to pressor effects.[216] Another found tolerance to neither.[217] Panic attacks following cocaine snorting have emerged after years of daily use, sometimes persisting after the drug was stopped.[218]

Signs of physical dependence are difficult to demonstrate, and abrupt discontinuation of cocaine is not dangerous. Chronic use causes abstinence symptoms, however, and these have been divided into three phases.[49] In phase one—the "crash"—there is an abrupt decline in mood and energy, with depression, anxiety, agitation, and drug craving. Suspiciousness and paranoia are common. Over the next few hours, cocaine craving decreases, replaced by exhaustion and the desire for sleep. Users often take sedatives, ethanol, marijuana, or opioids at this point, and when sleep is achieved, there is rapid eye movement rebound and frequent awakening, with continued depressed mood and hunger.[62] Hypersomnolence may last several days. Phase two then emerges, a protracted period of dysphoria, lack of motivation, and a return of cocaine craving, which may be intensified by environmental (conditioned) cues. If abstinence is maintained, dysphoria lasts up to 12 weeks. During phase three, dysphoria clears, but intermittent conditioned cocaine craving can continue for months or years.[49]

Depression in cocaine users thus has several causes. It may be a preexisting condition being "treated" with cocaine, a psychological reaction to inability to overcome addiction, or a physiologic feature of cocaine withdrawal. Suicide by cocaine overdose is probably underreported.[190]

Patterns of cocaine use include experimental (short-term), recreational (in social settings), circumstantial (to stimulate work or relieve depression), intensified (3 to 20 times daily), and compulsive ("dominates the individual's life and precludes other social functioning").[112] Recreational intranasal users are usually able to titrate and control their doses without escalation, and although insomnia, lassitude, irritability, anxiety, rhinitis, and weight loss are common, toxic psychosis is not. Intravenous users and smokers are likely to escalate use—sometimes at a cost of thousands of dollars per week—and to develop psychopathology and impaired social functioning. Variably present are chronic headache, exhaustion, tremor, grimacing, paranoia, hallucinations (visual, auditory, olfactory, and tactile), panic attacks, and sometimes violent or suicidal behavior.[219] Psychosocial disruption is not dependent on route of administration, however. Before the appearance of "crack," it was estimated that the average duration from first cocaine use to functional deterioration was 4 years in adults and 18 months in adolescents.[220] A more recent survey of adolescent users found that more than half progressed to at least weekly use.[221]

Cocaine Substitutes

Local anesthetics have reinforcing effects in animals,[222] and in human volunteers, intravenous procaine produced a "high" and was misidentified as cocaine.[223] Intranasal lidocaine also reportedly caused a cocaine-like "high" in humans, but in that study a placebo effect could not be excluded.[224] Although such drugs do not appear to be deliberately abused by humans, they are commonly used to adulterate or even substitute for cocaine in street preparations and could contribute to complications such as psychosis or seizures.[111,225] They (and other adulterants) may be present in "crack."[226] Thallium poisoning occurred in three subjects after snorting what they believed was cocaine.[227]

Other "cocaine substitutes," legally sold in paraphernalia stores as incenses but usually taken intranasally, include such products as "Cocaine Snuff" (caffeine and citric acid), "Coca Leaf Incense" (procaine, tetracaine, and caffeine), "Cokesnuff" (ground tobacco, menthol), "Ma-Huang Incense" (ephedrine), and "Yocaine Snuff" (yohimbine hydrochloride, coryanthine).[228] Conversely, "Health Inca Tea" and "Mate De Coca," commercially available in health food stores, do contain cocaine (despite disclaimers by the sellers) and have been abused.[229,230]

Other Medical and Neurological Complications

Because of vasoconstriction, chronic intranasal cocaine causes rhinitis, anosmia, epistaxis, and rarely perforated nasal septum, cerebrospinal fluid rhinorrhea, iritis, midline nasopharyngeal ulceration, osteolytic sinusitis with bilateral optic neuropathy, and even brain abscess.[128,231–235] Wound botulism, with dysphagia, dysarthria, diplopia, and descending paralysis, has affected parenteral cocaine users;[238,239] in addition, botulism has accompainied maxillary sinusitis in intranasal users.[238,239] A contributing factor might be local vasoconstriction and reduced tissue oxygen tension.

"Crack" smokers develop hoarseness, tracheobronchitis with dark sputum, dyspnea, and impaired pulmonary function. Oropharyngeal and tracheal thermal injury have occurred, as have pneumomediastinum, pneumopericardium, bronchiolitis obliterans, organizing pneumonia, and alveolar hemorrhage.[240] A telltale sign of crack smoking is madarosis—loss of eyebrow and eyelash hair.[241]

Acute cocaine enhances sexual drive—indeed, such linkage was depicted in the sexually explicit pottery and sculpture of the Peruvian Moche culture 1000 years before the Incas.[242] Both men and women frequently combine cocaine with ethanol for sexual enhancement.[243] Chronic use, however, causes hyperprolactinemia, decreased libido, impotence, and gynecomastia, which can persist for months after abstinence.[244] In eight cocaine-using men, blood levels of prolactin were elevated, whereas levels of luteinizing hormone, testosterone, and cortisol were normal.[245] It is possible that hyperprolactinemia contributes not only to sexual dysfunction, but also to impaired immune function.[246]

Cocaine unmasked and then exacerbated myasthenia gravis in a young snorting woman.[247] The cause may have been cocaine's local anesthetic actions on motor nerves coupled with decreased end plate reserve.

Cocaine hepatotoxicity is probably secondary to the metabolite norcocaine, which binds to hepatic proteins; it is produced in greater amounts in subjects with pseudocholinesterase deficiency. Ethanol potentiates cocaine-induced liver disease.[2]

Cocaine precipitated acute symptoms in a patient with variegate porphyria.[248]

Cocaine is an immunosuppressant, and intravenous cocaine users are at greater risk for endocarditis than are parenteral abusers of other drugs.[249] Parenteral cocaine users are also at particular risk for acquired immunodeficiency syndrome (AIDS) and perhaps other retroviral infections, for the drug is often taken in "shooting galleries" with shared needles and paraphernalia.[250,251] In addition, "crack" smoking is a risk factor for AIDS and other sexually transmitted diseases, including syphilis, gonorrhea, chlamydia, herpes simplex, and hepatitis B.[252–255] "Crack dens" are centers of promiscuity; sexual services are exchanged for drugs, and genital ulcers facilitate transmission of human immunodeficiency virus (HIV).[250,256,257] Enormous increases in the prevalence of syphilis and other sexually transmitted diseases paralleled the crack epidemic of the 1980s.

Although acute chest pain after cocaine use is usually noncardiac in origin,[258] it signifies myocardial infarction in up to one-third of such patients, who are often young and lack other evidence of coronary artery disease.[259,260] By 1991, 114 cases of cocaine-induced myocardial infarction had been reported, and of the 92 who received angiography or autopsy, 35 (age range 21 to 60 years, average 32) had normal coronary arteries. Most were also moderate to heavy cigarette smokers.[261] In several cases, symptoms of cardiac ischemia recurred when cocaine use was resumed.[262] Cardiac catheterization studies demonstrate that cocaine causes coronary artery constriction in humans,[263] and in dogs, cocaine increases myocardial oxygen demand while simultaneously preventing compensatory coronary artery vasodilation.[126] Cocaine also promotes coronary thrombosis in the absence of coronary artery constriction.[264] Episodic electrocardiographic evidence of myocardial ischemia persisted for several weeks after cessation of heavy chronic cocaine use in 8 of 21 subjects.[265] A middle-aged man had a myocardial infarction 3 days after he stopped using cocaine.[266]

Cocaine users also develop myocardial contraction band necrosis, myocarditis, and dilated cardiomyopathy.[267–271] Cocaine also acutely depresses myocardial function, perhaps independently of ischemia. In dogs cocaine decreased coronary artery diameter and left ventricular ejection fraction; when ethanol was given, myocardial function decreased further without additional coronary vasoconstriction. Fatal arrhythmia, including asystole, ventricular tachycardia, and ventricular fibrillation, results from combinations of increased sympathetic tone, local anesthetic effects, myocardial ischemia, and myocarditis.[2,122,152,267,272,273] Syncope, which is common following acute cocaine use, is probably cardiogenic in many instances.[122] In dogs, cocaine's acute negative cardiac inotropic effects were prevented by pretreatment with nifedipine but not when nifedipine was given after cocaine administration.[274]

Acute aortic dissection and rupture have occurred.[275,276] Bowel ischemia and gangrene have followed both oral and intravenous cocaine,[277] and perforated gastric ulcer has followed crack smoking.[278] Renal and splenic infarction, limb gangrene, and rupture of a splenic aneurysm have also been reported.[279–282] Pulmonary artery hypertrophy affects chronic users,[283] and alveolar hemorrhage after freebase smoking could be secondary to pulmonary vasoconstriction and tissue hypoxia.[284]

Parenteral cocaine users are at risk for stroke related to infection: endocarditis, AIDS, and hepatitis. They also have strokes caused by the drug itself, whether taken intranasally, intravenously, or intramuscularly or smoked as "crack."[285] The first report of a cocaine-related stroke was in 1977 from Harlem Hospital Center: A middle-aged, mildly hypertensive man drank a bottle of wine and injected cocaine intramuscularly and an hour later abruptly developed aphasia and right hemiparesis; cerebrospinal fluid was normal, and cerebral angiography was refused.[286] The same year fatal rupture of a cerebral saccular aneurysm occurred in a young cocaine snorter.[287] Further cocaine strokes were not reported until the mid-1980s, but by the early 1990s, more than 300 cases had been described, about half occlusive and half hemorrhagic (Tables 4–3 and 4–4).[269,285–347c]

Ischemic strokes have included transient ischemic attacks and infarction of cerebrum, thalamus, brain stem, spinal cord, and retina.[304,305,323,337,341] Infarction has occurred in pregnant women and both antenatally and perinatally in newborns whose mothers used cocaine shortly before delivery.[285,291,334] In an ultrasound study of 26 newborns exposed to cocaine, 5 had "periventricular leukomalacia"; 8, cerebral infarction; 7, intraventricular hemorrhage; and 6, intracerebral hemorrhage.[326]

In some cases, cerebral infarction has been attributed to vasculitis on the basis of angiographic findings;[298] such changes, however, may have represented vasospasm following undiagnosed subarachnoid hemorrhage.[348] Autopsies have usually shown histologically normal cerebral vessels,[285,312] although in three cases mild cerebral vasculitis was observed at biopsy or autopsy.[332,344] Two strokes were likely embolic secondary to cocaine-related cardiomyopathy.[269,340] A 20-year-old with no other risk factors had superior cerebellar artery occlusion 6 months after last use, raising the possibility of delayed effects.[330] In a 27-year-old cocaine sniffer with "heaviness and paresthesias" in the legs and occasional "forgetfulness," magnetic resonance imaging (MRI) revealed multiple periventricular white matter lesions.[306]

Intracerebral or subarachnoid hemorrhage has occurred during or within hours of cocaine use or has had less clear temporal relationship. Often there has been other substance use, especially ethanol. More than half of those undergoing angiography have had saccular aneurysms or vascular malformations. Other hemorrhages include bleeding into embolic infarction or glioma.[297] Cerebral hemorrhages have occurred in newborns and postpartum women.[285,309,321,324,326,334] Autopsy on a patient with multiple cerebral hemorrhages after smoking "crack" revealed histologically normal cerebral vessels.[331] In a retrospective survey of 150 consecutive patients admitted for subarachnoid hemorrhage, 17 had used intravenous cocaine within 72 hours. Mortality and morbidity were worse among the cocaine users, perhaps a consequence of drug-aggravated vasospasm.[329]

The mechanisms of cocaine-related stroke are unclear. Striking, considering that cocaine and amphetamine have similar actions and effects, are the high frequency of underlying aneurysm or vascular malformation in hemorrhagic strokes of cocaine users compared with amphetamine users and, conversely, the frequency of vasculitis in amphetamine users compared with cocaine users. Cocaine hydrochloride is more often associated with hemorrhagic than occlusive stroke, whereas hemorrhagic and occlusive strokes occur with roughly equal frequency in

Table 4–3. Cocaine-Related Stroke—Reports

	Type (number of cases)	Special Features	Route
1977			
Brust, Richter	CI		IM
Lundberg	SAH (1)	Aneurysm	IN
1982			
Caplan et al	ICH (1)	Negative angiogram	IN
1984			
Schwartz, Cohen	CI (1)	Angiogram: narrow MCA, ACA; occluded PCA	IN
	SAH (1)	Aneurysm	IN
	ICH (1)	Negative angiogram	IN
Lichtenfeld et al	SAH (1)	Aneurysm	IN
	ICH (1)	AVM	IN
1986			
Chasnoff et al	CI (1)	Newborn, maternal use	IN
Golbe, Merlin	CI (1)	Angiogram: narrow ICA, distal branch occlusion	Crack
Rogers et al	SAH (1)	Aneurysm	Not stated
1987			
Altes-Capella et al	SAH (1)	Aneurysm	IV
Levine et al	Infarct (3)	Cerebral 1, VB 2	Crack 3
Wojak, Flamm	ICH (4)	Glioma 1, hemorrhagic infarct 1	IN 2, 2 not stated
	SAH (2)	Aneurysm 2	Free-base 1, IN
Kaye, Feinstat	SAH? (1)	Vasospasm?	IN
Cregler, Mark	SAH (1)	Angiogram not done	IN
Mittelman, Wetli	ICH (4)	AVM 2	Not stated
	SAH (1)	Aneurysm	Not stated
Lowenstein et al	TIA (8)		Freebase 3, IV 3, IN 2
	Infarct (1)		IN
	ICH (2)	AVM 2	IN 1, IV 1
	SAH (1)	Aneurysm	IV
Lehman	ICH (1)	Angiogram not done	IN
1988			
Mangiardi et al	ICH (4)	AVM 2	IV 2, crack 2
	SAH (5)	Aneurysm 1, angiogram not done 3	IV 3, crack 2
Devenyi	Infarct (1)	Central retinal artery occlusion	IV
Mody et al	TIA (2)	Cerebral 1, VB 1	Crack 2
	Infarct (3)	Cerebral 2, VB 1	IN 1, crack 1
	Infarct (1)	Anterior spinal artery	Crack
	ICH (3)	AVM (1)	Crack 3
Weingarten	Infarct? (1)	MRI white matter lesions	IN
Toler	Infarct (1)	3 months after last use: lupus anticoagulant present	IV
Devore, Tucker	Infarct (1)	Pontine	Not stated
Henderson, Torbey	SAH (1)	Aneurysm, during pregnancy	Crack
Tenorio et al	Infarct (1)	Intrauterine exposure	Not stated
1989			
Nalls et al	ICH (4)	AVM? 1, radiographic vasculitis? 3	Not stated
Peterson, Moore	SAH or ICH (13)	Aneurysm 3, AVM 2	Crack 13
Moore, Peterson	TIA or CI (21)		Not stated
Mast et al	Periventricular leukomalacia (5)	Newborn, maternal use	Not stated
	Infarct (8)		

Table 4–3. *Continued*

	Type (number of cases)	Special Features	Route
	Intraventricular hemorrhage (7)		Not stated
	ICH (6)		Not stated
Tardiff et al	SAH or ICH (9)	Aneurysm 6	Not stated
Klonoff et al	SAH or ICH (7)	Aneurysm 3	Crack 1, IN 3, IV 2, ? 1
Rowley et al	Infarct (2)		IN 2
	ICH (1)	Angiogram not done	IN 2
de Broucker et al	ICH (1)		IN
Jacobs et al	Infarct (8)		Crack 4, IN 1
	ICH (4)	AVM 1	Crack 2, IV 2
	SAH (4)	Aneurysm 2	Crack 3, IV 1
Mercado et al	ICH (1)	Postpartum, negative angiogram	Not stated
Nolte, Gelman	ICH (1)	Autopsy: no vasculitis	IV
Engstrand et al	Infarct (8)	Cerebral 5, VB 2, spinal cord 1	Crack 4, IN 1, IV 1, ? 2
Spires et al	ICH (1)	Newborn, maternal use	Not stated
Meza et al	Infarct (1)		IN
Dixon, Bejar	Infarct and/or hemorrhage (13)	Combinations of CI, SAH ICH, IVH	Not stated
1990			
Seaman	Infarct (1)		Not stated
Levine et al	Infarct (18)	VB 4; autopsy 1: no vasculitis	Crack
	ICH (5)	AVM 1	Crack
	SAH (5)	Aneurysm 1	Crack
Deringer et al	Infarct (1)	Last used 6 months before	Not stated
Green et al	ICH (1)	Negative	Crack
Krendel et al	Infarct (2)	Biopsy: vasculitis Autopsy: vasculitis	Crack 2
Hall	Infarct (1)		Not stated
Petty et al	Infarct (1)	Cardiomyopathy, embolic	Crack
Kaku, Lowenstein	Infarct (7)		Not stated
	ICH (10)	AVM 1	Not stated
	SAH (6)	Aneurysm 5	Not stated
Hoyme et al	SAH (1)	Neonatal	Not stated
	Infarct (1)	Antenatal	
Simpson et al	SAH (17)	Aneurysm 16, AVM 1	IV
Kramer et al	Infarct (1)	Perinatal, bilateral MCA	Crack
Guidotti, Zanesi	Infarct (2)		IN 1, crack 1
1991			
Harruff et al	ICH (2)		Not stated
Peterson et al	Infarct (19)		IN 1, freebase 2, crack 16
	ICH (7)	Pontine 1, spinal cord 1	Freebase 1, crack 6
	SAH (8)	Aneurysm 5	IN 1, crack 7
Ramadan et al	ICH (1)	Pontine	Crack
Sloan et al	Infarct (3)		IN 3
	SAH (2)	Aneurysm 2	IV 1, IN 1
Sauer	Infarct (1)	Cardiomyopathy, embolic	IV
Daras et al	Infarct (18)	Anterior spinal artery 2 Coexistent meningovascular syphilis 1	IN 4, IV 3, crack 9
Hamer et al	Infarct (1)		Not stated
	SAH (1)		Not stated
Heier et al	Infarct (17)	Antenatal	Not stated
Fredericks et al	Infarct (1)	Multifocal; biopsy: vasculitis	IN and IV
Dominguez et al	Infarct (5)	Antenatal	IV 2, crack 2, Not stated 1

Table 4–3. *Continued*

	Type (number of cases)	Special Features	Route
Chadan et al	SAH (1)	Aneurysm	IV
1992			
Sloan	Infarct (1)	Concurrent myocardial and cerebral infarcts	IN
Konzen et al	Infarct (3)	Autopsy 1: marked vasospasm, no vasculitis	Crack 3
Nwosu et al	Infarct (1)	Mitral valve prolapse	IN
1993			
Libman et al	TIA (1)	Transient monocular blindness	Not stated

CI, cerebral infarct; SAH, subarachnoid hemorrhage; ICH, intracerebral hemorrhage; IVH, interventricular hemorrhage; TIA, transient ischemic attack; MCA, middle cerebral artery; ACA, anterior cerebral artery; PCA, posterior cerebral artery; AVM, arteriovenous malformation; VB, vertebrobasilar; IM, intramuscular; IN, intranasal; IV, intravenous.

"crack" users, but the rising prevalence of stroke since the appearance of "crack" is probably attributable to wider use and higher dosage rather than to a peculiarity of "crack" itself.[349] By blocking reuptake of norepinephrine from sympathetic nerve endings (and probably also by affecting calcium flux), cocaine is a vasoconstrictor.[350,351] Acute hypertension can lead to intracranial hemorrhage, especially in subjects with underlying aneurysms or vascular malformations. Compared to controls newborns exposed to cocaine in utero had increased mean arterial blood pressure and cerebral blood flow velocity during the first day of life, with levels becoming normal on the second day; such changes

Table 4–4. Cocaine-Related Stroke—Types and Numbers of Reported Cases

Occlusive	181
TIA	11
Infarct	154
TIA or infarct	21
Occlusive and/or hemorrhagic	13
Hemorrhagic	163
ICH	66
SAH	62
ICH or SAH	29
Intraventricular hemorrhage	7
Hemorrhage and angiogram or autopsy done	125
Aneurysm	54
AVM	15
% with aneurysm or AVM	55%
Total stroke	347

TIA, Transient ischemic attack; ICH, intracerebral hemorrhage; SAH, subarachnoid hemorrhage; AVM, arteriovenous malformation.

would increase the risk of perinatal cerebral hemorrhage.[351a] Myocardial infarction, cardiac arrhythmia, and cardiomyopathy carry a risk for embolic stroke. Cerebral vasoconstriction might cause occlusive stroke, and it is perhaps significant that cocaine metabolites, which in some chronic users are detectable in urine for weeks, also cause cerebral vasospasm.[68,352] A 34-year-old woman had thrombosis of the internal carotid artery; at emergency thrombectomy, the arterial wall was grossly normal. A 32-year-old woman had multiple hemorrhagic infarcts; at autopsy, there was no vasculitis, but large cerebral arteries were markedly narrowed with infolded and frayed internal elastic lamina. In these two cases, thrombosis and infarction could have been the result of severe vasospasm, with hemorrhage occurring during reperfusion.[347] During an attack of transient monocular blindness in a heavy cocaine user, funduscopic examination revealed "diffuse severe narrowing of the retinal arterioles" in the affected eye.[347e] In volunteers using cocaine intranasally, transcranial Doppler ultrasound revealed increased cerebral blood velocities, consistent with increased distal arteriolar resistance.[353]

In addition to direct vasoconstriction and the secondary effects of hypertension and cardiac disease, cocaine affects the cerebral circulation in diverse ways. Although intraluminal cocaine constricted cat and rat pial vessels in vitro, topical cocaine dilated pial vessels in living cats.[351,352,354] Cocaine enhances the response of platelets to arachidonic acid, promoting aggregation.[355] Conversely, severe destructive thrombocytopenia responsive to corticosteroids or splenectomy was reported in six HIV-negative cocaine users (none of whom had a stroke).[356] In rabbits, repeated cocaine injections caused arteriosclerotic aortopathy.[357] In a cocaine user with symptoms of coronary artery disease, protein C and antithrombin III were depleted and returned to normal, with clearing of symptoms, when use was discontinued.[270] Anticardiolipin antibodies have been found in occasional cocaine users.[339]

As with amphetamine and other stimulants, it is unclear whether chronic cocaine use causes lasting mental abnormalities. Protracted depression in abstinent users has been attributed, without much evidence, to permanent depletion of limbic dopamine. Psychological impairment and poor work performance were described in South American coca leaf chewers, but these studies, like those involving other recreational drugs, did not account for precocaine cognitive capacity, acute drug effects, or other confounders.[358,359] Better designed but preliminary human studies using controls suggest that chronic cocaine use produces subtle impairment in short-term auditory recall, concentration, and reaction time.[359a–359c] Chronic cocaine users have diffuse electroencephalographic theta activity, which increases with continuous use.[360] In a computed tomography (CT) study, habitual cocaine users (at least twice weekly for 2 years or more) had significant degrees of cerebral atrophy (enlargement of the lateral ventricles and widening of the sylvian fissures) compared with first-time users and nonusers; subjects were between 20 and 40 years of age, and those with alcoholism, polydrug abuse, and HIV seropositivity were excluded.[361] If cerebral atrophy is secondary to cocaine (and not to malnutrition, head injury, or adulterants), it might be ischemic in origin. Studies with positron-emission tomography (PET) and single-photon emission tomography (SPECT) in chronic cocaine users demonstrated irregularly decreased blood flow in the cerebral cortex, especially frontotemporally. Some of these subjects had normal CT and MRI scans and no other evidence of neurological disease.[362,363] Of 18 subjects with abnormal brain perfusion patterns on SPECT, 13 had mild and 5 had moderate deficits on psychometric testing, especially spatial learning, organization, perseveration, set maintenance, verbal learning, and concept attainment.[364] In a PET study, decreased blood flow to the prefrontal cortex was still present 10 days after withdrawal.[363] In another PET study, glucose metabolism was reduced over the entire cerebral cortex, thalamus, and midbrain following the acute administration of cocaine.[365] Twenty-six of 57 neurologically normal chronic cocaine users had abnormal visual evoked responses.[366]

Cocaine-related violence accounts for considerable urban trauma, neurological and nonneurological.

In a report from Phoenix, Arizona, urine contained cocaine metabolites in 21% of patients admitted for "multiple trauma."[367] Familiar to municipal hospitals are adolescent cocaine runners with leg or spinal gunshot wounds incurred during territorial drug wars. Sometimes the spinal cord is deliberately cut ("pithing").[98] Paralleling the crack epidemic, reported child abuse deaths in the United States rose by 36%—from 899 in 1985 to 1223 in 1988.[368]

Obstetric and Pediatric Aspects

In the United States, cocaine use during pregnancy is common and underreported, and "crack babies" have received considerable media attention. At Parkland Hospital in Dallas, 10% of pregnant women reported cocaine use,[369] and at Boston City Hospital's prenatal unit, 17% of urine samples were positive for cocaine or its metabolites.[370] At several public and private prenatal facilities in Pinellas County, Florida, urine samples reflected cocaine use in 1.9% of white women and 7.5% of black women.[371] Cocaine-exposed newborns have filled pediatric hospital units ("crack boarders") and if projections are accurate will have a devastating societal impact. In 1990, it was estimated that more than 100,000 such infants had been born in the United States and that by the year 2000 the number of American children exposed prenatally to cocaine could be as high as 4 million, in some school districts constituting more than half of all classrooms. As these children have begun to enter nursery and primary schools, the media have publicized their functional disabilities and their custodial and educational costs. For example, in Los Angeles in 1990, it reportedly cost $3500 a year to educate each normal child in a regular classroom; the cost of each drug-exposed child was $15,000.[372] Such alarms mandate careful scientific study of cocaine's perinatal and neonatal effects.[373,373a]

Several reports describe increased spontaneous abortion,[374,375] abruptio placentae,[375–377] and premature delivery[377–379] among cocaine-using women. Others describe retarded fetal growth, low birth weight, and decreased head circumference.[375,377–381] Reported congenital malformations include genitourinary[377,382–384] and cardiovascular anomalies (pulmonary artery atresia or stenosis and atrial or ventricular septal defects),[334,374,385] midline skull defects,[374] spinal anomalies,[326] intestinal atresia or necrotizing enterocolitis,[386] congenital limb reduction defects,[334,387] iris vessel tortuosity,[388] and developmental retinopathy.[389]

Tremor, irritability, brisk tendon reflexes, and hypertonia have been observed in 38% to 80% of cocaine-exposed infants, clearing in a few days.[379] Neonatal "depression of interactive behavior and poor organizational response to environmental stimuli" are described,[377] and a study using the Bayley Mental and Motor Scales of Infant Development found that 63% of cocaine-exposed infants had scores below average, compared with 33% of controls, with differences increasing with age.[390] A neonatal "withdrawal syndrome" resembling heroin's but lacking gastrointestinal symptoms was reported in 33 of 49 infants with in utero exposure.[326] Cardiac arrhythmia and seizures have occurred,[374] and even in the absence of seizures, electroencephalograms have shown spikes and sharp waves lasting several months.[391] Sixteen infants exposed to cocaine in utero had seizures at birth, and 8 of them continued to have seizures after the first month of life.[391a] In a prospective study of 30 cocaine-exposed newborns at Harlem Hospital Center, intrauterine growth retardation, small head circumference, and diffuse or axial hypertonus severe enough to label "hypertonic tetraparesis" were significantly more common among patients than among controls.[392]

In contrast to the opioid neonatal withdrawal syndrome, these symptoms and signs, if they are attributable to cocaine per se, are likely the result of direct toxicity, not abstinence. Moreover, although neonatal opioid withdrawal is a frequently lethal emergency, signs of neonatal cocaine toxicity seldom require vigorous treatment.

As noted, strokes have occurred both perinatally and neonatally in cocaine-exposed infants. In an ultrasound study of neonates exposed in utero to cocaine or methamphetamine there was evidence of ischemic or hemorrhagic stroke in over one-third.[327] In another report of 49 exposed infants, CT or MRI in more than half suggested periventricular leukomalacia, cerebral infarction, intraventricular hemorrhage, or intraparenchymal hemorrhage.[326] Not all infants so diagnosed have displayed neonatal behavioral abnormalities.[327] Brain stem auditory evoked reponse testing revealed prolonged latencies indicative of brain stem or cerebral damage in 18 cocaine-exposed infants.[393]

In a radiologic review (sonography, CT, or MRI) of 43 consecutive newborns of cocaine-using mothers, cerebral infarction occurred in 17% and congenital anomalies in 12%, compared with 2% and 0% in controls. Malformations included encephalocele, holoprosencephaly, intraspinal lipoma, and hypoplastic cerebellum. The authors speculated that strokes were caused by placental and cerebral vasospasm in the third trimester and malformations by vasospasm in the first trimester.[343] Others, however, have expressed doubt that first-trimester malformations are ischemic in origin.[394]

Sudden infant death syndrome (SIDS) was reported in 15% of 66 infants exposed to cocaine in utero,[395] and abnormal cardiorespiratory patterns were described in exposed neonates whether or not they subsequently developed apnea.[376] Several subsequent studies, however, found only a small increase in SIDS among infants prenatally exposed to cocaine,[396] and a study of premature infants found that in utero cocaine exposure actually *decreased* the risk of respiratory distress syndrome.[397]

Cocaine-using mothers are likely to avoid prenatal care, to be malnourished, to underreport cocaine use, and to abuse other substances including ethanol and tobacco. They have a high prevalence of sexually transmitted disease, including HIV and syphilis, which they transmit to offspring.[398] They are socioeconomically impoverished. Such factors confound attempts to determine the true risk of in utero cocaine exposure.[396] Although most workers have concurred that cocaine causes spontaneous abortion, abruptio placentae, intrauterine growth retardation, and decreased head circumference, some have found no increase in prematurity,[375,380] congenital anomalies,[370,380,399] or abnormal neonatal behavior.[400] In one report, "social users" who stopped taking cocaine when they realized they were pregnant did not have an increased incidence of "adverse pregnancy outcome."[401] Investigations in Boston found cranial ultrasound abnormalities in nearly two-thirds of inner city neonates whether they had been exposed to cocaine or not, with no significant difference between the two groups, suggesting that abnormalities reported by others are not cocaine specific.[402] It has been charged that studies failing to find a causal relationship between maternal cocaine use and fetal health problems are frequently rejected by journal reviewers on ideological grounds.[403]

In 1991, 20 scientific reports of cocaine use during pregnancy were subjected to metaanalysis (Table 4–5).[404] Fifteen were prospective cohort studies, four were retrospective cohort studies, and one was a case-control study; case reports were excluded, as were studies that did not separate cocaine users from other drug users and studies without control groups. Although the odds ratios for such outcomes as spontaneous abortion, abruptio placentae, prematurity, low birth weight, and malformations were elevated in cocaine users compared with drug-free controls, statistically significant risk was identified only for genitourinary malformations and intrauterine death. Comparing polydrug users who used cocaine with polydrug users who did not use cocaine, only the

Table 4–5. Reproductive Effects of Cocaine in 20 Studies Comparing Cocaine Users to Drug-Free Controls

	n	Odds Ratio	95% Confidence Interval	
			Lower	Upper
Small for gestational age	3	5.31	0.24	118.3
Low birth weight	4	4.40	0.11	175.8
Prematurity	7	4.31	0.13	138.4
Male:female ratio	5	1.33	0.007	246.9
Premature membrane rupture	2	2.60	0.06	107.1
Abruptio placentae	8	5.82	0.71	47.8
Meconium staining	5	2.21	0.03	128.6
Fetal distress	3	2.01	0.11	37.8
Genitourinary malformation	5	4.97	1.05	23.6
Cardiac malformation	6	2.36	0.83	6.74
Spontaneous abortion	2	5.32	0.22	125.9
In utero death	2	6.17	1.21	31.5
Sudden infant death syndrome	1	4.04	0.18	95.8

Modified from Lutiger B, Graham K, Einarson TR, Koren G. Relationship between gestational cocaine use and pregnancy outcome. A meta-analysis. Teratology 1991; 44:405, with permission of the publisher.

odds ratio for genitourinary malformations was significant. The authors stressed the difficulty in defining the role of cocaine alone in adverse pregnancy outcomes.

Animal studies support the contention that cocaine damages fetuses. In utero cocaine exposure to mice or rats causes soft tissue and skeletal anomalies, reduced fetal weight, fetal edema, abruptio placentae, and intracranial hemorrhage.[405–409] Impaired learning has followed doses too small to produce grossly evident abnormalities.[407] In animals, cocaine decreases uterine and placental blood flow,[410–412] and serum cholinesterase levels are decreased during pregnancy.[413] Animal studies also suggest that males exposed to cocaine before mating have an increased incidence of offspring with developmental abnormalities.[414] Cocaine binds to spermatazoa, which could act as a vector to transport cocaine into an ovum.[415] In cultures of fetal rat mesencephalic neurons, the cocaine metabolite norcocaine—but not cocaine itself—was cytotoxic to dopaminergic neurons, and fetal brains of rats exposed to cocaine in utero had norcocaine concentrations capable of causing such cytotoxicity.[416]

Postnatal cocaine exposure carries its own hazards. Infants have had tremor or seizures during nursing by cocaine-using mothers.[417,418] A 9-month-old developed status epilepticus after accidental ingestion of cocaine powder,[419] and seizures occurred in an infant and a 2-year-old who passively inhaled "crack" smoke.[420] In a report from Boston City Hospital, cocaine metabolites were present in 6 of 250 (2.4%) urine assays of small children seen in the emergency room for problems unrelated to cocaine. Possible exposure routes included breastfeeding, intentional administration, accidental ingestion of the drug or of cocaine-contaminated dust, and passive inhalation of "crack" smoke.[421] Dramatically illustrating the spectrum of pediatric cocaine catastrophes, one report described six fatal cases: intrauterine death of a 35-week fetus, anoxic encephalopathy at birth with 3 months' vegetative survival, traumatic asphyxia in a 4-month-old, infectious cardiomyopathy at age 21 months following maternal cocaine abuse at birth, malnutrition and dehydration in a 7-week-old, and poisoning of a 6-week-old by his teenage brother.[422]

Long-term Treatment

The long-term treatment of cocaine addiction has been frustrating (Table 4–6). A logical approach, analogous to methadone or naltrexone treatment of heroin addiction, would be to use dopamine agonists or antagonists. In self-administering animals, bromocriptine suppressed cocaine responding but only at doses that caused stereotypic movements and "proconvulsant signs", and chlorpromazine decreased cocaine responding only at doses that reduced food responding as well.[423] In humans, phenothiazines and haloperidol do not completely block cocaine euphoria and may aggravate anhedonic withdrawal symptoms.[15] Several studies, some placebo controlled, found bromocriptine effective for up to several weeks in reducing cocaine craving,

Table 4–6. Long-Term Treatment

Agonists
  Tricyclic antidepressants
  Bromocriptine
  Amantadine
  Methylphenidate
  Mazindol
Antagonists
  Phenothiazines
  Haloperidol
Other
  Flupenthixol
  Carbamazepine
  Bupropion
  Fluoxetine
For preexisting psychiatric disorder
  Desipramine
  Lithium
  Methylphenidate
For methadone maintenance
  Buprenorphine
Acupuncture
Psychotherapy
Contingency contracts
Self-help groups

but side effects were often prominent.[424–426] In a double-blind, placebo-controlled trial, bromocriptine did not reduce cocaine craving,[427] and in another study, bromocriptine did not alter cocaine's acute autonomic or subjective effects.[428] Amantadine has also been used, alone or in conjunction with bromocriptine, lorazepam and tryptophan, or tryptophan and tyrosine.[424,429,430] In one report, cocaine users with antisocial personality disorder had good treatment responses to amantadine.[431] In another report, amantadine was initially effective during abstinence but by the end of 4 weeks was no better than placebo.[432] Pergolide reportedly reduced insomnia and craving during cocaine withdrawal without causing side effects as often as bromocriptine.[433] The monoamine oxidase inhibitor phenylzine has also been recommended.[434] Mazindol, a dopamine uptake blocker that appears free of abuse potential, was similarly promising in a preliminary study lasting 4 weeks.[435] By contrast, methylphenidate not only was ineffective but may have increased cocaine craving.[436]

Tricyclic antidepressants have been given specifically to relieve withdrawal depression, with varying results. They have also been given less specifically as indirect dopamine agonists. Desipramine, imipramine, maprotiline, and trazadone have reportedly reduced withdrawal craving and attenuated cocaine euphoria.[437–439] A limitation of such agents is the 1- or 2-week delay in their efficacy, leading some workers to recommend hospitalization for cocaine withdrawal.[440] Moreover, desipramine sometimes causes symptoms (the *early tricyclic jitteriness syndrome*) that resemble those of cocaine intoxication, leading, paradoxically, to increased craving.[441] Desipramine appears to be more useful in achieving abstinence than in maintaining it.[442] In a study of methadone maintenance patients, desipramine was no better than placebo in preventing either cocaine or ethanol use.[443] In another study, patients without antisocial personality disorder were helped by desipramine, whereas those with antisocial personality disorder were not.[431] In a study of volunteers given access to cocaine, desipramine did not affect the rate of cocaine self-administration but did increase reports of negative mood effects (anxiety or anger) induced by cocaine; cocaine-induced tachycardia and hypertension were more severe in subjects receiving desipramine.[443a] In rats, imipramine had no effect on cocaine's ability to lower threshold for brain stimulation reward.[444] A preliminary report suggested efficacy of flupenthixol, a rapidly acting xanthine antidepressant which at low doses selectively blocks supersensitive dopamine D-2 inhibitory autoreceptors, thereby increasing dopaminergic activity and reducing anhedonia.[445] Carbamazepine also seems to reverse dopamine autoreceptor supersensitivity as well as cocaine-induced kindling in animals; preliminary trials have been encouraging.[60,446,446a] So has a preliminary trial of the second-generation antidepressant bupropion.[447]

Consistent with studies of cocaine's serotonergic effects, fluoxetine in open trials sharply reduced cocaine use in methadone maintenance patients.[448] In rats, however, fluoxetine blocked amphetamine self-administration but had no effect on cocaine self-administration.[449]

Some cocaine users appear to be self-medicating preexisting psychiatric illness. Studies estimate that depressive disorders are present in 30% of users, bipolar disorders in 20%, and attention deficit disorder in 5%; it is obviously difficult in some instances to tell cause from effect.[450] Both favorable and unfavorable results have been reported on the use of desipramine in those with preexisting depression; lithium in those with bipolar disorder; and methylphenidate, pemoline, or bromocriptine in those with attention deficit disorder.[440,451–453] Cocaine use fluctuated with depressed mood in two patients with seasonal affective disorder.[454]

Anorexia nervosa and bulimia also occur with unexpected frequency among cocaine users.[455] So do alcoholism, anxiety disorders, antisocial personality, and sensation seeking.[450,456,457] In one report, alcoholism was currently present in 29% of cocaine users seeking treatment, with a lifetime prevalence of 62%, "nearly twice the rate of alcoholism seen in opioid addicts."[450] In contrast to opioid addicts, cocaine users tended to become alcoholic after abusing cocaine, perhaps as a means of reducing cocaine-induced anxiety and insomnia.

Among users of combined heroin and cocaine, methadone maintenance therapy often decreases cocaine use, yet it is not unusual for methadone maintenance patients to begin using cocaine after starting treatment.[458,459] In one study, buprenorphine plus naltrexone was more effective than methadone in treating combined heroin and cocaine use.[460] In another study, cocaine produced euphoria in subjects receiving methadone but dysphoria in those receiving buprenorphine.[461] In another study, buprenorphine blocked the subjective effects of heroin and reduced craving, but although some subjects reported a decrease in cocaine euphoria, others reported an increase.[462] In rats, buprenorphine and cocaine were additive both in conditioned place preference studies and in producing increased extracellular dopamine in the NA, suggesting that buprenorphine might enhance rather than reduce the rewarding properties of cocaine.[463] Daily buprenorphine suppressed cocaine self-administration by monkeys in a dose-dependent fashion and independent of generalized behavioral suppression.[464] Naltrexone also reduced cocaine self-administration in monkeys but to a lesser extent than buprenorphine.[465]

As with other substance abuse, psychotherapy may have adjunctive benefit but is of little value used alone.[466] The notion that pavlovian conditioning contributes to craving is the basis for extinction therapy: presenting cocaine-associated stimuli until they lose their ability to provoke conditioned responses.[467] Whatever approach or medication is used, outpatients require regular physician visits, urine testing, counseling, and education (which should include other family members). Medication can be given for 4 to 6 months, with retreatment for relapse. Given the frustrations of medical therapy, it is not surprising that self-help and peer groups (Cocaine Anonymous) have proliferated.

References

1. Bozarth MA. New perspectives on cocaine addiction: recent findings from animal research. Can J Physiol Pharmacol 1989; 67:1158.

2. Johanson C-E, Fischman MW. The pharmacology of cocaine related to its abuse. Pharmacol Rev 1989; 41:3.

3. Post RM, Rose H. Increasing effects of repetitive cocaine administration in the rat. Nature 1976; 260:731.

4. Karler R, Petty C, Calder L, Turkanis SA. Proconvulsant and anticonvulsant effects in mice of acute and chronic treatment with cocaine. Neuropharmacology 1989; 28:709.

5. Reith MEA, Benuck M, Lajtha A. Cocaine disposition in the brain after continuous or intermittent treatment and locomotor stimulation in mice. J Pharmacol Exp Ther 1987; 243:281.

6. Steketee JD, Kalivas PW. Sensitization to cocaine produced by injection of pertussis toxin into the A-10 dopamine region. In: Harris LD, ed. Problems of Drug Dependence 1990. Rockville, MD: NIDA Research Monograph 105, DHHS, 1991:545.

7. Henry DJ, Greene MA, White FJ. Electrophysiological effects of cocaine in the mesoaccumbens dopamine system: repeated administration. J Pharmacol Exp Ther 1989; 251:833.

8. Post RM, Weiss SRB. Psychomotor stimulant vs local anesthetic effects of cocaine: role of behavioral sensitization and kindling. In: Clouet D, Asghar K, Brown R, eds. Mechanisms of Cocaine Abuse and Toxicity. Washington, DC: NIDA Research Monograph 88, DHHS, 1988:217.

9. Reith MEA, Meisler BE, Lajtha A. Locomotor effects of cocaine, cocaine congeners and local anesthetics in mice. Pharmacol Biochem Behav 1985; 23:831.

10. Witkin JM, Tortella FC. Modulators of N-methyl-D-aspartate protect against diazepam- or phenobarbital-resistant cocaine convulsions. Life Sci 1991; 48:PL51.

11. Karler R, Calder LD, Chaudhry IA, Turkanis SA. Blockade of "reverse tolerance" to cocaine and amphetamine by MK-801. Life Sci 1989; 45:599.

12. Ambre JJ, Belknap SM, Nelson J, et al. Acute tolerance to cocaine in humans. Clin Pharmacol Ther 1988; 44:1.

13. Aigner TC, Balster RL. Choice behavior in rhesus monkeys: cocaine versus food. Science 1978; 201:534.

14. Johanson CE. Assessment of the dependence potential of cocaine in animals. In: Grabowski J, ed. Cocaine: Pharmacology, Effects, and Treatment of Abuse. Washington, DC: NIDA Research Monograph 50, DHHS, 1984:54.

15. Wise RA. Neural mechanisms of the reinforcing action of cocaine. In: Grabowski J, ed. Cocaine: Pharmacology, Effects, and Treatment of Abuse. Washington, DC: NIDA Research Monograph 50, DHHS, 1984:15.

16. Bozarth MA, Wise RA. Toxicity associated with long-term intravenous heroin and cocaine self-administration in the rat. JAMA 1985; 254:81.

17. Johanson C-E, Balster RL, Bonese K. Self-administration of psychomotor stimulant drugs: the effects of unlimited access. Pharmacol Biochem Behav 1976; 4:45.

18. Winger GD, Woods JH. Comparison of fixed-ratio and progressive ratio schedules of maintenance of stimulant

drug-reinforced responding. Drug Alcohol Depend 1985; 15:123.

19. Yanagita T. An experimental framework for evaluation of dependence liability in various types of drugs in monkeys. Bull Narc 1973; 25:57.

20. Lakoski JM, Cunningham KA. Cocaine interaction with central monoaminergic systems: electrophysiological approaches. Trends Pharmacol Sci 1988; 9:177.

21. Ritz MC, Lamb RJ, Goldberg SR, Kuhar MJ. Cocaine receptors on dopamine transporters are related to self-administration of cocaine. Science 1987; 237:1219.

22. Madras BK, Fahey MA, Bergman J, et al. Effects of cocaine and related drugs in nonhuman primates. 1. [3-H]cocaine binding sites in caudate-putamen. J Pharmacol Exp Ther 1989; 251:131.

23. Shimada S, Kitayama S, Lin C-L, et al. Cloning and expression of a cocaine-sensitive dopamine transporter complementary DNA. Science 1991; 254:576.

24. Kilty JE, Lorang D, Amara SG. Cloning and expression of a cocaine-sensitive rat dopamine transporter. Science 1991; 254:578.

25. Pacholczyk T, Blakely RD, Amara SG. Expression cloning of a cocaine- and antidepressant-sensitive human noradrenaline transporter. Nature 1991; 350:350.

26. Seiden LS, Kleven MS. Lack of toxic effects of cocaine on dopamine or serotonin neurons in the rat brain. In: Clouet D, Arghar K, Brown R, eds. Mechanisms of Cocaine Abuse and Toxicity. Rockville, MD: NIDA Research Monograph 88, DHHS, 1988:276.

27. Wood DM, Emmett-Oglesby MW. Substitution and cross-tolerance profiles of anorectic drugs in rats trained to detect the discriminative stimulus properties of cocaine. Psychopharmacology 1988; 95:364.

28. McKenna ML, Ho BT. The role of dopamine in the discriminative stimulus properties of cocaine. Neuropharmacology 1980; 19:297.

29. Callahan PM, Appel JB, Cunningham KA. Dopamine D1 and D2 mediation of the discriminative stimulus properties of d-amphetamine and cocaine. Psychopharmacology 1991; 103:50.

30. Kleven MS, Anthony EW, Goldberg LI, Woolverton WL. Blockade of the discriminative stimulus effects of cocaine in rhesus monkeys with the D1 dopamine antagonist SCH 23390. Psychopharmacology 1988; 95:427.

31. Colpaert FC, Niemegeers CJE, Janssen PAJ. Evidence that a preferred substrate for type B monoamine oxidase mediates stimulus properties of MAO inhibitors: a possible role for beta-phenylethylamine in the cocaine cue. Pharmacol Biochem Behav 1980; 13:513.

32. de la Garza R, Johanson C-E. Discriminative stimulus properties of cocaine in pigeons. Psychopharmacology 1985; 85:23.

33. Huang J, Wilson MC. Comparative stimulus properties of cocaine and other local anesthetics in rats. Res Commun Subst Abuse 1982; 3:120.

34. Yokel RA, Wise RA. Amphetamine-type reinforcement by dopaminergic agonists in the cat. Psychopharmacology 1978; 58:289.

35. Baxter BL, Gluckman MI, Stein L, Scerni RA. Self-injection of apomorphine in the rat. Positive reinforcement by a dopamine receptor stimulant. Pharmacol Biochem Behav 1974; 2:387.

36. Woolverton WL, Goldberg LI, Ginos JZ. Intravenous self-administration of dopamine receptor agonists by rhesus monkeys. J Pharmacol Exp Ther 1984; 230:678.

37. Woolverton WL. Evaluation of the role of norepinephrine in the reinforcing effects of psychomotor stimulants in rhesus monkeys. Pharmacol Biochem Behav 1987; 26:835.

38. Risner ME, Jones BE. Role of noradrenergic and dopaminergic processes in amphetamine self-administration. Pharmacol Biochem Behav 1976; 5:477.

39. Ritz MC, Lamb RJ, Goldberg SR, Kuhar MJ. Cocaine receptors on dopamine transporters are related to self-administration of cocaine. Science 1987; 237:1219.

40. Pettit HD, Justice JB. Effect of dose on cocaine self-administration behavior and dopamine levels in the nucleus accumbens. Brain Res 1991; 539:94.

41. Dworkin SI, Smith JE. Neurobehavioral pharmacology of cocaine. In: Clouet D, Asghar K, Brown R, eds. Mechanisms of Cocaine Abuse and Toxicity. Washington, DC: NIDA Research Monograph 88, DHHS, 1988:185.

42. Roberts DCS, Koob GF. Disruption of cocaine self-administration following 6-hydroxydopamine lesions of the ventral tegmental area in rats. Pharmacol Biochem Behav 1982; 17:901.

43. Hubner CB, Koob GF. Ventral pallidal lesions produce decreases in cocaine and heroin self-administration in the rat. Soc Neurosci Abst 1987; 13:1717.

44. Goeders NE, Smith JE. Reinforcing properties of cocaine in the medial prefrontal cortex: primary action on presynaptic dopaminergic terminals. Pharmacol Biochem Behav 1986; 25:191.

45. Goeders NE, Dworkin SI, Smith JE. Neuropharmacological assessment of cocaine self-administration into the medial prefrontal cortex. Pharmacol Biochem Behav 1986; 24:1429.

46. Kornetsky C, Esposito RV. Reward and detection thresholds for brain stimulation: dissociative effects of cocaine. Brain Res 1981; 209:496.

46a. Stein EA, Fuller SA. Selective effects of cocaine on regional cerebral blood flow in the rat. J Pharmacol Exp Ther 1992; 262:327.

47. Spealman RD, Madras BK, Bergman J. Effects of cocaine and related drugs in nonhuman primates. II. Stimulant effects on schedule-controlled behavior. J Pharmacol Exp Ther 1989; 251:142.

48. Woolverton WL, Johnson KM. Neurobiology of cocaine abuse. Trends Pharmacol Sci 1992; 13:193.

49. Gawin FH. Cocaine addiction: psychology and neurophysiology. Science 1991; 251:1580.

50. DiChiara G, Imperato A. Drugs abused by humans preferentially increase synaptic dopamine concentra-

tions in the mesolimbic system of freely moving rats. Proc Natl Acad Sci USA 1988; 85:5274.

51. Bain GT, Kornetsky C. Naloxone attenuation of the effect of cocaine on rewarding brain stimulation. Life Sci 1987; 40:1119.

52. Devry J, Donselaar I, Van Ree JM. Food deprivation and acquisition of intravenous cocaine self-administration in rats: effect of naltrexone and haloperidol. J Pharmacol Exp Ther 1989; 251:735.

53. Houdi AA, Bardo MT, Van Loon GR. Opioid mediation of cocaine-induced hyperactivity and reinforcement. Brain Res 1989; 497:195.

54. Unterwald EM, Tempel A, Koob GF, Zukin RS. Characterization of opioid receptors in dopaminergic lesions. Brain Res 1989; 505:111.

55. Koob GF, Vaccarino FJ, Amalric M, Swerdlow NR. Neural substrates for cocaine and opiate reinforcement. In: Fischer S, Raskin A, Uhlenhuth EH, eds. Cocaine: Clinical and Biobehavioral Aspects. New York: Oxford University Press, 1987:80.

56. Yoburn BC, Luffy K, Sierra V. In vitro d-amphetamine and cocaine increase opioid binding in mouse brain homogenate. In: Harris L, ed. Problems of Drug Dependence 1990. Washington, DC: NIDA Research Monograph 105, DHHS, 1991:522.

57. Misra AL, Pontani RB, Vadlamani NL. Blockade of tolerance to morphine analgesia by cocaine. Pain 1989; 38:77.

58. Trulson ME, Babb S, Joe JC, et al. Chronic cocaine administration depletes tyrosine hydroxylase immunoreactivity in the rat brain nigrostriatal system: quantitative light microscopic studies. Exp Neurol 1986; 94:744.

59. Wyatt RJ, Karoum F, Suddath R, et al. Persistently decreased brain dopamine levels and cocaine. JAMA 1988; 259:2996.

60. Gawin F, Ellinwood E. Cocaine and other stimulants. N Engl J Med 1988; 318:1173.

61. Young ST, Porrino LJ, Iadarola MJ. Cocaine induces striatal c-fos-immunoreactive proteins via dopaminergic D1 receptors. Proc Natl Acad Sci USA 1991; 88:1291.

62. Jones RT. The pharmacology of cocaine. In: Grabowski J, ed. Cocaine: Pharmacology, Effects, and Treatment of Abuse. Washington, DC: NIDA Research Monograph 50, DHHS, 1984:34.

63. Russell RD, Stripling JS. Monoaminergic and local anesthetic components of cocaine's effects on kindled seizure expression. Pharmacol Biochem Behav 1987; 22:427.

64. Eidelberg E, Long M, Miller MK. Spectrum analysis of EEG changes induced by psychotomimetic agents. Int J Neuropharmacol 1965; 4:255.

65. Javaid JI, Musa MN, Fischman MW, et al. Kinetics of cocaine in humans after intravenous and intranasal administration. Biopharm Drug Dispos 1983; 4:9.

66. Busto U, Bendayan R, Sellers EM. Clinical pharmacokinetics of non-opiate abused drugs. Clin Pharmacokin 1989; 16:1.

67. Siegel RK. Cocaine free base use. J Psychoact Drugs 1982; 14:311.

68. Weiss RD, Gawin FH. Protracted elimination of cocaine metabolites in long-term, high dose cocaine abusers. Am J Med 1988; 85:879.

69. Devenyi P. Cocaine complications and cholinesterase. Ann Intern Med 1989; 110:167.

70. Graham K, Koren G, Klein J, et al. Determination of gestational cocaine exposure by hair analysis. JAMA 1989; 262:3328.

71. Bailey DN. Drug screening in an unconventional matrix: hair analysis. JAMA 1989; 262:3331.

72. Petersen RC. Cocaine: an overview. In: Petersen RC, Stillman RC, eds. Cocaine, 1977. Washington, DC: NIDA Research Monograph 13, DHEW, 1977:17.

73. Cartmell LW, Aufderhide A, Weems C. Cocaine metabolites in pre-Columbian mummy hair. J Okla State Med Assoc 1991; 84:11.

74. Schoenberg BS. Coke's the one: the centennial of the "ideal brain tonic" that became a symbol of America. South Med J 1988; 81:70.

75. Freud S. Uber Coca. Zentbl Ther 1884; 2:289.

76. Goldberg MF. Cocaine: the first local anesthetic and the "third scourge of humanity." Arch Ophthalmol 1984; 102:1143.

77. Gay P. Freud. A Life for Our Time. New York: WH Norton Co, 1988.

78. Penfield W. Halsted of Johns Hopkins. The man and his problem as described in the secret records of William Osler. JAMA 1969; 210:2215.

79. Nicholi AM. The nontherapeutic use of psychoactive drugs. A modern epidemic. N Engl J Med 1983; 308:925.

80. Adams EH, Durell J. Cocaine: a growing public health problem. In: Grabowski J, ed. Cocaine: Pharmacology, Effects and Treatment of Abuse. Washington, DC: NIDA Research Monograph 50, DHHS, 1984:9.

81. O'Malley PM, Bachman JG, Johnson LD. Period, age, and cohort effects on substance use among American youth, 1976–1982. Am J Public Health 1984; 74:682.

82. Van Dyck C, Byck R. Cocaine. Sci Am 1982; 246:128.

83. Barnes DM. Drugs: running the numbers. Science 1988; 240:1729.

84. Pollock DA, Holmgreen P, Lui K-J, Kirk ML. Discrepancies in the reported frequency of cocaine-related deaths, United States, 1983 through 1988. JAMA 1991; 266:2233.

85. Rogers JN, Henry TE, Jones AM, et al. Cocaine-related deaths in Pima County, Arizona, 1982–1984. J Forens Sci 1986; 31:1404.

86. Sander R, Ryser MA, Lamoreaux TC, Raleigh K. An epidemic of cocaine-associated deaths in Utah. J Forens Sci 1985; 30:478.

87. Cornwell PD, Valentour JC. Cocaine deaths in Virginia. Med Leg Bull 1986; 35:1.

88. Tardiff K, Gross E, Wu J, et al. Analysis of cocaine positive fatalities. J Forens Sci 1989; 34:53.

89. Bailey DN, Shaw RF. Cocaine- and methamphetamine-related deaths in San Diego County (1984): homicides and accidental overdoses. J Forens Sci 1989; 34:407.

90. Hood I, Ryan D, Monforte J, Valentour J. Cocaine in Wayne County medical examiner's cases. J Forens Sci 1990; 35:591.
91. McKelway R, Vieweg V, Westerman P. Sudden death from acute cocaine intoxication in Virginia in 1988. Am J Psychiatry 1990; 147:1667.
92. Tardiff K, Gross EM, Messner SF. A study of homicides in Manhattan. Am J Public Health 1986; 76:139.
93. Marshall E. Testing urine for drugs. Science 1988; 214:150.
94. Nadelmann EA. Drug prohibition in the United States: costs, consequences, and alternatives. Science 1989; 245:939.
95. Hanzlick R, Gowitt GT. Cocaine metabolite detection in homicide victims. JAMA 1991; 265:760.
96. Haruff RC, Francisco JT, Elkins SK, et al. Cocaine and homicide in Memphis and Shelby County: an epidemic of violence. J Forens Sci 1988; 33:1231.
97. Goldstein PJ. The drugs-violence nexus: a tripartite conceptual framework. J Drug Issues 1985; 15:493.
98. De La Rosa M, Lambert EY, Gropper B, eds. Drugs and Violence: Causes, Correlates, and Consequences. Rockville, MD: NIDA Research Monograph 103, DHHS, 1990.
99. Marzuk PM, Tardiff K, Leon AC, et al. Prevalence of recent cocaine use among motor vehicle fatalities in New York City. JAMA 1990; 263:250.
100. Shenon P. The score on drugs: it depends on how you see the figures. NY Times, April 22, 1990.
101. Lane C, Waller D, Larmer B, Katel P. The newest war. Newsweek, January 6, 1992.
102. Lewin NA, Goldfrank LR, Weisman RS. Cocaine. In: Goldfrank LR, Flomenbaum NE, Lewin NA, et al, eds. Toxicologic Emergencies, ed. 4. Norwalk, CT: Appleton & Lange, 1990:499.
103. Stone M. Coke Inc. New York Magazine, July 16, 1990.
104. Kleber HD. Tracking the cocaine epidemic. JAMA 1991; 266:2272.
105. Massing M. Whatever happened to the "War on Drugs"? New York Review of Books, June 11, 1992.
106. Treaster JB. Drop in youths' cocaine use may reflect a societal shift. NY Times, January 25, 1991.
107. Jarvik ME. The drug dilemma: manipulating the demand. Science 1990; 250:387.
108. Gelb LH. Yet another summit. NY Times, November 3, 1991.
108a. Treaster JB. Emergency rooms' cocaine cases rise. N.Y. Times, October 24, 1992.
109. Baldwin DC, Hughes PH, Conrad SE, et al. Substance use among senior medical students. A survey of 23 medical schools. JAMA 1991; 265:2074.
110. ElSohly MA, Brenneisen R, Jones AB. Coca paste: chemical analysis and smoking experiments. J Forens Sci 1991; 36:93.
111. Shannon M. Clinical toxicity of cocaine adulterants. Ann Emerg Med 1988; 17:1243.
112. Siegel RK. Changing patterns of cocaine use: longitudinal observations, consequences, and treatments. In:

Grabowski J, ed. Cocaine: Pharmacology, Effects, and Treatment of Abuse. Washington, DC: NIDA Research Monograph 50, DHHS, 1984:92.
113. DesJarlais DC, Friedman SR. Intravenous cocaine, crack, and HIV infection. JAMA 1988; 259:1945.
114. Wesson DR, Washburn P. Current patterns of drug abuse that involve smoking. In: Chiang CN, Hawks RL, eds. Research Findings on Smoking of Abused Substances. Rockville, MD: NIDA Research Monograph 99, DHHS, 1990:5.
115. Perez-Reyes M, DiGuiseppi S, Ondrusek G, et al. Freebase cocaine smoking. Clin Pharmacol Ther 1982; 32:459.
116. Mahler JC, Perry S, Sutton B. Intraurethral cocaine administration. JAMA 1988; 259:3126.
117. Ettinger TB, Stine RJ. Sudden death temporally related to vaginal cocaine abuse. Am J Emerg Med 1989; 7:129.
118. Doss PL, Gowitt GT. Investigation of a death caused by rectal insertion of cocaine. Am J Forens Med Pathol 1988; 9:336.
119. Tripp M, Dowd DD, Eitel DR. TAC toxicity in the emergency department. Ann Emerg Med 1991; 20:106.
120. Wilkinson P, Van Dyke C, Jatlow P, et al. Intranasal and oral cocaine kinetics. Clin Pharmacol Ther 1980; 27:386.
121. Caruana DS, Weinbach B, Goerg D, Gardner LB. Cocaine packet ingestion. Diagnosis, management, and natural history. Ann Intern Med 1984; 100:73.
122. Goldfrank LR, Hoffman RS. The cardiovascular effects of cocaine. Ann Emerg Med 1991; 20:165.
123. Fischman MW, Schuster CR. Acute tolerance to cocaine in humans. In: Harris LS, ed. Problems of Drug Dependence 1980. Washington, DC: NIDA Research Monograph 34, DHHS, 1981, 241.
124. Fischman MW, Schuster CR, Resnekov L, et al. Cardiovascular and subjective effects of intravenous cocaine administration in humans. Arch Gen Psychiatry 1976; 33:983.
125. Jones RT. The pharmacology of cocaine smoking in humans. In: Chiang CN, Hawks RL, eds. Research Findings on Smoking of Abused Substances. Rockville, MD: NIDA Research Monograph 99, DHHS, 1990:30.
126. Wilkerson RD. Cardiovascular effects of cocaine in conscious dogs: importance of fully functional autonomic and central nervous systems. J Pharmacol Exp Ther 1988; 246:466.
126a. Knuepfer MM, Branch CA. Cardiovascular responses to cocaine are initially mediated by the central nervous system in rats. J Pharmacol Exp Ther 1992; 263:734.
126b. Branch CA, Knuepfer MM. Adrenergic mechanisms underlying cardiac and vascular responses to cocaine in conscious rats. J Pharmacol Exp Ther 1992; 263:742.
127. Brody SL, Slovis CM, Wrenn KD. Cocaine-related medical problems: consecutive series of 233 patients. Am J Med 1990; 88:325.

128. Gay GR. Clinical management of acute and chronic cocaine poisoning. Ann Emerg Med 1982; 11:562.

129. Merab J. Acute dystonic reaction to cocaine. Am J Med 1988; 84:564.

130. Brower KJ, Blow FC, Beresford TP. Forms of cocaine and psychiatric symptoms. Lancet 1988; 1:50.

131. Derlet RW, Albertson TE. Emergency department presentation of cocaine intoxication. Ann Emerg Med 1989; 18:542.

132. Garland JS, Smith DS, Rice TB, Siker D. Accidental cocaine intoxication in a nine-month-old infant. Presentation and treatment. Pediatr Emerg Care 1989; 5:245.

133. Roth D, Alarcon FJ, Fernandez JA, et al. Acute rhabdomyolysis associated with cocaine intoxication. N Engl J Med 1988; 319:673.

134. Herzlich BC, Arsura EL, Pagala M, Grob D. Rhabdomyolysis related to cocaine abuse. Ann Intern Med 1988; 109:335.

135. Menashe PI, Gottlieb JE. Hyperthermia, rhabdomyolysis, and myoglobinuric renal failure after recreational use of cocaine. South Med J 1988; 81:379.

136. Anand V, Siami G, Stone WJ. Cocaine-associated rhabdomyolysis and acute renal failure. South Med J 1989; 82:67.

137. Pogue VA, Nurse HM. Cocaine-associated acute myoglobinuric renal failure. Am J Med 1989; 86:183.

138. Rubin RB, Neugarten J. Cocaine-induced rhabdomyolysis masquerading as myocardial ischemia. Am J Med 1989; 86:551.

139. Singhal P, Horowitz B, Quinnones MC, et al. Acute renal failure following cocaine abuse. Nephron 1989; 52:76.

140. Howard RL, Kaehny WD. Cocaine and rhabdomyolysis. Ann Intern Med 1989; 110:90.

141. Horst E, Bennett RL, Barrett O. Recurrent rhabdomyolysis in association with cocaine use. South Med J 1991; 84:269.

142. Campbell BG. Cocaine abuse and hyperthermia, seizures, and fatal complications. Med J Aust 1988; 149:387.

143. Lipton RB, Choy-Kwong M, Solomon S. Headaches in hospitalized cocaine users. Headache 1989; 29:225.

144. Satel SL, Gawin FH. Migraine-like headache and cocaine use. JAMA 1989; 261:2995.

145. Cunningham KA, Lakoski JM. Electrophysiological effects of cocaine and procaine on dorsal raphe serotonin neurons. Eur J Pharmacol 1988; 148:457.

146. Brower KJ. Self-medication of migraine headaches with freebase cocaine. J Subst Abuse Treat 1988; 5:23.

147. Sherer MA, Kumor KM, Cone EJ, Jaffe JH. Suspiciousness induced by four-hour infusions of cocaine. Arch Gen Psychiatry 1988; 45:673.

148. Satel SL, Southwick SM, Gawin FH. Clinical features of cocaine-induced paranoia. Am J Psychiatry 1991; 148:495.

149. Manschreck TC, Allen DF, Neville M. Freebase psychosis: cases from a Bahamian epidemic of cocaine abuse. Comp Psychiatry 1987; 28:555.

150. Jeri FR, Sanchez CC, del Pozo T, et al. Further experience with the syndromes produced by coca paste smoking. Bull Narc 1978; 30:1.

151. Lesko LM, Fischman MW, Javaid JR, Davis JM. Iatrogenous cocaine psychosis. N Engl J Med 1982; 307:1153.

152. Jonnson S, O'Meara M, Young JB. Acute cocaine poisoning. Importance of treating seizures and acidosis. Am J Med 1983; 75:1061.

153. Lowenstein DH, Massa SM, Rowbotham MC, et al. Acute neurologic and psychiatric complications associated with cocaine abuse. Am J Med 1987; 83:841.

154. Myers JA, Earnest MP. Generalized seizures and cocaine abuse. Neurology 1984; 34:675.

155. Choy-Kwong M, Lipton RB. Seizures in hospitalized cocaine users. Neurology 1989; 39:425.

156. Schwartz RH, Estroff T, Hoffman NG. Seizures and syncope in adolescent cocaine abusers. Am J Med 1988; 85:462.

157. Harden CL, Montjo RE, Tuchman AJ, Daras M. Seizures provoked by cocaine use. Ann Neurol 1990; 28:263.

158. Alldredge BK, Lowenstein DH, Simon RP. Seizures associated with recreational drug abuse. Neurology 1989; 39:1037.

159. Pascual-Leone A, Dhuna A, Altafullah I, Anderson DC. Cocaine-induced seizures. Neurology 1990; 40:404.

159a. Kramer LD, Locke GE, Ogunyemi A, Nelson L. Cocaine-related seizures in adults. Am J Drug Alcohol Abuse 1990; 16:307.

159b. Dhuna A, Pascual-Leone A, Langendorf F, Anderson DC. Epileptogenic properties of cocaine in humans. Neurotoxicology 1991; 16:621.

160. Washton AM, Tatarsky A. Adverse effects of cocaine abuse. In: Harris L, ed. Problems of Drug Dependence 1983. Washington, DC: NIDA Research Monograph 49, DHHS, 1984:247.

161. Schwartz RH, Luxenberg MG, Hoffman NG. Crack use by American middle-class adolescent polydrug abusers. J Pediatr 1991; 118:150.

162. Ng SKC, Brust JCM, Hauser WA, Susser M. Illicit drug use and the risk of new-onset seizures. Am J Epidemiol 1990; 132:47.

163. Ogunyemi AO, Locke GE, Kramer LD, Nelson L. Complex partial status epilepticus provoked by "crack" cocaine. Ann Neurol 1989; 26:785.

163a. Konkol RJ, Erickson BA, Doerr JK, et al. Seizures induced by the cocaine metabolite benzoylecgonine in rats. Epilepsia 1992; 33:420.

164. Rebischung D, Daras M, Tuchman AJ. Dystonic movements associated with cocaine use. Ann Neurol 1990; 28:267.

165. Kumor K. Cocaine withdrawal dystonia. Neurology 1990; 40:863.

166. Farrell PE, Diehl AK. Acute dystonic reaction to crack cocaine. Ann Emerg Med 1991; 20:322.

167. Choy-Kwong M, Lipton RB. Dystonia related to cocaine withdrawal: a case report and pathogenic hypothesis. Neurology 1989; 39:996.

167a. Cardoso F, Jankovic J. Movement disorders. In: Brust JCM, ed. Neurologic Complications of Drug and Alcohol Abuse. Neurol Clin 1993, in press.

168. Kumor K, Sherer M, Jaffe J. Haloperidol-induced dystonia in cocaine addicts. Lancet 1986; 2:1341.

169. Mesulam M-M. Cocaine and Tourette's syndrome. N Engl J Med 1986; 315:398.

170. Pascual-Leone A, Dhuna A. Cocaine-associated multifocal tics. Neurology 1990; 40:999.

171. Factor SA, Sanchez-Ramos JR, Wiener WJ. Cocaine and Tourette's syndrome. Ann Neurol 1988; 23:423.

172. Scharf D. Opsoclonus-myoclonus following the intranasal usage of cocaine. J Neurol Neurosurg Psychiatry 1989; 52:1447.

173. Welch RD, Todd K, Krause GS. Incidence of cocaine-associated rhabdomyolysis. Ann Emerg Med 1991; 20:154.

174. Parks JM, Reed G, Knochel JP. Case report: cocaine-associated rhabdomyolysis. Am J Med 1989; 297:334.

175. Steingrub JS, Sweet S, Teres D. Crack-induced rhabdomyolysis. Crit Care Med 1989; 17:1073.

176. Guerin JM, Lustman C, Barbotin-Larrieu F. Cocaine-associated acute myoglobinuric renal failure. Am J Med 1989; 87:248.

177. Zamora-Quezada JC, Dinerman H, Stadecker MJ, Kelly J. Muscle and skin infarction after free-basing cocaine (crack). Ann Intern Med 1988; 108:564.

178. Wetli CV, Wright RK. Deaths caused by recreational cocaine use. JAMA 1979; 241:2519.

179. Smart RG, Anglin L. Do we know the lethal dose of cocaine? J Forens Sci 1987; 32:303.

180. Amon CA, Tate LG, Wright RK, Matusiak W. Sudden death due to ingestion of cocaine. J Anal Toxicol 1986; 10:217.

181. Loghmanee F, Tobak M. Fatal malignant hyperthermia associated with recreational cocaine and ethanol abuse. Am J Forens Pathol 1986; 7:246.

182. Wetli CV, Fishbain DA. Cocaine induced psychosis and sudden death in recreational cocaine users. J Forens Sci 1985; 30:873.

183. Roberts JR, Quattrocchi E, Howland MA. Severe hyperthermia secondary to intravenous drug abuse. Am J Emerg Med 1984; 2:373.

184. Kosten TR, Kleber HD. Sudden death in cocaine abusers: relation to neuroleptic malignant syndrome. Lancet 1987; 1:1198.

185. Robin ED, Wong RJ, Ptashne KA. Increased lung water and ascites after massive cocaine overdosage in mice and improved survival related to beta-adrenergic blockage. Ann Intern Med 1989; 110:202.

186. Clarke MJ. Suicide and cocaine. JAMA 1988; 260:2506.

187. Honer WG, Gewirtz G, Turey M. Psychosis and violence in cocaine smokers. Lancet 1987; 2:451.

188. Mittleman RE, Wetli CV. Death caused by recreational cocaine use: an update. JAMA 1984; 252:1889.

189. Press S. Crack and fatal child abuse. JAMA 1988; 260:3132.

190. Sperry K. Suicide with, and because of, cocaine. JAMA 1988; 259:2995.

191. Randell T. Cocaine, alcohol mix in body to form even longer lasting, more lethal drug. JAMA 1992; 267:1043.

192. Catravas JD, Waters IW. Acute cocaine intoxication in the conscious dog: studies on the mechanism of lethality. J Pharmacol Exp Ther 1981; 217:350.

193. Derlet RW, Albertson TE. Diazepam in the prevention of seizures and death in cocaine-intoxicated rats. Ann Emerg Med 1989; 18:542.

194. Spivey WH, Schoffstall JM, Kirkpatrick, et al. Comparison of labatelol, diazepam, and haloperidol for the treatment of cocaine toxicity in the swine model. Ann Emerg Med 1990; 19:467.

195. Guinn MM, Bedford JA, Wilson JC. Antagonism of intravenous cocaine lethality in nonhuman primates. Clin Toxicol 1980; 16:499.

196. Catravas JD, Waters IW, Walz MA, et al. Acute cocaine intoxication in the conscious dog: pathophysiologic profile of acute lethality. Arch Int Pharmacodyn Ther 1978; 235:328.

197. Witkin JM, Goldberg SR, Katz JL. Lethal effects of cocaine are reduced by the dopamine-1 receptor antagonist SCH 23390 but not by haloperidol. Life Sci 1989; 44:1285.

198. Mercuro G, Gessa G, Rivano CA, et al. Evidence for a dopaminergic control of sympathoadrenal catecholamine release. Am J Cardiol 1988; 62:827.

199. Romoska E, Sacchetti AD. Propranolol-induced hypertension in the treatment of cocaine intoxication. Ann Emerg Med 1985; 14:1112.

200. Dusenberry SJ, Hicks MJ, Mariani PJ. Labetalol treatment of cocaine toxicity. Ann Emerg Med 1987; 16:235

201. Gay GR, Luperka KA. Control of cocaine-induced hypertension with labetolol. Anesth Analg 1988; 67:92.

202. Lathers CM, Tyau LSY, Spino MM, Agarwal L. Cocaine-induced seizures, arrhythmias and sudden death. J Clin Pharmacol 1988; 28:584.

203. Gay GR, Loper KA. The use of labatalol in the management of cocaine crisis. Ann Emerg Med 1988; 17:282.

204. Sand IC, Brody SL, Wrenn KD, Slovis CM. Experience with esmolol for the treatment of cocaine-associated cardiovascular complications. Am J Emerg Med 1991; 9:161.

205. Nahas G, Trouve R, Demus JF, von Sitbon M. A calcium-channel blocker as antidote to the cardiac effects of cocaine intoxication. N Engl J Med 1985; 313:520.

206. Derlet RW, Albertson TE. Potentiation of cocaine toxicity with calcium channel blockers. Am J Emerg Med 1989; 7:464.

206a. Shukla VK, Goldfrank LR, Turndorf H, Bansinath M. Antagonism of acute cocaine toxicity by buprenorphine. Life Sci 1991; 49:1887.

207. Antelman SM, Kocan D, Rowland N, et al. Amitriptyline provides long-lasting immunization against sudden cardiac death from cocaine. Eur J Pharmacol 1981; 69:119.

208. Derlet RW, Albertson T. Lidocaine potentiation of cocaine toxicity. Ann Emerg Med 1991; 20:135.

209. Miller NS, Gold MS, Belkin BM. The diagnosis of alcohol and cannabis dependence in cocaine dependence. Adv Alcohol Subst Abuse 1990; 8:33.

210. Hearn WL, Flynn DD, Hime GW, et al. Cocaethylene: a unique cocaine metabolite displays high affinity for the dopamine transporter. J Neurochem 1991; 56:698.

210a. Foltin RW, Fischman MW. The cardiovascular and subjective effects of intravenous cocaine and morphine combinations in humans. J Pharmacol Exp Ther 1992; 261:623.

211. Cushman P. Cocaine use in a population of drug abusers on methadone. Hosp Community Psychiatry 1988; 39:1205.

212. Kosten TA. Cocaine attenuates opiate withdrawal in human and rat. In: Harris L, ed. Problems of Drug Dependence 1989. Washington, DC: NIDA Research Monograph 95, DHHS, 1990: 361.

213. Sherer MA. Intravenous cocaine: psychiatric effects, biological mechanisms. Biol Psychiatry 1988; 24:865.

214. Zahniser NR, Peris J, Dwoskin LP, et al. Sensitization to cocaine in the nigrostriatal dopamine system. In: Clouet D, Asghar K, Brown R, eds. Mechanisms of Cocaine Abuse and Toxicity. Rockville, MD: NIDA Research Monograph 88, DHHS, 1988: 55.

215. Fischman MW, Schuster CR, Javaid J, et al. Acute tolerance development to the cardiovascular and subjective effects of cocaine. J Pharmacol Exp Ther 1985; 235:677.

216. Foltin RW, Fischman MW, Pedroso JJ, Pearlson GD. Repeated intranasal cocaine administration. Lack of tolerance to pressor effects. Drug Alcohol Depend 1988; 22:169.

217. Kumor K, Sherer M, Thompson L, et al. Lack of cardiovascular tolerance during intravenous cocaine infusions in human volunteers. Life Sci 1988; 42:2063.

218. Louie AK, Lannon RA, Kettler TA. Treatment of cocaine-induced panic disorder. Am J Psychiatry 1989; 146:40.

219. Schwartz RH, Luxenberg MG, Hoffman NG. "Crack" use by American middle-class adolescent polydrug abusers. J Pediatr 1991; 118:150.

220. Washton AM, Gold MS, Pottash AC, Semitz L. Adolescent cocaine abusers. Lancet 1984; 2:746.

221. Smith DE, Schwartz RH, Martin DM. Heavy cocaine use by adolescents. Pediatrics 1989; 83:539.

222. Johanson CE. The reinforcing properties of procaine, chloroprocaine, and proparacaine in rhesus monkeys. Psychopharmacology 1980; 67:189.

223. Fischman MW, Schuster CR, Rajfer S. A comparison of the subjective and cardiovascular effects of cocaine and procaine in humans. Pharmacol Biochem Behav 1983; 18:711.

224. Van Dyck C, Jatlow P, Ungerer J, et al. Cocaine and lidocaine have similar psychological effects after intranasal application. Life Sci 1979; 24:271.

225. Klatt EC, Montgomery S, Namiki T, Noguchi TT. Misrepresentation of stimulant street drugs: a decade of experience in an analysis program. J Toxicol Clin Toxicol 1986; 24:441.

226. Shannon M, Lacouture PG, Roa J, Woolf A. Cocaine exposure among children seen at a pediatric hospital. Pediatrics 1989; 83:337.

227. Insley BM, Grufferman S, Ayliffe HE. Thallium poisoning in cocaine abusers. Am J Emerg Med 1986; 4:545.

228. Siegel RK. Herbal intoxication. Psychoactive effects from herbal cigarettes, tea, and capsules. JAMA 1976; 236:473.

229. Siegel RK, Elsohly MA, Plowman T, et al. Cocaine in herbal tea. JAMA 1986; 255:40.

230. Engelke BF, Gentner WA. Determination of cocaine in "Mate de Coca" herbal tea. J Pharmaceut Sci 1991; 80:96.

231. Sawicka EH, Trosser A. Cerebrospinal fluid rhinorrhea after cocaine sniffing. BMJ 1983; 284:1476.

232. Wang ES. Cocaine-induced iritis. Ann Emerg Med 1991; 20:192.

233. Becker GD, Hill S. Midline granuloma due to illicit cocaine use. Arch Otolaryngol Head Neck Surg 1988; 114:90.

234. Newman NM, DiLoreto DA, Ho JT, et al. Bilateral optic neuropathy and osteolytic sinusitis. Complications of cocaine abuse. JAMA 1989; 259:72.

235. Rao AN. Brain abscess: a complication of cocaine inhalation. NY State J Med 1988; 88:548.

236. MacDonald KL, Cohen ML, Blake PA. The changing epidemiology of adult botulism in the United States. Am J Epidemiol 1986; 124:794.

237. Rapoport S, Watkins PB. Descending paralysis resulting from occult wound botulism. Ann Neurol 1984; 16:359.

238. Kudrow DB, Henry DA, Haake DA, et al. Botulism associated with Clostridium botulinum sinusitis after intranasal cocaine use. Ann Intern Med 1988; 109:984.

239. MacDonald KL, Rutherford GW, Friedman SM, et al. Botulism and botulism-like illness in chronic drug abusers. Ann Intern Med 1985; 102:616.

240. Ettinger NA, Albin RJ. A review of the respiratory effects of smoking cocaine. Am J Med 1989; 87:664.

241. Tames SM, Goldenring JM. Madarosis from cocaine use. N Engl J Med 1986; 314:1324.

242. Siegel RK. Cocaine and sexual dysfunction: the curse of Mama Coca. J Psychoact Drugs 1982; 14:71.

243. Smith DE, Wesson DR, Apter-Marsh M. Cocaine- and alcohol-induced sexual dysfunction in patients with addictive disease. J Psychoact Drugs 1984; 16:359.
244. Concores JA, Dackis CA, Gold MS. Sexual dysfunction secondary to cocaine abuse in two patients. J Clin Psychiatry 1986; 47:384.
245. Mendelson JH, Teoh SK, Lange U, et al. Anterior pituitary, adrenal, and gonadal hormones during cocaine withdrawal. Am J Psychiatry 1988; 145:1094.
246. Mendelson JH, Mello NK, Teoh SK, et al. Cocaine effects on pulsatile secretion of anterior pituitary, gonadal, and adrenal hormones. J Clin Endocrinol Metab 1989; 69:1256.
247. Berciano J, Oterino A, Rebollo M, Pascual J. Myasthenia gravis unmasked by cocaine abuse. N Engl J Med 1991; 325:892.
248. Dick AD, Prentice MG. Cocaine and acute porphyria. Lancet 1987; 2:1150.
249. Chambers HF, Morris DL, Tauber MG, Modin G. Cocaine use and the risk for endocarditis in intravenous drug users. Ann Intern Med 1987; 106:833.
250. Chaisson RE, Bacchetti P, Osmond D, et al. Cocaine use and HIV infection in intravenous drug users in San Francisco. JAMA 1989; 261:561.
251. Schoenbaum EE, Hartel D, Selwyn PA, et al. Risk factors for human immunodeficiency virus infection in intravenous drug users. N Engl J Med 1989; 321:874.
252. Lerner WD. Cocaine abuse and acquired immunodeficiency syndrome: a tale of two epidemics. Am J Med 1989; 87:661.
253. Fullilove RE, Fullilove MT, Bowser BP, Gross SA. Risk of sexually transmitted disease among black adolescent crack users in Oakland and San Francisco, Calif. JAMA 1990; 263:851.
254. Comer GM, Mittal MK, Donelson SS, Lee TP. Cluster of fulminant hepatitis B in crack users. Am J Gastroenterol 1991; 86:331.
255. Alternative case-finding methods in a crack-related syphilis epidemic—Philadelphia. MMWR 1991; 40:77.
256. Weiss RD. Links between cocaine and retroviral infection. JAMA 1989; 261:607.
257. DesJarlais DC, Abdul-Quader A, Minkoff H, et al. Crack use and multiple AIDS risk behaviors. J AIDS 1991; 4:446.
258. Gitter MJ, Goldsmith SR, Dunbar DN, Sharkey SW. Cocaine and chest pain: clinical features and outcome of patients hospitalized to rule out myocardial infarction. Ann Intern Med 1991; 115:277.
259. Amin M, Gabelman G, Kaspel J, Buttrick P. Acute myocardial infarction and chest pain syndromes after cocaine use. Am J Cardiol 1990; 66:1434.
260. Isner JM, Chokshi SK. Cardiovascular complications of cocaine. Curr Prob Cardiol 1991; 16:89.
261. Minor RL, Scott BD, Brown DD, Winniford MD. Cocaine-induced myocardial infarction in patients with normal coronary arteries. Ann Intern Med 1991; 115:797.

262. Zimmerman FH, Gustafson GM, Kemp HG. Recurrent myocardial infarction associated with cocaine abuse in a young man with normal coronary arteries: evidence for coronary artery spasm culminating in thrombosis. J Am Coll Cardiol 1987; 9:964.
263. Lange RA, Cigarroa RG, Yancy CW, et al. Cocaine-induced coronary-artery vasoconstriction. N Engl J Med 1989; 321:1558.
264. Gardezi N. Cardiovascular effects of cocaine. JAMA 1987; 257:979.
265. Nadamanee K, Gorelick DA, Josephson MA, et al. Myocardial ischemia during cocaine withdrawal. Ann Intern Med 1989; 111:876.
266. Del Aguila C, Rosman H. Myocardial infarction during cocaine withdrawal. Ann Intern Med 1990; 112:712.
267. Isner JJM, Estes NAM, Thompson PD, et al. Acute cardiac events temporally related to cocaine abuse. N Engl J Med 1986; 315:1438.
268. Karch SB, Billingham ME. The pathology and etiology of cocaine-induced heart disease. Arch Pathol Lab Med 1988; 112:225.
269. Petty GW, Brust JCM, Tatemichi TK, Barr ML. Embolic stroke after smoking "crack" cocaine. Stroke 1990; 21:1632.
270. Chokshi SK, Moore R, Pandian NG, Isner JM. Reversible cardiomyopathy associated with cocaine intoxication. Ann Intern Med 1989; 111:1039.
271. Peng SK, French WJ, Pelikan PC. Direct cocaine cardiotoxicity demonstrated by endomyocardial biopsy. Arch Pathol Lab Med 1989; 113:842.
271a. Uszenski RT, Gillis RA, Schaer GL, et al. Additive myocardial depressant effects of cocaine and ethanol. Am Heart J 1992; 124:1276.
272. Kabas JS, Blanchard SM, Matsuyama Y, et al. Cocaine-mediated impairment of cardiac conduction in the dog: a potential mechanism for sudden death after cocaine. J Pharmacol Exp Ther 1990; 252:185.
273. Jain RK, Jain MK, Bachenheimer LC, et al. Factors determining whether cocaine will potentiate the cardiac effects of neurally released norepinephrine. J Pharmacol Exp Ther 1990; 252:147.
274. Hale SL, Alker KJ, Rezkalla SH, et al. Nifedipine protects the heart from the acute deleterious effects of cocaine if administered before but not after cocaine. Circulation 1991; 83:1437.
275. Edwards J, Rubin RN. Aortic dissection and cocaine abuse. Ann Intern Med 1987; 107:779.
276. Barth CW, Bray M, Roberts WC. Rupture of the ascending aorta during cocaine intoxication. Am J Cardiol 1986; 57:496.
277. Freudenberger RS, Cappell MS, Huff DA. Intestinal infarction after intravenous cocaine administration. Ann Intern Med 1990; 113:715.
278. Abramson DL, Gertler JP, Lewis T, Kral JG. Crack-related perforated gastropyloric ulcer. J Clin Gastroenterol 1991; 13:17.
279. Sharff JA. Renal infarction associated with intravenous cocaine use. Ann Emerg Med 1984; 13:1145.

280. Novielli KD, Chambers CV. Splenic infarction after cocaine use. Ann Intern Med 1991; 114:251.

281. Berger JL, Nimier M, Desmonts JM. Continuous axillary plexus block in treatment of accidental intraarterial injection of cocaine. N Engl J Med 1988; 318:930.

282. Mines D. Splenic artery aneurysm rupture. Am J Emerg Med 1991; 9:74.

283. Murray R, Simialek J, Golle M, et al. Pulmonary artery medial hypertrophy without foreign particle microembolization in cocaine users. Chest 1988; 94S:48.

284. Godwin JE, Hasle RA, Miller KS, et al. Cocaine, pulmonary hemorrhage, and hemoptysis. Ann Intern Med 1989; 110:843.

285. Levine SR, Brust JCM, Futrell N, et al. Cerebrovascular complications of the use of the "crack" form of alkaloidal cocaine. N Engl J Med 1990; 323:699.

286. Brust JCM, Richter RW. Stroke associated with cocaine abuse? NY State J Med 1977; 77:1473.

287. Lundberg GD, Garriott JC, Reynolds PC, et al. Cocaine-related death. J Forens Sci 1977; 22:402.

288. Caplan LR, Hier DB, DeCruz I. Cerebral embolism in the Michael Reese Stroke Registry. Stroke 1983; 14:530.

289. Schwartz ICA, Cohen JA. Subarachnoid hemorrhage precipitated by cocaine snorting. Arch Neurol 1984; 41:705.

290. Lichtenfield PJ, Rubin DB, Feldman RS. Subarachnoid hemorrhage precipitated by cocaine snorting. Arch Neurol 1984; 41:223.

291. Chasnoff IJ, Bussey ME, Savich R, Stack CM. Perinatal cerebral infarction and maternal cocaine use. J Pediatr 1986; 108:456.

292. Golbe LI, Merkin MD. Cerebral infarction in a user of free-base cocaine ("crack"). Neurology 1986; 36:1602.

293. Cregler LL, Mark H. Medical complications of cocaine abuse. N Engl J Med 1986; 315:1495.

294. Rogers JN, Henry TE, Jones AM, et al. Cocaine-related deaths in Pima County, Arizona, 1982–1984. J Forens Sci 1986; 31:1404.

295. Altes-Capella J, Cabezudo-Artero JM, Forteza-Rei J. Complications of cocaine abuse. Ann Intern Med 1987; 107:940.

296. Levine SR, Washington JM, Jefferson MF, et al. "Crack" cocaine-associated stroke. Neurology 1987; 37:1849.

297. Wojak JC, Flamm ES. Intracranial hemorrhage and cocaine use. Stroke 1987; 18:712.

298. Kaye BR, Fainstat M. Cerebral vasculitis associated with cocaine abuse. JAMA 1987; 258:2104.

299. Cregler LI, Mark H. Relation of stroke to cocaine abuse. NY State J Med 1987; 87:128.

300. Mittleman RE, Wetli CV. Cocaine and sudden "natural" death. J Forens Sci 1987; 32:11.

301. Lowenstein DH, Massa SM, Rowbotham MC, et al. Acute neurologic and psychiatric complications associated with cocaine abuse. Am J Med 1987; 83:841.

302. Lehman LB. Intracerebral hemorrhage after intranasal cocaine use. Hosp Phys 1987; 7:69.

303. Mangiardi JR, Daras M, Geller ME, et al. Cocaine-related intracranial hemorrhage: report of nine cases and review. Acta Neurol Scand 1988; 77:177.

304. Devenyi P, Schneiderman JF, Devenyi RG, Lawby L. Cocaine-induced central retinal artery occlusion. Can Med Assoc J 1988; 138:129.

305. Mody CK, Miller BL, McIntyre HB, et al. Neurologic complications of cocaine abuse. Neurology 1988; 38:1189.

306. Weingarten KO. Cerebral vasculitis associated with cocaine abuse or subarachnoid hemorrhage? JAMA 1988; 259:1658.

307. Toler KA, Anderson B. Stroke in an intravenous drug user secondary to the lupus anticoagulant. Stroke 1988; 19:274.

308. Devore RA, Tucker HM. Dysphagia and dysarthria as a result of cocaine abuse. Otolaryngol Head Neck Surg 1988; 98:174.

309. Henderson CE, Torbey M. Rupture of intracranial aneurysm associated with cocaine use during pregnancy. Am J Perinatol 1988; 5:142.

310. Tenorio GM, Nazvi M, Bickers GH, Hubbird RH. Intrauterine stroke and maternal polydrug abuse. Clin Pediatr 1988; 27:565.

311. Rowbotham MC. Neurologic aspects of cocaine abuse. West J Med 1988; 149:442.

312. Levine SR, Welch KM. Cocaine and stroke. Stroke 1988; 19:779.

313. Nalls G, Disher A, Darabagi J, et al. Subcortical cerebral hemorrhages associated with cocaine abuse. CT and MR findings. J Comput Assist Tomogr 1989; 13:1.

314. Peterson PL, Moore PM. Hemorrhagic cerebrovascular complications of crack cocaine abuse. Neurology 1989; 39(suppl 1):302.

315. Moore PM, Peterson PL. Nonhemorrhagic cerebrovascular complications of cocaine abuse. Neurology 1989; 39(suppl 1):302.

316. Tardiff K, Gross E, Wu J, et al. Analysis of cocaine-positive fatalities. J Forens Sci 1989; 34:53.

317. Klonoff DC, Andrews BT, Obana WG. Stroke associated with cocaine use. Arch Neurol 1989; 46:989.

318. Rowley HA, Lowenstein DH, Rowbotham MC, Simon RP. Thalamomesencephalic strokes after cocaine abuse. Neurology 1989; 39:428.

319. DeBroucker, Verstichel P, Cambier J, DeTruchis P. Accidents neurologiqes apres prise de cocaine. Presse Med 1989; 18:541.

320. Jacobs IG, Roszler MH, Kelly JK, et al. Cocaine abuse: Neurovascular complications. Radiology 1989; 170:223.

321. Mercado A, Johnson G, Calver D, Sokol RJ. Cocaine, pregnancy, and postpartum intracerebral hemorrhage. Obstet Gynecol 1989; 73:467.

322. Nolte KB, Gelman BB. Intracerebral hemorrhage associated with cocaine abuse. Arch Pathol Lab Med 1989; 113:812.

323. Engstrand BC, Daras M, Tuchman AJ, et al. Cocaine-related ischemic stroke. Neurology 1989; 39(suppl 1):186.

324. Spires MC, Gordon EF, Choudhuri M, et al. Intracranial hemorrhage in a neonate following prenatal cocaine exposure. Pediatr Neurol 1989; 5:324.

325. Meza I, Estrad CA, Montalvo JA, et al. Cerebral infarction associated with cocaine use. Henry Ford Hosp Med J 1989; 37:50.

326. Mast J, Carpanzamo CR, Hier L. Maternal cocaine use: neurologic effects on offspring. Neurology 1989; 30(suppl 1):187.

327. Dixon SD, Bejar R. Echoencephalographic findings in neonates associated with maternal cocaine and methamphetamine use: incidence and clinical correlates. J Pediatr 1989; 115:770.

328. Seaman ME. Acute cocaine abuse associated with cerebral infarction. Ann Emerg Med 1990; 19:34.

329. Simpson RK, Fischer DK, Narayan RK, et al. Intravenous cocaine abuse and subarachnoid hemorrhage: effect on outcome. Br J Neurosurg 1990; 4:27.

330. Deringer PM, Hamilton LL, Whelan MA. A stroke associated with cocaine use. Arch Neurol 1990; 47:502.

331. Green R, Kelly KM, Gabrielson T, et al. Multiple intracerebral hemorrhages after smoking "crack" cocaine. Stroke 1990; 21:957.

332. Krendel DA, Ditter SM, Frankel MR, Ross WK. Biopsy-proven cerebral vasculitis associated with cocaine abuse. Neurology 1990; 40:1092.

333. Kaku DA, Lowenstein DH. Emergence of recreational drug abuse as a major risk factor for stroke in young adults. Ann Intern Med 1990; 113:821.

334. Hoyme HE, Jones KL, Dixon SD, et al. Prenatal cocaine exposure and fetal vascular disruption. Pediatrics 1990; 85:743.

335. Kramer LD, Locke GE, Ogunyemi A, Nelson L. Neonatal cocaine-related seizures. J Child Neurol 1990; 5:60.

336. Harruff RC, Phillips AM, Fernandez GS. Cocaine-related deaths in Memphis and Shelby County. Ten-year history, 1980–1989. J Tenn Med Assoc 1991; 84:66.

337. Peterson PL, Roszler M, Jacobs I, Wilner HI. Neurovascular complications of cocaine abuse. J Neuropsychiatr 1991; 3:143.

338. Ramadan N, Levine SR, Welch KMA. Pontine hemorrhage following "crack" cocaine use. Neurology 1991; 41:946.

339. Sloan MA, Kittner SJ, Rigamonti D, Price TR. Occurrence of stroke associated with use/abuse of drugs. Neurology 1991; 41:1358.

340. Sauer CM. Recurrent embolic stroke and cocaine-related cardiomyopathy. Stroke 1991; 22:1203.

341. Daras M, Tuchman AJ, Marks S. Central nervous system infarction related to cocaine abuse. Stroke 1991; 22:1320.

342. Hamer JJ, Kamphuis DJ, Rico RE. Cerebral hemorrhages and infarcts following use of cocaine. Ned Tijdschr Geneeskd 1991; 135:333.

343. Heirt LA, Carpanzano CR, Mast J, et al. Maternal cocaine abuse: the spectrum of radiologic abnormalities in the neonatal CNS. Am J Roentgenol 1991; 157:1105.

344. Fredericks RK, Lefkowitz DS, Challa VER, Troost BT. Cerebral vasculitis associated with cocaine abuse. Stroke 1991; 22:1437.

345. Dominguez R, Vila-Coro AA, Slopis JM, Bohan TP. Brain and ocular abnormalities in infants with in utero exposure to cocaine and other street drugs. Am J Dis Child 1991; 145:688.

346. Sloan MA, Mattioni TA. Concurrent myocardial and cerebral infarctions after intranasal cocaine use. Stroke 1992; 23:427.

347. Konzen JP, Levine SR, Charbel FT, Garcia JH. The mechanisms of alkaloidal cocaine-related stroke. Neurology 1992; 42(suppl 3):249.

347a. Guidotti M, Zanasi S. Cocaine use and cerebrovascular disease: Two cases of ischemic stroke in young adults. Ital J Neurol Sci 1990; 11:153.

347b. Hall JAS: Cocaine-induced stroke: First Jamaican case. J Neurol Sci 1990; 98:347.

347c. Chadan N, Thierry A, Sautreaux JL, et al. Rupture aneurysmale et toxicomanie a la cocaine. Neurochirurgie 1990; 37:403.

347d. Nwosu CM, Nwabueze AC, Ikeh VO. Stroke at the prime of life: A study of Nigerian Africans between the ages of 16 and 45 years. E Afr Med J 1992; 69:384.

347e. Libman RB, Masters SR, de Paola A, Mohr JP. Transient monocular blindness associated with cocaine abuse. Neurology 1993; 43:228.

348. Levine SR, Welch KMA, Brust JCM. Cerebral vasculitis associated with cocaine abuse or subarachnoid hemorrhage. JAMA 1988; 259:1648.

349. Levine SR, Brust JCM, Futrell N, et al. A comparative study of the cerebrovascular complications of cocaine: alkaloidal versus hydrochloride—a review. Neurology 1991; 41:1173.

350. Isner JM, Chokshi SK. Cocaine and vasospasm. N Engl J Med 1989; 321:1604.

351. Huang QF, Gebrewold A, Altura BT, Altura BM. Cocaine-induced cerebral vascular damage can be ameliorated by Mg2+ in rat brain. Neurosci Lett 1990; 109:113.

351a. van de Bor M, Walther FJ, Sims ME. Increased cerebral blood flow velocity in infants of mothers who abuse cocaine. Pediatrics 1990; 85:733.

352. Powers RH, Madden JA. Vasoconstrictive effects of cocaine, metabolites and structural analogs on cat cerebral arteries. FASEB 1990; 4:A1095.

353. Fayad PB, Price LH, McDougle CJ, et al. Acute hemodynamic effects of intranasal cocaine on the cerebral and cardiovascular systems. Stroke 1992; 23:26.

354. Dohi S, Jones D, Hudak ML, Traystman RJ. Effects of cocaine on pial arterioles in cats. Stroke 1990; 21:1710.

355. Togna G, Tempesta E, Togna AR, et al. Platelet responsiveness and biosynthesis of thromboxane and

prostacyclin in response to in vitro cocaine treatment. Haemostasis 1985; 15:100.

356. Leissinger CA. Severe thrombocytopenia associated with cocaine use. Ann Intern Med 1990; 112:708.

357. Langner RO, Bement CL, Perry LE. Arteriosclerotic toxicity of cocaine. In: Clouet D, Asghar K, Brown R, eds. Mechanisms of Cocaine Abuse and Toxicity. Washington, DC: NIDA Research Monograph 88, DHHS, 1987:325.

358. Buck AA, Sasaki TT, Hewitt JJ, Macrae AA. Coca chewing and health. An epidemiologic study among residents of a Peruvian village. Am J Epidemiol 1968; 88:159.

359. Negrete JC, Murphy HBM. Psychological deficit in chewers of coca leaf. Bull Narc 1967; 19:11.

359a. Weinrieb RM, O'Brien CP. Persistent cognitive deficits attributed to substance abuse. In Brust JCM, ed. Neurological Complications of Drug and Alcohol Abuse. Neurol Clin 1993, in press.

359b. Ardila A, Roselli M, Strumwasser S. Neuropsychological deficits in chronic cocaine abusers. Int J Neurosci 1991; 57:73.

359c. O'Malley S, Adamse M, Heaton RK, Gawin FH. Neuropsychological impairment in chronic cocaine abusers. Am J Drug Alcohol Abuse 1992; 18:131.

360. Pascual-Leone A, Dhuna A. EEG in cocaine addicts. Ann Neurol 1990; 28:250

361. Pascual-Leone A, Dhuna A, Anderson DC. Cerebral atrophy in habitual cocaine abusers: a planimetric CT study. Neurology 1991; 41:34.

362. Tumeh SS, Nagel JS, English RJ, et al. Cerebral abnormalities in cocaine abusers: demonstration by SPECT perfusion brain scintigraphy. Radiology 1990; 176:821.

363. Volkow ND, Fowler JS, Wolf AP, Gillespi H. Metabolic studies of drugs of abuse. In: Harris L, ed. Problems of Drug Dependence 1990. Washington, DC: NIDA Research Monograph 105, DHHS, 1991:47.

364. Holman BL, Carvalho PA, Mendelson J, et al. Brain perfusion is abnormal in cocaine-dependent polydrug users: a study using technetium-99m-HMPAO and ASPECT. J Nucl Med 1991; 32:1206.

365. London ED, Cascella NG, Wong DF, et al. Cocaine-induced reduction of glucose utilization in human brain. Arch Gen Psychiatry 1990; 47:567.

366. Levisohn PM, Kramer RE, Rosenberg NL. Neurophysiology of chronic cocaine and toluene abuse. Neurology 1992; 42(suppl 3):434.

367. Clark RF, Harchelroad F. Toxicology screening of the trauma patient: a changing profile. Ann Emerg Med 1991; 20:151.

368. Hinds MD. The instincts of parenthood become part of crack's toll. NY Times, March 17, 1990.

369. Little BB, Snell LM, Klein VR, Gilstrap LC. Cocaine abuse during pregnancy: maternal and fetal implications. Obstet Gynecol 1989; 73:157.

370. Frank DA, Zuckerman BS, Amaro H, et al. Cocaine use during pregnancy: prevalence and correlates. Pediatrics 1988; 82:888.

371. Chasnoff IJ, Landress HJ, Barrett ME. The prevalence of illicit-drug or alcohol use during pregnancy and discrepancies in mandatory reporting in Pinellas County, Florida. N Engl J Med 1990; 322:1202.

372. Chira S. Crack babies turn 5 and schools brace. NY Times May 25, 1990.

373. Heagarty M. Crack cocaine: a new danger for children. Am J Dis Child 1990; 144:756.

373a. Chiriboga CA. Fetal effects. In: Brust JCM, ed. Neurologic Complications of Drug and Alcohol Abuse. Neurol Clin 1993, in press.

374. Bingol H, Fuchs M, Diaz V, et al. Teratogenicity of cocaine in humans. J Pediatr 1987; 110:93.

375. Hadeed AJ, Siegel SR. Maternal cocaine use during pregnancy: effect on the newborn infant. Pediatrics 1989; 84:205.

376. Chasnoff IJ, Burns WJ, Schnoll SH, Burns KA. Cocaine use in pregnancy. N Engl J Med 1985; 313:666.

377. Chasnoff IJ, Griffiths DR, MacGregor S, et al. Temporal patterns of cocaine use in pregnancy. Perinatal outcome. JAMA 1989; 261:1741.

378. Chouteau M, Brickner P, Namerow PB, Leppert P. The effect of cocaine abuse on birth weight and gestational age. Obstet Gynecol 1988; 72:351.

379. Cherukuri R, Minkoff H, Feldman J, et al. A cohort study of alkaloidal cocaine ("crack") in pregnancy. Obstet Gynecol 1988; 72:147.

380. Zuckerman B, Frank DA, Hingson R, et al. Effects of marijuana and cocaine use on fetal growth. N Engl J Med 1989; 320:762.

381. Fulroth R, Phillips B, Durand BJ. Perinatal outcome of infants exposed to cocaine and/or heroin in utero. Am J Dis Child 1989; 143:905.

382. Ryan L, Ehrlich S, Finnegan L. Cocaine abuse in pregnancy: effects on the fetus and newborn. Neurotoxicol Teratol 1987; 9:295.

383. Chasnoff IJ, Chisum GM, Kaplan WE. Maternal cocaine use and genitourinary tract malformations. Teratology 1988; 37:201.

384. Urogenital anomalies in the offspring of women using cocaine during early pregnancy—Atlanta, 1968–1980. MMWR 1989; 38:536.

385. Lipschultz SE, Frassica JJ, Orav EJ. Cardiovascular abnormalities in infants prenatally exposed to cocaine. J Pediatr 1991; 118:44.

386. Downing GJ, Horner SR, Kilbride HW. Characteristics of perinatal cocaine-exposed infants with necrotizing enterocolitis. Am J Dis Child 1991; 145:26.

387. Bays J. Fetal vascular disruption with prenatal exposure to cocaine or methamphetamine. Pediatrics 1991; 87:416.

388. Spierer A, Isenberg SJ, Inkelis SH. Characteristics of the iris in 100 neonates. J Pediatr Ophthalmol Strabismus 1989; 26:28.

389. Teske MP, Trese MT. Retinopathy of prematurity-like fundus and persistent hyperplastic primary vitreous associated with maternal cocaine use. Am J Ophthalmol 1987; 103:719.

390. Singer L, Arendt R, Yamashita, et al. Development of infants exposed in utero to cocaine. Pediatr Res 1992; 31:260A.

391. Doberczak TM, Shanzer S, Senie RT, Kandall SR. Neonatal neurologic and electroencephalographic effects of intrauterine cocaine exposure. J Pediatr 1988; 113:354.

391a.Kramer LD, Locke GE, Ogunyemi A, Nelson L. Neonatal cocaine-related seizures. J Child Neurol 1990; 5:60.

392. Chiriboga CA, Bateman O, Brust JCM, Hauser WA. Neurological outcome of neonates exposed in-utero to cocaine. Ped Neurol, in press.

393. Shih L, Cone-Wesson B, Reddix B. Effects of maternal cocaine abuse on neonatal auditory system. Int J Pediatr Otorhinolaryngol 1988; 15:245.

394. Volpe BJ. Effect of cocaine use on the fetus. N Engl J Med 1992; 327:399.

395. Chasnoff IJ, Hunt CE, Kletter R, Kaplan D. Prenatal cocaine exposure is associated with respiratory pattern abnormalities. Am J Dis Child 1989; 143:583.

396. Mayes LC, Granger RH, Bornstein RH, Zuckerman B. The problem of prenatal cocaine exposure. JAMA 1992; 267:406.

397. Zuckerman B, Maynard EC, Cabral H. A preliminary report of prenatal cocaine exposure and respiratory distress syndrome in premature infants. Am J Dis Child 1991; 145:696.

398. Congenital syphilis—New York City, 1986–1988. MMWR 1989; 38:825.

399. Madden JD, Payne TF, Miller S. Maternal cocaine abuse and effect on the newborn. Pediatrics 1986; 77:209.

400. Neuspiel DR, Hamel SC, Hochberg E, et al. Maternal cocaine use and infant behavior. Neurotoxicol Teratol 1991; 13:229.

401. Graham K, Dimitrakoudis D, Pellegrini E, Koren G. Pregnancy outcome following first trimester exposure to cocaine in social users in Toronto, Canada. Vet Hum Toxicol 1989; 31:143.

402. Frank DA, McCarten K, Cahral H, et al. Cranial ultrasounds in term newborns: failure to replicate excess abnormalities in cocaine exposed. Pediatr Res 1992; 31:247A.

403. Koren G, Shear H, Graham K, Einarson T. Bias against the null hypothesis: the reproductive hazards of cocaine. Lancet 1989; 2:440.

404. Lutiger B, Graham K, Einarson TR, Koren G. Relationship between gestational cocaine use and pregnancy outcome: a meta-analysis. Teratology 1991; 44:405.

405. Mahalik MP, Gautieri RF, Mann DE. Teratogenic potential of cocaine hydrochloride in CF-1 mice. J Pharmacol Sci 1980; 69:703.

406. Fantel AG, Macphail T. The teratogenicity of cocaine. Teratology 1982; 26:17.

407. Spear LP, Kirstein C, Bell J, et al. Effects of prenatal cocaine on behavior during the early postnatal period in rats. Teratology 1987; 35:BTS12.

408. Church MW, Dintcheff BA, Gessner PK. Dose-dependent consequences of cocaine on pregnancy outcome in the Long-Evans rat. Neurotoxicol Teratol 1988; 10:51.

409. el-Bizri H, Guest I., Varma DR. Effects of cocaine on rat embryo development in vivo and in cultures. Pediatr Res 1991; 29:187.

410. Woods J, Plessinger M, Clark KE. Effects of cocaine on uterine blood flow and fetal oxygenation. JAMA 1987; 257:957.

411. Moore T, Sorg J, Miller L, et al. Hemodynamic effects of intravenous cocaine on the pregnant ewe and fetus. Am J Obstet Gynecol 1986; 155:883.

412. Morgan MA, Silavin SL, Randolf M, et al. Effect of intravenous cocaine on uterine blood flow in the gravid baboon. Am J Obstet Gynecol 1991; 164:1021.

413. Stewart DJ, Inaba T, Lucassen M, et al. Cocaine metabolism: cocaine and novocaine hydrolysis by liver and serum esterases. Clin Pharmacol Ther 1979; 25:464.

414. Abel EL, Moore C, Waselewsky D, et al. Effects of cocaine hydrochloride on reproductive function and sexual behavior of male rats and on the behavior of their offspring. J Androl 1989; 10:17.

415. Yazigi RA, Odem RR, Polakoski KL. Demonstration of specific binding of cocaine to human spermatozoa. JAMA 1991; 266:1956.

416. Sanchez-Ramos J, Song S, Weiner W, Busto R. Potential cytotoxicity of norcocaine for developing dopaminergic neurons. Neurology 1992; 42(suppl 3):406.

417. Chasnoff IJ, Lewis DE, Squires L. Cocaine intoxication in a breast-fed infant. Pediatrics 1987; 80:836.

418. Chaney NE, Franke J, Wadlington WB. Cocaine convulsions in a breast-feeding baby. J Pediatr 1988; 112:134.

419. Rivkin M, Gilmore HE. Generalized seizures in an infant due to environmentally acquired cocaine. Pediatrics 1989; 84:1100.

420. Bateman DA, Heagarty MC. Passive freebase cocaine ("crack") inhalation by infants and toddlers. Am J Dis Child 1989; 143:25.

421. Kharasch SJ, Glotzer D, Vinci R, et al. Unsuspected cocaine exposure in young children. Am J Dis Child 1991; 145:204.

422. Sturner WQ, Sweeney KG, Callery RT, Haley NR. Cocaine babies: the scourge of the '90s. J Forens Sci 1991; 36:34.

423. Winger G. Pharmacological modifications of cocaine and opioid self-administration. In: Clouet D, Asghar K, Brown R, eds. Mechanisms of Cocaine Abuse and Toxicity. Rockville, MD: NIDA Research Monograph 88, DHHS, 1988:125.

424. Tennant FS, Sagherian AA. Double-blind comparison of amantadine and bromocriptine for ambulatory withdrawal from cocaine dependence. Arch Intern Med 1987; 147:109.

425. Kosten TR, Schumann B, Wright D. Bromocriptine treatment of cocaine abuse in patients maintained on methadone. Am J Psychiatry 1988; 145:381.

426. Extein IL, Gross DA, Gold MS. Bromocriptine treatment of cocaine withdrawal symptoms. Am J Psychiatry 1989; 146:403.

427. Kranzler HR, Bauer LO. Effects of bromocriptine on subjective and autonomic responses to cocaine-associated stimuli. In: Harris LS, ed. Problems of Drug Dependence 1990. Rockville, MD: NIDA Research Monograph 105, DHHS, 1991:505.

428. Preston KL, Sullivan JT, Strain EC, Bigelow GE. Effects of cocaine alone and in combination with bromocriptine in human cocaine abusers. In: Harris LS, ed. Problems of Drug Dependence 1990. Rockville, MD: NIDA Research Monograph 105, DHHS, 1991:507.

429. Handelsman L, Chordia PL, Escovar IL, et al. Amantadine for treatment of cocaine dependence in methadone-maintained patients. Am J Psychiatry 1988; 145:533.

430. Pike RF. Cocaine withdrawal. An effective three-drug regimen. Postgrad Med 1989; 85:115.

431. Kosten TR, Morgan CH, Schottenfeld RS. Amantadine and desipramine in the treatment of cocaine abusing methadone maintenance patients. In: Harris LS, ed. Problems of Drug Dependence 1990. Rockville, MD: NIDA Research Monograph 105, DHHS, 1991:510.

432. Giannini AJ, Folts DJ, Feather JN, Sullivan BS. Bromocriptine and amantadine in cocaine detoxification. Psychiatr Res 1989; 29:11.

433. Malcolm R, Hutto BR, Phillips JD, Ballenger JC. Pergolide mesylate treatment of cocaine withdrawal. J Clin Psychiatry 1991; 52:39.

434. Golwyn DH. Cocaine abuse treated with phenylzine. Int J Addict 1988; 23:897.

435. Berger P, Gawin F, Kosten TR. Treatment of cocaine abuse with mazindol. Lancet 1989; 1:283.

436. Kleber H. Psychopharmacological trials in cocaine abuse treatment. Am J Drug Alcohol Abuse 1986; 12:235.

437. Gawin FH, Kleber HD, Byck R, et al. Desipramine facilitation of initial cocaine abstinence. Arch Gen Psychiatry 1989; 46:117.

438. Brotman AW, Witkie SM, Gelenberg AJ, et al. An open trial of maprotiline for the treatment of cocaine abuse: a pilot study. J Clin Psychopharmacol 1988; 8:125.

439. Giannini AJ, Billett W. Bromocriptine-desipramine protocol in treatment of cocaine addiction. J Clin Pharmacol 1987; 27:549.

440. Giannini AJ, Malone DA, Giannini MC, et al. Treatment of depression in chronic cocaine and phencyclidine abuse with desipramine. J Clin Pharmacol 1986; 26:211.

441. Weiss RD. Relapse to cocaine abuse after initiating desipramine teatment. JAMA 1988; 260:2545.

442. McElroy SL, Weiss RD, Mendelson JH, et al. Desipramine treatment for relapse prevention in cocaine dependence. In: Harris LS, ed. Problems of Drug Dependence 1989. Washington, DC: NIDA Research Monograph 95, DHHS, 1990:57.

443. Arndt I, Dorozynsky L, Woody G, et al. Desipramine treatment of cocaine abuse in methadone maintenance patients. In: Harris LS, ed. Problems of Drug Dependence 1989. Washington, DC: NIDA Research Monograph 95, DHHS, 1990:322.

443a.Fischman MW, Foltin RW, Nestadt G, Pearlson GD. Effects of desipramine maintenance on cocaine self-administration by humans. J Pharmacol Exp Ther 1990; 253:760.

444. Frank RA, Zubrycki E. Chronic imipramine does not block cocaine-induced increases in brain stimulation reward. Pharmacol Biochem Behav 1989; 33:725.

445. Gawin FH, Allen D, Humblestone B. Outpatient treatment of "crack" cocaine smoking with flupenthixol decanoate. A preliminary report. Arch Gen Psychiatry 1989; 46:322.

446. Halikas J, Kemp K, Kuhn K, et al. Carbamazepine for cocaine addiction? Lancet 1989; 1:623.

446a.Halikas JA, Kuhn KL, Crea FS, et al. Treatment of crack-cocaine use with carbamazepine. Am J Drug Alcohol Abuse 1992; 18:45.

447. Margolin A, Kosten T, Petrakis I, et al. Bupropion reduces cocaine abuse in methadone-maintained patients. Arch Gen Psychiatry 1991; 48:87.

448. Batki SL, Manfredi LB, Sorensen JL. Fluoxetine for cocaine abuse in methadone patients: preliminary findings. In: Harris LS, ed. Problems of Drug Dependence 1990. Rockville, MD: NIDA Research Monograph 105, DHHS, 1991:516.

449. Porrino LJ, Ritz MC, Goodman NL, et al. Differential effects of the pharmacological manipulation of serotonin systems on cocaine and amphetamine self-administration in rats. Life Sci 1989; 45:1529.

450. Rounsaville BJ, Anton SF, Carroll K, et al. Psychiatric diagnosis of treatment-seeking cocaine abusers. Arch Gen Psychiatry 1991; 48:43.

451. Weiss RD, Pope HS, Mirin SM. Treatment of chronic cocaine abuse and attention deficit disorder, residual type, with magnesium pemoline. Drug Alcohol Depend 1985; 15:69.

452. Concores JA, Davies RK, Mueller PS, Gold MS. Cocaine abuse and adult attention deficit disorder. J Clin Psychiatry 1987; 48:376.

453. Nunes EV, McGrath PJ, Wager S, Quitkin FM. Lithium treatment for cocaine abusers with bipolar spectrum disorders. Am J Psychiatry 1990; 147:655.

454. Satel SL, Gawin FH. Seasonal cocaine abuse. Am J Psychiatry 1989; 146:534.

455. Jonas JM, Gold MS, Sweeney D, Pottash AL. Eating disorders and cocaine abuse: a survey of 259 cocaine abusers. J Clin Psychiatry 1987; 48:47.

456. Walfish S, Massey R, Krone A. MMPI profiles of cocaine-addicted individuals in residential treatment: implications for practical treatment planning. J Subst Abuse Treatment 1990; 7:151.

457. Weiss RD, Mirin SM. Subtypes of cocaine abusers. Psychiatr Clin North Am 1986; 9:491.

458. Hanbury R, Sturiano V, Cohen M, et al. Cocaine use in persons on methadone maintenance. Adv Alcohol Subst Abuse 1986; 6:97.

459. Kosten TR, Rounsaville BJ, Kleber HD. A 2.5 year follow-up of cocaine use among treated opioid addicts: have our treatments helped? Arch Gen Psychiatry 1987; 44:281.

460. Kosten TR, Kleber HD, Morgan C. Role of opioid antagonists in treating intravenous cocaine abuse. Life Sci 1989; 44:887.

461. Kosten TR, Kleber MD, Morgan C. Treatment of cocaine abuse with buprenorphine. Biol Psychiatry 1989; 26:637.

462. Mendelson JH, Mello NK, Teoh SK, et al. Buprenorphine treatment for concurrent heroin and cocaine dependence: phase 1 study. In: Harris LS, ed. Problems of Drug Dependence 1990. Rockville, MD: NIDA Research Monograph 105, DHHS, 1991:196.

463. Brown EE, Finlay JM, Wong JT, et al. Behavioral and neurochemical interactions between cocaine and bu-prenorphine: implications for the pharmacotherapy of cocaine abuse. J Pharmacol Exp Ther 1991; 256:119.

464. Mello NK, Mendelson JH, Bree MP, Lukas SE. Buprenorphine suppresses cocaine self-administration by rhesus monkeys. Science 1989; 245:859.

465. Mello NK. Preclinical evaluation of the effects of buprenorphine, naltrexone and desipramine on cocaine self-administration. In: Harris LS, ed. Problems of Drug Dependence 1990. Rockville, MD: NIDA Research Monograph 105, DHHS, 1991:189.

466. Kang SY, Kleinman PH, Woody GE, et al. Outcomes for cocaine abusers after once-a-week psychosocial therapy. Am J Psychiatry 1991; 148:630.

467. O'Brien CP, Childress AR, Arndt ID, et al. Pharmacological and behavioral treatments of cocaine dependence: controlled studies. J Clin Psychiatry 1988; 49(suppl):17.

Chapter 5
Barbiturates and Other Hypnotics and Sedatives

Nor all the drowsy syrups of the world
Shall ever medicine thee to that sweet sleep
Which thou ow'dst yesterday.
                    —*William Shakespeare*, Othello

There was a pill for everything—for tranquility, for sleep,
for death.   —*Barbara Gordon*

They got the President to stop taking Halcion. That was
the year's bright spot for the war on drugs.
         —*Unnamed U.S. drug enforcement official, 1992*

A hypnotic drug ". . . produces drowsiness and facilitates the onset and maintenance of a state of sleep that resembles natural sleep in its electroencephalographic characteristics and from which the recipient may be easily aroused."[1] A sedative drug ". . . decreases activity, moderates excitement, and calms the recipient." In high enough doses, most sedative or hypnotic drugs—benzodiazepines are an exception—induce general anesthesia, and a broad classification would include alcohols and volatile anesthetics. This chapter addresses commercially available substituted barbituric acid compounds and nonbarbituric hypnotics and sedatives.

Pharmacology and Animal Studies

Barbiturates and benzodiazepines potentiate the effects of gamma-aminobutyric acid (GABA), an inhibitory neurotransmitter that acts by facilitating chloride conductance. Stereospecific receptors for GABA, barbiturates, and benzodiazepines form parts of a supramolecular *GABA-A-benzodiazepine-chloride ion channel complex*, which consists of protein subunits (alpha, beta, and gamma).[2–4] The GABA receptor resides on the beta subunit and the benzodiazepine receptor on the alpha subunit.[5,6] The barbiturate recognition site is at or close to the chloride channel. The different receptors are allosterically coupled, and the molecular composition of their subunits varies with different brain regions.[7] Benzodiazepines enhance GABA binding, GABA enhances benzodiazepine binding, and barbiturates increase the binding of both GABA and benzodiazepines in a chloride-dependent manner.[8] The convulsant bicuculline antagonizes GABA, perhaps by competing with it at its receptor. The convulsant picrotoxin also antagonizes GABA but acts at the barbiturate site. The effects of GABA, benzodiazepines, and barbiturates on each other's receptors and ultimately on chloride channels appears to be through allosteric modification.

Barbiturates in high enough doses ". . . depress the activity of all excitable tissues."[1] In sedative or hypnotic doses, their actions are largely confined to the central nervous system (CNS), and certain barbiturates have selective anticonvulsant properties at even lower doses. This dissociation between sedative and anticonvulsant properties is the result of barbiturates' dual actions—indirect and direct—at inhibitory synapses: They not only potentiate GABA, but also have their own direct effects on chloride channels, the latter antagonized by picrotoxin. Barbiturates also antagonize glutamate excitatory postsynaptic transmission.[9] Selectively anticonvulsant barbiturates (e.g., phenobarbital) modulate GABA and glutamate responses at doses too low to cause direct inhibitory actions, whereas anesthetic barbiturates (e.g., pentobarbital) at low doses are both modulatory and directly inhibitory.[10] Barbiturates facilitate chloride conductance by prolonging the duration of channel openings rather than by increasing their frequency.[11]

Barbiturates are strongly reinforcing in dogs and monkeys, which self-inject them to the point of unconsciousness.[12] By inducing their own metabolism through stimulation of cytochrome P450, barbiturates produce pharmacokinetic tolerance that peaks within a few days.[1] More important is pharmacodynamic tolerance, which continues to develop over weeks or months. Tolerance is greater to sedative than to anticonvulsant effects, and cross-tolerance (albeit incomplete) exists between barbiturates and other sedatives, including benzodiazepines and ethanol.[13]

In contrast to barbiturates, benzodiazepines are not general neuronal depressants. Acting at the CNS, they produce sedation, sleep, decreased anxiety, anterograde amnesia, and muscle relaxation, and they are anticonvulsant. Benzodiazepines are considered (especially by their manufacturers) to have greater anxiolytic and lesser hypnotic properties than barbiturates; such dissociation is difficult to prove, either in humans or in putative animal models of anxiety.[1,14]

Benzodiazepines occupy stereospecific receptors on the GABA-benzodiazepine macromolecular complex and exert their effects on chloride conductance only indirectly—by allosterically influencing GABA receptor binding.[2,15–17] They increase the frequency rather than the duration of chloride channel openings.[11] Although benzodiazepine agonists do not affect chloride conductance in the absence of GABA, they do have other actions, including enhancement of calcium-dependent potassium conductance and inhibition of certain sodium and calcium channels.[18] It is possible that these effects are secondary to benzodiazepine inhibition of adenosine uptake.[19]

Compounds that bind to the benzodiazepine receptor produce a continuum of effects.[20] Partial agonists produce more limited effects then full agonists, compete with full agonists for receptor binding, and thereby antagonize their actions. By contrast, full and partial *inverse agonists*—among which are a variety of nonbenzodiazepine beta-carboline compounds—produce effects opposite to those of benzodiazepines: inhibition of GABA-induced chloride currents, proconflict behavior, and seizures.[21,22] Full antagonists—for example, flumazenil—block the actions of both agonists and inverse agonists and have little biologic activity of their own.[23]

In animal models, low concentrations of benzodiazepine agonists are anxiolytic, and this action seems to be at least partly independent of GABA. (Interestingly, benzodiazepine withdrawal anxiety in a rat model is blocked by pretreatment with the calcium channel blocker verapamil.[24]) Higher benzodiazepine concentrations, acting through GABA, are anticonvulsant. Still higher concentrations produce sedation and then muscle relaxation.[20,25] Signs of benzodiazepine withdrawal—anxiety, seizures—resemble the effects of inverse agonists, suggesting a shift in the set-point of the receptor toward inverse agonism. Such a rearrangement might also explain the observations that the activity of flumazenil then changes from antagonist to weak inverse agonist and that pretreatment with flumazenil reduces the severity of benzodiazepine withdrawal.[26]

At least two benzodiazepine receptor subtypes, called type I and type II, have different regional distributions in the CNS. Type I receptors are especially prominent in lamina IV of the cerebral cortex, the nucleus basalis, the substantia nigra, the amygdala, and the molecular layer of the cerebellum; type II receptors are more prevalent in the striatum, the olfactory bulb, and the hippocampus.[27] Genetic manipulation of the alpha subunits of benzodiazepine receptors produces marked differences in their binding affinities; such subunit diversity provides a structural explanation for receptor subtypes and possibly for genetic differences.[28] Comparable to genetically different responses to ethanol, some strains of mice are either sensitive or resistant to benzodiazepine-induced ataxia, and these strains differ in the responsiveness of membrane chloride conductance to the GABA agonist muscimol.[29]

A very different *peripheral benzodiazepine receptor* is found on the outer mitochondrial membrane in various tissues, including adrenal, testis, and ovary. Present in low concentrations in brain, peripheral benzodiazepine receptors are most concentrated in proliferating glia. Their function is unknown.[30]

Stereospecific benzodiazepine receptors imply the existence of endogenous ligands, analogous to endorphins. One candidate is a polypeptide called *diazepam binding inhibitor* (DBI).[31] Injected intraventricularly into animals, DBI blocks the anticonflict actions of diazepam and by itself elicits proconflict behavior, an effect antagonized by flumazenil. A fragment of DBI, *octadecaneuropeptide* (ODN), has similar actions, suggesting that DBI is a precursor molecule. DBI's distribution in brain overlaps but is not identical to that of GABA. Other possible benzodiazepine receptor ligands include beta-carboline compounds isolated from mammalian CNS and having pharmacological and behavioral effects similar to those of DBI.[25] Still another possible ligand is *tribulin*, an endogenous monoamine oxidase (MAO) inhibitor and benzodiazepine receptor ligand found in the urine of patients with panic attacks and the urine of rats subjected to stress.[25] Finally, a true benzodiazepine, N-desmethyldiazepam (an active metabolite of diazepam), is present in animal and human brain and in contrast to the aforementioned ligands functions as an agonist.[32] N-desmethyldiazepam might be biosynthesized by microorganisms or plants and reach the CNS through diet.

It is thus possible that there are both *anxiogenic* and *anxiolytic* endogenous ligands for benzodiazepine receptors, serving the biologic role of adjusting *vigilance/alertness homeostasis.*[25] Perhaps there is even a common precursor for agonist and inverse agonist compounds.

Animals self-administer benzodiazepines but much less vigorously than barbiturates, psychostimulants, or opioids.[33,34] Orally administered benzodiazepines have little if any reinforcing effects in rats or monkeys. Intravenous administration is modestly reinforcing, with short-acting drugs such as triazolam or midazolam preferred over longer-acting agents such as diazepam or chlordiazepoxide.[35]

In contrast to barbiturates, benzodiazepines do not induce their own enzymatic metabolism, and the tolerance that develops to their effects is entirely pharmacodynamic. It is controversial whether different benzodiazepine actions have different degrees of tolerance. The widespread clinical impression—emphasized by the pharmaceutical industry—that tolerance develops to sedative but not to anxiolytic effects is supported by rather sparse animal data. As with other drugs, the basis of tolerance is unclear. It seems to require benzodiazepine receptor binding—flumazenil blocks it—and may involve receptor downregulation through changes in gene expression, but it is independent of duration or dose.[36-38] (Interestingly, chronic exposure to inverse agonists causes receptor up-regulation.[39]) Benzodiazepines are cross-tolerant with other sedatives and with ethanol, and in mice chronic ethanol administration causes decreased benzodiazepine-receptor binding.[40]

Barbiturates

In 1900, the only commercially available hypnotic-sedatives were bromides, chloral hydrate, paraldehyde, urethan, and Sulfonal, and reports of abuse of bromide, chloral hydrate, and paraldehyde had already appeared.[1,41-43] Barbital was introduced in 1903, and a report of abuse appeared a year later.[44]

Phenobarbital appeared in 1912, followed by a large number of long-acting, short-acting, and ultra–short-acting preparations (Table 5–1; Figure 5–1).

It was soon recognized that tolerance developed rapidly to sedation induced by barbiturates, rendering them ineffective as long-term sleeping pills,[45] and that chronic use could lead to severe abstinence symptoms.[46] Nonetheless, by 1962 over a million pounds of barbiturates were sold in the United States, equivalent to 24 100 mg doses for every man, woman, and child in the country.[47] Although legitimate use of barbiturates subsequently declined with the emergence of benzodiazepines,[48] abuse and overdose today are by no means rare. In 1985, barbiturates accounted for 4.2% of Drug Abuse Warning Network (DAWN) reports (compared with 7.7% in 1981).[35] They are abused by patients who obtain them through physician prescription and by street users who procure them illegally. In either setting, barbiturates—"goof balls," "downers," "barbs," "red devils" (secobarbital), "yellow-jackets" (pentobarbital), "blue angels," "blue birds," "blue devils" (amobarbital), "rainbows" (Tuinal)—are usually taken orally, but street addicts also administer them intravenously or intramuscularly. The abuse potential is greatest for short-acting agents, but none is exempt; abuse and symptomatic withdrawal have even been reported for the analgesic preparation Fiorinal, tablets of which contain butalbital.[49] Barbiturate addicts are often physically dependent on opioids and ethanol as well.[50]

The acute effects of barbiturates are similar to those of ethanol.[51] A single dose of 200 to 400 mg

Table 5–1. Barbiturates Currently or Recently Available in the United States

Amobarbital (Amytal, and in Tuinal)
Aprobarbital (Alurate)
Butabarbital (Butisol)
Butalbital (in mixtures only, e.g., Esgic, Fiorinal, Fioricet, Medigesic, Pacaps, Phrenilin, Repan, Sedapap, Tencet, Tencon)
Mephobarbital (Mebaral)
Metharbital (Gemonil)
Methohexital (Brevital)
Pentobarbital (Nembutal)
Phenobarbital (Luminal, and in mixtures, e.g., Bellergal, Donnatal, Gustase, Kinesed, Primatene, Quadrinal, Tedral)
Secobarbital (Seconal, and in Tuinal)
Talbutal (Lotusate)
Thiamylal (Surital)
Thiopental (Pentothal)

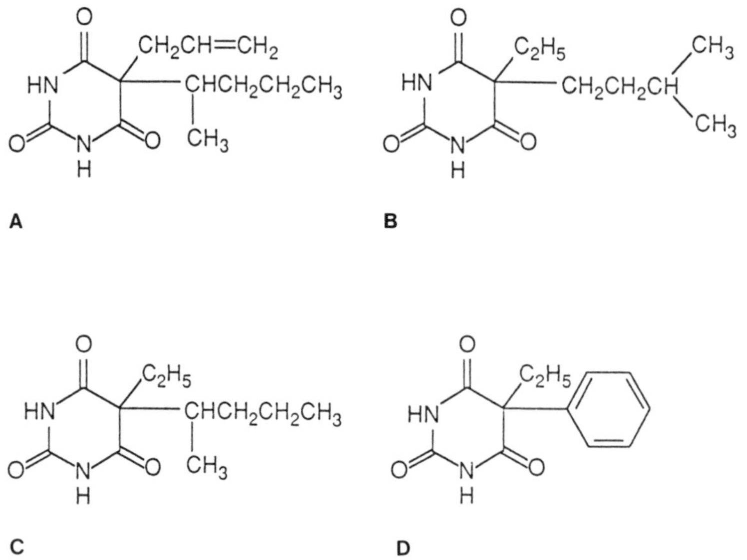

Figure 5–1. Secobarbital (A), amobarbital (B), pentobarbital (C), and phenobarbital (D).

secobarbital or 200 to 600 mg amobarbital in a novice produces a few hours of lightheadedness, euphoria, distortion of time sense, decreased attention and intellectual performance, sedation, ataxia, slurred speech, nystagmus, and diplopia.[52] There may be excitement, particularly as the sedative effect wears off after a few hours. Marked variations in response occur in subjects taking the same dose repeatedly, with either euphoria, depression, or hostility. There is decrease in the amount of sleep spent in the rapid eye movement (REM) phase. The electroencephalogram shows increased fast activity (15 to 35 Hz), most prominent frontally. Higher doses cause respiratory depression; carbon dioxide–sensitive areas of the medulla are more affected than oxygen receptors in the aortic and carotid bodies.

Barbiturate poisoning follows suicide attempts, accidental ingestion by children, and overdose by addicts. *Drug automatism*, unwitting repetition of hypnotic doses because of impaired memory, is probably infrequent.[1] Ethanol often aggravates symptoms; fatalities have occurred with combined blood concentrations of only 0.5 mg/dL for secobarbital and 100 mg/dL for ethanol.[53] Severe poisoning causes coma and respiratory depression. In milder cases, respirations may be rapid and shallow or of Cheyne-Stokes type. Hypotension is secondary to hypoxia, venous vasodilation, and hypovolemia from vomiting, diarrhea, or dehydration during prolonged coma. Very high doses of barbiturates directly depress the myocardium and brain stem vasomotor centers. Hypothermia, sometimes marked, can lead to dangerous cardiac arrhythmias.[54] Tendon reflexes may be

depressed, and flexor or extensor posturing has been observed.[55] Bullous skin eruptions result from a direct toxic action of barbiturates on the epidermis.[53,56] Deep vein thrombosis follows sustained immobility. Aspiration pneumonia is common. Very severe barbiturate poisoning can result in absent pupillary and other brain stem reflexes and an isoelectric (flat-line) electroencephalogram—the clinical picture of brain death—yet such patients may fully recover.

Treatment of barbiturate overdose begins with assessment of cardiorespiratory status, endotracheal intubation, oxygen, and intravenous fluids.[53,54,57] Because barbiturates decrease gastrointestinal motility, the stomach is evacuated by emesis or lavage, followed by activated charcoal and a cathartic.[58] Artificial ventilation and blood pressure support may be necessary. Fluid replacement is preferable to pressors, which aggravate hypotension by reducing cardiac output.[53] If shock persists despite normal central venous pressure, dopamine or dobutamine can be given. For long-acting barbiturates (e.g., phenobarbital), forced diuresis with mannitol and urinary alkalinization are instituted unless there is anuria secondary to shock.[57] Hemodialysis works faster than peritoneal dialysis and is more effective for long-acting agents. CNS stimulant drugs are contraindicated.

Tolerance to barbiturate sedation develops rapidly (in fact, can be seen after a single dose) and reaches a maximum level that varies among individuals. Although tolerance has allowed physically dependent subjects to ingest 2.5 g of short-acting barbiturates daily, there is, in contrast to opioids or amphetamines, less increase in the lethal dose, and someone with little intoxication on a high fixed daily dose of barbiturate may become severely symptomatic with an additional small increment.[47] As in animals, degrees of cross-tolerance exist between barbiturates, other hypnotic-sedatives, and ethanol.

Physical dependence is manifested by withdrawal symptoms similar to ethanol's: insomnia, anxiety, tremor, hyperreflexia, weakness, anorexia, nausea, vomiting, abdominal cramps, mydriasis, postural hypotension, tachypnea, and tachycardia. Rebound REM sleep produces frequent dreaming and nightmares.[57] Hallucinations occur, often auditory (and persecutory), less often visual; they usually clear within 1 or 2 weeks but can persist longer.[57,58] Seizures are most likely to occur on the second or third day following withdrawal of short-acting agents. Symptoms resembling delirium tremens, with confusion, disorientation, delusions, hallucinations, hyperthermia, and cardiovascular instability, begin on the second to fifth day and last from 1 day to several weeks. Electroencephalographic slowing and paroxysmal discharges occur during the first few days of withdrawal and are provoked (with myoclonic jerks) for much longer with photic stimulation.[46]

Abrupt withdrawal from oral pentobarbital or secobarbital taken in a daily dose of 400 mg for several months produced paroxysmal electroencephalographic changes without symptoms in one-third of subjects. Withdrawal from 600 mg/day caused minor symptoms in half the subjects and a seizure in 10%. Of those taking 900 mg or more daily, three-fourths had seizures and two-thirds delirium tremens.[59]

Treatment or prevention of barbiturate withdrawal can be accomplished with short-acting barbiturates (e.g., pentobarbital) given in doses (preferably oral) of 200 to 400 mg every 4 to 6 hours until mild signs of intoxication appear. After 2 or 3 days of stabilization at this dose, the drug is slowly withdrawn at a rate of no more than 100 mg daily. If abstinence symptoms appear, withdrawal is stopped until they subside; it is then resumed at the same or at a slower rate. If the initial 200 mg dose of pentobarbital produces gross signs of intoxication, it is unlikely that the subject is physically dependent on barbiturates. Severe withdrawal symptoms call for higher doses and more rapid stabilization. Some investigators believe that phenobarbital produces smoother withdrawal with less risk of overdose and recommend substituting 30 mg phenobarbital for each "equivalent" 100 mg amobarbital, secobarbital, or pentobarbital (up to 500 mg phenobarbital

per day.)[60] As with ethanol withdrawal, delirium tremens is a medical emergency requiring intensive sedation and supportive therapy and carrying substantial mortality; once such symptoms appear, they are not readily reversible with barbiturate administration.[50]

A neonatal withdrawal syndrome affects infants of mothers taking barbiturates, sometimes at customary hypnotic or anticonvulsant doses. Symptoms resemble those of neonatal opioid abstinence but occur later than with heroin (up to a week after delivery) and can last several months. Low birth weight has not been an associated feature.[61]

Cerebral infarction can follow barbiturate overdose and decreased brain perfusion, but occlusive or hemorrhagic strokes have not otherwise been convincingly demonstrated. Coma with right hemiplegia occurred in a 20-year-old man taking orally a combination of secobarbital and strychnine ("M and M's"). Cerebral angiography suggested arteritis, but he had been taking other drugs as well for at least 10 years.[62] Radiographic evidence of cerebral vasculitis was found in four other barbiturate abusers, two of whom also abused chlorpromazine and a third other unidentified drugs.[63] Monkeys receiving dissolved secobarbital capsules 1.5 mg/kg intravenously three times weekly for a year had widespread narrowing of cerebral arteries at angiography, and histologically there were scattered talc crystals in brain capillaries without cellular reaction. Frontal lobe microinfarction was seen in one animal.[64]

Chronic barbiturate abuse leads to psychological and social deterioration, with "poor grooming, lying, bizarre and paranoid thought processes, and erratic and suicidal behavior."[57] Volunteers and epileptics receiving phenobarbital have demonstrated impaired concentration and short-term memory.[65] In contrast to alcoholics, barbiturate-dependent subjects do not have abnormal computed tomography (CT) scans.[66] Barbiturates do reduce cerebral glucose metabolism, however.[67]

Of obvious importance is whether barbiturate exposure in utero or early in life causes long-lasting cognitive or behavioral alteration.[68] Such effects have been observed in some[69–71] but not all[72] studies of children receiving phenobarbital for febrile seizures; in one report, the mean IQ of children receiving phenobarbital was several points lower than the group receiving placebo 6 months after discontinuation of the drug.[73] Phenobarbital has reportedly caused morphologic abnormalities in neurons in culture and impaired brain growth and learning in animals exposed prenatally or postnatally.[74–76]

Benzodiazepines

The first available benzodiazepine was chlordiazepoxide in 1960, followed a year later by diazepam.[16] Marketed as antianxiety agents or *tranquilizers*, they soon became the most widely prescribed drugs in the United States. In the 1970s, flurazepam was marketed as a hypnotic and replaced barbiturates as the most-prescribed sleeping pill in the United States. In the 1980s, the shorter-acting triazolam became the most popular hypnotic. By the 1990s, eight benzodiazepines were promoted in the United States as tranquilizers, and five as hypnotics (Table 5–2; Figure 5–2). Clonazepam is used mainly as an anticonvulsant and for panic disorder, and midazolam is used for anesthesia induction.[14] Nitrazepam is available as both a hypnotic and an anticonvulsant in Europe. As with barbiturates, reports of abuse of individual benzodiazepines appeared within a few years of their introduction.[77–90] In 1981, a household survey found that 2% of adult Americans had used tranquilizers without appropriate prescription during the previous year.[35] Tranquilizer use among American high school seniors peaked in 1977 (10.8% within the previous year, 4.6% within the previous month), falling to 6.1% and 2.1% by 1985.[91] In 1991, a survey of American resident physicians and senior medical students revealed that of 11 drugs (including tobacco and ethanol), only benzodiazepines and ethanol (and, in the case of the medical students, "psychedelics other then LSD [lysergic acid diethylamide]") were taken more often than by national age-related comparison groups.[92,93]

The addictive liability of benzodiazepines is much less than that of barbiturates; there is slower onset of action, less euphoria, and a greater difference between a therapeutic dose and a dose producing physical dependence.[94] Although choice tests in sedative and ethanol abusers indicate a preference for benzodiazepines over placebo, similar tests in either normal or anxious subjects with no history of sedative abuse show no such preference.[95–97] Such findings are consistent with animal studies.[98] Drug-seeking behavior—obtaining prescriptions from several physicians or purchasing the drug on the street—and dosage escalation are therefore rarely encountered among the millions of current users.[96,99] In fact, in the surveys described here, although 2% of Americans took tranquilizers without proper prescription, only 0.1% did so for 30 days or more during the previous year, and the great majority of medical students and residents who used benzodiazepines did so for self-treatment rather than recreation.[92,93]

Although widespread overprescribing of benzodiazepines has been claimed, epidemiologic studies reveal that in the vast majority of instances they are prescribed and taken appropriately.[35,100–103] In fact, surveys indicate that most patients tend to take less than prescribed and for shorter periods.[96] About 15% of benzodiazepine users take the drug on a long-term basis and appear to benefit from doing so, again without dosage escalation or abuse. Abstinence symptoms are more likely to develop when treatment is abruptly discontinued in such patients, but as with opioids physical dependence is not the same as addiction or abuse.

Despite these considerations, the New York State Department of Health in 1989 decreed that benzodiazepines (which are schedule IV drugs) be prescribed on triplicate prescriptions for a maximum of 30 days, with each patient's, physician's, and pharmacist's name entered into a database.[104] The result was predictable. Because patients were required to return every 30 days for refills and physicians were reluctant to have their names on a computerized blacklist, needed treatment was denied. Moreover, although benzodiazepine prescribing did decline substantially, prescriptions for less effective and often more dangerous sedatives (meprobamate, methyprylon, ethchlorvynol, butalbital, chloral hydrate, hydroxyzine) rose sharply (even as their use was decreasing nationally). Whether the

Table 5–2. Benzodiazepines Available in the United States

Promoted as Tranquilizers
  Alprazolam (Xanax)
  Chlorazepate (Tranxene)
  Chlordiazepoxide (Librium)
  Diazepam (Valium)
  Halazepam (Paxipam)
  Lorazepam (Ativan)
  Oxazepam (Serax)
  Prazepam (Centrax)

Promoted as Hypnotics
  Estazolam (Prosom)
  Flurazepam (Dalmane)
  Quazepam (Doral)
  Temazepam (Restoril)
  Triazolam (Halcion)

Promoted as Anticonvulsant
  Clonazepam (Klonopin)

Promoted for Anesthesia Induction
  Midazolam (Versed)

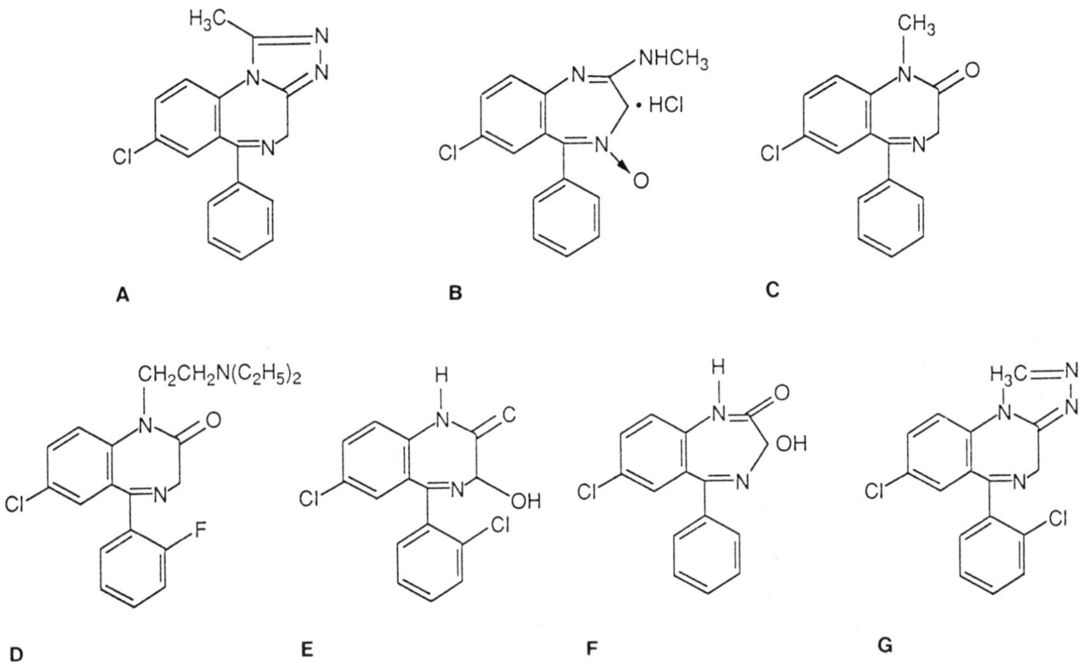

Figure 5–2. Alprazolam (A), chlordiazepoxide hydrochloride (B), diazepam (C), flurazepam (D), lorazepam (E), oxazepam (F), and triazolam (G).

reduced prescribing of benzodiazepines led to decreased street diversion is uncertain.[105,106]

Nearly all recreational benzodiazepine users also use other psychoactive drugs, especially ethanol.[35,107–111] Agents with rapid onset of action (e.g., diazepam) are more popular than agents with slower onset (e.g., oxazepam).[33,112] Parenteral use is rare.[113] Illicit use is especially frequent among patients in methadone maintenance programs,[35,114–116] perhaps reflecting drug interactions that enhance subjective opioid effects.[117]

Although some benzodiazepines are marketed as anxiolytics and others as hypnotics, the differences are "possibly insignificant."[14] Their effectiveness as muscle relaxants in usual oral doses has also been questioned. Differences do exist among benzodiazepines in rapidity of absorption after oral administration and in duration of action. For example, oxazepam requires hours to reach peak plasma concentrations, whereas diazepam reaches peak concentrations in about an hour; alprazolam, lorazepam, and chlordiazepoxide have intermediate rates of absorption. One reason triazolam replaced flurazepam as the nation's most popular prescription hypnotic was its shorter biologic half-life, reducing the likelihood of drowsiness (and traffic accidents) the following day. Some benzodiazepines such as diazepam

have biologically active metabolites. Of available benzodiazepines, only lorazepam is predictably absorbed after intramuscular injection.

If benzodiazepines are selectively anxiolytic, higher doses are also sedative and hypnotic. Their greatest advantage over barbiturates, however, is safety in overdose. Benzodiazepines are implicated in about 20% of DAWN reports and 15% of toxicologic fatalities, but in the vast majority, additional drugs—usually other sedatives or ethanol—have been taken.[35] Benzodiazepines alone seldom produce respiratory depression, and patients who have taken benzodiazepines with barbiturates do not appear more likely to have depressed respiration than patients who have taken barbiturates alone.[118] In mice, diazepam did not increase the LD-50 of ethanol.[119] It is extremely difficult to commit suicide with benzodiazepines. A review of 1239 deaths in which diazepam was implicated found that in only two was diazepam taken alone.[120] Even very large doses of benzodiazepines are more likely to produce somnolence, ataxia, and dysarthria than coma and respiratory depression. In a report of 60 cases of chlordiazepoxide poisoning, coma did not occur even with blood levels over 60 μg/mL; therapeutic doses of chlordiazepoxide usually produce levels of 0.5 to 3 μg/mL.[121]

When benzodiazepines are contributing to coma, the general management is the same as for barbiturate or ethanol poisoning. Overdose of benzodiazepines alone seldom requires ventilatory or blood pressure support, and hemodialysis is ineffective.[53,122] Intravenous flumazenil, a specific benzodiazepine antagonist, quickly reverses stupor or coma when benzodiazepines have been taken alone but because its duration of action is brief (20 to 45 minutes), it often must be given in repeated boluses or by continuous infusion.[23,123,124]

Benzodiazepines produce troublesome and potentially dangerous effects in addition to lethargy, especially in the elderly.[125,126] Psychomotor performance is impaired in a manner that mimics the effects of old age itself: Muscle strength and coordination are decreased, and impaired memory and confusion occur. Older subjects taking benzodiazepines are at increased risk for falls and fractures,[127,128] especially with agents such as nitrazepam or flurazepam, which are not only long acting themselves, but also have long-acting metabolites.[129] The risk is further increased when benzodiazepines are taken with ethanol, which enhances their absorption and has additive sedative and ataxic effects.[130]

Although tolerance develops rapidly to sedation and incoordination, it is less evident for anterograde amnesia,[131] a desirable feature when benzodiazepines are used for anesthesia induction, but decidedly undesirable for travelers who take benzodiazepines to sleep on airplanes.[132–134] The mechanisms underlying amnesia are unclear. Diazepam produces little amnesia given orally and rapid but brief amnesia given intravenously; lorazepam, by contrast, produces more delayed but longer lasting amnesia given orally or intravenously.[35]

Physical dependence does develop to benzodiazepines, and severe abstinence signs have been observed in rats, dogs, and baboons.[135–138] Rebound insomnia follows abrupt cessation of benzodiazepine hypnotics, and early morning awakening and daytime anxiety can emerge in chronic users of short-acting agents.[139,140] Similarly, withdrawal symptoms in patients taking benzodiazepine tranquilizers can either follow cessation of therapeutic doses[110,136,141–146] or emerge during chronic use (reflecting tolerance).[129]

Withdrawal symptoms usually occur 3 to 10 days after stopping long-acting agents and within 24 hours with short-acting agents.[147] The principal symptom, anxiety, can be difficult to distinguish from the patient's predrug state, but there may also be headache, muscle stiffness, tachycardia, sweating, anorexia, diarrhea, tremor, parethesias, psychosis, hallucinations, delirium, and seizures.[16,148–153] Unusual perceptual disturbances, with a false sense of movement and hypersensitivity to sensory stimuli—light, sound, and touch—are particularly characteristic of the benzodiazepine abstinence syndrome, which can last 1 to 6 weeks.[99] In a double-blind, placebo-controlled study, patients who abruptly discontinued therapeutic doses of benzodiazepines after at least 9 months of use developed symptoms that were clearly distinct from pretreatment anxiety, including tinnitus, muscle twitching, paresthesias, visual disturbances, and confusion; none had seizures, disorientation, or psychosis.[143] Withdrawal symptoms have also occurred in patients taking benzodiazepines for nonpsychiatric reasons such as muscle spasm.[138] Symptoms are most severe with short-acting agents and can be minimized by short treatment courses, low or intermittent flexible daily doses, and gradual dosage reduction.[99,152–154] The high doses of alprazolam recommended for panic attacks made long-term users especially vulnerable to physical dependence, an association that has received much medial attention.[154a] Propranolol, carbamazepine, and sedative and antidepressant drugs have reportedly relieved benzodiazepine withdrawal symptoms.[142,149,155]

Benzodiazepines cause paradoxical reactions that suggest withdrawal: anxiety, hyperactivity, irritability, hostility, agitation, depression, rage attacks, panic, delirium, hallucinations, and increased seizure frequency.[156,157] Aimless wandering and bizarre behavior lasting hours have affected patients who later had no recollection of the experience. Such symptoms are especially common with triazolam.[158] Data from the Food and Drug Administration (FDA) revealed that hyperexcitability, cognitive disturbance, "confusion," hallucinations, and depression occurred much more often with triazolam than with flurazepam or temazepam. In addition, triazolam was nearly as likely as flurazepam, and much more likely than temazepam, to cause daytime sedation. It was also more likely to cause withdrawal symptoms including seizures, and it was the only drug among the three to cause amnesia.[159] Similarly, a controlled study found "next-day amnesia" in 40% of triazolam users and 0% of temazepam users.[160] That study has been criticized on the grounds that equivalent doses were not compared, and the FDA spontaneous reporting system has been criticized as anecdotal.[161,162] Media attention, however, led to the withdrawal of triazolam from the market in the Netherlands and Britain [139,163,164] and by the 1990s had raised considerable concern over its availability in the United States.[165,166]

Long-term benzodiazepine treatment, with or without physical dependence, appears to be without permanent consequence.[35] Reports of psychological or cognitive impairment in long-term users are rare and, as with many other drugs, difficult to interpret.[167,168,168a,168b] So are descriptions of alleged fetal effects. A report from Sweden described dysmorphism, mental retardation, Dandy-Walker malformation, Moebius syndrome, seizures, or hemiplegia in several infants born to mothers taking benzodiazepines. The dysmorphism was considered similar but not identical to the fetal alcohol syndrome.[169] Animal studies have shown lowered threshold to bicuculline-induced but not pentylenetetrazol-induced seizures following in utero diazepam exposure.[170]

Nonbarbiturate, Nonbenzodiazepine Sedative-Hypnotics

A number of nonbarbiturate sedatives—ethinamate, ethchlorvynol, glutethimide, meprobamate, methaqualone, methyprylon—came on the market in the 1950s, each followed in short order by reports of abuse.[171–177] Although some of these agents have since been withdrawn, others are still widely sold (Table 5–3).[178]

Despite their chemical dissimilarity, nonbarbiturate, nonbenzodiazepine sedative-hypnotics produce symptoms of intoxication and withdrawal similar to those of barbiturates. In the 1970s, methaqualone

Table 5–3. Nonbarbiturate, Nonbenzodiazepine Sedative-Hypnotics

Bromide
Buspirone (Buspar)
Chloral hydrate (Noctec)
Chlormezanone (Trancopal)
Diphenhydramine (Benadryl, and in over-the-counter sleeping pills, e.g., Miles Nervine, Nytol, Sleep-eze, Sominex, Compoz)
Ethchlorvynol (Placidyl)
Ethinamate (Valmid, no longer produced in the U.S.)
Glutethimide (Doriden, after 1991 available only as generic)
Hydroxyzine (Vistaril, Atarax)
Meprobamate (Miltown, Equanil; in Equagesic with aspirin; in Deprol with benactyzine)
Methaqualone (Quaalude, Sopar, no longer produced in the U.S.)
Methyprylon (Nodular, no longer produced in the U.S.)
Paraldehyde
Triclofos (Triclos, no longer produced in the U.S.)

abuse became widespread among young people in the United States, West Germany, Japan, and Britain.[179] (A British commercial preparation, Mandrax, contains antihistamine.) Methaqualone—"Canadian blues," "quacks," "sopars," "ludes"—was often taken with wine or soft drinks in "juice bars" ("luding out") and was popular as a "downer" among cocaine users.[180,181] Poisoning causes delirium, hallucinations, hypertonicity, myoclonus, seizures, papilledema, coma, and death.[182–186] A tendency to congestive heart failure contraindicates forced diuresis.[185] There may be elevated prothrombin time and bleeding, and peripheral neuropathy has been reported.[187,188]

In the early 1970s, overdose accounted for most methaqualone fatalities; a decade later, as methaqualone abuse was becoming a nationwide epidemic, traumatic deaths (especially vehicular accidents) were more common.[189,190] "Counterfeit" methaqualone pills sold on the street contain unpredictable amounts of drug and other agents, including phencyclidine, barbiturates, or diazepam, either exclusively or as additives.[190] A man had seizures and coma after taking methaqualone with diphenhydramine; methaqualone blood levels were much lower then usually associated with coma, suggesting potentiation by the antihistamine.[191]

In the 1980s, production and distribution of methaqualone became illegal in the United States, and abuse subsequently declined. Illegally manufactured and imported methaqualone remains available, however.[192]

Of the sedatives discussed in this chapter, glutethimide probably has the least to recommend it. Its addiction liability is as great as the barbiturates, and its plasma half-life is as high as 100 hours following overdose, which is especially difficult to treat. Acute effects are barbiturate-like; overdose, however, causes less respiratory depression and more severe circulatory failure. There is also fever, muscle spasm, twitching, and even seizures. Coma can be prolonged with unpredictable fluctuations in depth.[193–196] Anticholinergic actions cause dilated unreactive pupils, xerostomia, ileus, and atonic bladder; in one report, pupillary dilation was unilateral.[197] In addition to its own prolonged half-life, glutethimide has active metabolites that accumulate with chronic use or after overdose. Management is supportive, as with barbiturates. Hemodialysis can shorten coma.

As a drug of abuse, glutethimide in the 1980s was often injected parenterally combined with codeine ("hits," "loads"), and numerous fatalities were reported (see Chapter 2).[198,199] Glutethimide abstinence symptoms, including seizures, occur in abusers taking large daily doses (0.5 to 3 g).[1] Glutethimide addicts have reportedly developed lasting peripheral neuropathy, cerebellar ataxia, and altered mentation.[200–202] Symptomatic hypocalcemia with elevated parathormone levels developed in a young man who had abused glutethimide for 15 years.[203]

Methyprylon has barbiturate-like effects, and its plasma half-life is increased following overdose.[1,53] As with glutethimide, methyprylon poisoning is less likely than barbiturates to cause respiratory depression and more likely to cause hypotension. Coma can last days and is shortened by hemodialysis. Methyprylon addiction produces an abstinence syndrome similar to that of barbiturates.

Acute effects of ethchlorvynol include dizziness, syncope, nausea, vomiting, facial numbness, and hypotension. Overdose causes severe respiratory depression with bradycardia and pulmonary edema. Hypothermia, nystagmus, and disconjugate eye movements are common, and coma tends to be deep, nonfluctuating, and prolonged.[204,205] Severe peripheral neuropathy, hemolysis, and thrombocytopenia have been reported.[205–207] Treatment includes forced diuresis, peritoneal dialysis, exchange transfusion, hemodialysis, and hemoperfusion with activated charcoal or amberlite resin.[205,208–210]

Similar to benzodiazepines, meprobamate does not produce general anesthesia, and it is uncertain if it has dissociable sedative and anxiolytic effects. Although its legitimate use has declined markedly over the past two decades, it is still widely abused, and studies of drug abusers reveal preference for meprobamate over benzodiazepines.[211–213] Overdose causes respiratory depression, hypotension, congestive heart failure, and pulmonary edema.[214] A tendency to relapse after apparent clearing of coma is a common feature of meprobamate overdose, perhaps the result of gastric hypomotility, undissolved tablets, and delayed absorption. Charcoal or resin filter hemoperfusion is more effective than hemodialysis in treating severe overdose.[215–218] Meprabromate withdrawal frequently produces hallucinations and seizures.[1]

Paraldehyde dependence sometimes occurs in alcoholics who receive it during withdrawal and then develop a preference for it. It can deteriorate in the bottle to acetic acid, producing metabolic acidosis; it also causes hemorrhagic gastritis and pulmonary damage.[219]

A popular drug of abuse in the 19th century, chloral hydrate is seldom taken illicitly today.[52] Following absorption, it is rapidly metabolized to trichloroethanol, which is pharmacologically active. It is widely believed (but difficult to prove) that chloral hydrate and ethanol are synergistic ("Mickey Finn"), perhaps because chloral hydrate inhibits ethanol metabolism, whereas ethanol enhances chloral hydrate metabolism.[1] Many clinicians also believe that elderly subjects tolerate chloral hydrate better than barbiturates. Acute intoxication, which resembles barbiturate poisoning, sometimes produces pinpoint pupils. Withdrawal can cause seizures, delirium, and death. Survivors often have liver and kidney damage with jaundice and proteinuria, and chronic users may develop acute toxicity because of impaired hepatic detoxification.

Since the early 1980s, bromide salts are no longer present in over-the-counter headache remedies and sedatives in the United States. Signs of chronic bromide intoxication include lethargy, inattentiveness, impaired memory, ataxia, dysarthria, and tremor; high doses cause delusions, delirium, hallucinations, and coma.[220,221] A rash (acneiform, nodular, or bullous) occurs in about one-third of intoxicated subjects. Serum bromide concentration is usually more than 19 mEq/L but may be lower. Serum chloride is correspondingly reduced, but if laboratory "chloride" determinations are actually for total halide, levels appear normal.[222] Treatment is with sodium chloride, 2 g three times daily, plus diuresis.[53]

The antihistamine/anticholinergic hydroxyzine is used as an anxiolytic, and diphenhydramine or other antihistamines are the principal ingredients in many over-the-counter sleeping pills (in some products replacing bromide or scopolamine). Their abuse potential is low, in part because of dose-related side effects (confusion, forgetfulness, anxiety, tremor, dizziness, dry mouth, paresthesias, muscle cramps). Case reports have appeared of cough syrup abuse by polydrug abusers, and tripelennamine combined with pentazocine ("T's and blues") was widely abused in the United States during the 1980s (see Chapter 2). In a study of volunteer sedative abusers, subjects frequently identified diphenhydramine as a barbiturate, benzodiazepine, or other hypnotic and at doses below 600 mg gave it favorable subjective ratings.[223]

Concerns about abuse and dependence and a desire for nonsedative anxiolytic agents led to the development of a novel class of nonbenzodiazepine drugs that act selectively at serotonin 5-HT$_{1A}$ receptors (which are especially prominent in limbic areas).[224] Buspirone, gepirone, and ipsapirone in several trials were as effective as benzodiazepines in relieving anxiety, yet did not cause sedation, motor incoordination, or impaired judgment and did not interact with ethanol.[224–226] Moreover, animal and human studies suggest that neither tolerance nor physical dependence develops and that addiction liability is minimal.[225-230]

The lexicon of abused drugs is of course replete with agents initially touted as nonaddicting (e.g., heroin and meperidine), but as of the early 1990s there were no reports of buspirone abuse. Perhaps related to actions at dopamine receptors, buspirone in high doses causes akathisia, tremor, rigidity, orofacial dyskinesia, myoclonus, and dystonia. In one case, dystonia persisted for several months after buspirone was discontinued.[231]

References

1. Rall TW. Hypnotics and sedatives; ethanol. In: Gilman AG, Rall TW, Nies AS, Taylor P, eds. The Pharmacological Basis of Therapeutics, ed 8. New York: Pergamon Press, 1990:345.

2. Pritchett D, Sontheimer H, Shivers B, et al. Importance of a novel GABA-A receptor subunit for benzodiazepine pharmacology. Nature 1989; 338:582.

3. Schofield PR. The GABA-A receptor: molecular biology reveals a complex picture. Trends Pharmacol Sci 1989; 10:476.

4. Luddens H, Killisch I, Seeburg PH. More than one alpha variant may exist in a GABA A/benzodiazepine receptor complex. J Recept Res 1991; 11:535.

5. Snyder SH, Trifiletti RR. Drug and neurotransmitter receptors: synaptic principles elucidated by GABA and benzodiazepines. Biogenic Amines 1988; 5:191.

6. Breier A, Paul SM. The GABA-A/benzodiazepine receptor: implications for the molecular basis of anxiety. J Psychiat Res 1990; 24:91.

7. Zimprich F, Zezula J, Sieghart W, Lassmann H. Immunohistochemical localization of the alpha 1, alpha 2, and alpha 3 subunit of the GABA-A receptor in the rat brain. Neurosci Lett 1991; 127:125.

8. Martin IL. The benzodiazepines and their receptors: 25 years of progress. Neuropharmacology 1987; 26:957.

9. Barker JL, Ransom BR. Pentobarbital pharmacology of mammalian neurons grown in tissue culture. J Physiol 1978; 280:331.

10. MacDonald RL, McLain MJ. Anticonvulsant drugs: mechanisms of action. Adv Neurol 1986; 44:713.

11. Twyman RE, Rogers CJ, MacDonald RL. Differential regulation of gamma-aminobutyric acid receptor channels by diazepam and phenobarbital. Ann Neurol 1989; 25:213.

12. Fraser HF, Jasinski DR. The assessment of the abuse potentiality of sedative/hypnotics (depressants): methods used in animals and man. In: Martin WR, ed. Drug Addiction. New York:Springer-Verlag, 1977:589.

13. Saunders PA, Ito Y, Baker ML, et al. Pentobarbital tolerance and withdrawal: correlation with effects on the GABA-A receptor. Pharmacol Biochem Behav 1990; 37:343.

14. Baldessarini RJ. Drugs and the treatment of psychiatric disorders. In: Gilman AG, Rall TW, Nies AS, Taylor P, eds. The Pharmacological Basis of Therapeutics, ed 8. New York: Pergamon Press, 1990:383.

15. Skolnick P, Paul SM. Benzodiazepine receptors in the central nervous system. Int Rev Neurobiol 1982; 23:103.

16. Greenblatt DJ, Shader RI, Abernethy DR. Current status of benzodiazepines. N Engl J Med 1983; 309:354.

17. Cook JM, Diaz-Arauzo H, Allen MS. Inverse agonists, probes to study the structure, topology and function of the benzodiazepine receptor. In: Harris L, ed. Problems of Drug Dependence 1990. Rockville, MD: NIDA Research Monograph 105, DHHS, 1991:133.

18. Rampe D, Triggle DJ. Benzodiazepines and calcium channel function. Trends Pharmacol Sci 1986; 7:461.

19. Phillis JW, O'Regan MH. Benzodiazepine interaction with adenosine systems explains some anomalies in GABA hypothesis. Trends Pharmacol Sci 1988; 9:153.

20. Gardner CR. Functional in vivo correlates of the benzodiazepine agonist-inverse agonist continuum. Prog Neurobiol 1988; 31:425.

21. Ninan PT, Insel TM, Cohen RM, et al. Benzodiazepine receptor-mediated experimental "anxiety" in primates. Science 1982; 218:1332.

22. Braestrup C, Schmiechen R, Neef G, et al. Interaction of convulsive ligands with benzodiazepine receptors. Science 1982; 216:1241.

23. Amrein R, Leishman B, Bentzinger C, Roncari G. Flumazenil in benzodiazepine antagonism. Med Toxicol 1987; 2:411.

24. Little HJ. The benzodiazepines: anxiolytic and withdrawal effects. Neuropeptides 1991; 19:11.

25. Polc P. Electrophysiology of benzodiazepine receptor ligands: multiple mechanisms and sites of action. Prog Neurobiol 1988; 31:349.

26. Nutt DJ. Pharmacological mechanisms of benzodiazepine withdrawal. J Psychiat Res 1990; 24:105.

27. Wamsley JK, Hunt MAE. Relative affinity of quazepam for type-1 benzodiazepine receptors in brain. J Clin Psychiatry 1991; 52(suppl):15.

28. Pritchett D, Luddens H, Seeburg PH. Type I and type II GABA$_A$-benzodiazepine receptors produced in transfected cells. Science 1989; 245:1389.

29. Allan AM, Gallaher EJ, Gionet SE, Harris RA. Genetic selection for benzodiazepine ataxia produces functional changes in the gamma-aminobutyric acid receptor chloride channel complex. Brain Res 1988; 452:118.

30. Verma A, Snyder SH. Peripheral type benzodiazepine receptors. Annu Rev Pharmacol Toxicol 1989; 29:307.

31. Costa E, Guidotti A. Diazepam binding inhibitor (DBI): a peptide with multiple biological actions. Life Sci 1991; 49:325.

32. Sangameswaran L, Fales HM, Friedrich P, DeBlas AL. Purification of a benzodiazepine from bovine brain and detection of benzodiazepine-like immunoreactivity in human brain. Proc Nat Acad Sci USA 1986; 83:9236.

33. Griffiths RR, McLeod DR, Bigelow GE, et al. Comparison of diazepam and oxazepam: preference, liking and extent of abuse. J Pharmacol Exp Ther 1984; 229:501.
34. Griffiths RR, Lamb RJ, Sannerud CA, et al. Self-injection barbiturates, benzodiazepines, and other sedative-anxiolytics in baboons. Psychopharmacology 1991; 103:154.
35. Woods JH, Katz JL, Winger G. Abuse liability of benzodiazepines. Pharmacol Rev 1987; 39:254.
36. File SE. Tolerance to the behavioral actions of benzodiazepines. Neurosci Biobehav Rev 1985; 9:113.
37. Kang I, Miller LG. Decreased GABA-A receptor subunit mRNA concentrations following lorazepam administration. Br J Pharmacol 1991; 103:1285.
38. Miller LG. Chronic benzodiazepine administration: from the patient to the gene. J Clin Pharmacol 1991; 31:492.
39. Pritchard GA, Galpern WR, Lumpkin M, Miller LG. Chronic benzodiazepine administration. VIII. Receptor upregulation produced by chronic exposure to the inverse agonist FG-7142. J Pharmacol Exp Ther 1991; 258:280.
40. Barnhill JG, Ciraulo DA, Greenblatt DJ, et al. Benzodiazepine response and receptor binding after chronic ethanol ingestion in a mouse model. J Pharmacol Exp Ther 1991; 258:812.
41. Kelp H. Chloral-wirkung in grossen dosen. Allg Z Psychiatr Ihre Grenzeb 1875; 31:389.
42. Seguin EC. The abuse and use of bromides. J Nerv Ment Dis 1877; 4:445.
43. Krafft-Ebbing RV. Ueber Paralehyde-Gebrauch und Missbrauch nebst einem Falle von Paraldehyde-Delirium. Z Ther 1887; 7:244.
44. Fernandez G, Clarke M. A case of "Veronal" poisoning. Lancet 1904; 1:223.
45. Kales A, Kales JD, Bixler EO, Scharf MB. Effectiveness of hypnotic drugs with prolonged use: flurazepam and pentobarbital. Clin Pharmacol Ther 1975; 18:356.
46. Wulff MH. The barbiturate withdrawal syndrome: a clinical and electrophysiologic study. Electroenceph Clin Neurophysiol 1959; 14(suppl):1.
47. AMA Committee on Alcoholism and Addiction and Council on Mental Health: Dependence on barbiturates and other sedative drugs. JAMA 1965; 193:673.
48. Wysowski DK, Baum C. Outpatient use of prescription sedative-hypnotic drugs in the United States, 1970 through 1989. Arch Intern Med 1991; 151:1779.
49. Preskorn S, Schwin RL, McKuelly WV. Analgesic abuse and the barbiturate abstinence syndrome. JAMA 1980; 244:369.
50. Jaffe JH. Drug addiction and drug abuse. In: Gilman AG, Rall TW, Nies AS, Taylor P, eds. The Pharmacological Basis of Therapeutics, ed 8. New York: Pergamon Press, 1990:522.
51. Guarino J, Roache JD, Kirk WT, Griffiths RR. Comparison of the behavioral effects and abuse liability of ethanol and pentobarbital in recreational sedative abusers. In: Harris L, ed. Problems of Drug Dependence 1989. Rockville, MD: NIDA Research Monograph 95, DHHS, 1990:453.
52. Mendelson WB. The Use and Misuse of Sleeping Pills. New York: Plenum, 1980.
53. Osborn H, Goldfrank LR, Howland MA, et al. Barbiturates and other sedative-hypnotics. In: Goldfrank LR, Flomenbaum NE, Lewin NA, et al, eds. Toxicologic Emergencies, ed 4. Norwalk, CT: Appleton & Lange, 1990:449.
54. Gary NE, Tresznewsky O. Barbiturates and a potpourri of other sedatives, hypnotics, and tranquilizers. Heart Lung 1983; 12:122.
55. Simon RP. Decorticate and decerebrate posturing in sedative drug-induced coma. Neurology 1982; 32:448.
56. Groschel D, Gerstein AR, Rosenbaum JM. Skin lesions as a diagnostic aid in barbiturate poisoning. N Engl J Med 1970; 283:409.
57. Khantzian EJ, McKenna GJ. Acute toxic and withdrawal reactions associated with drug use and abuse. Ann Intern Med 1979; 90:361.
58. Wikler A. Diagnosis and treatment of drug dependence of the barbiturate type. Am J Psychiatry 1968; 125:758.
59. Fraser HF, Wikler A, Essig CF, Isbell H. Degree of physical dependence induced by secobarbital or pentobarbital. JAMA 1958; 166:126.
60. Smith DE, Wesson DR. Phenobarbital technique for treatment of barbiturate dependence. Arch Gen Psychiatry 1971; 24:56.
61. Desmond MM, Schwaneche RP, Wilson GS, et al. Maternal barbiturate utilization and neonatal withdrawal symptomatology. J Pediatr 1972; 80:190.
62. Rumbaugh CL, Fang HCH. The effects of drug abuse on the brain. Medical Times, March 1980:37s.
63. Rumbaugh CL, Bergeron RT, Fang HCH, McCormick R. Cerebral angiographic changes in the drug abuse patient. Radiology 1971; 101:335.
64. Rumbaugh CL, Fang HCH, Higgins RE, et al. Cerebral microvascular injury in experimental drug abuse. Invest Radiol 1976; 11:282.
65. MacLeod CM, Dekaban AS, Hunt E. Memory impairment in epileptic patients: selective effects of phenobarbital on concentration. Science 1978; 202:1102.
66. Allgulander C, Borg S, Vikander B. A 4–6 year follow-up of 50 patients with primary dependence on sedative and hypnotic drugs. Am J Psychiatry 1984; 141:1580.
67. Theodore WA, DiChiro G, Margolin R, et al. Barbiturates reduce human cerebral glucose metabolism. Neurology 1986; 36:60.
68. Fishman RHB, Yanai J. Long-lasting effects of early barbiturates on central nervous system and behavior. Neurosci Biobehav Rev 1983; 7:19.
69. Camfield CS, Chaplin S, Doyle AB, et al. Side-effects of phenobarbital in toddlers: behavioral and cognitive aspects. J Pediatr 1979; 95:361.
70. Wolf SM, Forsythe A. Behavioral disturbance, phenobarbital, and febrile seizures. Pediatrics 1978; 61:728.
71. Vining EP, Mellitis ED, Dorsen MM, et al. Psychologic and behavioral effects of antiepileptic drugs in children: a double-blind comparison between phenobarbital and valproic acid. Pediatrics 1987; 80:165.

72. Wolf SM, Forsythe A, Stunden AA, et al. Long-term efffect of phenobarbital on cognitive function in children with febrile convulsions. Pediatrics 1981; 68:820.

73. Farwell JR, Lee YJ, Hirtz DG, et al. Phenobarbital for febrile seizures—effects on intelligence and on seizure recurrence. N Engl J Med 1990; 322:364.

74. Bergey GKK, Swaiman KF, Schrier BK, et al. Adverse effects of phenobarbital on morphological and biochemical development of fetal mouse spinal cord neurons in culture. Ann Neurol 1981; 9:584.

75. Diaz J, Schain RJ, Bailey BG. Phenobarbital-induced brain growth retardation in artificially reared rat pups. Biol Neonate 1977; 32:77

76. Reinisch JM, Sanders SA. Early barbituraate exposure: the brain, sexually dimorphic behavior and learning. Neurosci Biobehav Rev 1982; 6:311.

77. Guile LA. Rapid habituation to chlordiazepoxide "Librium." Med J Aust 1963; 2:56.

78. Czerwenka-Wenkstetten H, Hofman G, Krypsin-Exner K. Ein Fall von Valium-Entzugsdelir. Wien Med Wochenschr 1965; 47:994.

79. Selig JW. A possible oxazepam abstinence syndrome. JAMA 1966; 198:279.

80. Johnson L, Clift AD. Dependence on hypnotic drugs in general practice. BMJ 1968; 4:613.

81. Parry HJ, Butler MB, Mellinger GD, et al. National patterns of psychotherapeutic drug use. Arch Gen Psychiatry 1973; 28:769.

82. Swanson DW, Weddige RL, Morse RM. Abuse of prescription drugs. Mayo Clin Proc 1973; 48:359.

83. Rucker TD. Drug use: data, sources, and limitations. JAMA 1974; 230:888.

84. Korsgaard S. Misbrug av lorazepam. Vgeschrift for Laeger 1976; 135:164.

85. Lader M. Benzodiazepines: the opium of the masses? Neuroscience 1978; 3:159.

86. Allgulander C, Borg S. Case report: a delirious abstinence syndrome associated with chlorazepate "Tranxilen." Br J Addict 1978; 73:175.

87. Stark L, Sykes R, Mullin P. Temazepam abuse. Lancet 1987; 2:802.

88. Farrell M, Strang J. Misuse of temazepam. BMJ 1988; 297: 1402.

89. Juergens S, Morse R. Alprazolam dependence in seven patients. Am J Psychiatry 1988; 145:625.

90. Schmauss C, Apelt S, Emrich HM. Preference for alprazolam over diazepam. Am J Psychiatry 1989; 146:408.

91. Johnston LD, O'Malley PM, Bachman JG. Drug use among American high school students, college students, and other young adults: national trends through 1985. Rockville, MD: DHHS Publication (ADM) 86-1450, 1986.

92. Baldwin DC, Hughes PH, Conard SE, et al. Substance use among senior medical students. JAMA 1991; 265:2074.

93. Hughes PH, Conard SSE, Baldwin DC, et al. Resident physician substance use in the United States. JAMA 1991; 265:2069.

94. Ladewig D. Dependence liability of the benzodiazepines. Drug Alcohol Depend 1984; 13:139.

95. American Psychiatric Association Task Force on Benzodiazepine Dependency. Benzodiazepine Dependency, Abuse. Washington, DC: APA, 1990.

96. Woods JH, Katz JL, Winger G. Use and abuse of benzodiazepines. Issues relevant to prescribing. JAMA 1988; 260:3476.

97. Ciraulo DA, Barnhill JG, Greenblatt DJ, et al. Abuse liability and clinical pharmacokinetics of alprazolam in alcoholic men. J Clin Psychiatry 1988; 49:333.

98. Griffiths RR, Ator NA, Lukas SE, et al. Experimental abuse liability assessment of benzodiazepines. In: Usdin E, Skolnick P, Tallman JF, et al, eds. Pharmacology of Benzodiazepines. London: MacMillan Publishing, 1982:609.

99. Tyrer PJ. Benzodiazepines on trial. BMJ 1984; 288:1101.

100. Ballenger JC. Psychopharmacology of the anxiety disorders. Psychiatr Clin North Am 1984; 7:757.

101. Tennant FS, Pumphrey EA. Benzodiazepine dependence of several years duration: clinical profile and therapeutics. In: Harris LS, ed. Problems of Drug Dependence 1984. Washington, DC: NIDA Research Monograph 55, DHHS, 1984:211.

102. Ellis P, Carney MW. Benzodiazepine abuse and management of anxiety in the community. Int J Addict 1988; 23:1083.

103. Warneke LB. Benzodiazepines: abuse and new use. Can J Psychiatry 1991; 36:194.

104. Reidenberg MM. Effect of the requirement for triplicate prescriptions for benzodiazepines in New York State. Clin Pharmacol Ther 1991; 50:129.

105. Weintraub M, Singh S, Byrne L, et al. Consequences of the 1989 New York State triplicate benzodiazepine prescription regulations. JAMA 1991; 266:2392.

106. Glass RM. Benzodiazepine prescription regulation. Autonomy and outcome. JAMA 1991; 266:2431.

107. Abuse of benzodiazepines: the problems and solutions. A report of a Committee of the Institute for Behavior and Health, Inc. Am J Drug Alcohol Abuse 1988; 14(suppl 1):1.

108. Busto U, Sellers EM, Sisson B, Segal R. Benzodiazepine use and abuse in alcoholics. Clin Pharmacol Ther 1982; 31:207.

109. Chan AWK. Effects of combined alcohol and benzodiazepine: a review. Drug Alcohol Depend 1984; 13:315.

110. DuPont RL. A practical approach to benzodiazepine discontinuation. J Psychiatr Res 1990; 24(suppl 2): 81.

111. Cole JO, Chiarello RJ. The benzodiazepines as drugs of abuse. J Psychiatr Res 1990; 24(suppl 2):135.

112. Griffiths RR, Wolf B. Relative abuse liability of different benzodiazepines in drug abusers. J Clin Psychopharmacol 1990; 10:237.

113. Kaminer Y, Modai I. Parenteral abuse of diazepam: a case report. Drug Alcohol Depend 1984; 14:63.

114. Magura S, Goldsmith D, Casriel C, et al. The validity of methadone clients' self-reported drug use. Int J Addict 1987; 22:727.

115. Weddington WA, Carney A. Alprazolam abuse during methadone maintenance therapy. JAMA 1987; 257:3363.
116. Fraser A. Alprazolam abuse and methadone maintenance. JAMA 1987; 258:2061.
117. Preston KL, Griffiths RR, Stitzer ML, et al. Diazepam and methadone interactions in methadone maintenance. Clin Pharmacol Ther 1984; 36:534.
118. Greenblatt DJ, Allen MD, Noel BJ, Shader RI. Acute overdosage with benzodiazepine derivatives. Clin Pharmacol 1977; 21:497.
119. Vapaatalo H, Karppanen H. Combined toxicity of ethanol with chlorpromazine, diazepam, chlormethiazole, or pentobarbital in mice. Agents Actions 1969; 1:43.
120. Finkle BS, McClosky KL, Goodman LS. Diazepam and drug-associated deaths: a survey in the United States and Canada. JAMA 1979; 242:429.
121. Cate JC, Jatlow PI. Chlordiazepoxide overdose: interpretation of serum drug concentrations. Clin Toxicol 1973; 6:553.
122. Gaudreault P, Guay J, Thivierge RL, Verdy I. Benzodiazepine poisoning. Clinical and pharmacological considerations and treatment. Drug Safety 1991; 6:247.
123. Brogden RN, Goa KL. Flumazenil. A preliminary review of its benzodiazepine antagonist properties, intrinsic activity and therapeutic use. Drugs 1988; 25:448.
124. Geller E, Crome P, Schaller MD, et al. Risks and benefits of therapy with flumazenil (Anexate) in mixed drug intoxications. Eur Neurol 1991; 31:241.
125. Prinz PN, Vitiello MV, Raskind MA, Thorpy MJ. Geriatrics: sleep disorders and aging. N Engl J Med 1990; 323:520.
126. Greenblatt DJ, Harmatz JS, Shapiro L, et al. Sensitivity to triazolam in the elderly. N Engl J Med 1991; 324:1691.
127. Ray WA, Griffin MR, Schaffner W, et al. Psychotropic drug use and the risk of hip fracture. N Engl J Med 1987; 316:363.
128. Larson EB, Kukull WA, Buchner D, Reifler BV. Adverse drug reactions associated with global cognitive impairment in elderly persons. Ann Intern Med 1987; 107:169.
129. Ashton H. Benzodiazepine withdrawal: an unfinished story. BMJ 1984; 288:1135.
130. Hayes SL, Pablo G, Radomski T, Palmer RF. Ethanol and oral diazepam absorption. N Engl J Med 1977; 296:186.
131. Lucki I, Rickels K, Geller AM. Chronic use of benzodiazepines and psychomotor and cognitive test performance. Psychopharmacology 1986; 88:426.
132. Juhl RP, Daugherty VM, Kroboth PD. Incidence of next-day anterograde amnesia caused by flurazepam hydrochloride and triazolam. J Clin Psychopharmacol 1984; 3:622.
133. Shader RI, Greenblatt DJ. Triazolam and anterograde amnesia: all is not well in the Z-zone. J Clin Psychopharmacol 1983; 3:273.
134. Morris HH, Estes ML. Traveler's amnesia. Transient global amnesia secondary to triazolam. JAMA 1987; 258:945.
135. McNicholas LF, Martin WR, Cherian S. Physical dependence on diazepam and lorazepam in the dog. J Pharmacol Exp Ther 1983; 226:783.
136. Owen RT, Tyrer P. Benzodiazepine dependence: a review of the evidence. Drugs 1983; 25:385.
137. Ryan GP, Boisse NR. Experimental induction of benzodiazepine tolerance and physical dependence. J Pharmacol Exp Ther 1983; 226:100.
138. Lader M, File S. The biological basis of benzodiazepine dependence. Psychol Med 1987; 17:539.
139. Griffiths RR, Lamb RJ, Ator NA, et al. Relative abuse liability of triazolam: experimental assessment in animals and humans. Neurosci Biobehav Rev 1985; 9:133.
140. Kales A, Scharf MB, Kales JD, Soldatos CR. Rebound insomnia: a potential hazard following withdrawal of certain benzodiazepines. JAMA 1979; 241:1692.
141. Rickels K, Case WG, Downing RW, Winokur A. Long-term diazepam therapy and clinical outcome. JAMA 1983; 250:767.
142. Tyrer PJ, Seivewright N. Identification and management of benzodiazepine dependence. Postgrad Med J 1984; 60(suppl 2):41.
143. Busto U, Sellers EM, Naranjo CA, et al. Withdrawal reaction after long-term therapeutic use of benzodiazepines. N Engl J Med 1986; 315:854.
144. Nutt D. Benzodiazepine dependence in the clinic: reason for anxiety? Trends Pharmacol Sci 1986; 7:457.
145. Schmauss C, Apelt S, Emrich HM. Characterization of benzodiazepine withdrawal in high- and low-dose dependent psychiatric inpatients. Brain Res Bull 1987; 19:393.
146. Dickinson B, Rush PA, Radcliffe AB. Alprazolam use and dependence. A retrospective analysis of 30 cases of withdrawal. West J Med 1990; 152:604.
147. Committee on the Review of Medicines. Systematic review of the benzodiazepines. BMJ 1980; 1:910.
148. Einarson TR. Lorazepam withdrawal seizures. Lancet 1980; 1:151.
149. Abernathy DR, Greenblatt DJ, Shader RI. Treatment of diazepam withdrawal syndrome with propranolol. Ann Intern Med 1981; 94:354.
150. Fialip J, Aumaitre O, Eschalier A, et al. Benzodiazepine withdrawal seizures. Analysis of 48 case reports. Clin Neuropharmacol 1987; 10:538.
151. Roy-Byrne PP, Hommer D. Benzodiazepine withdrawal: an overview and implications for the treatment of anxiety. Am J Med 1988; 84:1041.
152. Greenblatt DJ, Miller LG, Shader RI. Benzodiazepine discontinuation syndromes. J Psychiatr Res 1990; 24:73.
153. Harrison M, Busto U, Naranjo CA, et al. Diazepam tapering in detoxification for high-dose benzodiazepine abuse. Clin Pharmacol Ther 1984; 36:527.
154. Greenblatt DJ, Harmatz JS, Zinny MA, Shader RI. Effect of gradual withdrawal on the rebound sleep

disorder after discontinuation of triazolam. N Engl J Med 1987; 317:722.

154a. High anxiety. Consumer Reports, January 1993:19.

155. Klein E, Uhde TW, Post RM. Preliminary evidence for the utility of carbamazepine in alprazolam withdrawal. Am J Psychiatry 1986; 143:235.

156. Karch FE. Rage reaction associated with chlorazepate dipotassium. Ann Intern Med 1979; 91:62.

157. Fouilladieu J-L, D'Engert J, Conseiller C. Benzodiazepines. N Engl J Med 1984; 310:464.

158. Oswald I. Triazolam syndrome 10 years on. Lancet 1989; 2:451.

159. Bixler EO, Kales A, Brubaker BH, Kales JD. Adverse reactions to benzodiazepine hypnotics: spontaneous reporting system. Pharmacology 1987; 35:286.

160. Bixler EO, Kales A, Manfredi RL, et al. Next-day memory impairment with triazolam use. Lancet 1991; 337:827.

161. Gillin JC. The long and short of sleeping pills. N Engl J Med 1991; 324:1735.

162. Greenblatt DJ, Shader RI, Harmatz JS. Triazolam in the elderly. N Engl J Med 1991; 325:1744.

163. Trappler B, Bezeredi T. Triazolam intoxication. Can Med Assoc J 1982; 126:893.

164. van der Kroef C. Reactions to triazolam. Lancet 1979; 2: 526.

165. Cowley G, Springen K, Iarovici D, Hagee M. Sweet dreams or nightmare? Newsweek, August 19, 1991.

166. Kolata G. Maker of sleeping pill hid data on side effects, researchers say. NY Times, January 20, 1992.

167. Lader M. Benzodiazepines, psychological functioning, and dementia. In: Trimble MR, ed. Benzodiazepines Divided: A Multidisciplinary Review. Chichester: Wiley, 1983:309.

168. Brooker AE, Wiens AN, Wiens DA. Impaired brain functions due to diazepam and meprobamate abuse in a 53-year-old male. J Nerv Ment Dis 1984; 142:498.

168a. Golombok S, Moodley P, Lader M. Cognitive impairment in long-term benzodiazepine users. Psychol Med 1988; 18:365.

168b. Bergman H, Borg S, Engelbrektson K, et al. Dependence on sedative-hypnotics: Neuropsychological impairment, field dependence and clinical course in a 5-year followup study. Br J Addict 1989; 84:547.

169. Laegreid L, Olegard R, Wahlstrom J, Conradi N. Abnormalities in children exposed to benzodiazepines in utero. Lancet 1987; 1:108.

170. Bitran D, Primus RJ, Kellogg CK. Gestational exposure to diazepam increases sensitivity to convulsants that act at the GABA/benzodiazepine receptor complex. Eur J Pharmacol 1991; 196:223.

171. Lemere F. Habit-forming properties of meprobamate. Arch Neurol Psychiatry 1956; 76:205.

172. Brouschek R, Feuerlein M. Valamin als suchtmittel. Nervenarzt 1956; 27:115.

173. Battegay R. Sucht nach Abusus von Doriden. Praxis 1957; 46:991.

174. Cahn CH. Intoxication to ethchlorvynol (Placidyl). Can Med Assoc J 1959; 81:733.

175. Jensen GR. Addiction to "Noludar." N Z Med J 1960; 59:431.

176. Tengblad K-F. Heminevrin-enformani. Lahartidingen 1961; 58:1936.

177. Ewart RBL, Priest RG. Methaqualone addiction and delirium tremens. BMJ 1967; 3:92.

178. Gillin JC, Byerley WF. The diagnosis and management of insomnia. N Engl J Med 1990; 322:239.

179. Falco M. Methaqualone misuse: foreign experience and United States drug control policy. Int J Addict 1976; 11:597.

180. Fishburne PM, Abelson HI, Cisin I. National Survey on Drug Abuse: Main Findings: 1979. Washington, DC: DHHS Publication No (ADM) 80-976, 1980.

181. Inaba DS, Gay GR, Newmeyer JA, Whitehead C. Methaqualone abuse. "Luding out." JAMA 1973; 224:1505.

182. Sanderson JH, Cowdell RH, Higgins G. Fatal poisoning with methaqualone and diphenhydramine. Lancet 1966; 2:803.

183. Wallace MR, Allen E. Recovery after massive overdose of diphenhydramine and methaqualone. Lancet 1968; 2:1247.

184. Gerald MC, Schwirian PM. Non-medical use of methaqualone. Arch Gen Psychiatry 1973; 28:627.

185. Pascarelli EF. Methaqualone abuse, the quiet epidemic. JAMA 1973; 224:1512.

186. Abboud RT, Freedman MT, Rogers RM, Daniele RP. Methaqualone with muscular hyperactivity necessitating the use of curare. Chest 1974; 65:204.

187. Marks P. Methaqualone and peripheral neuropathy. Practitioner 1974; 212:721.

188. Hoaken PCS. Adverse effects of methaqualone. Can Med Assoc J 1975; 112:685.

189. Methaqualone abuse implicated in injuries and death nationwide. JAMA 1981; 246:813.

190. Wetli CV. Changing patterns of methaqualone abuse. JAMA 1983; 249:621.

191. Coleman JR, Barone JA. Abuse potential of methaqualone-diphenhydramine combination. Am J Hosp Pharm 1981; 38:160.

192. O'Malley PM, Bachman JG, Johnson LD. Period, age, and cohort effects on substance use among young Americans: a decade of change, 1976–86. Am J Public Health 1988; 78:1315.

193. Mayer JF, Schreiner GE, Westervelt FB. Acute glutethimide intoxication. Am J Med 1962; 33:70.

194. Caplan JL. Recovery in severe glutethimide poisoning. Postgrad Med J 1967; 43:611.

195. Myers RR, Stockard JJ. Neurologic and electroencephalographic correlates in glutethimide intoxication. Clin Pharmacol Ther 1975; 17:212.

196. Hansen AR, Kennedy KA, Ambre JJ, Fischer LJ. Glutethimide poisoning. N Engl J Med 1975; 292:250.

197. Brown DG, Hammill JF. Glutethimide poisoning: unilateral pupillary abnormalities. N Engl J Med 1971; 285:806.

198. Feuer E, French J. Descriptive epidemiology of mortality in New Jersey due to combinations of codeine and glutethimide. Am J Epidemiol 1984; 119:202.

199. Bender FH, Cooper JV, Dreyfus R. Fatalities associated with an acute overdose of glutethimide (Doriden) and codeine. Vet Hum Toxicol 1988; 30:332.
200. Lingl FA. Irreversible effects of glutethimide addiction. Am J Psychiatry 1966; 123:349.
201. Nover R. Persistent neuropathy following chronic use of glutethimide. Clin Pharmacol Ther 1967; 8:283.
202. Haas DC, Marassigan A. Neurological effects of glutethimide. J Neurol Neurosurg Psychiatry 1968; 31:561.
203. Ober RP, Hennessy JF, Hellman RM. Severe hypocalcemia associated with chronic glutethimide addiction. A case report. Am J Psychiatry 1981; 138:1239.
204. Westervelt FB. Ethchlorvynol (Placidyl) intoxication. Ann Intern Med 1966; 64:1229.
205. Teehan BP, Maher JF, Carey JJH, et al. Acute ethchlorvynol (Placidyl) intoxication. Ann Intern Med 1970; 72:875.
206. Ogilvie RI, Douglas DE, Lochead JR, et al. Ethchlorvynol (Placidyl) intoxication and its treatment by hemodialysis. Can Med Assoc J 1966; 95:954.
207. Klock JC. Hemolysis and pancytopenia in ethchlorvynol overdose. Ann Intern Med 1974; 81:131.
208. Hyde JS, Lawrence GI, Moles JB. Ethchlorvynol intoxication: successful treatment by exchange transfusion and peritoneal dialysis. Clin Pediatr 1968; 4:739.
209. Tozer TN, Witt LD, Gee L, et al. Evaluation of hemodialysis for ethchlorvynol (Placidyl) overdose. Am J Hosp Pharm 1974; 31:986.
210. Lynn RI, Honig CL, Jatlow PI, Kliger AS. Resin hemoperfusion for treatment of ethchlorvynol overdose. Ann Intern Med 1979; 91:549.
211. Essig CF, Ainslie JD. Addiction to meprobamate. JAMA 1957; 164:1382.
212. Haizlip TM, Ewing JA. Meprobamate habituation: a controlled clinical study. N Engl J Med 1958; 258:1181.
213. Roache JD, Griffiths RR. Lorazepam and meprobamate dose effects in humans: behavioral effects and abuse liability. J Pharmacol Exp Ther 1987; 243:978.
214. Kintz P, Tracqui A, Mangin P, Lugnier AA. Fatal meprobamate self-poisoning. Am J Forens Med Pathol 1988; 9:139.
215. Maddock RK, Bloomer HA. Meprobamate overdosage, evaluation of its severity and methods of treatment. JAMA 1967; 201:999.
216. Jenis EH, Payne RJ, Goldbaum LR. Acute meprobamate poisoning. A fatal case following a lucid interval. JAMA 1969; 207:361.
217. Hoy WE, Rivero A, Marin MG, Rieders F. Resin hemoperfusion for treatment of a massive meprobamate overdose. Ann Intern Med 1980; 93:455.
218. Jacobsen D, Wiik-Larson E, Saltvedt E, Bredesen JE. Meprobamate kinetics during and after terminated hemoperfusion in acute intoxications. Clin Toxicol 1987; 25:317.
219. Hayward JN, Boshell BR. Paraldehyde intoxication with metabolic acidosis. Am J Med 1957; 23:965.
220. Kunze U. Chronic bromide intoxication with a severe neurological deficit. J Neurol 1976; 213:149.
221. Trump DL, Hochberg MC. Bromide intoxication. Johns Hopkins Med J 1976; 138:119.
222. Palatucci DM. Paradoxical levels in bromide intoxication. Neurology 1978; 28:1189.
223. Wolf B, Guarino JJ, Preston KL, Griffiths RR. Abuse liability of diphenhydramine in sedative abusers. In: Harris L, ed. Problems of Drug Dependence 1989. Rockville, MD: NIDA Research Monograph 95, DHHS, 1990:486.
224. Traber J, Glaser T. 5-HT$_{1A}$ receptor-related anxiolytics. Trends Pharmacol Sci 1987; 8:432.
225. Smiley A, Moskowitz H. Effects of long-term administration of buspirone and diazepam on driver steering control. Am J Med 1986; 80:22.
226. Taylor DP, Moon SL. Buspirone and related compounds as alternative anxiolytics. Neuropeptides 1991; 19(suppl):15.
227. File SE. The search for novel anxiolytics. Trends Neurosci 1987; 10:461.
228. Griffith JD, Jasinski DR, Casten GP, McKinney GR. Investigation of the abuse liability of buspirone in alcohol-dependent subjects. Am J Med 1986; 80:30.
229. Schnabel T. Evaluation of the safety and side-effects of antianxiety agents. Am J Med 1987; 82:7.
230. Lader M. Assessing the potential for buspirone dependence or abuse and effects of its withdrawal. Am J Med 1987; 82:20.
231. Boylan K. Persistent dystonia associated with buspirone. Neurology 1990; 40:1904.

Chapter 6
Marijuana

"This will be deducted from your share in paradise," he
said, as he handed me my portion.   —*Theophile Gautier*

La cucaracha, la cucaracha
Ya no puede caminar
Porque no tiene, porque no tiene
Marijuana que fumar.
                              —*Pancho Villa*
                              marching song

Man, they can say what they want about us vipers, but
you just dig them lushhounds with their old antique
jive . . . that come uptown juiced to the gills, crackin' out
of line and passin' out in anybody's hallway. Don't
nobody come up thataway when he picks upon some
good grass.   —*Mezz Mezzrow*

Marijuana is derived from the hemp plant, *Cannabis sativa*. A resin covering the flowers and leaves of the female plant contains the active substances. Preparations made mainly from this resin—called "hashish" in the Middle East and "charas" in India—are several times more potent than marijuana, which is made from cut tops and leaves or whole plants and called "bhang," "kif," "dagga" (low resin content), or "ghanja" (high resin content).[1,2] The resin protects the plant from heat and dryness and is most abundant in plants grown in tropical climates; for that reason, marijuana from Latin America or Southeast Asia is likely to be more potent than marijuana from the continental United States. It weakens with aging. Among the plant's many cannabinoid compounds (cannabinols) are several isomers of tetrahydrocannabinol (THC), of which delta-9-THC is the principal psychoactive agent (Figure 6–1). Delta-8-THC has similar effects but is present in only minute amounts. Cannabichromene also has euphoriant activity, and cannabigerol has sedative properties. Cannabinol and cannabidiol are anticonvulsant, but cannibinol is only mildly psychoactive, and cannabidiol is not psychoactive at all. 9-beta-hydroxyhexahydrocannabinol is a potent analgesic, and cannabidolic acid has both sedative and antimicrobial actions. The 11-hydroxy metabolites of delta-9-THC and delta-8-THC are as psychically active as their parent compounds.[3]

Pharmacology and Animal Studies

Psychoactive cannabinoids, as exemplified by delta-9-THC, have unique effects in animals. In mice, low doses produce simultaneous depression and stimulation termed the *popcorn effect*.[1,2] The animals appear sedated until one mouse is stimulated, causing it to jump hyperreflexly; as it falls on another mouse, that animal then jumps, and the subsequent chain reaction throughout the cage resembles corn popping in a pan. Higher doses of delta-9-THC produce more typical sedation, as do both low and high doses of nonpsychoactive cannabinoids. In contrast to barbiturates and ethanol, however, even high doses of cannabinoids do not produce general anesthesia.[2] Accompanying the stimulatory effect of delta-9-THC is increased aggressiveness in rodents (an observation that is not predictive of its effect on humans). Delta-9-THC in animals also produces hypothermia and—again in contrast to its effects in humans—bradycardia and decreased food intake. It impairs memory and interferes with performance on sensory informatic.

Animal studies of the reinfor... ...f psychoactive cannabinoids have been contlic g; the physical properties of the drugs—gummy and water insoluble—make injectable preparations difficult (and indeed they are hardly ever abused parenterally by humans). Generally, animals are disinclined to self-administer delta-9-THC.[6-9] Tolerance develops to the psychoactive and hypothermic effects; it is pharmacodynamic in type and striking in its duration: Dogs receiving delta-9-THC for a week and then not treated for 11 days had little behavioral change when rechallenged.[10] Cross-tolerance exists between different cannabinoids and to a degree between delta-9-THC and ethanol (sedation) and delta-9-THC and morphine (analgesia and bradycardia).[1] The ability of delta-9-THC to relieve opioid abstinence symptoms in animals has been claimed and denied.[11] Delta-9-THC (but not cannabidiol) reportedly suppressed opioid withdrawal signs in mice and rats but not in monkeys.[12,13] Animal studies to determine if cannabinoids produce an abstinence syndrome of their own have been similarly conflicting. Increased gross movements and teeth-baring were described in monkeys,[14] and writhes, kicks, and "wet shakes" were described in rats,[15] but others either failed to observe such behavior or if they did were unable to interrupt it by giving more cannabinoid.[1]

Perhaps paralleling combined stimulatory and sedative effects, delta-9-THC in animals can be proconvulsant at low doses and anticonvulsant at high doses, with tolerance developing to its anticonvulsant effects. By contrast, cannabidiol is more consistently anticonvulsant at both low and high doses, and, relevant to its potential as a pharmaceutical, there is little tolerance to this action.[1,2,4] The proconvulsant and anticonvulsant actions of cannabinoids vary with species, seizure model, and route of administration.[16-19] Delta-9-THC protected chickens from photic-induced but not pentylenetetrazol-induced seizures.[20] In mice, delta-9-THC was anticonvulsant for maximal electroshock seizures but proconvulsant for pentylenetetrazol-induced and

chnine-induced seizures.[21] In cats, delta-9-THC ...ented kindled amygdaloid seizures if given ...y but not if given after seizures were developed.[22] ...baboons, delta-9-THC blocked established kin...d amygdaloid seizures but not photic-induced ...zures.[23] In seizure-prone gerbils, THC was ...nticonvulsant.[24] A strain of New Zealand rabbits is uniquely susceptible to seizures induced by psychoactive cannabinoids in doses equivalent to these consumed by humans, and these seizures are blocked by pretreatment with cannabidiol.[25,26] In studies of transcallosal cortical-evoked responses in rats and spinal monosynaptic reflexes in cats, low doses of delta-9-THC enhanced synaptic transmission, whereas higher doses of delta-9-THC and all doses of cannabidiol caused only depression.[27] In rats, cannabidiol was anticonvulsant for both maximal electroshock and audiogenic seizures and enhanced the anticonvulsant potency of phenytoin (although it antagonized that of ethosuximide, clonazepam, and trimethadione).[28] Although cannabidiol and phenytoin are effective against similar types of seizures, electrophysiologic studies suggest they have different mechanisms of action.[29]

In some animal models, delta-9-THC and other psychoactive cannabinoids have been as potently analgesic as morphine. Other workers have not found comparable analgesic efficacy. As with actions on seizures, cannabinoid analgesia varies with the particular agent, species, pain model, and route of administration.[4,30]

Cannabinoids affect a number of neurotransmitter systems. Delta-9-THC accelerates the synthesis, neuronal uptake, and storage of norepinephrine and dopamine; increases the affinity of dopamine D-2 receptors for dopamine agonists; and enhances the coupling of beta-adrenergic receptors to adenylyl cyclase. Delta-9-THC increases dopaminergic transmission in the nucleus accumbens[31] and medial prefrontal cortex,[32] and the dopaminergic effects of different cannabinoids correlate with their psychoactive potency.[2]

Delta-9-THC inhibits synaptosomal uptake of serotonin; in rats, the anticonvulsant efficacy of cannabis resin against maximal electroshock seizures was inhibited by reserpine, and this inhibition was reversed by the serotonin precursor 5-hydroxytryptophan.[33] In cats, parachlorophenylalanine, which decreases serotonin synthesis, lowers the threshold of delta-9-THC-induced seizures.[34] Delta-9-THC reduces the firing rate of acetylcholine neurons, including those in the hippocampus, perhaps relevant to its effects on memory. At low doses, it reduces gamma-aminobutyric acid (GABA) turnover, but at high doses it increases it. The anticonvulsant actions of cannabinoids have been attributed to these effects on GABA; in fact, cannabidiol in mice prevented seizures caused by the GABA inhibitors picrotoxin, pentylenetetrazol, and bicuculline but not those induced by the glycine antagonist strychnine.[35] Others have found that the anticonvulsant properties of cannabinoids correlate with their ability to inhibit depolarization-dependent synaptic uptake of calcium.[36]

Cannabinoids raise blood levels of prostaglandins, and this action might contribute to some of its effects. In human volunteers, the prostaglandin synthesis inhibitor indomethacin attenuated the subjective "high" induced by delta-9-THC as well as its effect on time estimation but did not affect impairment of cognitive tasks such as word recall.[37]

The dose-dependent biphasic nature of the effects of delta-9-THC implies more than one mode of action, and indeed low doses appear to act at stereospecific receptors, whereas higher doses may act less specifically—similar to ethanol—on neuronal membranes.[38] Cannabinoid receptors are G-protein coupled and inhibit adenylyl cyclase dose dependently and stereospecifically.[39,40] They are present in brain, with highest levels in cerebral cortex, basal ganglia, cerebellum, and hippocampus, and they are most responsive to psychoactive cannabinoids.[41-42] In 1990, the cDNA for the cannabinoid receptor was cloned;[43,44] in humans, it resides on the short arm of chromosome 6.[45] The diverse pharmacological actions of cannabinoids suggest the existence of receptor subtypes, and the fact that delta-9-THC is a less potent inhibitor of adenylyl cyclase than other synthetic cannabinoids suggests that it acts as a mixed agonist-antagonist.[46] Rat and human cannabinoid receptors display 97.3% sequence conservation,[46a] and in 1992 an endogenous ligand for the cannabinoid receptor was identified in porcine brain. Named "anandamide" (from the Sanskrit word *ananda,* meaning bliss), it is arachidonylethanolamide, a C-20 fatty acid derivative.[46b]

Historical Background and Epidemiology

Marijuana was described in China in the third millenium BC.[47] The hemp fiber was used for clothing, bowstrings, and paper, and although recreational intoxication was frowned on in the Taoist culture, marijuana was used medicinally and in religious and magical rites. As an intoxicant, marijuana played a more prominent role in ancient India; according to the Hindu *Vedas,* the god Siva discovered cannabis and concocted the liquid refreshment from it called *bhang* (which additionally contains poppyseeds, ginger, cloves, cardamon, nutmeg, and milk). A more potent brew made from the flowers and upper leaves is called *ganja,* and an even stronger concoction made with high resin content is called *charas.* For at least 3000 years, marijuana, ingested or smoked, has been as popular in India as ethanol is in the West.

In the 5th century BC, Herodotus described the Scythian Cult of the Dead: Hemp was placed on red-hot stones in a closed room producing an intoxicating vapor.[48] Pliny and Dioscorides also described marijuana intoxication, and possible Old Testament references include the "honeycomb" of Song of Solomon and the "honeywood" of I Samuel.[49]

In the Middle East during the 11th century, members of the Sufi Islamic sect used hashish—comparable in potency to charas and either eaten as a paste or mixed with sesame and chewed like gum—to achieve religious ecstasy.[47] The association of cannabis with this despised and economically downtrodden minority launched the drug's false reputation as an inspirer of violence. The Arab reference to hashish users as *ashishin* became transcribed during the Crusades to the word *assassin.*

Introduced into Europe, cannabis was cultivated for its fiber. (In the 16th century, Rabelais described many marvelous uses of cannabis—he called it "pantagruelian"—but intoxication was not one of them.[50]) During this time, it was used as a folk medicine (including seizure prevention); nonmedicinal ingestion was largely restricted to religious cults.[47]

Marijuana smoking has long been popular in Africa; Dutch settlers observed the custom among the Hottentots, who called the cannabis plant *dagga.* Napolean's invasion of Egypt familiarized a new generation of Europeans to hashish, and in mid-19th century Paris, the celebrated "Club des Hachichins" included among its members Theophile Gautier, Victor Hugo, Alexandre Dumas, Eugene Delacroix, and Charles Baudelaire.[51]

In the United States during the 18th century, cannabis was also grown for its fiber. In the mid-19th century, it was listed in the U.S. Dispensatory for treating "neuralgia, gout, tetanus, hydrophobia, epidemic cholera, convulsions, chorea, hysteria, mental depression, insanity, and uterine hemorrhage." William Osler considered marijuana the treatment of choice for migraine.[52] In 1905, cannabis was offered by Sears, Roebuck as a cure for morphine addiction. Unrecognized as a euphoriant, cannabis was not included in the Harrison Narcotics Act of 1914. Its use among Mexicans, however, led to popular associations with disreputable behavior, and just as

America's antiopioid attitudes arose out of fear and distrust of Chinese immigrants, by the 1920s several western states had passed antimarijuana laws. During this time, cannabis continued to be present in both prescription and over-the-counter pharmaceuticals, and smoked "reefers" became popular with the Black urban jazz culture (inspiring such works as Louis Armstrong's "Muggles," Cab Calloway's "Reefer Man," and Fats Waller's "Viper's Drag"). To what extent racism contributed to the Marijuana Tax Act of 1937 is still debated, but that federal legislation—vigorously opposed by the American Medical Association on the grounds that serious ill effects of cannabis had never been demonstrated—banned its nonmedicinal possession or sale.[53] Draconian state laws soon followed: Penalties included life imprisonment for first-offense selling (Utah) and death for selling to minors (Missouri).[49]

Despite such measures, marijuana today is the most widely used illicit drug in the United States. Domestic production is greatest in California, and Colombia and Mexico are the leading exporters (although by the mid-1980s governmental spraying of Mexican marijuana with the herbicide paraquat had not only reduced supplies from that country, but also made the product less desirable than marijuana from other sources).[54] The bulkiness of marijuana makes interdiction easier than with cocaine or heroin; ironically, however, the success of such programs has resulted in the United States itself becoming one of the world's leading marijuana producers.[55] In 1980, 32% of Americans aged 12 to 17 and 68% aged 18 to 25 had used marijuana, 40% of the latter group more than 100 times.[56,57] Use then steadily declined during the 1980s.[58] In 1990, the National Youth Risk Behavior Survey, sampling more than 11,000 high school students in the 50 states, reported that 31% of all students had used marijuana at least once and 14% had used it within 30 days of the survey.[59] (For seniors, the numbers were 42% and 18.5%.) A similar survey in 1989, found that marijuana use among high school seniors within the preceding 12 months ranged from 17% to 44% depending on sex and race (Table 6–1).[60] According to the National Household Survey on Drug Abuse, the number of current marijuana users in the United States fell from 18.2 million in 1985 to 11.6 million[61] in 1988, and the number of at least weekly users fell from 9.2 million to 6.6 million.[61] In 1990, 66 million Americans had tried marijuana at least once, and 10.2 million had used it within the preceding month. The potency of commercially available marijuana is much higher than a decade ago, but so is the retail price—often over $250 an

Table 6–1. Marijuana Use within Preceding 12 Months by U.S. High School Seniors, 1985–1989

White male	40.2%
Black male	29.8
Mexican American male	37.3
Puerto Rican/Latin American male	30.6
Asian male	19.6
Native American male	42.0
White female	36.0
Black female	18.4
Mexican American female	26.0
Puerto Rican/Latin American female	21.3
Asian female	17.1
Native American female	44.0

Source: Bachman JG, Wallace JM, O'Malley PM, et al. Racial/ethnic differences in smoking, drinking, and illicit drug use among American high school seniors, 1976–89. Am J Publ Health 1991; 81:372.

ounce (compared with $800 to $1200 an ounce for cocaine and more than $5000 an ounce for heroin).[62]

A puzzling aspect of marijuana's allegedly declining popularity is that during this same period other data imply increased consumption. Estimated nondomestic and domestic production of marijuana actually increased during the late 1980s, and emergency room visits associated with Drug Abuse Warning Network (DAWN) reports of marijuana use more than doubled.[61] Such discrepancies reflect the difficulties in obtaining reliable epidemiologic data on substance abuse, especially with a drug as politically charged as marijuana.

American marijuana users come from all age groups, socioeconomic classes, and geographic regions. The major period of risk for initiation to marijuana use—similar to tobacco and ethanol—is before age 20, and those who have not experimented with it by then are unlikely to do so. Similar to ethanol, but in contrast to tobacco, the prevalence of marijuana use declines after age 21.[63,64]

Acute Effects

In the United States, marijuana ("grass," "pot," "tea," "reefer," "weed," "hash," "skunk," "sens," "Mary Jane," "MJ," "Colombian gold," "Acapulcan gold," "Panama red," "Thai sticks," "Cambodian red") is usually smoked. As with other psychoactive agents, effects vary not only with dose, but also with social setting and expectation. An average good quality cigarette ("joint") delivers 2.5 to 5 mg delta-9-THC. Effects begin within 10 to 20 minutes and last 2 to 3 hours. Ingested marijuana is only about one-third as potent, but the effects last up to 12 hours.[65]

During the first few minutes, smoked marijuana may produce jitteriness, anxiety, or fear. There then ensues a relaxed, dreamy euphoria ("stoned"), often with jocularity or silliness. If a user is alone, sleepiness is more likely. There is disinhibition or depersonalization, subjective slowing of time, and a sensation of altered body proportion.[66–68] In contrast to the dulled thinking associated with ethanol, users report increased awareness of events or stimuli; objective testing, however, reveals decreased auditory signal detection, impaired visual acuity for detecting small moving targets or discriminating colors, and no change in cutaneous sensitivity.[69–72] Familiar objects or relationships may appear novel or profound, yet there are decreased empathy and perception of the emotions of others.[73] Paranoid feelings are common but usually of minor concern.[74] The limbs feel numb, weak, or floating, and there is a sensation of pressure in the head or dizziness. Speech may be rapid or flighty. At high doses, memory and problem solving are impaired.[75,76] There is also difficulty in digit repetition, serial subtraction, concept formation, reading comprehension, and coherent speaking.[77–79] Although subjective effects and tachycardia resolve within a few hours of use, impaired performance on cognitive tasks can last for more than 24 hours.[80] Balance and hand steadiness are also impaired, compromising complex motor tasks such as driving.[81,82] In contrast to ethanol, however, there is rarely gross ataxia or nystagmus.[67]

Marijuana causes conjunctival injection, decreased salivation, urinary frequency, tachycardia, and increased systolic blood pressure and urinary epinephrine; it also causes postural hypotension and faintness (Table 6–2).[63,83] Propranolol prevents tachycardia induced by marijuana, but not its subjective or behavioral effects.[84] Alpha-methyltyrosine, which reduces brain dopamine and norepinephrine, similarly does not prevent marijuana-induced psychological effects.[85] Marijuana reduces urinary methoxyhydroxyphenylglycol levels and increases homovanillic acid, consistent with altered turnover of norepinephrine and dopamine.[86]

Appetite and thirst increase. There is decreased intraocular pressure, long-lasting bronchodilation, and analgesia to both traumatic and experimental pain.[69,87] If sleep occurs, there is less time spent in the rapid eye movement phase, and the subject awakens with little sense of "hangover."[88]

Except for a slight shift toward slower alpha frequencies, the electroencephalogram in humans

Table 6–2. Marijuana: Acute Effects

Anxiety, jitteriness, paranoia
Euphoria, relaxation, jocularity
Depersonalization
Subjective time-slowing
Dizziness, sensation of floating
Impaired memory and problem solving
Impaired balance and hand steadiness
Conjunctival injection
Decreased salivation
Urinary frequency
Tachycardia
Systolic hypertension with postural hypotension
Increased appetite and thirst
Decreased intraocular pressure
Analgesia
Auditory and visual illusions and hallucinations
Psychotic excitement or depression
Bradycardia, hypotension
Acute dysphoria, panic

shows no gross changes during a conventional "high."[89] Visual, auditory, and somatosensory evoked response amplitudes are depressed.[90] While smoking marijuana, a patient with implanted brain electrodes developed euphoria and high-voltage-delta waves in the septal region but not in other areas, including the amygdala, thalamus, hippocampus, or caudate.[91] Similar changes in monkeys persisted after the drug was stopped.[92]

High doses cause auditory and visual illusions or hallucinations that consist of flashes of light or color, geometric figures, human faces, or complex pictures.[93] Bizarre illusions include loss of depth perception, a "strobe light effect" (seeing a moving object as if it were a series of still pictures), the appearance of people talking with their mouths and voices unsynchronized, and "streaking" (moving light sources in a dark environment becoming long streaks as in a time-exposed photograph).[94] Fantastic complex hallucinations with extraordinary dilation of subjective time were vividly described by 19th century users.[95] Anecdotal reports suggest that marijuana improves night vision.[96]

Still higher doses cause confusion, disorientation, markedly impaired memory, anxiety, and psychotic depression or excitement.[93] Bradycardia and hypotension occur.[97] Fatal overdose has not been documented. A 23-year-old was found dead from no apparent cause, and cannabinoids were identified in the urine.[98] A man attempted suicide by smoking hashish and was comatose for 4 days.[99] A small child after ingesting 1.5 g cannabis resin had hypothermia, alternating stupor and excitement, ataxia, and decreased respiratory rate; recovery occurred after several hours.[100] A young man smuggled Moroccan hashish oil into the United States by swallowing drug-filled balloons; he developed euphoria and then 48 hours of sleepiness, tachycardia, disorientation to place, and, unexpectedly, anisocoria.[101]

Without other signs of toxicity, marijuana sometimes causes acute adverse reactions consisting of intense emotional upset, confusion, paranoia, delusions, depression, or panic ("freaking out"). Such symptoms can last hours or days.[93,102,103] They are rare, usually follow first use, and are more often associated with ingestion than smoking—probably because the effects of smoked marijuana are so short-lived, and doses of 20 to 70 mg delta-9-THC are required.[67,104] Especially vulnerable to anxiety or psychosis are subjects whose ingestion has been inadvertent—for example, unknowingly eating laced brownies or cookies. Claims of "acute cannabis psychosis" lasting 6 weeks or longer were not confirmed in several field studies.[105,106] Marijuana has been reported to trigger psychosis in people with previous psychotic histories or hallucinogenic drug use, and acute dysphoric reactions are more common in patients with chronic pain and depression. They can occur, however, in otherwise normal users.[107-109] Two small children repeatedly given oral marijuana by their parents developed manic psychosis requiring antipsychotic medication; they eventually recovered.[110] Mania, paranoia, and auditory hallucinations also affected several Jamaican adults who increased their usual dose.[111] Manic psychosis developed in a marijuana user who was also taking fluoxetine.[112] In this and other similar reports, recovery was complete with abstinence.[113,114]

"Flashbacks" refer to the spontaneous experience weeks to months after using marijuana of hallucinations or other feelings associated with the original use.[115,116] However—despite the claim that marijuana is an independent risk factor for the development of schizophrenia,[117]—there is little evidence that it causes lasting violent or psychotic behavior. (For a taste of antimarijuana propaganda at its most droll, the interested reader is recommended the 1930s cult film classic, Reefer Madness.) Acute marijuana panic states and toxic psychoses can usually be managed with calm reassurance. Benzodiazepines or haloperidol relieve severe symptoms.[67,118,119]

Within a few minutes of smoking a marijuana cigarette, plasma levels of delta-9-THC reach about 100 ng/mL, falling to 10 ng/mL at 1 hour, 1 ng/mL at 4 hours and 0.1 ng/mL at 24 hours.[67,120] The rapid drop in plasma concentrations is the result of tissue distribution and accounts for the relatively short subjective effects compared with the elimination half-life, which averages 59 hours in novices and 28 hours in chronic smokers.[121] Absorption of oral delta-9-THC is slow and erratic, with peak plasma levels after 1 hour.[120] Ingested delta-9-THC results in higher plasma levels of the active metabolite 11-hydroxy-THC than of the parent compound; smoked marijuana produces barely detectable levels of this metabolite. In first-time or irregular users, cannabinoid metabolites are detectable in urine for several days.[4] Frequent users accumulate delta-9-THC and continue to shed metabolites for more than a week; an incarcerated heavy user had a positive urine sample for 2 months.[122]

Tolerance develops to marijuana's cardiovascular, motor, and psychic effects and is more pharmacodynamic than pharmacokinetic.[97,123] Very high doses are taken in many countries, and American soldiers in Germany consumed up to 2000 mg hashish daily.[124] The possibility of sensitization or reverse tolerance to stimulatory effects is controversial. In a study of human volunteers, experienced marijuana smokers obtained a "high" more readily than did novices,[66] but alternative explanations include greater skill at efficiently inhaling marijuana smoke and a conditioned placebo effect based on expectation.[125] In favor of dissociative tolerance—unmasking of stimulant effects by the development of tolerance to depressant effects—are chronic users who are not as functionally impaired as novices yet report a subjective "high."[66]

Dependence and Withdrawal

The question of physical dependence to marijuana is also controversial. Monkeys given high doses of delta-9-THC for several weeks had several days of abstinence signs when the drug was stopped: irritability, aggression, yawning, tremor, photophobia, piloerection, and penile erections.[126] Similarly, humans withdrawing from several weeks of high-dose marijuana have displayed various combinations of emotional lability, anxiety, restlessness, insomnia, anorexia, nausea, vomiting, diarrhea, tremor, hyperreflexia, sweating, and salivation.[123,127-129] Such symptoms are rare, however, and most chronic users, if they have symptoms at all, describe simply jitteriness, anorexia, headache, and mild gastrointestinal upset without exhibiting objective abstinence signs. Addictive craving is common, however.

Marijuana and Other Drugs

Street preparations of marijuana may be contaminated with oregano, stramonium leaves, lysergic acid diethylamide (LSD), methamphetamine, or other agents, and marijuana is often deliberately taken with other drugs such as heroin, cocaine, or phencyclidine ("supergrass").[130-132] Barbiturates or ethanol and marijuana have additive or synergistic subjective and psychomotor effects.[133,134] In humans, marijuana does not potentiate opioid effects,[135] and studies of its influence on opioid withdrawal are unavailable. Marijuana use usually precedes "harder" drugs, but a cause and effect relationship is difficult to establish.[136] The illegality of marijuana, of course, brings users into contact with purveyors of other illicit substances.

Medical and Neurological Complications

Whether marijuana use produces lasting mental abnormalities is uncertain and controversial.[136a] Reports from India and Morocco were the first to describe personality change with chronic cannabis use, an *antimotivational syndrome* consisting of diminished drive and ambition, apathy and flat affect, decreased attentiveness, and impaired recent memory.[124,137,138] Such symptoms were reported in Americans taking chronic high doses, and cerebral atrophy was observed by pneumoencephalography.[139] Others have been unable to confirm these reports. Studies with computerized tomography (CT) have shown normal cerebral ventricular size in users, and several studies have failed to demonstrate neuropsychological differences between cannabis users and controls.[140-149] In Jamaica, where marijuana is smoked, chewed, added to food, and used as a medicinal in tea from early childhood, a National Institute of Mental Health study found no evidence of antimotivational syndrome and no significant physical abnormalities.[105] That study, however, included only 30 daily cannabis users, and many of the controls sometimes used cannabis tea. Moreover, subjects were farmers and laborers, and so subtle intellectual impairment could have gone undetected. In Costa Rica, where marijuana is widely used, no differences on physical examination, neuropsychological assessment, or laboratory testing were evident between 80 users and 80 nonusers.[148] In Greece, 47 hashish users were compared with 40 nonusers, and no differences in cognitive function were observed.[89]

In a study with volunteers, high doses (210 mg) of delta-9-THC were given daily for 30 days. The most striking finding was the rapid development of tolerance and lack of psychotomimetic effects.[150] Similarly, volunteers who smoked 35 to 198 mg delta-9-THC daily for 78 days had no untoward mental effects.[151] (That was the study that identified the ability of cannabis to lower intraocular pressure. In addition, serum testosterone was decreased, and pulmonary airways were eventually narrowed, but there were no abnormalities of chromosomes or immune response.)

Neuropsychological studies comparing heavy marijuana users with nonusers have been confounded by the absence of any measure of intellectual functioning before drug use. One study that provided such data found no adverse effects of chronic marijuana use.[142] Another found impairments in verbal expression and mathematical skills but only in very heavy users.[152] A study comparing "cannabis-dependent" adolescents with occasional users and nonusers found abnormal visual and verbal memory in the heavy users, with "significant improvement" after 6 weeks of abstinence.[153]

An Egyptian study found impaired psychomotor and visual-motor performance and impaired memory for designs in cannabis users compared with controls.[154] Other studies found decreased work output among cannabis smokers,[155-157] and the Greek study found that hashish users were more likely than nonusers to have personality disorders.[89] There appears to be no relation between marijuana use and crime independent of the drug's illegality.[158] Thus, if marijuana causes lasting cognitive or behavioral change in humans, it must be very subtle; moreover, a personality disorder could be the cause of marijuana use rather than its consequence.

Mice or rats receiving high doses of delta-9-THC daily for several weeks or months and then tested after several months of abstinence had impaired learning.[136a,158a] Chimpanzees receiving comparable doses of delta-9-THC, however, did not display residual cognitive impairment[158b] In rats, chronic cannabinoid administration reportedly reduced the cell volume and shortened the dendritic spines of hippocampal neurons.[159,160] In rats and monkeys, however, chronic delta-9-THC did not produce any lasting alterations of cannabinoid receptor function or of binding to several neurotransmitter receptors, including dopamine, serotonin, acetylcholine, GABA, opioid, and benzodiazepine.[161]

Marijuana causes bronchial and laryngeal damage, with hoarseness, cough, and impaired pulmonary function.[57,162] Hydrocarbon tars in marijuana smoke are more carcinogenic than those in tobacco smoke,[163] and users have developed cancer of the mouth, larynx, and lung.[164-166] Compared with tobacco smoking, marijuana is associated with nearly fivefold greater increments in blood carboxyhemoglobin levels.[167] Digital clubbing has been observed in hashish users without other evidence of pulmonary disease.[168] Contamination of cannabis plants with the herbicide paraquat adds further potential danger to the respiratory system,[57] as does the presence in most marijuana samples of pathogenic inhalable *Aspergillus*, a particular risk to users infected with human immunodeficiency virus (HIV).[169,170] A multistate outbreak of salmonella enteritis was traced to contamination of marijuana samples.[171] Four Puerto Rican policemen assigned to uprooting illegally cultivated marijuana developed acute pulmonary histoplasmosis.[172]

Anaphylactic reaction to marijuana has been reported;[173] less convincingly, marijuana has been linked to cirrhosis,[174] gastroenteritis,[175] and obliterative arteritis of the legs.[176]

Reported abnormalities of cellular immunity include inhibition of phytohemagglutinin-stimulated lymphocyte blastogenesis, decreased numbers of T lymphocytes, impaired macrophage function, reduced cytokine secretion, altered killer cell activity, delayed allogenic skin graft rejection, and enhanced susceptibility of mice to gram-negative bacterial infection.[129,177,178] Some workers, while confirming marijuana's effects on T cell function, found such abnormalities to be transitory. Others, studying skin tests for cellular immunity or cultured lymphocyte responses to mitogens, did not detect abnormalities attributable to marijuana smoking.[129] Marijuana users, in contrast to heavy ethanol users, do not seem to be especially vulnerable to infection independent of direct contamination; in particular, marijuana has not hastened the development of acquired immunodeficiency syndrome (AIDS) in HIV-infected users.[179]

Marijuana inhibits secretion of luteinizing hormone (LH), follicle-stimulating hormone (FSH), and testosterone. In men, there is decreased sperm count, gynecomastia, and impotence and in women menstrual irregularity and anovulatory menstrual cycles.[129,180,181] These changes are reversible; permanently impaired potency or fertility have not been reported in chronic marijuana users. A 16-year-old boy who had smoked marijuana since age 11 had pubertal arrest; with abstinence, growth resumed, and testosterone levels became normal.[182]

In humans, marijuana depresses growth hormone and cortisol response to insulin hypoglycemia.[183] In animals, it depresses thyroid gland function and plasma prolactin levels and raises levels of plasma adrenocorticotropic hormone (ACTH) and adrenocortical steroids.[184] Tolerance develops to these hormone changes. In rats, delta-9-THC suppression of LH was attributed to blocked release of LH-releasing hormone, whereas suppression of growth hormone

release was secondary to stimulation of somatostatin release.[185] One report, cautioning against too readily extrapolating animal endocrine effects to humans, found no change in plasma prolactin levels among marijuana-smoking men. Another study found no effects of moderate short-term marijuana use on plasma prolactin, ACTH, cortisol, LH, and testosterone in men.[186] In other reports, moderate short-term marijuana use had no effect on plasma prolactin, ACTH, cortisol, LH, and testosterone,[187] and chronic marijuana use had no effect on blood levels of testosterone, LH, FSH, prolactin, or cortisol.[188]

In subjects with angina pectoris, marijuana decreases exercise performance by increasing myocardial oxygen demand and decreasing myocardial oxygen delivery.[189] Fatal myocardial infarction occurred in a 32-year-old man who had smoked marijuana the same evening; coronary atherosclerosis was present at autopsy.[190]

There have been several reports of alleged occlusive stroke in young marijuana users.[191–195] Some are more convincing than others. In two young men, the only abnormality was conjugate deviation of the eyes for days or weeks after marijuana use.[191,194] Another young man awoke with hemiparesis and dysarthria the morning after smoking marijuana.[194] Imaging studies were not performed in these patients. Better documented were two young men—both hypertensive cigarette smokers—who developed hemiparesis during marijuana smoking and whose CT scans demonstrated cerebral infarction.[195] A 30-year-old chronic smoker of marijuana and tobacco had three episodes suggestive of transient ischemia and then a striatocapsular infarct with hemiparesis and aphasia.[196] In one, platelet function was normal after using marijuana, and the proposed mechanism of stroke was drug-induced hypotension and possible vasospasm in the setting of high blood pressure. In rats, delta-9-THC has vasoconstrictor actions.[197] In humans, marijuana has unpredictable effects on cerebral blood flow, either increasing or decreasing it.[198]

Marijuana smokers are overrepresented in highway fatalities.[57,199] Studies with volunteers have confirmed impairment in driving ability for up to 150 minutes after smoking enough marijuana to achieve a "high."[200]

In a case-control study from Harlem Hospital Center, marijuana use was protective against new-onset seizures in men; use was significantly less for cases than controls (28.9% versus 40.6%), and the protective effect persisted after controlling in multivariate analysis for heroin, ethanol, and other confounders (Table 6–3).[201] Among women, a smaller

Table 6–3. Adjusted Odds Ratio of Marijuana Use and New-Onset Seizures

	Men: Odds Ratio (95% Confidence Interval)	Women: Odds Ratio (95% Confidence Interval)
Unprovoked Seizures		
Marijuana use ever	0.42 (0.22–0.82)	1.09 (0.35–3.40)
Marijuana use within 3 months of admission	0.36 (0.18–0.74)	1.87 (0.56–6.20)
Provoked Seizures		
Marijuana use ever	1.03 (0.36–2.89)	0.79 (0.14–4.37)
Marijuana use within 3 months of admission	0.18 (0.04–0.84)	1.08 (0.12–9.79)

From Ng SKC et al. Illicit drug use and the risk of new onset seizures. Am J. Epidemiol 1990; 132:47.

nonsignificant difference existed in the same direction (11.7% versus 15.2%). Frequency and duration of marijuana use was similar among cases and controls. About one-third were daily users, and two-thirds were weekly users; 70% had used marijuana for at least 2 years and 50% for at least 5 years. Of special interest is that although marijuana smoked within 90 days conferred maximal protection, the risk was reduced for unprovoked seizures (unaccompanied by an additional potential precipitant such as metabolic derangement or head trauma) even in those who had last smoked it more remotely.

These findings are consistent with animal studies demonstrating the anticonvulsant properties of some cannabinoids. Marijuana was recommended for the treatment of epilepsy as far back as the 15th century,[202] yet few trials have been conducted in humans.[203–211] Five mentally retarded, poorly controlled epileptic children were switched from conventional anticonvulsants to "isomeric homologs of THC"; three responded "at least as well as to previous therapy," one was much improved, and one became entirely seizure free.[206] In a single case report, marijuana smoking was necessary for seizure control.[203] A New Mexico survey of 42 epileptics under age 30 found that 29% used marijuana; one subject reported that marijuana decreased seizures and another that it "caused" them.[208] In another case report, intravenous cannabidiol did not alter (and maybe even increased) the electroencephalographic spike and wave abnormalities of a young man with well-controlled "tonic-clonic seizures."[210] A young man who abused ethanol and smoked marijuana daily developed episodic olfactory hallucinations, confusion, urinary incontinence, and electroencephalographic temporal lobe spikes when he stopped using marijuana; symptoms cleared with resumption and recurred when he again discontinued the drug.[212]

There has been only one prospectively designed treatment study, a double-blind, placebo-controlled trial of patients refractory to other drugs. Cannabidiol, given to 8 of the 16 patients, acutely exacerbated electroencephalographic but not behavioral seizures. After 4 to 5 months, however, seven of eight patients receiving cannabidiol were electroencephalographically and behaviorally seizure free compared with one of eight controls. The only sign of toxicity was somnolence.[211] These observations imply that marijuana's cannabinoid compounds include potentially useful anticonvulsant drugs.

Trochlear nerve dysfunction, with superior oblique muscle paresis, was reported in 20 "medium to heavy" marijuana users; if the drug was causal, the mechanism is obscure.[213] Electromyographic studies of peripheral nerves in cannabis users have shown no abnormalities.[214]

Rarely water infusions of cannabis plant material have been injected intravenously; complications seem to be from the crude plant material rather than from cannabinoid effects and include gastroenteritis, hypoalbuminemia, hepatitis, hypovolemia, renal insufficiency, thrombocytopenia, and rhabdomyolysis.[215–217]

A report from Texas described smoking of tobacco or marijuana dipped in formaldehyde to produce hallucinations. A patient who smoked and ingested such cigarettes developed confusion, agitation, pulmonary edema, and then coma and rhabdomyolysis.[218]

Obstetric and Pediatric Aspects

In the United States, marijuana is used by up to one-third of pregnant women.[219] Studies of effects on offspring have been conflicting in part because use is often underreported.[220–228] In a study that performed urine assays—without which 16% of marijuana users would have been unidentified—marijuana smoking during pregnancy was associated with decreased birth weight and length.[229] The newborns had reduced nonfat mass and normal fat stores, similar to what is found in the offspring of tobacco smokers and implicating hypoxia or other nonnutritional causes of impaired fetal growth. Cannabinoids easily cross the placenta, especially early in gestation, and fetal abnormalities could be the consequence of direct toxicity, abnormal maternal ventilation-perfusion, or inhalation of carbon monoxide.[230]

Whether these changes lead to neurobehavioral abnormalities is uncertain. Offspring of moderate to heavy marijuana users have reportedly had tremor, decreased responsiveness to stimuli during sleep, abnormally high-pitched cries, and altered sleep patterns;[231–233] others have found no such abnormalities.[224] Neurobehavioral development was normal among 1-year-olds and 2-year-olds exposed prenatally to marijuana,[234] yet at age 4 the same children performed poorly on verbal and memory tests.[235] Infants exposed to marijuana through breast-feeding had delayed motor development compared with controls.[236] As with other drugs, the effects of marijuana on fetal and later development are difficult to separate from confounding variables such as maternal nutrition, other substance abuse, and home environment.

In human lymphocytes, cannabinoids reportedly prevented normal chromosome segregation and induced chromosomal breakage.[237,238] Not all workers have been able to confirm such effects.[239] In rodents, cannabinoids caused morphologically abnormal ova, fetal wastage, and increased mortality at birth, especially among female offspring.[224,240–242] Also reported are liver, kidney, and vascular abnormalities; hydrocephalus; and delayed postnatal growth and brain protein synthesis.[242–246] In a study with rats, maternal exposure to cannabinoids altered the development of nigrostriatal, mesolimbic, and tuberoinfundibular dopaminergic neurons.[247] Other workers could not confirm cannabinoid effects on either protein synthesis or development.[248]

As with humans, neurobehavioral abnormalities in animals have been elusive, especially in properly controlled studies.[249,250] When pair-fed controls and surrogate fostering were employed, there were neither short-term nor long-term effects of marijuana on nipple attachment, locomotion, activity level, avoidance, water maze learning, or auditory startle.[251–253]

A case-control study of abruptio placentae in humans revealed that weekly use of marijuana during pregnancy carried a risk ratio of 2.8.[254]

Therapeutic Uses

In addition to their potential as anticonvulsants, cannabinoids might someday play a useful role as antiemetics, analgesics, and euphoriants in cancer patients;[255,256] as bronchodilators in asthmatics;[257] and in the treatment of glaucoma.[258] Cannabinoids have been tested for their antiemetic properties in patients receiving cancer chemotherapy, and the oral agents dronabinol (delta-9-THC) and nabilone (a synthetic cannabinoid) are commercially available.[259,260] Anecdotal reports suggest that such preparations are less effective than metoclopramide, domperidone, or smoked marijuana.[129,261] In a 1991 survey of more than 1000 oncologists, nearly half said they would prescribe marijuana if it were legal. Soon afterward a federal appeals court declared that the Drug Enforcement Agency (DEA) was using illogical criteria in prohibiting marijuana use for medical purposes.[262] In 1992, the DEA refused to reconsider its position.[263] Marijuana's illegality, of course, constrains scientific efforts to determine its effectiveness.

Marijuana reportedly relieved spasticity and postural tremor in patients with multiple sclerosis.[264,265] In another study, however, marijuana impaired motor performance in both multiple sclerosis patients and controls.[266] In the late 19th century, Gowers[267] reported that cannabis relieved parkinsonian tremor. In a study of five patients with idiopathic Parkinson's disease and tremor sensitive to levodopa, the claim was not borne out.[268] An anecdotal report suggested that marijuana might ameliorate the symptoms of ulcerative colitis.[269]

Long-term Treatment

The silliness of U.S. marijuana policy does not negate the potentially harmful consequences of its use, including addiction. Of the more than 10 million current users in the United States, more than a million are psychologically dependent—that is, addicted—and many seek treatment.[270,271] The vast majority of marijuana-dependent subjects use other drugs as well, especially cocaine, ethanol, and tobacco. In contrast to heroin, no effective pharmacotherapy for marijuana dependence exists. In contrast to ethanol or cocaine, potentially useful pharmacotherapies have not even been studied. Of 110 adults who received intensive group therapy over 12 weeks, only 30% reported complete abstinence from marijuana during the month following treatment.[270] Such an outcome practically defines addiction.

References

1. Dewey WL. Cannabinoid pharmacology. Pharmacol Rev 1986; 38:151.
2. Pertwee RG. The central neuropharmacology of psychotropic cannabinoids. Pharmacol Ther 1988; 36:189.
3. Perez-Reyes M, Timmons MC, Lipton MA, et al. Intravenous injection in man of delta-9-tetrahydrocannabinol and 11-hydroxy-delta-9-tetrahydrocannabinol. Science 1972; 177:633.
4. Seth R, Sinha S. Chemistry and pharmacology of cannabis. Prog Drug Res 1991; 36:71.
5. Deadwyler SA, Heyser CJ, Michaelis RC, Hampson RE. The effects of delta-9-THC on mechanisms of learning and memory. In: Erinoff L, ed. Neurobiology of Drug Abuse: Learning and Memory. Rockville, MD: NIDA Research Monograph 97, DHHS, 1990:79.
6. Compton DR, Dewey WL, Martin BR. Cannabis dependence and tolerance production. Adv Alcohol Subst Abuse 1990; 9:129.
7. Harris RT, Waters W, McLendon D. Evaluation of reinforcing capability of delta-9-tetrahydrocannibinol in rhesus monkeys. Psychopharmacology 1979; 37:23.
8. Takahashi RN, Singer G. Self-administration of delta-9-tetrahydrocannabinol by rats. Pharmacol Biochem Behav 1979; 11:737.
9. Jones RT. What have we learned from nicotine, cocaine, and marijuana about addiction. In: O'Brien CP, Jaffe JH, eds. Addictive States. Res Publ Assoc Res Nerv Ment Dis 1992; 70:109.
10. McMillan DE, Dewey WL, Harris LS. Characteristics of tetrahydrocannabinol tolerance. Ann NY Acad Sci 1971; 191:83.
11. Bloom AS, Dewey WL. A comparison of some pharmacologic actions of morphine and delta-9-tetrahydrocannabinol in the mouse. Psychopharmacology 1978; 57:243.
12. Bhargava HN. Time course of the effects of naturally occurring cannabinoids on morphine abstinence syndrome. Pharmacol Biochem Behav 1978; 8:7.
13. Hine B, Friedman E, Torrelio M, Gershon S. Morphine dependent rats. Blockade of precipitated abstinence by tetrahydrocannabinol. Science 1974; 187:443.
14. Fredericks AB, Benowitz NL. An abstinence syndrome following chronic administration of delta-9-tetrahydrocannabinol in rhesus monkeys. Psychopharmacology 1980; 71:201.
15. Taylor DA, Fennessy MR. Time-course of the effects of chronic delta-9-tetrahydrocannabinol on behavior, body temperature, brain amines, and withdrawal-like behavior in the rat. J Pharm Pharmacol 1981; 34:240.
16. Colasanti BK, Lindamood C, Craig CR. Effects of marijuana cannabinoids on seizure activity in cobalt-epileptic rats. Pharmacol Biochem Behav 1982; 16:573.
17. Karler R, Turkanis SA. Subacute cannabinoid treatment: anticonvulsant activity and withdrawal excitability in mice. Br J Pharmacol 1980; 68:479.
18. Consroe P, Benedito MA, Leite JR, et al. Effects of cannabidiol on behavioral seizures caused by convulsant drugs or current in mice. Eur J Pharmacol 1982; 83:293.
19. Consroe P, Martin A, Singh V. Antiepileptic potential of cannabidiol. J Clin Pharmacol 1981; 21(suppl): 428S.
20. Johnson DD, McNeill JR, Crawford RD, Wilcox WC. Epileptiform seizures in domestic fowl. V. The anticonvulsant activity of delta-9-tetrahydrocannabinol. Can J Physiol Pharmacol 1975; 53:1007.
21. Sofia RD, Solomon TA, Barry H. Anticonvulsant activity of delta-9-tetrahydrocannabinol compared with three other drugs. Eur J Pharmacol 1976; 35:7.
22. Wada JA, Wake A, Sato M, Corcoran ME. Antiepileptic and prophylactic effects of tetrahydrocannabinols in amygdaloid kindled rats. Epilepsia 1975; 16:503.
23. Wada JA, Osawa T, Corcoran ME. Effects of tetrahydrocannabinols on kindled amygdaloid seizures in Senegalese baboons, Papio papio. Epilepsia 1975; 16:439.
24. Ten-harn M, Laskota WJ, Lumak P. Acute and chronic effects of beta-9-tetrahydrocannabinol on seizures in the gerbil. Eur J Pharmacol 1975; 31:148.
25. Consroe P, Fish BS. Rabbit behavioral model of marijuana psychoactivity in humans. Med Hypotheses 1981; 7:1079.
26. Consroe P, Martin P, Eisenstein D. Anticonvulsant drug antagonism of delta-9-tetrahydrocannabinol-induced seizures in rabbits. Res Commun Chem Pathol Pharmacol 1977; 16:1.
27. Turkanis SA, Karler R. Electrophysiologic properties of the cannabinoids. J Clin Pharmacol 1981; 21(suppl):449S.
28. Consroe P, Wolkin A. Cannabidiol—antiepileptic drug comparisons and interactions in experimentally induced seizures in rats. J Pharmacol Exp Ther 1977; 20:26.
29. Karler R, Turkanis SA. The cannabinoids as potential antiepileptics. J Clin Pharmacol 1981; 21:437S.
30. Martin BR. Structural requirements for cannabinoid-induced anti-nociceptive activity in mice. Life Sci 1985; 36:1523.
31. Chen JP, Paredes W, Li J, et al. Delta-9-tetrahydrocannabinol produces naloxone-blockable enhancement of presynaptic basal dopamine efflux in nucleus accumbens of conscious, freely-moving rats as measured by intracerebral microdialysis. Psychopharmacology 1990; 102:156.

32. Chen J, Paredes W, Lowinson JH, Gardner EL. Delta-9-tetrahydrocannabinol enhances presynaptic dopamine efflux in medial prefrontal cortex. Eur J Pharmacol 1990; 190:259.
33. Ghosh P, Bhattacharya SK. Anticonvulsant action of cannabis in the rat: role of brain monoamines. Psychopharmacology 1978; 59:293.
34. Adams PM, Barrett ES. Role of biogenic amines in the effects of marijuana on electroencephalographic patterns in cats. Electroencephalogr Clin Neurophysiol 1986; 39:621.
35. Consroe P, Benedito MA, Leite JR, et al. Effects of cannabidiol on behavioral seizures caused by convulsant drugs or current in mice. Eur J Pharmacol 1982; 83:293.
36. Harris RA, Stokes JA. Cannabinoids inhibit calcium uptake by brain synaptosomes. J Neurosci 1982; 2:443.
37. Perez-Reyes M, Burstein SH, White WR, et al. Antagonism of marijuana effects by indomethacin in humans. Life Sci 1991; 48:507.
38. Martin BR. Cellular effects of cannabinoids. Pharmacol Rev 1986; 38:45.
39. Abood ME, Martin BR. Neurology of marijuana abuse. Trends Pharmacol Sci 1992; 13:201.
40. Bidaut-Russell MR, Devane WA, Howlett AC. Cannabinoid receptors and modulation of cyclic AMP accumulation in the rat brain. J Neurochem 1990; 55:21.
41. Herkenham M, Lynn AB, Little MD, et al. Cannabinoid receptor localization in the brain. Proc Natl Acad Sci USA 1990; 87:1932.
42. Howlett AC, Bidaut-Russell M, Devane WA, et al. The cannabinoid receptor: biochemical, anatomical and behavioral characterization. Trends Neurosci 1990; 13:420.
43. Marx J. Marijuana receptor gene cloned. Science 1990; 249:624.
44. Matsuda LA, Lolait SJ, Brownstein MJ, et al. Structure of a cannabinoid receptor and functional expression of the cloned cDNA. Nature 1990; 346:561.
45. Hoehe MR, Caenazzo L, Martinez MM, et al. Genetic and physical mapping of the human cannabinoid receptor gene to chromosome 6q14-q15. New Biol 1991; 3:880.
46. Snyder SH. Planning for serendipity. Nature 1990; 346:508.
46a. Gerard CM, Mollereau C, Brownstein MJ, et al. Molecular cloning of a human cannabinoid receptor which is also expressed in testis. Biochem J 1991; 279:129.
46b. Devane WA, Hanus L, Breuer A, et al. Isolation and structure of a constituent that binds to the cannabinoid receptor. Science 1992; 258:1946.
47. Abel EL. Marijuana, The First Twelve Thousand Years. New York: Plenum Press, 1980.
48. Herodotus. The Histories. Book Four. Harmondsworth, UK, Penguin Books, 1954.
49. Brecher EM. Licit and Illicit Drugs. Boston, Little, Brown, 1972.
50. Rabelais F. The Histories of Gargantua and Pantagruel, Book Three. Harmondsworth, UK, Penguin Books, 1955.
51. Gautier T. Hachich. Revue des Deux Mondes, February 1, 1846. Reprinted in: Ebin D, ed. The Drug Experience. New York, Orion Press, 1961:1.
52. Osler W, MacCrae T. Principles and Practice of Medicine, ed 8. New York: D. Appleton, 1916:1089.
53. Federal regulation of the medicinal use of cannabis (edit.). JAMA 1937; 108:1543.
54. Schwartz RH. Marijuana. a crude drug with a spectrum of under-appreciated toxicity. Pediatrics 1984; 73:455.
55. Nadelmann EA. Drug prohibition in the United States: costs, consequences, and alternatives. Science 1989; 245:939.
56. Fishburne PM, Abelson HI, Cisin I. National Survey on Drug Abuse: Main Findings: 1979. Washington, DC: DHHS Publication No (ADM) 80-976, 1980.
57. Nicholi AM. The nontherapeutic use of psychoactive drugs. A modern epidemic. N Engl J Med 1983; 308:925.
58. O'Malley PM, Bachman JG, Johnson LD. Period, age, and cohort effects on substance use among young Americans: a decade of change, 1976-86. Am J Publ Health 1988; 78:1315.
59. Alcohol and other drug use among high school students—United States, 1990. MMWR 1991; 40:776.
60. Bachman JG, Wallace, JM, O'Malley PM, et al. Racial/ethnic differences in smoking, drinking, and illicit drug use among American high school seniors, 1976–89. Am J Public Health 1991; 81:372.
61. Sidney S. Evidence of discrepant data regarding trends in marijuana use and supply, 1985–1988. J Psychoact Drugs 1990; 22:319.
62. Treaster JB. Costly and scarce, marijuana is a high most are rejecting. NY Times, October 29, 1991.
63. Marijuana and Health. Ninth Annual Report to the U.S. Congress from the Secretary of Health and Human Services. Rockville, MD: NIDA, DHHS Publication No (ADM) 82-1216, 1982.
64. Kandel DB, Logan JA. Patterns of drug use from adolescence to young adulthood. I. Periods of risk for initiation, continued use, and discontinuation. Am J Publ Health 1984; 74:660.
65. Lieberman CM, Lieberman BW. Marihuana—a medical review. N Engl J Med 1971; 284:88.
66. Weil AT, Zineberg NE, Nelsen JM. Clinical and psychological effects of marijuana in man. Science 1968; 162:1234.
67. Goldfrank LR, Melinek M. Marijuana. In: Goldfrank LR, Flomenbaum NE, Lewin NA, et al, eds. Toxicologic Emergencies, ed 4. Norwalk, CT: Appleton & Lange, 1990:529.
68. Borg J, Gershon S. Dose effects of smoked marihuana on human cognitive and motor functions. Psychopharmacologia 1975; 42:211.
69. Milstein SL, MacCannell KL, Karr G, Clark S. Marijuana-produced changes in cutaneous sensitivity

and affect: users and non-users. Pharmacol Biochem Behav 1974; 2:367.

70. Moskowitz H, McGlothlin W. Effects of marijuana on auditory signal detection. Psychopharmacologia 1974; 40:137.

71. Adams AJ, Brown B, Flom MC, et al. Alcohol and marijuana effects on static visual acuity. Am J Optom Physiol Opt 1975; 52:729.

72. Brown B, Adams AJ, Hagerstrom-Portnoy G, et al. Effects of alcohol and marijuana on dynamic visual acuity. I. Threshold measurements. Percept Psychophysiol 1975; 18:441.

73. Clopton PL, Janowsky DS, Clopton JM, et al. Marihuana and the perception of affect. Psychopharmacology 1979; 61:203.

74. Keeler MH, Moore E. Paranoid reactions while using marijuana. Dis Nerv Syst 1974; 35:535.

75. Sharma S, Moskowitz H. Effects of two levels of attention demand on vigilance performance under marijuana. Percept Motor Skills 1974; 38:967.

76. Roth WT, Rosenbloom MJ, Darley CF, et al. Marijuana effects on TAT form and content. Psychopharmacologia 1975; 43:261.

77. Belmore SM, Miller LL. Levels of processing acute effects of marijuana on memory. Pharmacol Biochem Behav 1980; 13:199.

78. Melges FT, Tinklenberg JR, Hollister LE, Gillespie HK. Marijuana and the temporal span of awareness. Arch Gen Psychiatry 1971; 24:564.

79. Klonhoff H, Low M, Marcus A. Neuropsychological effects of marijuana. Can Med Assoc J 1973; 108:150.

80. Heishman SJ, Huestis MA, Henningfield JE, Cone EJ. Acute and residual effects of marijuana: profiles of plasma THC levels, physiological, subjective and performance measures. Pharmacol Biochem Behav 1990; 37:561.

81. Janowsky DS, Meacham MP, Blaine JD, et al. Marijuana effects on simulated flying ability. Am J Psychiatry 1976; 133:384.

82. Kvalseth TO. Effects of marijuana on human reaction time and motor control. Percept Motor Skills 1977; 45:935.

83. Schaefer CF, Cunn CG, Dubowski KM. Marihuana dosage control through heart rate. N Engl J Med 1975; 293:101.

84. Bachman JA, Benowitz NL, Herning RI, Jones RT. Dissociation of autonomic and cognitive effects of THC in man. Psychopharmacology 1979; 61:171.

85. Hollister LE. Interactions in man of delta-9-tetrahydrocannabinol. I. Alphamethylparatyrosine. Clin Pharmacol Ther 1974; 15:18.

86. Markianos M, Vakis A. Effects of acute cannabis use on urinary neurotransmitter metabolites and cyclic nucleotides in man. Drug Alcohol Depend 1984; 14:175.

87. Tashkin DP, Soares JR, Hepler RS, et al. Cannabis, 1977. Ann Intern Med 1978; 89:539.

88. Tassinari CA, Peraita-Adrados MR, Ambrosetto G, Gastaut H. Effects of marijuana and delta-9-THC at high doses in man. A polygraphic study. Electroencephalogr Clin Neurophysiol 1974; 36:94.

89. Fink M, Volavka J, Panagiotopoulos CP, Stafanis C. Quantitative EEG studies of marijuana, delta-9-THC and hashish in man. In: Braude MC, Szara S, eds. Pharmacology of Marijuana. New York: Raven Press, 1976:383.

90. Herning RI, Jones RT, Peltzman DJ. Changes in human event related potentials with prolonged delta-9-tetrahydrocannabinol (THC) use. Electroencephalogr Clin Neurophysiol 1979; 47:556.

91. Heath RG. Marijuana effects on deep and surface electroencephalographs of man. Arch Gen Psychiatry 1972; 26:577.

92. Heath RG. Marihuana and delta-9-THC: acute and chronic effects on brain function of monkeys. In: Braude M, Szara S, eds. Pharmacology of Marihuana. New York: Raven Press, 1976:345.

93. Bromberg W. Marijuana intoxication. Am J Psychiatry 1934; 91:303.

94. Levi L, Miller NR. Visual illusions associated with previous drug abuse. J Clin Neuroophthalmol 1990; 10:103.

95. Ludlow F. The Hasheesh Eater: Being Passages from the Life of a Pythagorean, 1857. Reprinted in: Ebin D, ed. The Drug Experience. New York: Orion Press, 1961.

96. West ME. Cannabis and night vision. Nature 1991; 351:703

97. Benowitz NL, Jones RT. Cardiovascular effects of prolonged delta-9-tetrahydrocannabinol ingestion. Clin Pharmacol Ther 1975; 18:287.

98. Heyndrickx A, Scheiris C, Schepens P. Toxicological study of a fatal intoxication in man due to cannabis smoking. J Pharm Belg 1970; 24:37.

99. Gourves J, Viallard C, LeLuan D, et al. Case of coma due to Cannabis sativa. Presse Med 1971; 79:1389.

100. Bro P, Shou J, Topp G. Cannabis poisoning with analytical verification. N Engl J Med 1975; 293:1049.

101. Lopez HH, Goldman SM, Liberman II, Barnes DT. Cannabis—accidental peroral intoxication. JAMA 1974; 227:1041.

102. Weil AT. Adverse reactions to marijuana: classification and suggested treatment. N Engl J Med 1970; 282:997.

103. Imade AG, Ebie JC. A retrospective study of symptom patterns of cannabis-induced psychosis. Acta Psychiatr Scand 1991; 83:134.

104. Thacore VR, Shukla SRP. Cannabis psychosis and paranoid schizophrenia. Arch Gen Psychiatry 1976; 33:383.

105. Rubin V, Comitas L. Ganja in Jamaica: A Medical Anthropological Study of Chronic Marijuana Use. The Hague: Mouton, 1975.

106. Thornicroft G. Cannabis and psychosis. Is there epidemiological evidence for an association? Br J Psychiatry 1990; 157:25.

107. Treffert DA. Marijuana use in schizophrenia: a clear hazard. Am J Psychiatry 1978; 135:1213.

108. Ablon SL, Goodwin FK. High frequency of dysphoric reactions to tetrahydrocannabinol among depressed patients. Am J Psychiatry 1974; 131:448.

109. Knudson P, Vilmar T. Cannabis and neuroleptic agents in schizophrenia. Acta Psychiatr Scand 1984; 69:162.

110. Binitie A. Psychosis following ingestion of hemp in children. Psychopharmacologia 1975; 44:301.

111. Harding T, Knight F. Marijuana-modified mania. Arch Gen Psychiatry 1973; 29:635.

112. Stoll AL, Cole JO, Lukas SF. A case of mania as a result of fluoxetine-marijuana interaction. J Clin Psychiatry 1991; 52:280.

113. Rottanburg D, Robins AH, Ben-Arie O, et al. Cannabis-associated behavior with hypomanic features. Lancet 1982; 2:1364.

114. Palsson A, Thulin SO, Tunving KK. Cannabis psychosis in South Sweden. Acta Psychiatr Scand 1982; 66:311.

115. Keeler M, Reifler CB, Lipzin MB. Spontaneous recurrence of marijuana effect. Am J Psychiatry 1968; 125:384.

116. Stanton MD, Mintz J, Franklin RM. Drug flashbacks II. Some additional findings. Int J Addict 1976; 11:53.

117. Andreasson S, Allebeck P, Eugstrom A, Rydberg U. Cannabis and schizophrenia: a longitudinal study of Swedish conscripts. Lancet 1987; 2:1483.

118. Khantzian EJ, McKenna GJ. Acute toxic and withdrawal reactions associated with drug use and abuse. Ann Intern Med 1979; 90:361.

119. Chaudry HR, Moss HB, Bashir A, Suliman T. Cannabis psychosis following bhang ingestion. Br J Addict 1991; 86:1075.

120. Agurell S, Halldin M, Lindgren J-E, et al. Pharmacokinetics and metabolism of delta-1-tetrahydrocannabinol and other cannabinoids with emphasis on man. Pharmacol Rev 1986; 38:21.

121. Busto U, Bendayan R, Sellers EM. Clinical pharmacokinetics of non-opiate abused drugs. Clin Pharmacokinetics 1989; 16:1.

122. Morgan JP. Marijuana metabolism in the context of urine testing for cannabinoid metabolites. J Psychoact Drugs 1988; 20:107.

123. Jones RT, Benowitz N. The 30-day trip—clinical studies of cannabis tolerance and dependence. In: Braude MC, Szara S, eds. Pharmacology of Marihuana. New York: Raven Press, 1976:627.

124. Tennant FS, Groesback CJ. Psychiatric effects of hashish. Arch Gen Psychiatry 1972; 27:133.

125. Jones RT. Marijuana-induced "high": influence of expectation, setting, and previous drug experience. Pharmacol Rev 1971; 23:359.

126. Kaymakcalan S. Tolerance to and dependence on cannabis. Bull Narc 1973; 25:39.

127. Bensusan SD. Marijuana withdrawal symptoms. BMJ 1971; 1:112.

128. Mendelson JH, Mello NK, Lex BW, Bavli S. Marijuana withdrawal syndrome in a woman. Am J Psychiatry 1984; 141:1289.

129. Hollister LE. Health aspects of cannabis. Pharmacol Rev 1986; 38:1.

130. Miller NS, Klahr AL, Gold MS, et al. The prevalence of marijuana (cannabis) use and dependence in cocaine dependence. NY State J Med 1990; 90:491.

131. Saxon AJ, Calsyn DA, Blaes PA, et al. Marijuana use by methadone maintenance patients. In: Harris L, ed. Problems of Drug Dependence 1990. Rockville, MD: NIDA Research Monograph 105, DHHS, 1991:306.

132. Miller NS, Giannini AJ. Drug misuse in alcoholics. Int J Addict 1991; 26:851.

133. MacAvoy MG, Marks DF. Divided attention performance of cannabis users and non-users following cannabis and alcohol. Psychopharmacologia 1975; 44:147.

134. Dalton WS, Martz R, Lemberger L, et al. Effects of marijuana combined with secobarbital. Clin Pharmacol Ther 1975; 18:298.

135. Johnstone RE, Lief PL, Kulp RA, Smith TC. Combination of delta-9-tetrahydrocannabinol with oxymorphone or pentobarbital: effects on ventilatory control and cardiovascular dynamics. Anesthesiology 1974; 42:674.

136. Yamaguchi K, Kandel DB. Patterns of drug use from adolescence to young adulthood. II. Sequences of progression. Am J Publ Health 1984; 74:668.

136a. Weinreb RM, O'Brien CP. Persistent cognitive deficits attributed to substance abuse. In Brust JCM, ed. Neurological Complications of Drug and Alcohol Abuse. Neurol Clin 1993, in press.

137. Kolansky H, Moore WT. Marijuana: can it hurt you? JAMA 1975; 232:923.

138. Cohen S. Adverse effects of marijuana: selected issues. Ann NY Acad Sci 1981; 362:119.

139. Campbell AMG, Evans M, Thomson JLG, Williams MJ. Cerebral atrophy in young cannabis smokers. Lancet 1971; 2:1219.

140. Mendelson J, Meyere R. Behavioral and biological concomitants of chronic marijuana use by heavy and casual users. In: National Commission on Marijuana and Drug Abuse: Marijuana: A Signal of Misunderstanding, Appendix, Vol 1. Washington, D.C., US Government Printing Office, 1972:68.

141. Beaubrun MH, Knight F. Psychiatric assessment of 30 chronic users of cannabis and 30 matched controls. Am J Psychiatry 1973; 130:309.

142. Culver CM, King FW. Neuropsychological assessment of undergraduate marijuana and LSD users. Arch Gen Psychiatry 1974; 31:707.

143. Connell PH, Dorn N, eds. Cannabis and Man. New York: Churchill Livingstone, 1975.

144. Bruhn P, Maage N. Intellectual and neuropsychological functions in young men with heavy and long-term patterns of drug abuse. Am J Psychiatry 1975; 132:397.

145. Satz R, Fletcher JM, Sutker L. Neuropsychological, intellectual, and personality correlates of marijuana use in native Costa Ricans. Ann NY Acad Sci 1976; 282:266.

146. Co BT, Goodwin DW, Gado M, et al. Absence of cerebral atrophy in chronic cannabis users by computerized transaxial tomography. JAMA 1977; 237:1299.

147. Kuehnle J, Mendelson JH, Davis KR, New PFJ. Computerized tomographic examination of heavy marijuana smokers. JAMA 1977; 237:1231.

148. Carter WE. Cannabis in Costa Rica. Philadelphia: ISHI Press, 1980.

149. Hannertz J, Hinmarsh T. Neurological and neuroradiological examination of chronic cannabis smokers. Ann Neurol 1983; 13:207.

150. Kolansky H, Moore WT. Toxic effects of chronic marijuana use. JAMA 1972; 222:35.

151. Cohen S, Lessin PJ, Hahn PM, Tyrell ED. A 94-day cannabis study. In: Braude MC, Szara S, eds. Pharmacology of Marihuana. New York: Raven Press, 1976:621.

152. Block RI, Farnham S, Braverman K, et al. Long-term marijuana use and subsequent effects on learning and cognitive functions related to school achievement: preliminary study. In: Spencer JW, Boren JJ, eds. Residual Effects of Abused Drugs on Behavior. Rockville, MD: NIDA Research Monograph 101, DHHS, 1990:96.

153. Schwartz RH, Gruenewald PJ, Klitzner M, Fedio P. Short-term memory impairment in cannabis-dependent adolescents. Am J Dis Child 1989; 143:1214.

154. Soueif MI. Chronic cannabis users: further analysis of objective test results. Bull Narc 1975; 27:1.

155. Miles CG, Congreve GRS, Gibbins RJ, et al. An experimental study of the effects of daily cannabis smoking on behavior patterns. Acta Pharmacol Toxicol 1974; 34(suppl 1):1.

156. Sharma BP. Cannabis and its users in Nepal. Br J Psychiatry 1975; 127:550.

157. Mendelson JH, Koehnle JC, Greenberg I, Mello N. The effects of marijuana use on human operant behavior; individual data. In: Braude M, Szara S, eds. Pharmacology of Marihuana. New York: Raven Press, 1976:643.

158. Goode E. The criminogenics of marijuana. Addict Dis 1974; 1:279.

158a. Radvoco-Thomas S, Magnan F, Grove RN, et al. Effect of chronic administration of delta-1-tetrahydrocannabinol on learning and memory in developing mice. In Braude MC, Szara S, eds. Pharmacology of Marihuana. New York: Raven Press, 1976:487.

158b. Ferraro DP, Grilly DM. Effects of chronic exposure to delta-9-tetrahydrocannabinol on delayed matching-to-sample in chimpanzees. Psychopharmacologia 1974; 37:127.

159. Scallet AC, Vemura E, Andrews A, et al. Morphometric studies of the rat hippocampus following chronic delta-9-tetrahydrocannabinol (THC). Brain Res 1987; 436:193.

160. Landfield PW, Cadwallader LB, Vinsant S. Quantitative changes in hippocampal structure following long-term exposure to delta-9-tetrahydrocannabinol: possible mediation by glucocorticoid systems. Brain Res 1988; 443:47.

161. Westlake TM, Howlett AC, Ali SF, et al. Chronic exposure to delta-9-tetrahydrocannabinol fails to irreversibly alter brain cannabinoid receptors. Brain Res 1991; 544:145.

162. Tashkin DP. Pulmonary complications of smoked substance abuse. West J Med 1990; 152:525.

163. Sparacino CM, Hyldburg PA, Hughes TJ. Chemical and biological analysis of marijuana smoke condensate. In: Chiang CN, Hawks RL, eds. Research Findings on Smoking Abused Substances. Rockville, MD: NIDA Research Monograph 99 DHHS, 1990:121.

164. Fergeson RP. Metastatic lung cancer in a young marijuana smoker. JAMA 1989; 261:41.

165. Donald PJ. Advanced malignancy in the young marijuana smoker. Adv Exp Med Biol 1991; 288:33.

166. Almadori G, Palutetti G, Cerullo M, et al. Marijuana smoking as a possible cause of tongue carcinoma in young patients. J Laryngol Otol 1990; 104:896.

167. Wu T-C, Tashkin DP, Djahed B, Rose JE. Pulmonary hazards of smoking marijuana as compared with tobacco. N Engl J Med 1988; 318:347.

168. Baris YI, Tan E, Kalyoncu F, et al. Digital clubbing in hashish addicts. Chest 1990; 98:1545.

169. Levitz SM, Diamond RD. Aspergillosis and marijuana. Ann Intern Med 1991; 115:578.

170. Denning DW, Follansbee SE, Scolaro M, et al. Pulmonary aspergillosis in the acquired immunodeficiency syndrome. N Engl J Med 1991; 324:654.

171. Taylor DN, Wachsmuth IK, Shangkuan Y-H, et al. Salmonellosis associated with marijuana. N Engl J Med 1982; 306:1249.

172. Ramirez RJ. Acute pulmonary histoplasmosis: newly recognized hazard of marijuana plant hunters. Am J Med 1990; 88:60N.

173. Liskow B, Liss JL, Parker CW. Allergy to marijuana. Ann Intern Med 1971; 85:571.

174. Kew MC, Bersohn L, Siew S. Possible hepatotoxicity of cannabis. Lancet 1969; 1:578.

175. Tennant FS, Preble M, Prendergast TJ, Ventry P. Medical manifestations associated with hashish. JAMA 1971; 216:1965.

176. Sterne J, Ducasting C. Les arterites du cannabis indica. Arch Mal Coeur 1960; 53:143.

177. Watzl B, Scuderi P, Watson RR. Influence of marijuana components (THC and CBD) on human mononuclear cell cytokine secretion in vitro. Adv Exp Med Biol 1991; 288:63.

178. Specter S, Lancz G. Effects of marijuana on human natural killer cell activity. Adv Exp Med Biol 1991; 288:47.

179. Coates RA, Farewell VT, Rabovd J, et al. Cofactors of progression to acquired immunodeficiency syndrome in a cohort of male sexual contacts of men with human immunodeficiency virus disease. Am J Epidemiol 1990; 132:717.

180. Smith CG, Asch RH. Acute, short-term and chronic effects of marijuana on the female primate reproductive function. In: Braude MC, Ludford JP, eds. Marijuana Effects on the Endocrine and Reproductive Systems. Washington, DC: NIDA Research Monograph 44, DHHS, 1984:82.

181. Mueller BA, Daling JR, Weiss NS, Moore DE. Recreational drug use and the risk of primary infertility. Epidemiology 1990; 1:189.

182. Copeland KC, Underwood LC, Van Wyk JJ. Marijuana smoking and pubertal arrest. J Pediatr 1980; 96:1079.

183. Benowitz NL, Jones RT, Lerner CB. Depression of growth hormone and cortisol response to insulin-induced hypoglycemia after prolonged oral delta-9-tetrahydrocannabinol administration in man. J Clin Endocrinol Metab 1976; 42:938.

184. Harclerode J. Endocrine effects of marijuana in the male: preclinical studies. In: Braude MC, Ludford JP, eds. Marijuana Effects on the Endocrine and Reproductive Systems. Washington, DC: NIDA Research Monograph 44, DHHS, 1984:46.

185. Rettori V, Aguila MC, Gimeno MF, et al. In vitro effect of delta-9-tetrahydrocannabinol to stimulate somatostatin release and block that of luteinizing hormone-releasing hormone by suppression of the release of prostaglandin E2. Proc Natl Acad Sci 1990; 87:10063.

186. Mendelson JH, Ellingboe J, Mello NK. Acute effects of natural and synthetic cannabis compounds on prolactin levels in human males. Pharmacol Biochem Behav 1984; 20:103,

187. Dax EM, Pilotte NS, Adler WH, et al. Short-term delta-9-tetrahydrocannabinol (THC) does not affect neuroendocrine or immune parameters. In: Harris L, ed. Problems of Drug Dependence 1990. Rockville, MD: NIDA Research Monograph 105, DHHS, 1990:567.

188. Block RI, Farinpour R, Schlechte JA. Effects of chronic marijuana use on testosterone, luteinizing hormone, follicle stimulating hormone, prolactin and cortisol in men and women. Drug Alcohol Depend 1991; 28:121.

189. Aronow WS, Cassidy J. Effect of smoking marijuana and of a high-nicotine cigarette on angina pectoris. Clin Pharmacol Ther 1975; 17:549.

190. MacInnes DC, Miller KM. Fatal coronary artery thrombosis associated with cannabis smoking. JR Coll Gen Pract 1984; 34:575.

191. Mohan H, Sood GC. Conjugate deviation of the eyes after cannabis intoxication. Br J Ophthalmol 1964; 48:160.

192. Garrett CP, Braithwaite RA, Teale JD. Unusual case of tetrahydrocannabinol intoxication confirmed by radioimmunoassay. BMJ 1977; 2:166.

193. Wilkins MR, Kendall MJ. Stroke affecting young men after alcoholic binges. BMJ 1985; 291:1392.

194. Cooles P. Stroke after heavy cannabis smoking. Postgrad Med J 1987; 63:511.

195. Zachariah SB. Stroke after heavy marijuana smoking. Stroke 1991; 22:406.

196. Barnes D, Palace J, O'Brien MD. Stroke following marijuana smoking. Stroke 1992; 23:1381.

197. Adams MD, Earhardt JT, Dewey WL, Harris LS. Vasoconstrictor actions of delta-8 and delta-9-tetrahydrocannabinol in the rat. J Pharmacol Exp Ther 1976; 196:649.

198. Mathew RJ, Wilson WH. Substance abuse and cerebral blood flow. Am J Psychiatry 1991; 148:292.

199. Cimbura G, Lucas DM, Bennett RC, Donelson AC. Incidence and toxicological aspects of cannabis detected in 1394 fatally injured drivers and pedestrians in Ontario (1982–1984). J Forens Sci 1990; 35:1035.

200. Hollister LE, Gillespie HK, Ohlsson A, et al. Do plasma concentrates of delta-9-tetrahydrocannabinol reflect the degree of intoxication? J Clin Pharmacol 1981; 21:1715.

201. Ng SKC, Brust JCM, Hauser WA, Susser M. Illicit drug use and the risk of new onset seizures. Am J Epidemiol 1990; 132:47.

202. Mechoulam R, Carlini EA. Toward drugs derived from cannabis. Naturwissensschaften 1978; 65:174.

203. Consroe PF, Wood GC, Buchsbam H. Anticonvulsant nature of marijuana smoking. JAMA 1975; 234:306.

204. O'Shausghnessy WB. On the preparation of Indian hemp or ganja. Trans Med Phys Soc Bombay 1842; 8:421.

205. Reynolds JR. Therapeutic uses and toxic effects of *Cannabis indica*. Lancet 1980; 1:637.

206. Davis JP, Ramsey HH. Antiepileptic actions of marijuana-active substances. Fed Proc 1949; 8:284.

207. Karler R, Turkanis SA. Cannabis and epilepsy. Adv Biosci 1978; 22–23:619.

208. Feeney DM. Marijuana use among epileptics. JAMA 1976; 235:1105.

209. Feeney DM. Marijuana and epilepsy: paradoxical anticonvulsant and convulsant effects. Adv Biosci 1978; 22–23:643.

210. Perez-Reyes M, Wingfield M. Cannabidiol and electroencephalographic epileptic activity. JAMA 1974; 230:1635.

211. Cunha JM, Carlini EA, Pereira AE, et al. Chronic administration of cannabidiol to healthy volunteers and epileptic patients. Pharmacology 1980; 21:175.

212. Ellison JM, Gelwan E, Ogletree J. Complex partial seizure symptoms affected by marijuana abuse. J Clin Psychiatry 1990; 51:439.

213. Coleman JH, Tacker HL, Evans WE, et al. Neurological manifestations of chronic marihuana intoxication. Part I: paresis of the fourth cranial nerve. Dis Nerv Syst 1976; 37:29.

214. DiBendetto M, McNammee HB, Kuehnle JC, Mendelson JH. Cannabis and the peripheral nervous system. Br J Psychiatry 1977; 131:361.

215. Lundberg GD, Adelson J, Prosnitz EH. Marijuana-induced hospitalization. JAMA 1971; 215:121.

216. Payne RJ, Brand SN. The toxicity of intravenously used marijuana. JAMA 1975; 233:351.

217. Farber SJ, Huertas VE. Intravenously injected marijuana syndrome. Arch Intern Med 1976; 136:337.
218. Schulz P, Jones JL, Patten BM. Encephalopathy and rhabdomyolysis from ingesting formaldehyde-dipped cigarettes. Neurology 1988; 38(suppl):207.
219. Zuckerman B, Bresnahan K. Developmental and behavioral consequences of prenatal drug and alcohol exposure. Pediatr Clin North Am 1991; 38:1387.
220. Hingson R, Alpert JJ, Day N, et al. Effects of maternal drinking and marijuana use on fetal growth and development. Pediatrics 1982; 70:539.
221. Linn S, Schoenbaum SC, Monson RR, et al. The association of marijuana use with outcome of pregnancy. Am J Publ Health 1983; 73:1161.
222. Gibson GT, Bayhurst PA, Colley DP. Maternal alcohol, tobacco, and cannabis consumption on the outcome of pregnancy. Aust NZ Obstet Gynaecol 1983; 25:15.
223. Fried PA, Watkinson B, Willan A. Marijuana use during pregnancy and decreased length of gestation. Am J Obstet Gynecol 1984; 150:23.
224. Tennes K, Avitable N, Blackard A, et al. Marijuana: prenatal and postnatal exposure in the human infant. In: Pinkert TM, ed. Current Research on the Consequences of Maternal Drug Use. Washington, DC: NIDA Research Monograph 59, DHHS, 1985:48.
225. Hatch EE, Bracken MB. Effect of marijuana use in pregnancy on fetal growth. Am J Epidemiol 1986; 124:986.
226. Kline J, Stein Z, Hutzler M. Cigarettes, alcohol, and marijuana: varying associations with birthweight. Int J Epidemiol 1987; 16:44.
227. Fried PA. Marijuana use during pregnancy: consequences for the offspring. Semin Perinatol 1991; 15:280.
228. Hingson R, Zuckerman B, Amaro H, et al. Maternal marijuana use and neonatal outcome: uncertainty posed by self-reports. Am J Publ Health 1986; 76:667.
229. Zuckerman B, Frank DA, Hingson R, et al. Effects of marijuana and cocaine use on fetal growth. N Engl J Med 1989; 320:762.
230. Frank DA, Bauchner H, Parker S, et al. Neonatal body proportionality and body composition after in utero exposure to cocaine and marijuana. J Pediatr 1990; 117:622.
231. Fried PA, Makin JE. Neonatal behavioral correlates of prenatal exposure to marijuana, cigarettes, and alcohol in a low risk population. Neurobehav Toxicol Teratol 1987; 9:1.
232. Lester BM, Dreher M. Effects of marijuana use during pregnancy on newborn cry. Child Dev 1989; 60:765.
233. Sher MS, Richardson GA, Coble PA, et al. The effects of prenatal alcohol and marijuana exposure: disturbances in neonatal sleepcycling and arousal. Pediatr Res 1988; 24:101.
234. Fried PA, Watkinson B. 12- and 24-month neurobehavioral follow-up of children prenatally exposed to

marijuana, cigarettes, and alcohol. Neurotoxicol Teratol 1988; 10:305.
235. Fried PA, Watkinson B. 36- and 48-month neurobehavioral follow-up of children prenatally exposed to marijuana, cigarettes, and alcohol. J Dev Behav Pediatr 1990; 11:49.
236. Astley SJ, Little RE. Maternal marijuana use during lactation and infant development at one year. Neurotoxicol Teratol 1990; 12:161.
237. Stenchever MA, Kunysz TJ, Allen MA. Chromosome breakage in users of marijuana. Am J Obstet Gynecol 1974; 118:106.
238. Zimmerman S, Zimmerman AM. Genetic effects of marijuana. Int J Addict 1990–91; 25:19.
239. Matsuyama SS, Jarvik LF, Fu TK, Yen FS. Chromosomal studies before and after supervised marijuana smoking. In: Braude MC, Szara S, eds. Pharmacology of Marihuana. New York: Raven Press, 1976:723.
240. Persaud TVN, Ellington AC. Cannabis in early pregnancy. Lancet 1967; 2:1306.
241. Morishima A. Effects of cannabis and natural cannabinoids on chromosomes and ova. In: Braude MC, Ludford JP, eds. Marijuana Effects on the Endocrine and Reproductive Systems. Washington, DC: NIDA Research Monograph 44, DHHS, 1984:25.
242. Hutching DE, Morgan B, Brake SC, et al. Delta-9-tetrahydrocannabinol during pregnancy in the rat. I. Differential effects on maternal nutrition, embryotoxicity, and growth in the offspring. Neurotoxicol Teratol 1987; 9:39.
243. Wright PL, Smith SH, Keplinger ML, et al. Reproductive and teratological studies of delta-9-tetrahydrocannabinol and crude marijuana extract. Toxicol Appl Pharmacol 1976; 38:223.
244. Fried PA, Charlebois A. Effects upon rat offspring following cannabis inhalation before and/or after mating. Can J Psychology 1979; 33:125.
245. Hingson R, Alpert JJ, Day N, et al. Effects of maternal drinking and marijuana use on fetal growth and development. Pediatrics 1982; 70:539.
246. Morgan B, Brake SC, Hutchings DE, et al. Delta-9-tetrahydrocannabinol during pregnancy in the rat: effects on development of RNA, DNA, and protein in offspring brain. Pharmacol Biochem Behav 1988; 31:365.
247. Rodriguez-de-Fonseca F, Cabeira M, Fernandez-Ruiz JJ, et al. Effects of pre- and perinatal exposure to hashish extracts on the ontogeny of brain dopaminergic neurons. Neuroscience 1991; 43:713.
248. Fleischman RW, Hayden DW, Rosenkrantz H, Braude M. Teratologic evaluation of delta-9-tetrahydrocannabinol in mice, including a review of the literature. Teratology 1975; 12:47.
249. Hutchings DE, Brake SC, Morgan B. Animal studies of prenatal delta-9-tetrahydrocannabinol: female embryolethality and effects on somatic and brain growth. Ann NY Acad Sci 1989; 562:133.
250. Abel EL, Rockwood GA, Riley EP. The effects of early marijuana exposure. In: Riley E, Vorhees C, eds.

Handbook of Behavioral Teratology. New York: Plenum Press, 1986:267.

251. Brake S, Hutchings DE, Morgan B, et al. Delta-9-tetrahydrocannabinol during pregnancy in the rat. II. Effects on ontogeny of locomotor activity and nipple attachment in the offspring. Neurotoxicol Teratol 1987; 9:45.

252. Hutchings DE, Miller N, Gamagaris Z, Fico TA. The effects of prenatal exposure to delta-9-tetrahydrocannabinol on the rest-activity cycle of the preweanling rat. Neurotoxicol Teratol 1989; 11:353.

253. Hutchings DE, Brake SC, Banks AN, et al. Prenatal delta-9-tetrahydrocannabinol in the rat: effects on auditory startle in adulthood. Neurotoxicol Teratol 1991; 13:413.

254. Williams MA, Lieberman E, Mittendorf R, et al. Risk factors for abruptio placentae. Am J Epidemiol 1991; 134:965.

255. Bloom AS, Dewey WL, Harris LS, Brosius KK. 9-nor-9-betahydroxyhexahydrocannabinol, a cannabinoid with potent antinociceptive activity. Comparisons with morphine. J Pharmacol Exp Ther 1977; 200:263.

256. Chang AE, Shiling DO, Stillman RL, et al. Delta-9-tetrahydrocannabinol as an antiemetic in cancer patients receiving high-dose methotrexate. Ann Intern Med 1979; 91:819.

257. Gong H, Tashkin DP, Simmons MS, et al. Acute and subacute bronchial effects of oral cannabinoids. Clin Pharmacol Ther 1984; 35:26.

258. Liu JHK, Dacas AC. Central nervous system and peripheral mechanisms in ocular hypotensive effect of cannabinoids. Arch Ophthalmol 1987; 105:245.

259. Abramowicz M, ed. Nabilone and other antiemetics for cancer patients. Med Lett 1988; 29:1.

260. Plasse TF. Clinical use of dronabinol. J Clin Oncol 1991; 9:2079.

261. Doblin R, Kleinman MAR. Medical use of marijuana. Ann Intern Med 1991; 114:809.

262. Court tells the US to reconsider its ban on marijuana therapy. NY Times, April 28, 1991.

263. Treaster JB. Agency says marijuana is not proven medicine. NY Times, March 19, 1992.

264. Ellenberger C, Petro DJ. Treatment of human spasticity with delta-9-tetrahydrocannabinol. Neurology 1979; 29:551.

265. Clifford DB. Tetrahydrocannabinol for tremor in multiple sclerosis. Ann Neurol 1983; 13:669.

266. Greenberg HS, Pugh JE, Anderson DJ, et al. Marijuana and its effect on postural stability in spastic multiple sclerosis patients and controls. Neurology 1990; 40(suppl 1):259.

267. Gowers WR. A Manual of Diseases of the Nervous System, Vol II. London: Churchill, 1888:589.

268. Frankel JP, Hughes A, Lees AJ, Stern GM. Marijuana for parkinsonian tremor. J Neurol Neurosurg Psychiatry 1990; 53:436.

269. Baron JA. Ulcerative colitis and marijuana. Ann Intern Med 1990; 112:471.

270. Roffman RA, Stephens RS, Simpson EE, Whitaker DL. Treatment of marijuana dependence: preliminary results. J Psychoact Drugs 1988; 20:129.

271. Zweben JE, O'Connell K. Strategies for breaking marijuana dependence. J Psychoact Drugs 1988; 20:121.

Chapter 7
Hallucinogens

... the visit to the World's Biggest Drug Store safely
behind us, ... I had returned to that reassuring but
profoundly unsatisfactory state known as 'being in one's
right mind.'
                                    —*Aldous Huxley*

Picture yourself in a boat on a river
With tangerine trees and marmalade skies.
Somebody calls you, you answer quite slowly
A girl with kaleidoscope eyes.   —*John Lennon*

Tune in, turn on, drop out.   —*Timothy Leary*

Hallucinogens are chemicals that in low doses alter perception, thought, or mood, while preserving alertness, attentiveness, memory, and orientation. They cause auditory, visual, and tactile distortions and hallucinations—that is, dream-like episodes—in awake humans.[1,2] Also known as *psychedelics* ("mind revealing"), most of these agents are indole-containing ergot derivatives (e.g., lysergic acid diethylamide [LSD]), indolealkylamines (e.g., psilocybin), or phenylalkylamines (e.g., mescaline)(Table 7–1). Not classified as hallucinogens are marijuana, anticholinergics, bromides, phencyclidine, cocaine, and amphetamine, which produce confusion, delirium, or psychosis at hallucinogenic doses.

Pharmacology and Animal Studies

How hallucinogens produce their effects is unknown.[3] LSD's Schedule I classification has restricted human research,[4] and animal studies, which obviously require end points other than altered perception, cannot easily be extrapolated to human experience. LSD, mescaline, or psilocybin have caused hyperactivity in rats, catatonia in pigeons and salamanders, agitation in fish, aggressive behavior in ants, disorganized web-spinning in spiders, aimless crawling in worms, surface detachment in snails, and status epilepticus in an elephant.[5–10] Attempts to define biochemical similarities among these agents have focused on central nervous system (CNS) serotonergic (5-HT) pathways, a task made additionally complex by the existence of excitatory and inhibitory receptor subtypes for this neurotransmitter.[11,12]

In animals, hallucinogens can either augment or depress spinal reflexes by interacting with 5-HT systems in the dorsal or ventral horns.[13] In rats, LSD initially suppresses locomotor activity and then stimulates it; suppression is prevented by the serotonin antagonist ritanserin and stimulation by the beta-adrenergic antagonist propranolol.[14] In guinea pigs, LSD, mescaline, and other hallucinogenic agents cause myoclonus, whereas the nonhallucinogenic drug 2-bromo-LSD does not.[15]

Phenylalkylamine hallucinogens possess the same chemical skeleton as amphetamine, and structure-activity studies have identified a behavioral continuum among these chemically related compounds. At one end are psychostimulants, such as amphetamine, which exert their actions primarily through dopaminergic mechanisms. At the other end are hallucinogens such as mescaline or 2,4-dimethoxy-4-methylamphetamine (DOM), which act through serotonergic pathways. Animals trained to discriminate amphetamine from saline do not generalize to DOM and vice versa. In the middle of the continuum are drugs such as 3,4-methylenedioxyamphetamine (MDA), which are both stimulatory and hallucinogenic. Animals trained to discriminate MDA from

149

Table 7–1. Hallucinogenic Compounds

Ergot-Derived
d-Lysergic acid diethylamide (LSD)

Indolealkylamines
Psilocybin
Psilocin
N,N-dimethyltryptamine (DMT)
N,N-diethyltryptamine (DET)

Phenylalkylamines
Mescaline
2,4-Dimethoxy-4-methylamphetamine (DOM)
3,4,5-Trimethoxyamphetamine (TMA)
4-Bromo-2,5-dimethoxyamphetamine (DOB)
2,5-Dimethoxy-4-ethylamphetamine (DOET)
3-Methoxy-4,5-methylenedioxyamphetamine (MMDA)
3,4-Methylenedioxyamphetamine (MDA; see Chapter 3)
3,4-Methylenedioxymethamphetamine (MDMA; see Chapter 3)
3,4-Methylenedioxyethamphetamine (MDEA; see Chapter 3)

saline generalize to both amphetamine and DOM (see Chapter 3).[16,17]

LSD and hallucinogenic indolealkylamines also act through serotonergic pathways; in drug discrimination studies, animals generalize from LSD to mescaline, psilocybin, and other indolealkylamine and phenylalkylamine hallucinogens, and this generalization is blocked by pretreatment with serotonin antagonists.[18,19] Two different actions have been proposed for the psychic effects of these drugs. One is inhibition of serotonergic neurons in the brain stem raphe nuclei.[2,12] Behavioral tolerance to LSD, however, occurs without any abatement of this inhibition.[20] Moreover, although LSD and indolealkylamine hallucinogens inhibit raphe neurons, mescaline and DOM do not,[21] and destruction of the raphe nuclei, which should decrease LSD's behavioral effects, actually increases them.[12]

The other proposed mechanism is direct action on postsynaptic 5-HT receptors.[22] The behavioral effects of these drugs are blocked by serotonin antagonists,[23] and their hallucinogenic potency in humans strongly correlates with their binding affinities to serotonin receptors.[24]

Mammalian brain contains at least six serotonin receptor subtypes: 5-HT_{1A}, 5-HT_{1B}, 5-HT_{1C}, 5-HT_{1D}, 5-HT_2, and 5-HT_3.[25] LSD binds to several of these receptor subtypes as well as to dopaminergic and alpha-adrenergic receptors.[25] On the basis of behavioral, electrophysiologic, and radioligand binding studies, workers in the 1980s considered activation of 5-HT_2 receptors as the likely basis of LSD's hallucinatory effects.[26–30] In rat cerebral cortex slices,

LSD is a partial agonist at 5-HT_2 receptors. However, LSD and indolalkylamine hallucinogens are also agonists at 5-HT_{1C} receptors, which share 51% sequence homology with 5-HT_2 receptors (and probably should be subclassified with 5-HT_2 rather than 5-HT_1 receptors).[25] Both are coupled to G proteins and ultimately to hydrolysis of phosphoinositide. In studies using rat choroid plexus, which contains 5-HT_{1C} but not 5-HT_2 receptors, LSD stimulates phosphoinositide hydrolysis, an effect maximally blocked by 5-HT_{1C} antagonists; by contrast, nonhallucinogenic congeners of LSD (2-bromo-LSD and lisuride) have no such effect, although, like LSD, they are partial agonists at 5-HT_2 receptors.[31] Further, agents that antagonize both 5-HT_2 and 5-HT_{1C} receptors block LSD discrimination in animals,[30] whereas spiperone, a relatively selective 5-HT_2 antagonist, does not.[32] In rats, LSD and psilocybin decrease 5-HT_2 receptor binding in cerebral cortex, and this down-regulation parallels behavioral tolerance, but mescaline, which is cross-tolerant with LSD and psilocybin, produces no such down-regulation.[33] Such studies implicate 5-HT_{1C} receptors as mediators of LSD's major behavioral effects.[34] In addition to choroid plexus, 5-HT_{1C} receptors are most abundant in basal ganglia, hypothalamus, hippocampus, and spinal cord.[25]

Retinal as well as cortical actions may contribute to LSD and mescaline hallucinations. In rats, systemic LSD or mescaline suppresses the primary component of the flash-evoked cortical potential (FEP), consistent with reduced conduction through the retinogeniculocortical system, and this suppression is blocked by the serotonin receptor antagonists cyproheptadine and methysergide. Intraocular mescaline or LSD also attenuates the FEP, and topical or intraocular atropine antagonizes the effects of systemic mescaline on the FEP.[35]

Animals do not self-administer LSD, mescaline, or psilocybin.[18,36,37] They rapidly develop tolerance to these and other hallucinogens, with cross-tolerance between LSD, phenylalkylamines, and indolealkylamines, but withdrawal signs have not been observed.[18,19,38]

Historical Background and Epidemiology

Of the world's more than 700,000 species of plants, nearly 100 have been identified as hallucinogenic (Table 7–2), and human ingestion, intentional and unintentional, goes back as far as recorded history.[1] The parasitic fungus ergot (*Claviceps* sp) infests a variety of grains, especially rye, and contains a large

Table 7–2. Miscellaneous Hallucinogenic Plants

Plant	Active substances
Peyote cactus (*Lophophora williamsii*)	Mescaline
Psilocybe mushroom	Psilocybin, psilocin
Panaeolus mushroom	Psilocybin, psilocin
Gymnopilus mushroom	Psilocybin, psilocin
Amanita muscaria mushroom	Ibotenic acid
Morning glory (*Ipomoea* sp)	d-Lysergic acid amide
Nutmeg (*Myristica fragrans*)	Myristicin, elemicin
Periwinkle (*Catharanthus roseus*)	Indole alkaloids
Catnip (*Nepeta cataria*)	Nepetalactone
Yohimbe (*Corynanthe yohimbe*)	Yohimbine (see Chapter 3)
Juniper (*Juniperus macropoda*)	Unknown
Kava (*Piper methysticum*)	Unknown
Passion flower (*Passiflora caerulea*)	Harmine alkaloids
Virola (*Virola calophylla*)	Indolealkylamines
Iboga (*Tabernanthe iboga*)	Ibogaine

number of pharmacologically active ergot alkaloids, including isoergine (lysergic acid amide), a hallucinogen about 10% as potent as LSD. Hallucinogenic ergot alkaloids may have been the source of the ancient Greek Mysteries of Eleusis, at which initiates sought a glimpse of the hereafter.[39] (Participants included Aeschylus, Sophocles, Plato, and Aristotle.) Similar plant ergots—especially the morning glory ololiuqui (*Rivea corymbosa*)—were used for religious purposes by the Aztecs, as was the indoleamine-containing mushroom Teonanacatl (*Psilócybe* sp).[40,41] In fact, it has been argued that the religions of mankind began with neolithic exposure to mushroom-induced ecstasy.[42]

In medieval Europe (and in 1951 in France), accidental ingestion of the rye fungus *Claviceps purpurea* produced epidemics of gangrenous and convulsive ergotism with hallucinations (*St. Anthony's fire*).[43] Similar poisoning may have accounted for outbreaks of "witchcraft" throughout the Middle Ages and, in 1692, in Salem, Massachusetts. The Salem tragedy, which resulted in the torture or hanging of at least 20 innocent people, began with the sudden appearance in the community of bizarre behavior, including terrifying hallucinations.[44]

For thousands of years, American Indians of Mexico and the southwestern United States have used the peyote cactus (*Lophophora williamsii*) and the San Pedro cactus (*Trichocercus pachanoi*) to induce visions in religious ceremonies. The psychoactive ingredient is mescaline (3,4,5-trihydroxy-phenylethylamine), named after the Mescalaro Apaches and present in much higher concentration in peyote than in the easier to find San Pedro cactus.[45,46] Either the raw peyote plant itself is eaten, or dried powdered cactus "buttons" are taken orally (or in enemas). Celebrated 19th century users of mescaline were S. Weir Mitchell and Havelock Ellis. Each described the experience enthusiastically.

Mitchell: "A white spear of grey stone grew up to huge height, and became a tall, richly finished Gothic tower of very elaborate and definite design.... Every projecting angle, cornice, and even the face of the stones ... were covered or hung with clusters of what seemed to be huge precious stones.... These were green, purple, red, and orange.... All seemed to possess an interior light."[47,48]

Ellis: "I would see thick glorious fields of jewels, solitary or clustered, sometimes brilliant and sparkling, sometimes with a dull rich glow. Then they would spring up into flower-like shapes, then seem to turn into gorgeous butterfly forms or endless fields of glistening, iridescent wings of wonderful insects."[49]

These descriptions led to an editorial in the *British Medical Journal* proclaiming that "... such eulogy for any drug is a danger to the public."[50] Peyote is still used sacramentally in the United States by members of the Native American Church,[51] and less orthodox users have recommended it as a means to self-transcendence and cosmic revelation.[52] (A less rhapsodic description of a mescaline experience, by a Professor of Eastern Religions and Ethics, referred to "transcendence into a world of farcical meaninglessness."[53])

Mexican Indians have worshipfully eaten hallucinogenic mushrooms, especially *Psilocybe mexicana* and other *Psilocybe* species, which contain the indoles psilocybin (4-phosphoryl-N,N-dimethyltryptamine) and psilocin (4-hydroxy-N,N-dimethyltryptamine).[51] Natives of Siberia and northwestern Canada have employed the mushroom *Amanita muscaria* (fly agaric) in shamanistic practices; active ingredients include ibotenic acid—a glutamate receptor agonist—and its metabolite muscimol—a gamma-aminobutyric acid (GABA) agonist.[41] There is evidence that *Amanita muscaria* was the original basis of the Rigveda deity Soma and the Greek god Dionysius (until geographic separation from the mushroom's northern source led to southern replacement by the fermented grape).[54]

Natives of the Orinoco and Amazon basins make hallucinogenic snuffs from a number of plants, including *Anadenanthera* seeds, which contain dimethyltryptamine (DMT), and *Virola* bark, which contains 5-methoxy-N,N-dimethyltryptamine.[1] The beta-carbolines, harmine and harmaline, are present in seeds of *Peganum harmala,* which are chewed as intoxicants in India; the same hallucinogenic compounds are found in *Banisteriopsis caapi,* used in psychotropic beverages ("yage") and snuffs by Amazonian Indians.[51,55] West African natives chew the roots of *Tabernanthe iboga,* a shrub containing the hallucinogen ibogaine, and the bark of *Corynanthe yohimbe,* which contains yohimbine (see Chapter 3).[51] Other naturally occurring hallucinogenic agents include nepetalactone in *Nepeta cataria* ("catnip"), d-lysergic acid amide and d-isolysergic acid amide in seeds of the Mexican morning glory, *Rivea corymbosa,* and myristicin in seeds of *Myristica fragans* (nutmeg).[51]

Lysergic acid, the nucleus of psychoactive ergot alkaloids, is not hallucinogenic, but in 1943 it was discovered that a semisynthetic derivative, d-lysergic acid diethylamide (LSD), produced striking mental symptoms (Figure 7–1). Albert Hofmann, a pharmacologist at Sandoz Laboratories in Basel, was working with LSD when he developed "kaleidoscope-like" hallucinations. He then deliberately ingested 250 μg of LSD and experienced several hours of grotesque illusions and hallucinations accompanied by depersonalization and a sense of demonic possession. When his symptoms cleared, he felt well and had total recall of the experience.[56]

In the years that followed, LSD was studied as a possible model for schizophrenia[57] and as a psychotherapeutic agent.[58] Neither venture was successful, but the ensuing publicity soon led to recreational use. Referred to as "acid," "purple haze," "purple hearts," "window pane," and "sunshine," it was especially popular with American college students, and, associated with such cult figures as Timothy Leary, became a symbol of the counterculture of the 1960s. LSD and other hallucinogenic drugs were soon banned by federal statute. (In 1978, the American Indian Religious Freedom Act made an exception in the sacramental use of peyote, a First

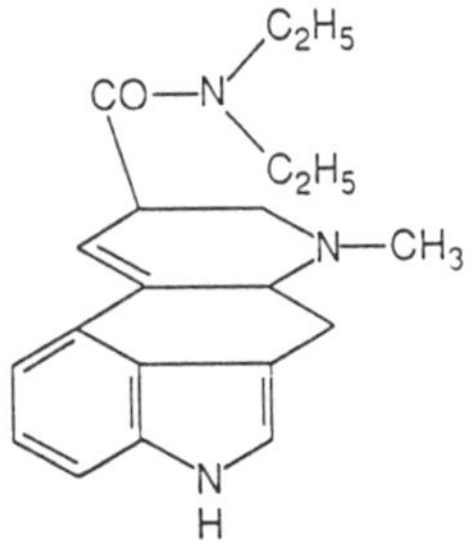

Figure 7–1. Lysergic acid diethylamide (LSD).

Amendment protection that lasted until 1990, when the U.S. Supreme Court ruled that states may prohibit use of peyote for religious purposes.[59,60])

In 1979, hallucinogenic drugs had been used by 25% of Americans aged 18 to 25, by 13% of American high school seniors, and by 7% of children aged 12 to 17.[61] Twelve years later, while use of ethanol, marijuana, and cocaine was declining among high school seniors, LSD use was rising: 5.4% reported using LSD within the preceding 12 months, compared with 4.9% the year before. About 10 million Americans have tried LSD at least once.[62] Of 105 children admitted to a Montreal hospital during 1983 through 1986 for acute poisoning, 8% had taken "hallucinogens." (The specific agents were not disclosed.)[63]

Most LSD sold in the United States is clandestinely manufactured in San Francisco. One of the cheapest illegal drugs, it sold in 1991 at $2 to $3 for a dose of 80 to 100 μg, enough to produce effects lasting 8 to 12 hours.[62] Available in impregnated blotting paper, in sugar cubes, and as tablets, it is nearly always taken orally. Alternate routes include snorting and injecting.[64]

During the 1980s, mushroom abuse also became increasingly popular in the United States and Europe.[65–69] In a 1985 survey of 1500 American college students, 15% had abused mushrooms compared with only 5% who had used LSD.[70] A 1986 survey of California high school students revealed that psilocybin-containing mushrooms had been eaten by 3.4% of seventh graders, 5.8% of ninth graders, and 8.8% of eleventh graders.[71] Among middle to upper class adolescents in a substance abuse program in Virginia during 1988, 26% had abused psilocybin-containing mushrooms.[71]

Acute Effects

Hallucinogenic drugs produce three major kinds of effects: (1) perceptual (distortions or hallucinations), (2) psychological (depersonalization or altered mood), and (3) somatic (dizziness, paresthesias, or tremor).

Within a few minutes of ingestion, 0.5 to 3 μg/kg of LSD produces dizziness, sleepiness, weakness, blurred vision, paresthesias, chilliness, headache, nausea, and either euphoria or anxiety.[72] In the second or third hour, visual illusions appear, including micropsia, macropsia, and altered body image. Hearing seems keener, afterimages are prolonged (palinopsia), and there may be synesthesias (stimuli in one modality producing perceptions in another;

e.g., colors are heard). Somewhat later hallucinations occur, usually visual. They consist at first of brightly colored geometric designs and later of formed images—faces, animals, buildings, or landscapes, often elaborately beautiful or grotesque. Subjective time is prolonged. Familiar surroundings seem strange (derealization), and there are peculiar alterations of self-awareness (depersonalization), hypervigilance, or autistic withdrawal. Concentrating on inner feelings or the seemingly profound significance of trivial objects, the subject appears cataleptic. Memories intrude vividly, giving the sensation of events occurring in the wrong order. Mystical elation may alternate with anxiety or paranoia. Insight is usually but not always retained.[73]

The number and variety of symptoms are greater when the subject is alone, especially in the dark. Subjective effects usually last 6 to 12 hours, but fragments of the syndrome tend to recur spontaneously in "waves" of progressively shorter duration and diminished intensity for several hours longer.[74]

Hyperreflexia, fever, ataxia, tremor, pupillary dilation (with preserved light reflex), increased blood pressure, tachycardia, and piloerection parallel or precede the subjective symptoms.[75,76] Electroencphalographic changes consist of slightly increased alpha frequency and decreased alpha amount.[77] Initial insomnia is followed by sleep with enhanced rapid eye movement phase out of proportion to sleep deprivation.[78]

Symptoms and signs are dose-related between 1 and 16 µg/kg; pretreatment with reserpine enhances and prolongs an LSD response.[64,72] Tolerance develops rapidly to pupillary and psychic effects, and there is cross-tolerance to mescaline and psilocybin but not to amphetamine or delta-9-tetrahydrocannibinol.[64,79–82] Withdrawal symptoms do not occur after chronic use, which even among "acid heads" is infrequently more than weekly.[77,83]

Adverse reactions ("bad trips") consist of marked paranoia or panic. They can occur in users who have previously had only "good trips" and can lead to homicide or suicide.[83–86] Ocular injuries have included self-enucleation and retinal burns from staring at the sun.[87,88] Such symptoms usually clear within 24 hours and can be managed with "talking down"; if the patient is unmanageable, benzodiazepines are preferable to phenothiazines, which have caused paradoxical reactions.[72,89–92] There is sometimes prolonged depression, paranoia, or psychosis, and it is then uncertain if LSD was causal or simply exacerbated a preexisting mental disturbance.[92–96] Prolonged adverse reactions have occurred in apparently normal individuals, however, and although LSD has

reportedly caused persistent polymodal hallucinosis in schizophrenic patients,[97] most schizophrenics are no more sensitive than others to LSD's psychotomimetic effects.[64,98]

Of a different nature are "flashbacks," which consist of spontaneous recurrence of LSD symptoms without taking the drug.[72,99] Their reported frequency ranges from 15% to 77% and may increase with repeated LSD use, but they have occurred after single exposure.[83,92,100,101] Precipitants include a dark environment, marijuana, fatigue, anxiety, ethanol, amphetamine, and intention.[102] Symptoms may last only a few seconds and are perceptual or emotional.[18] Visual phenomena include heightened imagery, palinopsia, perceptual distortions, illusions of movement, "streaking" (moving lights in a dark environment resembling long streaks as in a time-exposed photograph), "disjointed movements" (as with a strobe light), and geometric or formed hallucinations.[102,103] The tenuous view that these phenomena are epileptic is based on mild electroencephalographic abnormalities.[72] Flashbacks usually respond to sedatives and diminish in duration, intensity, and frequency over months or years.[92] Chlorpromazine can exacerbate them.[89,102]

Very high doses of LSD cause hypertension, obtundation, and convulsions.[103a,104] Hyperactivity following large doses of LSD can produce severe hyperthermia.[105,106] A violent patient restrained in a straightjacket developed a temperature of 41.6°C, hypotension, rhabdomyolysis, and fatal renal failure.[107] In animals, LSD causes dose-related hyperthermia independent of other behavioral responses.[108] Fatalities among LSD users have usually resulted from accidents or suicide, however.[72]

Medical and Neurological Complications

Many ergot agents are vasoconstrictors, and cerebral vessel strips undergo spasm when immersed in solution containing LSD, an effect blocked by methysergide.[109] Following ingestion of LSD, a 14-year-old boy developed seizures and, 4 days later, left hemiplegia; carotid angiography showed progressive narrowing of the internal carotid artery from its origin to the siphon, with occlusion at its bifurcation.[110] A young woman developed sudden left hemiplegia 1 day after using LSD; at angiography, there was marked vasoconstriction of the internal carotid artery at the siphon, which 9 days later was occluded.[111] A 19-year-old with acute aphasia and cerebral angiographic findings consistent with arteritis had used both LSD and heroin, but the temporal relationship of drug use to stroke was uncertain.[112] Another patient with angiographic evidence of "vasculitis" had used both LSD and "diet pills."[113]

Controversial is whether repeated LSD use causes permanent mental change, such as paranoia, depression, psychosis, or memory disturbance. Passivity, tangential thinking, and a tendency to ascribe special significance to everyday events have been described, but as with other drugs, a causal relationship is difficult to establish, and the weight of evidence is against long-term damage to cognition or behavior.[83,92,114–118]

Hepatitis has followed intravenous LSD use.[119]

Chromosomal breakage was reported in human leukocytes incubated with LSD and in leukocytes from LSD users.[120,121] Human spontaneous abortion and infant deformity were attributed to maternal LSD use, and teratogenicity was described in animals.[122–126] A number of investigators failed to find such association, however.[127–129] In one study, chromosomal aberrations disappeared within a few months of discontinuing LSD use; in other studies they were not found at all.[130–132] Chromosomal abnormalities were similarly absent in lymphocytes of Mexican Huichol Indians, generations of whom had used mescaline.[133]

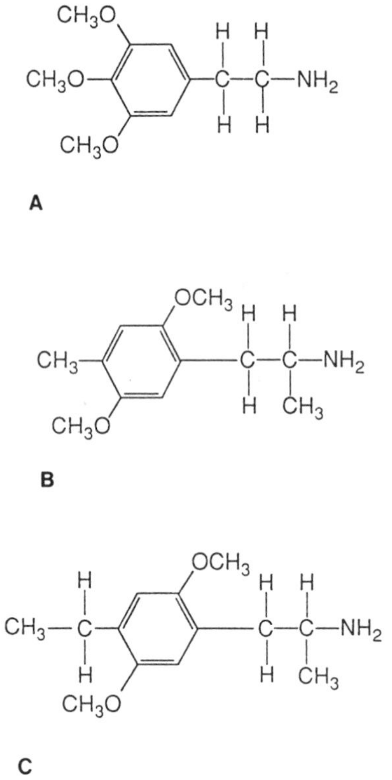

Other Hallucinogenic Agents

Mescaline (Figure 7–2), infrequently abused as a street drug, is taken orally as peyote buttons ("tops," "moon," "cactus," "mesc," "the bad seed," "peyote," "p") or as mescaline powder in capsules or dissolved in water.[46] (Most alleged street mescaline powder is really LSD or phencyclidine.) Five milligrams per kilogram of mescaline is hallucinogenic, and 20 to 60 mg/kg causes bradycardia, hypotension, and respiratory depression.[41] One peyote button contains about 45 mg mescaline; synthetic mescaline usually comes in doses of 200 to 500 mg. As with LSD, side effects include nausea, vomiting, abdominal cramps, and diarrhea. There may also be flushing, sweating, and piloerection.[134] Psychic effects include olfactory, tactile, auditory, visual, or gustatory hallucinations; distortions of space and time; and paranoia, panic, or suicidal ideation. Symptoms last 6 to 12 hours.[41]

Psilocybin and psilocin (Figure 7–3) are present in both Central American *Psilocybe* species of mushrooms ("magic mushrooms," "blue legs," "liberty caps") and in *Panaeolus* species native to the United States.[135–137] Mushrooms are usually dried or fro-

Figure 7–2. Mescaline (A), 2,5-dimethoxy-4-methylamphetamine (DOM) (B), 2,5-dimethoxy-4-ethylamphetamine (DOET) (C).

zen; even cooking does not destroy the hallucinogenic compounds. Two to 6 mushrooms cause symptoms, and as many as 100 have been taken at one time. There is much variability in response: Agitation and hallucinations have followed 10 mushrooms and gastritis without psychic effects has followed 200.[138] Other effects include anticholinergic symptoms and seizures.[139–143] Hallucinations usually last a few hours but have lasted several days. Intravenous injection of mushroom extracts causes vomiting, cyanosis, fever, arthralgia, abnormal liver function, and methemoglobinemia.[139,144]

LSD, mescaline, and psilocybin differ in potency, time to peak action, and duration of effects. One microgram LSD is equivalent to 5 to 6 mg mescaline and 150 to 200 µg psilocybin. LSD's hallucinogenic effects begin after 1 to 1.5 hours, mescaline's after 2 to 2.5 hours, and psilocybin's after 30 minutes. The psychic and physiological effects of the three drugs are indistinguishable even to experienced users.[72,76,145]

Rarely abused in the United States is *Amanita muscaria*, which produces euphoria, mania, delirium, ataxia, and both liliputian and brobdingnagian illusions. Less often there are frank visual hallucina-

A

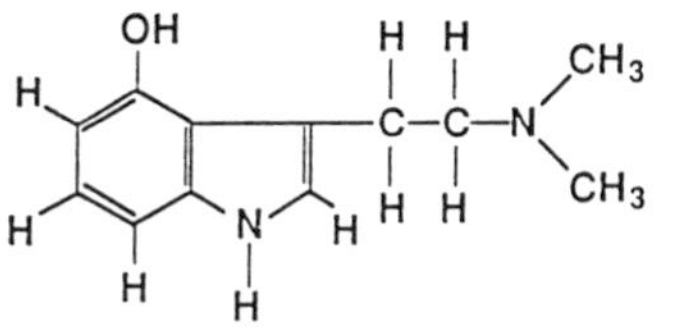

B

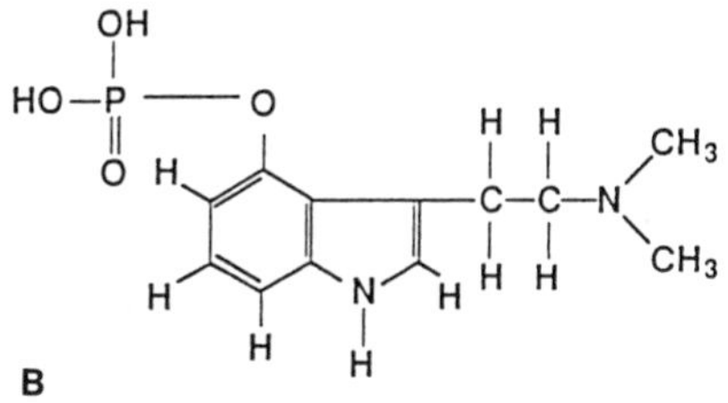

Figure 7–3. Psilocin (A) and psilocybin (B).

tions. Seizures, coma, and death have followed ingestion.[146] Unidentified hallucinogens are present in native American *Gymnopilus* species mushrooms.[147,148] How often they are taken recreationally is unknown, as is the prevalence of abuse of many other native and imported hallucinogenic plants, any of which, in this era of easy travel, could produce confounding symptoms in patients brought to unsuspecting emergency rooms (Table 7–2).

N,N-Dimethyltryptamine (DMT) and N,N-diethyltryptamine (DET) are easily synthesized and available on the illicit street market. DMT is inactive orally and is therefore injected, smoked, or taken as a snuff. It produces LSD-like effects, including adverse reactions.[85,149,150]

Also abused as street drugs are DOM (nicknamed "STP" after a commercial oil additive said to increase the power of automobile engines) (Figure 7–2), 4-bromo-2,5-dimethoxyamphetamine (DOB), 2,5-dimethoxy-4-ethylamphetamine (DOET) (Figure 7–2), 3,4,5-trimethoxyamphetamine (TMA), and 3-methoxy-4,5-methylenedioxyamphetamine (MMDA).[72,85,151–153] Panic, violent behavior, seizures, and death have followed abuse of DOB,[154] as have diffuse vascular spasm and limb ischemia, resulting in bilateral above-the-knee amputations.[155] As noted in Chapter 3, MDA and 3,4-methylenedioxymethamphetamine (MDMA, nicknamed "ecstasy") can be taken to induce hallucinations.[156]

Psychosis lasting 3 weeks occurred in an amateur chemist who snorted and injected isosafrole (4-propenyl-1,2-methylenedioxybenzene) because of its resemblance to MDA; such a reaction had not followed his use of amphetamine, marijuana, or LSD.[157]

Seeds of the morning glory (*Ipomoea* sp) or the related Mexican plant ololiuqui (*Rivea corymbosa*) are popular hallucinogens in the United States. In one case, emotional lability, fixed dilated pupils, and increased awareness of colors followed ingestion of 250 seeds.[158] In another case, ingestion of 300 seeds produced vivid visual and tactile hallucinations, fantasies, and depersonalization, and 3 weeks later suicide occurred during a flashback hallucinatory psychosis.[159] Other acute effects include nausea, vomiting, diarrhea, muscle tightness, and paresthesias of the limbs.[41] Ololiuqui is still used for religious purposes in Mexico, and teas made from morning glory seeds (e.g., "Panacea Tea") are available in American "health food" stores.[160] Of the many ergot alkaloids present in morning glory seeds, the most psychoactive appears to be d-lysergic acid amide (ergine).[161]

In the United States, nutmeg abuse is common among prison inmates.[51,162] (It is so described in *The Autobiography of Malcolm X*.[163]) Effects are the result of several phenylalkylamines—myristicin, elemicin, eugenol, safrole, and borneal—and their active metabolites MMDA and TMA.[41,162,164] One to three nutmegs (5 to 30 g ground powder, or 1 to 4 tbsp) produce psychic effects that resemble those of marijuana. After a delay of up to several hours, there is giddiness, anxiety, and excitement; euphoria; depersonalization; and distortions of space and time. Higher doses cause visual illusions and hallucinations. Fear of death or panic may ensue, followed by lethargy for more than 24 hours. Anticholinergic signs include flushing, tachycardia, and urinary retention, yet miosis is seen more often than mydriasis. Nausea, vomiting, abdominal pain, and hypotension limit nutmeg's popularity among the nonincarcerated.[165–170]

Kava (or kava-kava) is a beverage made by Pacific islanders from roots of the shrub *Piper methysticum*. Used both socially and in religious ceremonies, it induces sedation and euphoria. High doses are hallucinogenic, and chronic users develop yellow skin discoloration, drowsiness, ataxia, liver damage, and malnutrition (the result of dysphagia secondary to oropharyngeal numbness caused by contact with the beverage). The pharmacological basis of kava's effects has not been identified. Herbal teas containing kava are sold in American "health food" stores, and toxicity has been reported.[171–173]

Other herbal teas sold in American "health food" stores often contain more than a dozen different types of leaves, seeds, and berries. Some, for example hydrangea or lobelia teas, are taken for psychostimulation and euphoria and do not cause hallucinations except in situations of obvious toxicity. Others, for example yohimbe bark or periwinkle teas, more readily produce hallucinations. Still others, such as those containing morning glory seeds, juniper, or catnip, are frankly sold for their hallucinogenic properties (Table 7–2).[160,173]

Bizarre even by the often rococo standards of substance abuse is "toad licking." Skin glands of the Australian cane toad secrete the hallucinogen bufoterine; as a consequence, this creature has become a popular pet in the United States. Undesired side effects include sweating, palpitations, vomiting, and fecal incontinence.[174]

References

1. Siegel RK. The natural history of hallucinogens. In: Jacobs BL, ed. Hallucinogens: Neurochemical, Behavioral, and Clinical Perspectives. New York: Raven Press, 1984:1.
2. Hamon M. Common neurochemical correlates to the action of hallucinogens. In: Jacobs BL, ed. Hallucinogens: Neurochemical, Behavioral, and Clinical Perspectives. New York: Raven Press, 1984:143.
3. McKenna DJ, Towers GHN. Biochemistry and pharmacology of tryptamines and beta-carbolines. A minireview. J Psychoact Drugs 1984; 16:347.
4. Strassman EJ. Human hallucinogenic drug research in the United States: a present-day history and review of the process. J Psychoact Drugs 1991; 23:29.
5. Abramson HA, Evans LT. Lysergic acid diethylamide (LSD-25). II. Psychobiological effects on the Siamese fighting fish. Science 1954; 120:990.
6. Abramson HA, Jarvik ME. Lysergic acid diethylamide (LSD-25). IX. Effect on snails. J Psychol 1955; 40:337.
7. Witt PN. D-Lysergsäure-Diathylamid (LSD-25) im Spinnentest. Experientia 1951; 7:310.
8. West L, Pierce C, Thomas W. Lysergic acid diethylamide: its effect on a male Asiatic elephant. Science 1962; 138:1100.
9. Christiansen A, Baum R, Witt PN. Changes in spider webs brought about by mescaline, psilocybin, and an increase in body weight. J Pharmacol Exp Ther 1962; 136:31.
10. Siegel RK. Intoxication. Life in Pursuit of Artificial Paradise. New York: EP Dutton, 1989:57.
11. Jacobs BL. Postsynaptic serotonergic action of hallucinogens. In: Jacobs BL, ed. Hallucinogens: Neurochemical, Behavioral, and Clinical Perspectives. New York: Raven Press, 1984:183.
12. Jacobs BL. How hallucinogenic drugs work. Am Sci 1987; 75:386.
13. Nichols DE, Glennon RA. Medicinal chemistry and structure-activity relationships of hallucinogens. In: Jacobs BL, ed. Hallucinogens: Neurochemical, Behavioral, and Clinical Perspectives. New York: Raven Press, 1984:95.
14. Mittman SM, Geyer MA. Dissociation of multiple effects of acute LSD on exploratory behavior in rats by ritanserin and propranolol. Psychopharmacology 1991; 105:69.
15. Carvey P, Nausieda P, Weertz R, Klawans H. LSD and other related hallucinogens elicit myoclonic jumping behavior in the guinea pig. Prog Neuropsychopharmacol Biol Psychiatry 1989; 13:199.
16. Glennon RA. Phenylalkylamine stimulants, hallucinogens, and designer drugs. In: Harris L, ed. Problems of Drug Dependence 1990. Rockville, MD: NIDA Research Monograph 105, DHHS, 1991:154.
17. McKenna DJ, Guan XM, Shulgin AT. 3,4-Methylenedioxyamphetamine (MDA) analogues exhibit differential effects on synaptosomal release of 3H-dopamine and 3H-5-hydroxytryptamine. Pharmacol Biochem Behav 1991; 38:505.
18. Carroll ME. PCP and hallucinogens. Adv Alcohol Subst Abuse 1990; 9:167.
19. Appel JB, Rosecrans JA. Behavioral pharmacology of hallucinogens in animals: conditioning studies. In: Jacobs BL, ed. Hallucinogens: Neurochemical, Behavioral, and Clinical Perspectives. New York: Raven Press, 1984:77.
20. Trulson ME, Jacobs BL. Dissociations between the effects of LSD on behavior and raphe unit activity in freely moving cats. Science 1979; 205:515.
21. Trulson ME, Heym J, Jacobs BL. Dissociations between the effects of hallucinogenic drugs on behavior and raphe unit activity in freely moving cats. Brain Res 1981; 215:275.
22. Sloviter RS, Drust EG, Damiano DP, Connor JD. A common mechanism for lysergic acid, indolealkylamine and phenylethylamine hallucinogens: serotonergic mediation of behavioral effects in rats. J Pharmacol Exp Ther 1980; 214:231.
23. Heym J, Rasmussen K, Jacobs BL. Some behavioral effects of hallucinogens are mediated by a postsynaptic serotonergic action: evidence from single unit studies in freely moving cats. Eur J Pharmacol 1984; 101:57.
24. Glennon RA, Titeler M, McKenney JD. Evidence for 5HT$_2$ involvement in the mechanism of action of hallucinogenic agents. Life Sci 1984; 35:2505.
25. Schmidt AW, Peroutka SJ. 5-hydroxytryptamine receptor "families." FASEB J 1989; 3:2242.
26. Appel JB, Callahan PM. Involvement of 5-HT receptor subtypes in the discriminative stimulus properties of mescaline. Eur J Pharmacol 1989; 159:41.
27. McClue SJ, Brazell C, Stahl SM. Hallucinogenic drugs are partial agonists of the human platelet shape change response: a physiological model of the 5-HT$_2$ receptor. Biol Psychiatr 1989; 26:297.
28. Sadzot B, Baraban JM, Glennon RA, et al. Hallucinogenic drug interactions at human brain 5-HT$_2$ receptors: implications for treating LSD-induced hallucinogenesis. Psychopharmacology 1989; 98:495.
29. McKenna DJ, Repke DB, Lo L, Peroutka SJ. Differential interactions of indolealkylamines with 5-hydroxytryptamine receptor subtypes. Neuropharmacology 1990; 29:193.

30. Glennon RA. Do classical hallucinogens act as 5-HT_2 agonists or antagonists? Neuropsychopharmacology 1990; 3:509.

31. Burris KD, Breeding M, Sanders-Bush E. (+)Lysergic acid diethylamide, but not its nonhallucinogenic congeners, is a potent serotonin 5HT_{1C} receptor agonist. J Pharmacol Exp Ther 1991; 258:891.

32. Cunningham KA, Appel JB. Neuropharmacological reassessment of the discriminative stimulus properties of d-lysergic acid diethylamide (LSD). Psychopharmacology 1987; 91:67.

33. Buchholtz NS, Zhou DF, Freedman DX, Potter WZ. Lysergic acid diethylamide (LSD) administration selectively downregulates serotonin-2 receptors in rat brain. Neuropsychopharmacology 1990; 3:137.

34. Pierce PA, Peroutka SJ. Antagonist properties of d-LSD at 5-hydroxytryptamine-2 receptors. Neuropsychopharmacology 1990; 3:503.

35. Eells JT, Wilkison DM. Effects of intraocular mescaline and LSD on visual-evoked responses in the rat. Pharmacol Biochem Behav 1989; 32:191.

36. Brady JV, Griffith RR, Heinz RD, et al. Assessing drugs for abuse liability and dependence potential in laboratory primates. In: Bozarth MA, ed. Methods of Assessing the Reinforcing Properties of Abused Drugs. New York: Springer-Verlag, 1987:47.

37. Yokel RA. Intravenous self-administration: response rates, the effects of pharmacological challenges, and drug preference. In: Bozarth MA, ed. Methods of Assessing the Reinforcing Properties of Abused Drugs. New York: Springer-Verlag, 1987:1.

38. Schlemmer RF, David JM. A primate model for the study of hallucinogens. Pharmacol Biochem Behav 1986; 24:381.

39. Wasson RG, Ruck CAP, Hofmann A. The Road to Eleusis. New York: Harcourt Brace Jovonovich, 1978.

40. Elferink JGR. Some little-known hallucinogenic plants of the Aztecs. J Psychoact Drugs 1988; 20:427.

41. Spoerke DG, Hall AH. Plants and mushrooms of abuse. Emerg Med Clin North Am 1990; 8:579.

42. Wasson RG. Soma: Divine Mushroom of Immortality. New York: Harcourt Brace Jovonovitch, 1968.

43. Fuller JG. The Day of St. Anthony's Fire. New York: MacMillan, 1968.

44. Caporael LR. Ergotism: the satan loosed in Salem? Science 1976; 192:21.

45. Brecher EM. Licit and Illicit Drugs. Boston: Little, Brown, 1972.

46. Schwartz RH. Mescaline: a survey. Am Fam Phys 1988; 37:122.

47. Mitchell SW. Remarks on the effects of *Anhalonium lewinii* (the mescal button). BMJ 1896; 2:1625.

48. Metzer WS. The experimentation of S. Weir Mitchell with mescal. Neurology 1989; 39:303.

49. Ellis H. Mescal: a new artificial paradise. Reprinted in: Ebin D, ed. The Drug Experience. New York: Orion Press, 1961:223.

50. Paradise or inferno (edit.). BMJ 1898; 1:390.

51. Farnsworth NR. Hallucinogenic plants. Science 1968; 162:1086.

52. Huxley A. The Doors of Perception. New York: Harper & Row, 1954.

53. Zaehner RC. Mysticism, sacred and profane. Reprinted in: Ebin D, ed. The Drug Experience. New York: Orion Press, 1961:275.

54. Wohlberg J. Haoma-Soma in the world of ancient Greece. J Psychoact Drugs 1990; 22:333.

55. Sanchez-Ramos JR. Banisterine and Parkinson's disease. Clin Neuropharmacol 1991; 14:391.

56. Hoffmann A. How LSD originated. J Psychedelic Drugs 1979; 11:53.

57. Osmond H. A review of the clinical effects of psychotomimetic agents. Ann NY Acad Sci 1957; 66:418.

58. Abramson HA. The use of LSD as an adjunct to psychotherapy. Fact and fiction. In: Sankar DVS, ed. LSD: A Total Study. New York: PJD Publications Ltd, 1975.

59. Greenhouse L. Court is urged to rehear case on ritual drugs. NY Times, May 11, 1990.

60. Bullis RK. Swallowing the scroll: Legal implications of the recent Supreme Court peyote cases. J Psychoact Drugs 1990; 22:325.

61. Fishburne PM, Abelson HI, Cisin I. National Survey on Drug Abuse: Main Findings: 1979. Washington DC, DHHS, Publ (ADM) 80-976, 1980.

62. Treaster JB. Use of LSD, drug of allure and risk, is said to rise. NY Times, December 27, 1991.

63. Lacroix J, Gaudreault P, Gauthier M. Admission to a pediatric intensive care unit for poisoning: a review of 105 cases. Crit Care Med 1989; 17:748.

64. Freedman DX. LSD: the bridge from human to animal. In: Jacobs BL, ed. Hallucinogens: Neurochemical, Behavioral, and Clinical Perspectives. New York: Raven Press, 1984:203.

65. Hyde C, Glancy G, Omerod P, et al. Abuse of indigenous psilocybin mushrooms: a new fashion and some psychiatric complications. Br J Psychiatry 1978; 132:602.

66. Mills PR, Lesinskas D, Watkinson G. The danger of hallucinogenic mushrooms. Scott Med J 1979; 24:316.

67. Benjamin C. Persistent psychiatric symptoms after eating psilocybin mushrooms. BMJ 1979; 1:1319.

68. Young RE, Milroy R, Hutchinson S, et al. The rising price of mushrooms. Lancet 1982; 1:213.

69. Siegel RK. New trends in drug use among young in California. Bull Narc 1985; 37:7.

70. Thompson JP, Anglin MD, Emboden W, et al. Mushroom use by college students. J Drug Educ 1985; 15:111.

71. Schwartz RH, Smith DE. Hallucinogenic mushrooms. Clin Pediatr 1988; 27:70.

72. Hollister LE. Effects of hallucinogens in humans. In: Jacobs BL, ed. Hallucinogens: Neurochemical, Behavioral, and Clinical Perspectives. New York: Raven Press, 1984:19.

73. Moser P. LSD. In: Ebin D, ed. The Drug Experience. New York: Orion Press, 1961:353.

74. Jaffe JH. Drug addiction and drug abuse. In: Gilman AG, Rall TW, Nies AS, Taylor P, eds. The Pharmacological Basis of Therapeutics, ed 8. New York: Pergamon Press, 1990:522.

75. Isbell H, Belleville RE, Fraser HF, et al. Studies in lysergic acid diethylamide (LSD-25). I. Effects in former morphine addicts and development of tolerance during chronic administration. Arch Neurol Psychiatry 1956; 76:468.
76. Isbell H. Comparison of the reactions produced by psilocybin and LSD-25 in man. Psychopharmacologia 1959; 1:29.
77. Gastaut H, Ferrer S, Castells C. Action de la diethylamide de l'acide d-lysergique (LSD-25) sur les fonctions psychiques et l'electroencephalogramme. Confin Neurol 1953; 13:102.
78. Musio JN, Roffwarg HP, Kaufmann E. Alterations in the nocturnal sleep cycle resulting from LSD. Electroencephalogr Clin Neurophysiol 1966; 21:313.
79. Isbell H, Wolbach AB, Wikler A, Miner EJ. Cross tolerance between LSD and psilocybin. Psychopharmacologia 1961; 2:147.
80. Wolbach AB, Isbell H, Miner EJ. Cross tolerance between mescaline and LSD-25, with a comparison of the mescaline and LSD reactions. Psychopharmacologia 1962; 3:1.
81. Rosenberg DE, Wolbach AB, Miner EJ, Isbell H. Observations on direct and cross tolerance with LSD and d-amphetamine in man. Psychopharmacologia 1963; 5:1.
82. Isbell H, Jasinski DR. A comparison of LSD-25 with delta-9-tetrahydrocannabinol (THC) and attempted cross-tolerance between LSD and THC. Psychopharmacologia 1969; 14:115.
83. McGlothlin WH, Arnold DO. LSD revisited: a ten-year followup of medical LSD use. Arch Gen Psychiatry 1971; 24:35.
84. Cohen S. A classification of LSD complications. Psychosomatics 1966; 7:182.
85. Ungerleider JT, Fisher DD, Goldsmith SR, et al. A statistical survey of adverse reactions to LSD in Los Angeles County. Am J Psychiatry 1968; 125:352.
86. Klepfisz A, Racy J. Homicide and LSD. JAMA 1973; 223:429.
87. Thomas R, Fuller D. Self-inflicted ocular injury associated with drug use. J SC Med Assoc 1972; 68:202.
88. Fuller D. Severe solar maculopathy associated with use of lysergic acid diethylamide. Am J Ophthalmol 1976; 81:413.
89. Schwarz C. Paradoxical responses to chlorpromazine after LSD. Psychosomatics 1967; 8:210.
90. Ungerleider J, Fisher D, Fuller M, Caldwell A. The "bad trip": the etiology of the adverse LSD reaction. Am J Psychiatry 1968; 124:41.
91. Barnett BEW. Diazepam treatment for LSD intoxication. Lancet 1977; 2:270.
92. Strassman RJ. Adverse reactions to psychedelic drugs. J Nerv Ment Dis 1984; 172:577.
93. Frosh W, Robbins E, Stern M. Untoward reactions to lysergic acid diethylmide (LSD) resulting in hospitalization. N Engl J Med 1965; 273:1235.
94. Bewley T. Adverse reaction from the illicit use of lysergide. BMJ 1967; 3:28.
95. Baker A. Hospital admissions due to lysergic acid diethylamide. Lancet 1970; 1:714.
96. Decker W, Brandes W. LSD misadventures in middle age. J Forens Sci 1978; 23:3.
97. Scher M, Neppe V. Carbamazepine adjunct for nonresponsive psychosis with prior hallucinogenic abuse. J Nerv Ment Dis 1989; 177:755.
98. Hatrick J, Dewhurst K. Delayed psychoses due to LSD. Lancet 1970; 2:742.
99. Jacobs D. Psychiatric symptoms and hallucinogenic compounds. BMJ 1979; 2:49.
100. Nagitch M, Fenwick S. LSD flashbacks and ego functioning. J Abnorm Psychol 1977; 86:352.
101. Stanton M, Bardoni A. Drug flashbacks: reported frequency in a military population. Am J Psychiatry 1972; 129:751.
102. Abraham HD. Visual phenomenology of the LSD flashback. Arch Gen Psychiatry 1983; 40:884.
103. Levi L, Miller NR. Visual illusions associated with previous drug abuse. J Clin Neuroophthalmol 1990; 10:103.
103a. Fisher D, Ungerleider J. Grand mal seizures following ingestion of LSD. Calif Med 1976; 106:210.
104. Stimmel B. Cardiovascular Effects of Mood-altering Drugs. New York: Raven Press, 1979.
105. Friedman SA, Hirsch SE. Extreme hyperthermia after LSD ingestion. JAMA 1979; 217:1549.
106. Klock JC, Boerner V, Becker CE. Coma, hyperthermia, and bleeding associated with massive LSD overdose. A report of eight cases. West J Med 1973; 119:183.
107. Mercieca J, Brown EA. Acute renal failure due to rhabdomyolysis associated with use of a straightjacket in lysergide intoxication. BMJ 1984; 288:1949.
108. Horita A, Hamilton AE. Lysergic acid diethylamide: dissociation of its behavioral and hyperthermic actions by dl-alpha-methyl-paratyrosine. Science 1969; 164:78.
109. Altura B, Altura BM. Phencyclidine, lysergic acid diethylamide, and mescaline: cerebral artery spasms and hallucinogenic activity. Science 1981; 212:1051.
110. Sobel J, Espinas OE, Friedman SA. Carotid artery obstruction following LSD capsule ingestion. Arch Intern Med 1971;127:290.
111. Lieberman AN, Bloom W, Kishore PS, Lin JP. Carotid artery occlusion following ingestion of LSD. Stroke 1974; 5:213.
112. Lignelli GJ, Buchheit WA. Angitis in drug abusers. N Engl J Med 1971; 284:112.
113. Rumbaugh CL, Bergeron RT, Fang HCH, McCormick R. Cerebral angiographic changes in the drug abuse patient. Radiology 1971; 101:335.
114. McWilliams SA, Tuttle R. Long-term psychological effects of LSD. Psychol Bull 1973; 79:341.
115. Blacker KH, Jones RT, Stone GC, Pfefferbaum D. Chronic users of LSD: the "acidheads." Am J Psychiatry 1968; 125:97.
116. Wright M, Hogan T. Repeated LSD ingestion and performance on neuropsychological tests. J Nerv Ment Dis 1972; 154:432.

117. Tucker GJ, Quinlan D, Harrow M. Chronic hallucinogenic drug use and thought disturbance. Arch Gen Psychiatry 1972; 27:443.

118. Vardy MM, Kay SR. LSD psychosis or LSD-induced schizophrenia? A multi-method inquiry. Arch Gen Psychiatry 1983; 40:877.

119. Materson BJ, Barrett-Conner E. LSD "mainlining": a new hazard to health. JAMA 1967; 200:202.

120. Cohen MM, Marinello MJ, Back N. Chromosomal damage in human leukocytes induced by lysergic acid diethylamide. Science 1967; 155:1417.

121. Irwin S, Egozcue J. Chromosomal abnormalities in leukocytes from LSD-users. Science 1967; 157:313.

122. Auerback R, Rugowski JA. Lysergic acid diethylamide: effects on embryos. Science 1967; 157:1325.

123. Skakkebaek NE, Philip J, Rafelsen OJ. LSD in mice: abnormalities in meiotic chromosomes. Science 1968; 160:1246.

124. Alexander GJ, Miles B, Gold GM, Alexander RB. LSD: ingestion early in pregnancy produces abnormalities in offspring in rats. Science 1967; 157:459.

125. Eller JL, Morton JM. Bizarre deformities in offspring of user of lysergic acid diethylamide. N Engl J Med 1970; 283:395.

126. Chan CC, Fishman M, Egbert PR. Multiple ocular anomalies associated with maternal LSD ingestion. Arch Ophthalmol 1978; 96:282.

127. Loughman WD, Sargent TW, Isrealstein DM. Leukocytes of humans exposed to lysergic acid diethylamide: lack of chromosomal damage. Science 1967; 508:1967.

128. Sparkes RS, Melnyk J, Bozzetti LP. Chromosomal effect in vivo of exposure to lysergic acid diethylamide. Science 1968; 160:1343.

129. Warkany J, Takacs E. Lysergic acid diethyltryptamide (LSD): no teratogenicity in rats. Science 1968; 159:731.

130. Bender L, Siva-Sanker DV. Chromosome damage not found in children when treated with LSD. Science 1968; 159:749.

131. Hungerford DA, Tagler KM, Shagass C, et al. Cytogenic effects of LSD-25 therapy in man. JAMA 1968; 206:2287.

132. Corey MJ, Andrews JC, McLeod MJ, et al. Chromosome studies on patients (in vivo) and cells (in vitro) treated with lysergic acid diethylamide. N Engl J Med 1970; 282:939.

133. Cohen MM, Shiloh Y. Genetic toxicology of lysergic acid diethylamide (LSD-25). Mutat Res 1977–1978; 47:183.

134. Teitelbaum DT, Wingeleth DC. Diagnosis and management of recreational mescaline self-poisoning. J Anal Toxicol 1977; 1:36.

135. Jacobs KW. Hallucinogenic mushrooms in Mississippi. J Miss State Med Assoc 1975; 16:35.

136. Pollock SH. A novel experience with Panaeolus: a case study from Hawaii. J Psychedelic Drugs 1974; 6:85.

137. Pollock SH. *Psilocybian mycetismus* with special reference to Panaeolus. J Psychedelic Drugs 1976; 8:43.

138. Francis J, Murray VSG. Review of inquiries made to the NPIS concerning Psilocybe mushroom ingestion, 1973–1981. Hum Toxicol 1983; 2:349.

139. Curry SC, Rose MC. Intravenous mushroom poisoning. Ann Emerg Med 1985; 14:900.

140. McCormick DJ, Aubel AJ, Gibbons MC. Nonlethal mushroom poisoning. Ann Intern Med 1979; 90:332.

141. McCawley EL, Brummett RE, Dana GW. Convulsions from Psilocybe mushroom poisoning. Proc West Pharmacol Soc 1962; 5:27.

142. Harries AD, Evans V. Sequelae of a "magic mushroom banquet." Postgrad Med J 1981; 57:571.

143. Peden NR, Pringle SD, Crooks J. The problem of Psilocybin mushroom abuse. Hum Toxicol 1982; 1:417.

144. Sivyer C, Dorrington L. Intravenous injection of mushrooms. Med J Aust 1984; 140:182.

145. Wolbach AB, Miner EJ, Isbell H. Comparison of psilocin with psilocybin, mescaline, and LSD-25. Psychopharmacologia 1962; 3:219.

146. Spoerke DG, Spoerke SE, Jumack BH. Rocky Mountain high. Ann Emerg Med 1985; 14:162.

147. Waters MB. *Pholiota spectabilis*, hallucinogenic fungus. Mycologia 1965; 57:837.

148. Buck RW. Psychedelic effect of *Philiota spectabilis*. N Engl J Med 1967; 276:391.

149. Szara S, Rochland LH, Rosenthal D, Handlon JH. Psychological effects and metabolism of N,N-dimethyltryptamine in man. Arch Gen Psychiatry 1966; 15:320.

150. Rubin D. Dimethyltryptamine, a do-it-yourself hallucinogenic drug. JAMA 1967; 201:157.

151. Snyder SH, Failace L, Hollister L. 2,5-dimethoxy-4-methylamphetamine (STP): a new hallucinogenic drug. Science 1967; 158:669.

152. Snyder SH, Faillace LA, Weingartner H. DOM (STP), a new hallucinogenic drug, and DOET: effects in normal subjects. Am J Psychiatry 1968; 125:357.

153. Snyder SH, Weingartner H, Faillace LA. DOET (2,5-dimethoxy-4-ethylamphetamine), a new psychotropic drug. Arch Gen Psychiatry 1971; 24:50.

154. Winek CL, Collum WD, Bricker JD. A death due to 4-bromo-2,5-dimethoxyamphetamine. Clin Toxicol 1981; 18:267.

155. Bowen JS, Davis GB, Kearney TE, Bardin J. Diffuse vascular spasm associated with 4-bromo-2,5-dimethoxyamphetamine ingestion. JAMA 1983; 249:1477.

156. Seiden LS, Kleven MS. Methamphetamine and related drugs: toxicity and resulting behavioral changes in response to pharmacological probes. In: Arghar K, De-Souza E, eds. Pharmacology and Toxicology of Amphetamine and Related Designer Drugs. Rockville, MD: NIDA Research Monograph 94, DHHS, 1989:146.

157. Keitner GI, Sabaawi M, Haier RJ. Isosafrole and schizophrenia-like psychosis. Am J Psychiatry 1984; 141:997.

158. Ingram AL. Morning glory seed reaction. JAMA 1964; 190:1133.

159. Cohen S. Suicide following morning glory seed ingestion. Am J Psychiatry 1964; 120:1024.

160. Lewin NA, Holland MA, Goldfrank LR, Flomenbaum NE. Herbal preparations. In: Goldfrank LR, Flomenbaum NE, Lewin NA, et al, eds. Toxicologic Emergencies, ed 4. Norwalk, CT: Appleton & Lange, 1990:587.

161. Rice WB, Genest K. Acute toxicity of extracts of morning glory seeds in mice. Nature 1965; 207:302.

162. Weil AT. Nutmeg as a psychoactive drug. In: Efron DH, Holmstedt V, Kline NS, eds. Ethnopharmacologic Search for Psychoactive Drugs. New York: Raven Press, 1967:188.

163. Malcolm X, Haley A. The Autobiography of Malcolm X. New York: Grove Press, 1964.

164. Truitt EB, Callaway E, Braude MC, et al. The pharmacology of myristicin: a contribution to the psychopharmacology of nutmeg. J Neuropsychol 1961; 2:205.

165. Venables GS, Evered D, Hall R. Nutmeg poisoning. BMJ 1976; 1:96.

166. Payne RB. Nutmeg intoxication. N Engl J Med 1963; 269:36.

167. Shafran I. Nutmeg toxicology. N Engl J Med 1976; 294:849.

168. Painter JC, Shanor SP, Winek CL. Nutmeg poisoning—a case report. Clin Toxicol 1971; 4:1.

169. Lavy G. Nutmeg intoxication in pregnancy. A case report. J Reprod Med 1987; 32:63.

170. Green RC. Nutmeg poisoning. JAMA 1959; 171:1342.

171. Kava. Lancet 1988; 2:258.

172. Cawte J. Psychoactive substances of the South Seas: betel, kava, and pituri. Aust NZ J Psychiatry 1985; 19:83.

173. Siegel RK. Herbal intoxication: psychoactive effects from herbal cigarettes, tea, and capsules. JAMA 1976; 236:473.

174. Howard R, Foerstl H. Toad-licker's psychosis—a warning. Br J Psychiatry 1990; 157:779.

Chapter 8
Inhalants

Oh, Tom! Such a gas has Davy discovered! . . . It made
me laugh and tingle . . . It made one strong, and so
happy!
　　　　　　　　　　　　　　　　—*Robert Southey*

You're in outer space. You're Superman. You're floating
in air, seeing double, riding next to God. It's Kicksville.
　　　　　　　　　—*Anonymous juvenile glue sniffer*

A strong smell of turpentine prevails throughout.
　—*Oliver Wendel Holmes, describing his vision of heaven
while sniffing ether*

Before they were recognized as general anesthetics, nitrous oxide and diethyl ether were used recreationally. Today volatile substance abuse is a worldwide problem. The different products that are used often contain several psychically active compounds, yet the "highs" and "jags" produced are remarkably similar.

Pharmacology and Animal Studies

Among the several chemical classes of abused volatile compounds (Table 8–1), the aromatic hydrocarbon toluene and the halogenated hydrocarbon trichloroethane have been most extensively studied. Acute effects in animals are dose related and similar to those of sedatives and ethanol: Hyperactivity progresses to ataxia, sedation, coma, respiratory depression, and death.[1] In mice, toluene and xylene prevent pentylenetetrazol-induced seizures. In rats, toluene increases operant behavior that has been suppressed by electric shock.[2] In rodents and pigeons, low doses of toluene and xylene increase rates of operant responding, but high doses decrease them.[3,4] By contrast, halogenated hydrocarbons such as trichloroethane and ketones such as methyl-n-amylketone decrease response rates at both low and high doses.[1]

Animal evidence for the development of tolerance to these agents is equivocal. For toluene, it was found in rats but not in mice or monkeys.[5–7] For trichloroethane, it was not evident in mice.[8] Cross-tolerance has been demonstrated in mice between ethanol and several inhalational anesthetics, but such effects involving solvent compounds have not been reported.[1] Similarly, although mice develop withdrawal seizures following exposure to ethylene, diethyl ether, or cyclopropane and although chloroform can suppress the signs of barbiturate withdrawal, physical dependence to toluene, trichloroethane, or other solvent hydrocarbons has not been demonstrated in animals.[1]

Monkeys self-administer chloroform, diethyl ether, nitrous oxide, and toluene.[1,9,10] In drug discrimination studies, mice trained to identify barbiturate generalize to halothane, trichloroethane, and toluene.[11,12] In mice, ethanol enhances the behavioral and lethal effects of trichloroethane, and toluene and trichloroethane enhance the effects of ethanol and sedatives.[1,13] Whether solvent compounds such as toluene and trichloroethane, which like ethanol and volatile anesthetics are small, lipophilic molecules, similarly "perturb" cell membranes (see Chapter 11) is unknown.

Historical Background and Epidemiology

The inhalation of vapors to achieve religious ecstasy pre-dates recorded history; substances have included

Table 8–1. Chemical Classification of Abused Volatile Compounds

Aliphatic hydrocarbons
  n-Butane
  Isobutane
  n-Hexane
  Propane
  Pentane

Aromatic hydrocarbons
  Toluene
  Xylene
  Benzene

Esters
  Ethyl acetate

Ketones
  Acetone
  Butanone
  Methylethylketone
  Methylisobutylketone

Halogenated hydrocarbons
  Chloroform
  Halothane
  Enflurane
  Isoflurane
  Trichloroethane
  Dichloroethylene
  Trichloroethylene
  Tetrachloroethylene
  Dichloromethane
  Carbon tetrachloride
  Dichlorodifluoromethane
  Chlorodifluoromethane
  Bromochlorodifluoromethane
  Trichlorofluoromethane

Ethers
  Diethyl ether
Anesthetic gases
  Nitrous oxide
Nitrites
  Butyl nitrite
  Isobutyl nitrite
  Amyl nitrite

cannabis and ergot hallucinogens (see Chapters 6 and 7). The discovery of diethyl ether in the 13th century added a secular element to such activity. In the 18th century, diethyl ether was marketed as a medicinal tonic called "Anodyne," and whether drunk or sniffed it quickly became a popular recreational drug in Britain—cheaper than heavily taxed alcoholic beverages and producing short-lived effects without hangover.[14] In the 19th century, diethyl ether was promoted as an alternative to ethanol in Ireland ("ether frolics"), and it was widely used by American students well before its demonstration as a surgical anesthetic by William Morton in 1846. Diethyl ether was drunk as an alcohol substitute during American Prohibition (1920–1933) and in Germany during World War II.

Nitrous oxide was discovered by Sir Joseph Priestley in 1776 and later synthesized by Sir Humphrey Davy, who personally described both its intoxicating effects and its addiction liability. Dubbed "laughing gas," nitrous oxide was inhaled recreationally by Davy's friends, including the poets Samuel Taylor Coleridge and Robert Southey and the thesaurist Peter Roget.[14,15] In the early 19th century, nitrous oxide sniffing was widespread in the United States; it was not until 1845 that the Connecticut dentist Horace Wells began using it as a general anesthetic.[16]

Chloroform, like diethyl ether, is a readily vaporized liquid. It was discovered in 1831, and recreational use quickly followed. Although a tendency to sudden death limited its popularity, 19th century chloroform addicts were not rare; less odorous than diethyl ether or nitrous oxide, it was easily concealed, and users could sniff it throughout the day undetected. Horace Wells died a chloroform addict.[14]

In recent decades, inhalant abusers have turned to a wide variety of household products, especially glues, solvents, and fuels (Table 8–2).[17,18] The earliest reference to glue sniffing seems to have been a 1959 newspaper article describing children in several western American cities.[19] What ensued is instructional. A national chorus of alarm, intended to deter use, instead became a lure, and as exaggerated warnings led to legislation and arrests, glue sniffing became a nationwide epidemic.[20] Diversification to other substances soon followed, and today volatile substance abuse involves children throughout the world.

In 1979, inhalants had been used by 17% of Americans aged 18 to 25 and 10% of children aged 12 to 17.[21,22] Throughout the 1980s, this prevalence held steady, peaking during sixth and seventh grades.[23,24] In 1986, 20% of American high school seniors had abused inhalants, 3% within the previous 30 days.[25] Sniffing by much younger children is not unusual; reports include a 3-year-old gasoline addict.[26–28]

In Britain during 1984 through 1986, up to 10% of secondary school children had tried volatile substances, and 0.5% to 1% were current users.[29] In 1989, inhalant abuse in Britain accounted for 113 deaths, half in children 16 years old or younger.[25]

Table 8–2. Abused Products and Their Contents

Products	Contents
Aerosols (refrigerants, frying pan cleaners, antitussives, hair sprays, bronchodilators, shampoos, deodorants, antiseptics, pain killers)	Fluorinated hydrocarbons, propane, isobutane
Dry cleaning fluids, spot removers, furniture polish, degreasers	Chlorinated hydrocarbons, naphtha (gasoline hydrocarbons)
Glues, cements, rubber patching	Toluene, acetone, benzene, aliphatic acetates, n-hexane, cyclohexane, tri-chloroethylene, xylene, butyl alcohol, dichloroethylene, methylethylketone, methylethylisobutylketone, chloroform, ethanol, triorthocresyl phosphate
Lighter fluid	Aliphatic and aromatic hydrocarbons
Fire-extinguishing agents	Bromochlorodifluoromethane
Fingernail polish remover	Acetone, aliphatic acetates, benzene
Bottled fuel gas	Butane, propane
Typewriter correction fluid	Trichloroethane, trichloroethylene
Natural gas	Methane, ethane, propane, butane
Marker pens	Toluene, xylene
Paints, enamels, lacquers, lacquer and paint thinners	Toluene, methylene chloride, aliphatic acetates, benzene, ethanol
Petroleum (gasoline, naphtha gas, benzine)	Many aliphatic, aromatic, and other hydrocarbons (e.g., olefins, naphthanes), including butane, hexane, pentane, benzene, toluene, and xylene; tetraethyl lead
Anesthetics (surgical supply, whipped cream dispensers)	Nitrous oxide, diethyl ether, halothane, chloroform, enflurane, isoflurane, trichloroethylene
"Room odorizers"	Amyl, butyl, and isobutyl nitrite

The most common products used were gas fuels, especially butane for cigarette lighters (33%), antiperspirant or deodorant aerosols (21%), and glue (21%). (Many users had switched from glue because of its telltale odor, tendency to leave stains, and increasing scarcity on store shelves.) Similar experiences have been reported from other Western European countries, Hungary, Canada, Mexico, South America, Japan, South Africa, Israel, Australia, and Singapore.[30–36]

Among users in the United States, males outnumber females by 10:1, blacks are underrepresented, and Hispanics and Native Americans are overrepresented. Inhalant abusers are usually not part of a drug subculture, although many take other drugs as well. Regular users are most often children of low socioeconomic background, often neglected, abused, or from unstable homes.[24,27,37] Similar to alcoholics, many carry a diagnosis of antisocial personality disorder.[38] Gasoline sniffing is particularly common among Native Americans in the United States and Canada; in one community, 50% of children age 4 to 18 were chronic abusers.[17,39–41]

In the 1970s, it was discovered that fluorinated hydrocarbon propellants—which include the proprietary mixture Freon—adversely affect the earth's atmospheric ozone. A decline in abuse followed restrictions on their manufacture.[42]

In the United States, there are three main types of inhalant abusers: (1) inhalant-addicted adults, (2) adolescent polydrug users, and (3) younger inhalant users.[43] Most children eventually give up inhalants, but some become addicted and continue use through adulthood.[44] Overrepresented among adults are shoemakers and sandal makers, cabinetmakers, printers, painters, gas station attendants, automobile and bicycle repair shop workers, petroleum refinery workers, and workers in chemical plants.[45] Inhalant abuse is also common among military recruits and prison inmates.[27,46] The occupational risk of physicians and other medical workers for anesthesia abuse has been recognized for more than a century.[47]

Juvenile sniffers are not restricted to impoverished communities or broken homes; epidemics of solvent abuse have occurred in boarding schools. Obtaining products from home, school, grocery stores, hardware stores, or gas tanks, children sniff gasoline, glue, paint, lighter fluid, nail polish remover, marker pens, deodorants, kerosene, aerosols, typing correction fluid, school laboratory gas jets, nitrous oxide, lacquer thinner, transmission fluid, gun-cleaning solvents, and fire-extinguishing agents.[45]

Amidst this array are four major classes of inhalants: (1) volatile solvents such as glues, paint thinners, and gasoline; (2) aerosols such as hair sprays, deodorants, and spray paints; (3) volatile anesthetics such as diethyl ether or nitrous oxide; and (4) volatile nitrites.[48] Substances are usually sniffed (nasal) or "huffed" (oral inhalation) from a saturated rag (if liquid), a plastic bag (if viscous), or directly from a container.[22] A gently heated frying pan may be used. Sniffing can continue over hours, and chronic abusers might inhale 0.5 L daily for years. Infrequently the same substance is drunk, sometimes mixed with beer or chaser. Children have mixed nail polish remover with Coca-Cola.[35] Rarely volatile substances are injected intravenously.[49,50] A form of inhalant abuse carrying its own special hazard is propane or butane "fire breathing."[51]

Acute Effects

Whichever substance is used, the desired effects resemble ethanol intoxication: euphoria and relaxation with or without ataxia, diplopia, and slurred speech. As with ethanol, grandiosity and impulsiveness produce accidents and violence. There may be a feeling of "blankness" or "numbness," and consciousness may be briefly lost. Higher doses cause toxic psychosis. Delusions can lead to self-destructive behavior; during glue-sniffing, an 18-year-old enucleated his own eye.[52] Visual distortions or hallucinations can be either pleasant or terrifying— for example, savage animals, ghosts, or gory wounds.[27,53–55] The presence of hallucinations during intoxication is perhaps the symptom that most distinguishes inhalants from ethanol and sedatives.[35] High doses cause ataxia, nystagmus, dysarthria, and drowsiness progressing to coma and sometimes seizures.[56]

Dizziness, flushing, coughing, sneezing, increased salivation, nausea, and vomiting frequently accompany intoxication. Symptoms last only 15 to 30 minutes but can be sustained for hours by repeated use.[46,55] Except for occasional headache, most users do not experience "hangover."[57] Some have amnesia for the episode.[58]

Death occurs from vomiting and aspiration, suffocation by plastic bags, accidents, violence, or suddenly without apparent cause.[59–65] An epidemiologic survey in Britain attributed death to direct toxic effects in 51%, asphyxia in 21%, aspiration of vomitus in 18%, and trauma in 11%.[66] Some substances—for example, tricholoroethane, fluorinated hydrocarbons, and non-Freon aerosols such as isobutane and propane—cause cardiac arrhythmia, especially when there is hypoxia or exertion.[67] Directly spraying cold gases (e.g., butane or aerosol propellants) into the mouth stimulates the larynx

and can lead to reflexic vagal cardiac depression.[68] Many inhalants depress myocardial contractility and increase the sensitivity of the heart to catecholamines.[69] Ventricular fibrillation followed toluene sniffing in a 16-year-old boy, and inhalant-related sudden death has occurred during sexual intercourse.[70] A 15-year-old boy was successfully resuscitated after being found in cardiorespiratory arrest following inhalation of a typewriter correction fluid containing trichloroethylene and trichloroethane,[71] and respiratory depression has followed inhalation of glue,[72] paint,[73] and gasoline.[74] A 15-year-old boy collapsed and died after inhaling bromochlorodifluoromethane from a fire extinguisher.[75] An 11-year-old boy was found dead after sniffing butane cigarette lighter fuel, and a 15-year-old boy died from pulmonary burns during propane "torch breathing."[76] Of 282 inhalant deaths in Britain, 17% were associated with deliberate sexual asphyxia.[66]

Clues to inhalant abuse are the smell of solvent on the breath (which may last hours after use) and, in those sniffing from plastic bags, a characteristic "glue-sniffer's rash" around the nose and mouth.[35] With the exception of gasoline, gas chromatography identifies most volatile compounds in the blood within 10 hours of exposure. Urinary metabolites can be detected for toluene, xylene, trichloroethylene, trichloroethane, and tetrachloroethylene. Breath analysis by mass spectrometry is also used.[29]

Because symptoms are so short-lived, inhalant intoxication infrequently requires treatment unless there are cardiorespiratory complications. Cardiac arrhythmia, however, remains a risk for several hours after intoxication has subsided.

In contrast to some animals, human inhalant abusers experience tolerance to acute effects.[27,77] Abrupt discontinuation can produce mild symptoms resembling ethanol withdrawal,[78] but chronic inhalant abuse does not seem to be associated with any consistent abstinence syndrome.[77,79–81] (Reports of delirium, hallucinations, or seizures are so exceptional as to invite skepticism.[45]) Psychic dependence—that is, addiction—is common, however.[35]

Medical and Neurological Complications

Different volatile substances damage different organs. Fatal congestive heart failure occurred in a 24-year-old man who sniffed a shoe cleaning solvent containing trichloroethylene.[82] Massive pulmonary hemorrhages and cerebral edema were found at autopsy in a benzene sniffer.[61] Kidney, liver, and bone marrow damage follow exposure to many of these substances, especially benzene and chlorinated hydrocarbons.[83,84] (Because of its association with fatal liver, kidney, and cardiac disease, carbon tetrachloride is no longer present in household products, but it is still used in industry.[55]) Toluene causes metabolic acidosis with either a normal or increased anion gap; intoxication has been reported in association with severe diabetic ketoacidosis.[85]

Fatal aplastic anemia has affected glue sniffers.[86] Glue and solvent sniffers have developed emphysema and pulmonary hypertension.[87] A man mixed Vim and Ajax cleaning powders with water and deliberately sniffed the chlorine fumes produced; he developed reversible pulmonary insufficiency and cor pulmonale.[88]

A number of studies have found behavioral, cognitive, electroencephalographic, and computerized tomographic (CT) abnormalities in inhalant abusers (as well as in occupationally exposed subjects).[89–98] The milder the impairment, the more difficult it is to infer causality. Methodologic problems include small samples, lack of controls, lack of preexposure data, uncertainty regarding last use, and unblinded examiners. Certainly there are often other contributing factors, especially in emotionally deprived or physically abused children, and behavioral disturbance is as likely to be the cause of inhalant abuse as its result. Nonetheless, in some individuals, volatile substance abuse has devastating neuropsychiatric consequences.

Gasoline sniffing causes lead encephalopathy.[99–103] Tetraethyl lead poisoning in an adolescent gasoline sniffer led to progressive dementia, ataxia, and death, and another 14-year-old gasoline sniffer died with dementia, chorea, peripheral neuropathy, myopathy, and hepatic and renal damage.[104,105] A 27-year-old gasoline sniffer developed generalized myoclonus, agitation, and hallucinations; erythrocytes had basophilic stippling, and blood lead level was 104 μg/dL.[106] More subtle neurological abnormalities have been found in populations with a high prevalence of leaded gasoline abuse.[105] Symptomatic lead poisoning, with colic and anemia, occurred in a painter who ingested lead carbonate–containing paint deliberately to induce hallucinations.[107] Peripheral neuropathy in some gasoline sniffers has been attributed to triorthocresylphosphate in the product.[108]

Persistent encephalopathy and cerebellar ataxia follow chronic toluene exposure.[109–119] Of 25 adults with symptomatic toluene poisoning from spray paint sniffing, 9 had myopathic weakness, often severe and accompanied by hypokalemia, hypophosphatemia, and cardiac arrhythmia; 6 had gastrointestinal symptoms (nausea, vomiting, abdominal pain, hematemesis); and 10 had "neuropsychiatric syndromes".[120] Consistent with other reports,[121,122] renal tubular acidosis was common.

In a study of 20 young adults who had sniffed toluene-containing products for at least 2 years but had abstained for at least 4 weeks, 13 had neurological abnormalities, including cognitive (60%), pyramidal (50%), cerebellar (45%), and cranial nerve or brain stem (25%). Seven had disabling dementia, with apathy, poor concentration, memory loss, visuospatial dysfunction, and "impaired complex cognition." Oculomotor dysfunction included ocular flutter and opsoclonus. Four had anosmia, and two had bilateral sensorineural deafness.[123] Magnetic resonance imaging in demented toluene abusers has shown diffuse cerebral, cerebellar, and brain stem atrophy with loss of gray and white matter differentiation and increased periventricular white matter signal on T2-weighted images.[124,125] Autopsy in a demented patient revealed diffuse myelin pallor maximal in the cerebellar, periventricular, and deep cerebral white matter without neuronal loss, axonal swelling, or gliosis.[124] Autopsy on another toluene sniffer showed cerebral and cerebellar atrophy with degeneration and gliosis of long tracts.[117]

A study of house painters exposed to solvents for decades revealed cognitive abnormalities but little or no evidence of brain atrophy on CT scans; however, cerebral blood flow was significantly reduced compared with controls.[95] Positron-emission tomographic studies of workers chronically exposed to tetrabromoethane showed cortical and subcortical hypometabolism,[126] and subjects occupationally exposed to toluene and trichloroethylene had abnormally reduced amplitudes of the N100 and P300 event-related potentials.[127]

In young rodents, toluene impairs learning, high-frequency hearing, and coordination and is concentrated in central nervous system (CNS) white matter.[128–132] Pathological CNS changes have not been observed, however.

Toluene abusers have developed irreversible optic atrophy,[114,133] and a young man who had sniffed glue for 5 years developed progressive optic neuropathy accompanied by severe sensorineural hearing loss.[134] More subtle but persistent visual abnormalities were described in 12 adolescent glue sniffers.[135] Two young paint sniffers with optic neuropathy, dementia, and cerebellar ataxia had abnormal brain stem auditory evoked potentials and CT evidence of pontomedullary atrophy.[136] Horizontal and vertical pendular nystagmus in four chronic glue sniffers was attributed to brain stem and cerebellar white matter damage; all four additionally had visual impairment, and two had optic atrophy.[137]

A 15-year-old boy developed status epilepticus while sniffing glue and thereafter had chronic epilepsy and behavioral problems.[138] A 22-year-old man who had sniffed lacquer thinner for nearly a decade developed hypokalemic periodic paralysis; attacks of weakness and hypokalemic hyperchloremic metabolic acidosis correlated temporally with toluene exposure.[139] Toluene probably does not cause peripheral neuropathy.[97,123]

Combined carbon monoxide and methanol poisoning affected a 17-year-old boy who sniffed a carburetor cleaner containing toluene and methylene chloride (which is metabolized to carbon dioxide and carbon monoxide); marked metabolic acidosis and elevated blood carboxyhemoglobin levels cleared with oxygen and ethanol treatment.[140]

In contrast to toluene, carbon tetrachloride causes delirium, cerebellar ataxia, seizures, and coma after brief exposure. Patients often have several days of headache and myalgia and then develop jaundice, renal failure, congestive heart failure, and CNS symptoms. Autopsies show Purkinje cell loss and perivenous hemorrhages most prominent in the cerebellum and basis pontis.[141–143]

Well studied is peripheral neuropathy in glue and lacquer-thinner sniffers.[97,144–152] Paresthesias in the feet are followed by ascending weakness and atrophy, leading to quadriplegia over a few weeks. Trophic changes are common, and cranial neuropathies occur. Cerebrospinal fluid is normal, or there is mildly elevated protein content. Nerve conduction velocities are reduced, and nerve biopsy reveals segmental distention of axons by masses of neurofilaments and secondary demyelination. Incomplete improvement occurs with abstinence, and the occasional presence of spasticity during recovery suggests that CNS damage also occurs but is masked by the peripheral signs. The responsible toxin is n-hexane, the metabolic product of which, 2,5-hexane-dione, is also the metabolite of methyl-n-butyl-ketone, a cause of peripheral neuropathy in industrial workers.[153] Both n-hexane and 2,3-hexane-dione cause peripheral nerve and CNS axonal degeneration in rats,[154,155] and n-hexane is also probably the responsible toxin in peripheral neuropathy associated with naphtha sniffing.[156] That additional substances in glue are neurotoxic is suggested by an epidemic of peripheral neuropathy among Berlin glue sniffers after methyl-ethyl-ketone was added to the n-hexane-containing product.[157] Severe polyneuropathy also affects sniffers of lacquer thinners containing n-heptane, and in other cases of solvent-related

peripheral neuropathy trichloroethylene may contribute.[158,159] In the 1970s, oil of mustard, which irritates mucous membranes, was added to a number of glue products to discourage abuse.[160]

Parkinsonism followed years of occupational exposure to n-hexane in a middle-aged woman,[161] and rodents given n-hexane or 2,5-hexane-dione have reduced striatal levels of dopamine and homovanillic acid (but not norepinephrine or serotonin).[162] As with 1-methyl-4-phenyl-1,2,3,6-tetrahydropyridine (MPTP) (see Chapter 2), the association has raised the possibility that human Parkinson's disease is related to similar environmental toxins.[163]

Trichloroethylene, present in dry cleaning fluids, causes trigeminal neuropathy.[97,164] The mechanism is unclear, but the association led to its use earlier in this century to treat trigeminal neuralgia.

A 12-year-old habitual glue sniffer developed dense hemiparesis, and cerebral angiography showed occlusion of the middle cerebral artery. A proposed mechanism was vasospasm secondary to trichloroethylene-induced sensitization of vessel receptors to circulating catecholamines.[165] Radioisotope brain scan in a boy with status epilepticus after toluene sniffing showed several wedge-shaped areas of increased uptake in both cerebral hemispheres, consistent with infarcts.[166] Few studies in either animals or humans have addressed the effects of solvents on cerebral circulation. Chloroform, diethyl ether, and trichloroethylene are cerebral vasodilators, but chronic use leads to decreased cerebral blood flow.[167]

Popular among frequenters of disco-bars are amyl, butyl, and isobutyl nitrite ("snappers," "poppers," "pearls"). To circumvent Food and Drug Administration (FDA) regulations, butyl and isobutyl nitrite are sold in "head shops" as "room odorizers," "liquid aroma," or "liquid incense." Believed to enhance sexual pleasure, especially among homosexuals, they carry such trade names as "Rush," "Locker Room," "Heart On," "Bang," "Climax," and "Mama Poppers" and are often taken with ethanol, marijuana, or sedatives.[168] In 1986, 9% of American high school seniors reported having used alkyl nitrites at least once.[23] The euphoric "high" lasts only seconds to minutes. Cerebral vasodilation and increased intracranial pressure accompany the euphoria; headache and nausea are frequent. There is also peripheral vasodilation, flushing, and a feeling of warmth.[168–170] Irritating to skin and mucous membranes, nitrites cause crusty perioral and nasal lesions and tracheobronchitis.[170] Nitrites also cause methemoglobinemia, but syncope tends to limit the dosage when they are inhaled. Ingestion, however, has caused collapse, coma, and death despite treatment with methylene blue.[171–176]

Rupture of a basilar artery aneurysm occurred during sexual intercourse following nitrite inhalation in a 43-year-old man.[177]

Nitrites are immunosuppressive,[178] and among their metabolites are carcinogenic nitrosoamines.[168,179] It is possible that nitrites carry independent risk either for acquiring human immunodeficiency virus (HIV) infection during homosexual intercourse or for developing Kaposi's sarcoma once infected.[169,179] In an epidemiologic study of homosexual couples in Boston, the odds ratio (OR) for HIV infection was much greater among men who always used nitrites during unprotected receptive anal intercourse (OR = 31.8) than among men who sometimes (OR = 7.1) or never (OR = 9.0) used them.[180] A study of homosexual HIV-infected men from Vancouver found nitrites an independent risk factor for Kaposi's sarcoma.[181] A similar study from San Francisco did not.[182]

Not surprisingly, health care personnel are overrepresented among abusers of volatile anesthetics, especially nitrous oxide.[183–185] A survey at a leading American medical school revealed that up to 20% of medical and dental students used nitrous oxide recreationally, usually from whipped cream cans or cartridges, but sometimes from medical or commercial sources.[183] Anoxic brain damage, sometimes fatal, has been reported in nitrous oxide abusers.[186–188] Pneumomediastinum has resulted from inhalation of pressurized nitrous oxide,[189] and acute pulmonary insufficiency followed inhalation of homemade nitrous oxide contaminated by nitrogen dioxide.[190]

Myeloneuropathy after prolonged exposure to nitrous oxide clinically resembles subacute combined degeneration secondary to cobalamin (vitamin B_{12}) deficiency. At least 28 patients have been reported with varying combinations of peripheral neuropathy, myelopathy, and altered mentation.[191–201] Electrophysiologic studies have revealed abnormal somatosensory evoked responses and visual evoked responses.[200,201] Anemia has been conspicuously absent, and subtle hematological abnormalities—macrocytosis or neutrophil hypersegmentation—have been infrequent. In 16 patients whose serum cobalamin was measured, it was normal in 13 and slightly decreased in 3.[191,193,195,196,201] Shilling tests have been normal except in one patient with a low normal serum cobalamin level and malabsorption consistent with pernicious anemia.[201]

A similar syndrome with typical pathological findings affects monkeys and fruit bats (but not mice or rats) exposed to nitrous oxide for prolonged periods.[202,203] Briefer heavy human exposure to nitrous oxide, moreover, causes megaloblastic bone marrow changes,[204] and both anemia and myeloneuropathy have been precipitated or exacerbated in cobalamin deficient patients undergoing nitrous oxide anesthesia.[205–207] Nitrous oxide oxidizes cobalamin, rendering inactive the vitamin B_{12}-dependent enzymes methionine synthetase[208] and methylmalonyl-CoA mutase,[209] and in a nitrous oxide abuser methylmalonic acid levels were increased in serum and, to an even greater degree, in cerebrospinal fluid.[201] Methionine supplementation protects nitrous oxide–exposed animals from myelopathy.[210]

Fatal hepatitis and sudden death have occurred in hospital workers who deliberately inhaled, ingested, or injected halothane.[211–213] Among German adolescents, coma has followed chloroform sniffing.[214]

Reports from England describe abuse of the antiasthmatic aerosol preparation of salbutamol, a beta-2-adrenergic agonist.[215–217] Probably both salbutamol itself (which has amphetamine-like effects) and fluorocarbons in the mixture contribute to addiction liability.[218,219]

Effects in Pregnancy

Inhalant abuse before delivery causes neonatal depression.[44] Teratogenicity is more difficult to prove.[220] Congenital cerebellar ataxia was reported in offspring of mothers who abused toluene during pregnancy.[120,221] Some workers have claimed a "fetal solvent syndrome" similar to the "fetal alcohol syndrome," with microcephaly, craniofacial anomalies, and retarded growth.[222–226] Of nine women giving birth to children with sacral agenesis, five had been exposed to xylene, trichloroethylene, methyl chloride, acetone, or gasoline.[227] Two case-control studies from Finland found an association between in utero solvent exposure and congenital CNS anomalies;[220,228] another Finnish case-control study did not.[229] In other studies, in utero solvent exposure was implicated in cleft palate[230] and cardiovascular malformations.[231] In a cohort study from California, there was no difference in neurobehavioral development between children who were exposed in utero to solvents and those who were not.[232] The same study, however, found an association between solvent exposure and preeclampsia.[233]

Rats exposed in utero to toluene had decreased fetal weight and retarded skeletal growth.[234] In exposed fetal mice, inhaled toluene was not associated with specific malformations,[235] but ingested toluene produced cleft palate.[236]

Exposure of rats to large doses of nitrous oxide led to congenital malformations in offspring.[237] Exposure to small doses led to reduced fertility.[238] In a study of dental assistants, women exposed to high levels of nitrous oxide were less fertile than women who were unexposed or exposed only to low levels.[239]

Severe mental retardation, hypotonia, and microcephaly with a prominent occiput were present in two children born to gasoline-sniffing parents.[240]

Long-Term Treatment

Long-term treatment of inhalant abuse has special difficulties. No pharmacotherapy exists. Addicts, whether juvenile or adult, tend to be social isolates lacking the cognitive capacity to participate in a rehabilitation program. Many also abuse ethanol and other drugs. Others deny that inhalant use is a form of drug abuse: "I don't do drugs, I just do tywol" (toluene).[241]

References

1. Evans EB, Balster RL. CNS depressant effects of volatile organic solvents. Neurosci Biochem Rev 1991; 15:233.
2. Glowa JR, Dews PB. Behavioral toxicology of volatile organic solvents. IV. Comparisons of the rate-decreasing effects of acetone, ethyl acetate, methyl ethyl ketone, toluene, and carbon disulfide on schedule-controlled behavior of mice. J Am Coll Toxicol 1987; 6:461.
3. Hinman DJ. Biphasic dose-response relationship for effects of toluene on locomotor activity. Pharmacol Biochem Behav 1987; 26:65.
4. Wood RW, Coleman JB, Schuler R, Cox C. Anticonvulsant and antipunishment effects of toluene. J Pharmacol Exp Ther 1984; 230:407.
5. Rees DC, Wood RW, Laties VG. Evidence of tolerance following repeated exposure to toluene in the rat. Pharmacol Biochem Behav 1989; 32:283.
6. Moser VC, Balster RL. The effects of acute and repeated toluene exposure on operant behavior in mice. Neurobehav Toxicol Teratol 1981; 3:471.
7. Taylor JD, Evans HL. Effects of toluene inhalation on behavior and expired carbon dioxide in macaque monkeys. Toxicol Appl Pharmacol 1985; 80:487.
8. Moser VC, Scimeca JA, Balster RL. Minimal tolerance to the effects of 1,1,1-trichloroethane on fixed ratio responding in mice. Neurotoxicology 1985; 6:35.
9. Yanagita T, Takahashi S, Ishida K, Fumamoto H. Voluntary inhalation of volatile anesthetics and organic solvents by monkeys. Jpn J Clin Pharmacol 1970; 1:13.
10. Wood RW, Grubman J, Weiss B. Nitrous oxide self-administration by the squirrel monkey. J Pharmacol Exp Ther 1977; 202:491.
11. Rees DC, Coggeshall E, Balster RL. Inhaled toluene produces pentobarbital-like discriminative stimulus effects in mice. Life Sci 1985; 37:1319.
12. Rees DC, Knisely JS, Balster RL, et al. Pentobarbital-like discriminative stimulus properties of halothane, 1,1,1-trichloroethane, isoamyl nitrite, flurothyl and oxazepam in mice. J Pharmacol Exp Ther 1987; 241:507.
13. Woolverton WL, Balster RL. Behavioral and lethal effects of combinations of oral ethanol and inhaled 1,1,1-trichloroethane in mice. Toxicol Appl Pharmacol 1981; 59:1.
14. Nagle DR. Anesthetic addiction and drunkenness: a contemporary and historical survey. Int J Addict 1968; 3:25.
15. Cartwright FF. The English Pioneers of Anesthesia. Bristol: John Wright and Sons Ltd, London, 1952.
16. Layzer RB. Nitrous oxide abuse. In: Eger EI, ed. Nitrous Oxide/N$_2$O. New York: Elsevier, 1985:249.
17. Cohen S. Inhalant abuse: an overview of the problem. In: Sharp CW, Brehm MS, eds. Review of Inhalants: Euphoria to Dysfunction. Washington, DC: NIDA Research Monograph 15, DHEW, 1977:2.
18. Kerner K. Current topics in inhalant abuse. In: Crider REA, Rouse BA, eds. Epidemiology of Inhalant Abuse: An Update. Rockville, MD: NIDA Research Monograph 85, DHHS, 1988:8.
19. Lenore R, Kupperstein LR, Susman RM. Bibliography of the inhalation of glue fumes and other toxic vapors. Int J Addict 1968; 3:177.
20. Brecher EM. Licit and Illicit Drugs. Boston: Little, Brown, 1972.
21. Fishburne PM, Abelson HL, Cisin I. National Survey on Drug Abuse: Main Findings 1979. Washington, DC: DHHS Publication No(ADM) 80-976, 1980.
22. Barnes GE. Solvent abuse: a review. Int J Addict 1979; 14:1.
23. Johnston L, Bachman J, O'Malley P. Use of Licit and Illicit Drugs for America's High School Students, 1975–1986. Washington, DC: NIDA, DHHS Publication No(ADM) 85-1394, US Government Printing Office, 1987.
24. Nicholi AM. The nontherapeutic use of psychoactive drugs. A modern epidemic. N Engl J Med 1983; 308:925.
25. Johns A. Volatile substance abuse and 963 deaths. Br J Addict 1991; 86:1053.
26. Easson WM. Gasoline addiction in children. Pediatrics 1962; 29:250.
27. Press E, Done AK. Solvent sniffing. Physiologic effects and community control measures for intoxication from the intentional inhalation of organic solvents. I. Pediatrics 1967; 39:451.
28. Beauvais F, Oetting ER. Inhalant abuse by young children. In: Crider RA, Rouse BA, eds. Epidemiology of Inhalant Abuse: An Update. Rockville, MD: NIDA Research Monograph 85, DHHS, 1988:30.

29. Ramsey J, Anderson HR, Bloor K, Flanagan RJ. An introduction to the practice, prevalence, and chemical toxicology of volatile substance abuse. Hum Toxicol 1989; 8:261.

30. Nicholi AM. The inhalants: an overview. Psychosomatics 1983; 24:914.

31. Moosa A, Loening WEK. Solvent abuse in black children in Natal. S Afr Med J 1981; 59:509.

32. Eastwell HD, Thomas BJ, Thomas BW. Skeletal lead burden in Aborigine petrol sniffing. Lancet 1983; 2:524.

33. Davathasan G, Low D, Teoh PC, et al. Complications of chronic glue toluene abuse in adolescents. Aust NZ J Med 1984; 14:39.

34. Watson JM. Solvent abuse and adolescents. Practitioner 1984; 228:487.

35. Morton HG. Occurrence and treatment of solvent abuse in children and adolescents. Pharmacol Ther 1987; 33:449.

36. Tamura M. Japan: stimulant epidemics past and present. Bull Narc 1989; 41:83.

37. Bachrach KM, Sandler IN. A retrospective assessment of inhalant abuse in the barrio: implications for prevention. Int J Addict 1985; 20:1177.

38. Dinwiddie SH, Reich T, Cloninger CR. The relationship of solvent use to other substance use. Am J Drug Alcohol Abuse 1991; 17:173.

39. Kaufman A. Gasoline sniffing among children in a Pueblo Indian village. Pediatrics 1973; 51:1060.

40. Seshia SS, Rajani KR, Boeckx RL, Chow PN. The neurological manifestations of chronic inhalation of leaded gasoline. Dev Med Child Neurol 1978; 20:323.

41. Remington G, Hoffman BF. Gas sniffing as a form of substance abuse. Can J Psychiatry 1984; 29:31.

42. Garriott JJ, Petty CS. Death from inhalant abuse: toxicological and pathological evaluation of 34 cases. Clin Toxicol 1980; 16:305.

43. Oetting ER, Edwards RW, Beauvais F. Social and psychological factors underlying inhalant abuse. In: Crider RA, Rouse BA, eds. Epidemiology of Inhalant Abuse: An Update. Rockville, MD: NIDA Research Monograph 85, DHHS, 1988:172.

44. Ashton CH. Solvent abuse. BMJ 1990; 300:135.

45. Westermeyer J. The psychiatrist and solvent-inhalant abuse: recognition, assessment, and treatment. Am J Psychiatry 1987; 144:903.

46. Press E, Done AK. Solvent sniffing. Physiologic effects and community control measures for intoxication from the intentional inhalation of organic solvents. II. Pediatrics 1967; 39:611.

47. Kerr N. Ether inebriety. JAMA 1891; 17:791.

48. Crider RA, Rouse BA. Inhalant overview. In: Crider RA, Rouse BA, eds. Epidemiology of Inhalant Abuse: An Update. Rockville, MD: NIDA Research Monograph 85, DHHS, 1988:1.

49. Ferguson CA. Chemical abuse in the north. Univ Manitoba Med J 1975; 45:129.

50. Storms WW. Chloroform parties. JAMA 1973; 225:160.

51. Marsh WW. Butane firebreathing in adolescents: a potentially dangerous practice. J Adolesc Health Care 1984; 5:59.

52. Jones NP. Self-enucleation and psychosis. Br J Ophthalmol 1990; 74:571.

53. Ackerly WC, Gibson G. Lighter fluid "sniffing." Am J Psychiatry 1964; 120:1056.

54. Tolan EJ, Lingl FA. "Model psychosis" produced by inhalation of gasoline fumes. Am J Psychiatry 1964; 120:757.

55. Meredith TJ, Ruprah M, Liddle A, Flanagan RJ. Diagnosis and treatment of acute poisoning with volatile substances Hum Toxicol 1989; 8:277.

56. Watson JM. Solvent abuse and adolescents. Practitioner 1984; 228:487.

57. Cohen S. The hallucinogens and the inhalants. Psychiatr Clin North Am 1984; 7:681.

58. Herzberg JL, Wolkind SN. Solvent sniffing in perspective. Br J Hosp Med 1983; 29:72.

59. Bass M. Sudden sniffing death. JAMA 1970; 212:2075.

60. Musclow CE, Awen CF. Glue-sniffing. Report of a fatal case. Can Med Assoc J 1971; 104:315.

61. Winek CL, Collom WD. Benzene and toluene fatalities. J Occup Med 1971; 13:259.

62. Cohen S. Inhalants. In: DuPont RI, Goldstein A, O'Donnell JJ, eds. Handbook on Drug Abuse. Washington, DC: US Government Printing Office, 1979:213.

63. Edwards IR. Solvent abuse. NZ Med J 1982; 95:879.

64. Steadman C, Dorrington LC, Kay P, Stephens H. Abuse of a fire-extinguishing agent and sudden death in adolescents. Med J Aust 1984; 140:54.

65. McBride P, Busuttil A. A new trend in solvent abuse deaths? Med Sci Law 1990; 30:207.

66. Anderson HR, Macnair RS, Ramsey JD. Deaths from abuse of volatile substances: a national epidemiological study. BMJ 1985; 290:304.

67. Wason S, Gibler B, Hassan M. Ventricular tachycardia associated with non-Freon aerosol propellants. JAMA 1986; 256:78.

68. Shepherd RT. Mechanism of sudden death associated with volatile substance abuse. Hum Toxicol 1989; 8:287.

69. Garb S, Chenoweth MB. Studies on hydrocarbon epinephrine induced ventricular fibrillation. J Pharmacol 1948; 94:12.

70. Cunningham SR, Dalyell GWN, McGirr P, Khan MM. Myocardial infarction and primary ventricular fibrillation after glue sniffing. BMJ 1987; 294:739.

71. Wodka RM, Jeong EWS. Cardiac effects of inhaled typewriter correction fluid. Ann Intern Med 1989; 110:91.

72. Cronk SL, Barkley DEH, Farrell MF. Respiratory arrest after solvent abuse. BMJ 1985; 290:897.

73. Chowdhury JK. Acute ventilatory failure from sniffing paint. Chest 1977; 71:687.

74. Carroll H, Abel G. Chronic gasoline inhalation. South Med J 1973; 66:1429.

75. Heath MJ. Solvent abuse using bromochlorodifluoromethane from a fire extinguisher. Med Sci Law 1986; 26:33.
76. Siegel E, Wason S. Sudden death caused by inhalation of butane and propane. N Engl J Med 1990; 323:1638.
77. Cohen S. Glue sniffing. JAMA 1975; 231:653.
78. Merry J, Zachariades N. Addiction to glue-sniffing. BMJ 1962; 2:1448.
79. Crites J, Schukit MA. Solvent misuse in adolescents at a community alcohol center. J Clin Psychiatry 1979; 40:39.
80. Skuse D, Burrell S. A review of solvent abusers and their management by a child-psychiatric outpatient service. Hum Toxicol 1982; 1:321.
81. Sourindhrin I, Baird JA. Management of solvent misuse: a Glasgow community approach. Br J Addict 1984; 79:227.
82. Mee AS, Wright PL. Congestive (dilated) cardiomyopathy in association with solvent abuse. J R Soc Med 1980; 73:671.
83. Marjot R, McLeod AA. Chronic non-neurological toxicity from volatile substance abuse. Hum Toxicol 1989; 8:301.
84. Baerg RD, Kimberg DV. Centrolobular hepatic necrosis and acute renal failure in "solvent sniffers." Ann Intern Med 1970; 73:713.
85. Brown JH, Hadden DR, Hadden DS. Solvent abuse, toluene acidosis and diabetic ketoacidosis. Arch Emerg Med 1991; 8:65.
86. Powars D. Aplastic anemia secondary to glue sniffing. N Engl J Med 273; 700:1965.
87. Schikler KN, Lane EE, Seitz K, Collins WM. Solvent abuse associated with pulmonary abnormalities. Adv Alcohol Subst Abuse 1984; 3:75.
88. Rafferty P. Voluntary chlorine inhalation: a new form of self-abuse? BMJ 1980; 281:1178.
89. Chalupa B, Synkova J, Seveik M. The assessment of electroencephalographic changes and memory disturbances in acute intoxications with industrial poisons. Br J Indust Med 1960; 17:238.
90. Berry GJ. Neuropsychological assessment of solvent inhalants In: Sharp CW, Carroll LT, eds. First International Symposium on Voluntary Inhalation of Industrial Solvents. Washington, DC: DHHS Publication No (ADM) 79-779. US Government Printing Office, 1978.
91. Korman M, Matthews R, Lovitt R. Neuropsychological effects of abuse of inhalants. Percept Mot Skills 1981; 53:547.
92. Allison WM, Jerrom DW. Glue-sniffing: A pilot study of the cognitive effects of long-term use. Int J Addict 1984; 19:453.
93. Bigler ED. Neuropsychological evaluation of adolescent patients hospitalized with chronic inhalant abuse. Clin Neuropsychol 1979; 1:8.
94. Ron MA. Volatile substance abuse: a review of possible long-term neurological, intellectual, and psychiatric sequelae. Br J Psychiatry 1986; 148:235.
95. Arlien-Soborg P, Henriksen L, Gade A, et al. Cerebral blood flow in chronic toxic encephalopathy in house painters exposed to organic solvents. Acta Neurol Scand 1982; 66:34.
96. Chadwick OFD, Anderson HR. Neuropsychological consequences of volatile substance abuse: a review. Hum Toxicol 1989; 8:307.
97. Lolin Y. Chronic neurological toxicity associated with exposure to volatile substances. Hum Toxicol 1989; 8:293.
98. Zur J, Yule W. Chronic solvent abuse. 1. Cognitive sequelae. Child Care Health Dev 1990; 16:1.
99. Boeckx RL, Postle B, Coodin FJ. Gasoline sniffing and tetraethyl lead poisoning in children. Pediatrics 1977; 60:140.
100. Fortenberry JD. Gasoline sniffing. Am J Med 1985; 79:740.
101. Coulehan JL, Hirsh W, Brillman J, et al. Gasoline sniffing and lead toxicity in Navajo adolescents. Pediatrics 1983; 71:113.
102. Young RSK, Grzyb SE, Crisman L. Recurrent cerebellar dysfunction as related to chronic gasoline sniffing in an adolescent girl. Clin Pediatr 1977; 16:706.
103. Procop LD, Karampelas D. Encephalopathy secondary to abusive gasoline inhalation. J Fla Med Ass 1981; 68:823.
104. Robinson RO. Tetraethyl lead poisoning from gasoline sniffing. JAMA 1978; 240:1373.
105. Valpey R, Sumi S, Copass MK, Goble GJ. Acute and chronic progressive encephalopathy due to gasoline sniffing. Neurology 1978; 28:507.
106. Hansen KS, Sharp FR. Gasoline sniffing, lead poisoning, and myoclonus. JAMA 1978; 240:1375.
107. Chiba M, Toyada T, Inaba Y, et al. Acute lead poisoning in an adult from ingestion of paint. N Engl J Med 1980; 303:459.
108. Karani V. Peripheral neuritis after addiction to petrol. BMJ 1966; 2:216.
109. Grabski D. Toluene sniffing producing cerebellar degeneration. Am J Psychiatry 1961; 118:461.
110. Satran R, Dodson VN. Toluence habituation: report of a case. N Engl J Med 1963; 268:719.
111. Knox JW, Nelson JR. Permanent encephalopathy from toluene inhalation. N Engl J Med 1966; 275:1494.
112. Kelly T. Prolonged cerebellar dysfunction associated with paint-sniffing. Pediatrics 1975; 56:605.
113. Procop LD. Neuropathy in an artist. Hosp Pract 1978; 13:89.
114. Fornazzari L, Wilkinson D, Kapur B, Carlen P. Cerebellar, cortical and functional impairment in toluene abuse. Acta Neurol Scand 1983; 67:319.
115. King MD. Neurological sequelae of toluene abuse. Hum Toxicol 1982; 1:281.
116. Boor JW, Hurtig HI. Persistent cerebellar ataxia after exposure to toluene. Ann Neurol 1977; 2:440.
117. Escobar A, Aruffo C. Chronic thinner intoxication: clinicopathologic report of a human case. J Neurol Neurosurg Psychiatry 1980; 43:986.
118. Malm G, Lying-Tunell V. Cerebellar dysfunction related to toluene sniffing. Acta Neurol Scand 1980; 62:188.

119. Lazar RB, Ho SU, Melen O, Daghestani AN. Multifocal central nervous system damage caused by toluene abuse. Neurology 1983; 33:1337.

120. Streicher HZ, Gabow PA, Moss AH, et al. Syndromes of toluene sniffing in adults. Ann Intern Med 1981; 94:758.

121. Taher SM, Anderson RJ, McCartney R, et al. Renal tubular acidosis associated with toluene "sniffing." N Engl J Med 1974; 290:765.

122. Fischman CM, Oster JR. Toxic effects of toluene: a new cause of high anion gap metabolic acidosis. JAMA 1979; 241:1714.

123. Hormes JT, Filley CM, Rosenberg NL. Neurologic sequelae of chronic vapor abuse. Neurology 1986; 36:698.

124. Rosenberg NL, Kleinschmidt-DeMasters BK, Davis KA, et al. Toluene abuse causes diffuse central nervous system white matter changes. Ann Neurol 1988; 23:611.

125. Filley CM, Heaton RK, Rosenberg NL. White matter dementia in chronic toluene abuse. Neurology 1990; 40:532.

126. Morrow L, Callender T, Lottenberg S, et al. PET and neurobehavioral evidence of tetrabromoethane encephalopathy. J Neuropsychiatr Clin Neurosci 1990; 2:431.

127. Morrow L, Steinhauer SR, Hodgeson MJ. Delay in P300 latency in patients with organic solvent exposure. Arch Neurol 1992; 49:315.

128. Miyake H, Ikeda T, Maehara N, et al. Slow learning in rats due to long-term inhalation of toluene. Neurobehav Toxicol Teratol 1983; 5:541.

129. Lorenzana-Jiminez M, Salas M. Neonatal effects of toluene on motor behavior development of the rat. Neurobehav Toxicol Teratol 1983; 5:295.

130. Pryor GT, Dickinson J, Howd RA, Rebert CS. Neurobehavioral effects of subchronic exposure of weaning rats to toluene or hexane. Neurobehav Toxicol Teratol 1983; 5:47.

131. Pryor GT, Dickinson J, Howd RA, Rebert CS. Transient cognitive deficits and high-frequency hearing loss in weanling rats exposed to toluene. Neurobehav Toxicol Teratol 1983; 5:53.

132. Pryor GT. Persisting neurotoxic consequences of solvent abuse: a developing animal model for toluene-induced neurotoxicity. In: Spencer JW, Boren JJ, eds. Residual Effects of Abused Drugs on Behavior. Rockville, MD: NIDA Research Monograph 101, DHHS, 1990:156.

133. Keane JR. Toluene optic neuropathy. Ann Neurol 1978; 4:390.

134. Ehyai A, Freeman FR. Progressive optic neuropathy and sensorineural hearing loss due to chronic glue sniffing. J Neurol Neurosurg Psychiatry 1983; 46:349.

135. Cooper R, Newton P, Reed M. Neurophysiological signs of brain damage due to glue sniffing. Electroencephalogr Clin Neurophysiol 1985; 60:23.

136. Mettrick SA, Brenner RP. Abnormal brainstem auditory evoked potentials in chronic paint sniffers. Ann Neurol 1982; 12:553.

137. Maas FF, Ashe J, Spiegel P, et al. Acquired pendular nystagmus in toluene addiction. Neurology 1991; 41:282.

138. Allister C, Lush M, Oliver JS, Watson JM. Status epilepticus caused by solvent abuse. BMJ 1981; 283:1156.

139. Bennett RH, Forman HR. Hypokalemic periodic paralysis in chronic toluene exposure. Arch Neurol 1980; 37:673.

140. McCormick MJ, Mogabgab E, Adams SL. Methanol poisoning as a result of inhalational solvent abuse. Ann Emerg Med 1990; 19:639.

141. Cohen MM. Central nervous system in carbon tetrachloride intoxication. Neurology 1957; 7:238.

142. Luse SA, Wood WG. The brain in fatal carbon tetrachloride poisoning. Arch Neurol 1967; 17:304.

143. Johnson BP, Meredith TJ, Vale JA. Cerebellar dysfunction after acute carbon tetrachloride poisoning. Lancet 1983; 2:968.

144. Gonzalez E, Downey J. Polyneuropathy in a glue sniffer. Arch Phys Med 1972; 53:333.

145. Matsumura M, Inoue N, Ohnishi A. Toxic polyneuropathy due to glue sniffing. Clin Neurol 1972; 12:290.

146. Goto I, Matsumura M, Inoue N, et al. Toxic polyneuropathy due to glue-sniffing. J Neurol Neurosurg Psychiatry 1974; 7:848.

147. Shirabe T, Tsuda T, Terao AA, Araki S. Toxic polyneuropathy due to glue sniffing: report of two cases with a light and electron microscopic study of the peripheral nerves and muscles. J Neurol Sci 1974; 21:101.

148. Procop LD, Alt M, Tison J. Huffer's neuropathy. JAMA 1974; 229:1083.

149. Korobkin R, Asbury AK, Sumner AJ, Nielsen SL. Glue-sniffing neuropathy. Arch Neurol 1975; 32:158.

150. Oh S, Kim J. Giant axonal swelling in "huffer's neuropathy." Arch Neurol 1976; 33:583.

151. Means ED, Procop LD, Hooper GS. Pathology of lacquer thinner-induced neuropathy. Ann Clin Lab Sci 1976; 6:240.

152. Means ED, Tison J, Procop LD. Experimental lacquer thinner neuropathy. Neurology 1978; 28:333.

153. Mendell J, Saida K, Ganansi M. Toxic polyneuropathy produced by methyl-n-butyl ketone. Science 1974; 185:787.

154. Schaumburg H, Spencer P. Degeneration in central and peripheral nervous systems produced by pure n-hexane: an experimental study. Brain 1976; 99:183.

155. Spencer P, Schaumburg H. Experimental neuropathy produced by 2,5-hexanedione—a major metabolite of the neurotoxic industrial solvent methyl-n-butyl ketone. J Neurol Neurosurg Psychiatry 1975; 38:771.

156. Tenenbein M, DeGroot W, Rajamo KR. Peripheral neuropathy following intentional inhalation of naphtha. Can Med Assoc J 1984; 131:1077.

157. Altenkirch H, Mager J, Stoltenburg G, Helmbrecht J. Toxic polyneuropathies after sniffing a glue thinner. J Neurol 1977; 214:137.

158. Bruchner JV, Petersen RG. Toxicology of aliphatic and aromatic hydrocarbons. In: Sharp CW, Brehm ML, eds. Review of Inhalants: Euphoria to Dysfunction. Washington, DC: NIDA Research Monograph 15, DHEW, 1977:124.

159. Hayden J, Comstock E, Comstock B. The clinical toxicology of solvent abuse. Clin Toxicol 1976; 9:169.

160. Procop L. Neurotoxic volatile substances. Neurology 1979; 29:862.

161. Pezzoli G, Ferrante C, Barbieri S, et al. Parkinsonism due to n-hexane exposure. Lancet 1989; 2:874.

162. Pezzoli G, Ricciardi S, Masotto C, et al. n-hexane induces parkinsonism in rodents. Brain Res 1990; 531:355.

163. Pezzoli G, Perbellini L, Zecchinelli A, et al. n-hexane and parkinsonism. Neurology 1992; 42(suppl 3):283.

164. Mitchell ABS, Parsons-Smith BG. Trichloroethylene neuropathy. BMJ 1969; 1:422.

165. Parker MJ, Tarlow MJ, Milne-Anderson J. Glue sniffing and cerebral infarction. Arch Dis Child 1984; 59:675.

166. Lamont CM, Adams FG. Glue-sniffing as a cause of a positive radio-isotope brain scan. Eur J Nucl Med 1982; 7:387.

167. Mathew RJ, Wilson WH. Substance abuse and cerebral blood flow. Am J Psychiatry 1991; 148:292.

168. Sharp CW, Stillman RC. Blush not with nitrites. Ann Intern Med 1980; 92:700.

169. Newell GR, Spitz MR, Wilson MB. Nitrite inhalants: historical perspective. In: Haverkos HW, Dougherty JA, eds. Health Hazards of Nitrite Inhalants. Rockville, MD: NIDA Research Monograph 83, DHHS, 1988:1.

170. Wood RW. The acute toxicity of nitrite inhalants. In: Haverkos HW, Dougherty JA, eds. Health Hazards of Nitrite Inhalants. Rockville, MD: NIDA Research Monograph 83, DHHS, 1988:28.

171. Horne MK, Waterman MR, Simon LM, et al. Methemoglobinemia from sniffing butyl nitrite. Ann Intern Med 1979; 91:417.

172. Haley TJ. Review of the physiological effects of amyl, butyl, and isobutyl nitrites. Clin Toxicol 1980; 16:317.

173. Shesser RS, Dixon D, Allen Y, et al. Fatal methemoglobinemia from butyl nitrite ingestion. Ann Intern Med 1980; 92:131.

174. Wason S, Detsky AS, Platt OS, Lovejoy FH. Isobutyl nitrite toxicity by ingestion. Ann Intern Med 1980; 92:637.

175. Dixon DS, Reisch RF, Santinga PH. Fatal methemoglobinemia resulting from ingestion of isobutyl nitrite, a "room odorizer" widely used for recreational purposes. J Forens Sci 1981; 26:587.

176. Laaban JP, Bodenan P, Rochemaure J. Amyl nitrite poppers and methemoglobinemia. Ann Intern Med 1985; 103:804.

177. Nudelman RW, Salcman M. The birth of the blues. II: Blue movie. JAMA 1987; 257:3230.

178. Soderberg LS, Barnett JB. Exposure to inhaled isobutyl nitrite reduces T cell blastogenesis and antibody responsiveness. Fundam Appl Toxicol 1991; 17:821.

179. Haverkos HW. The search for cofactors in AIDS, including an analysis of the association of nitrite inhalant abuse and Kaposi's sarcoma. Prog Clin Biol Res 1990; 325:93.

180. Seage GR, Mayer KH, Horsburgh CR, et al. The relation between nitrite inhalants, unprotected receptive anal intercourse, and the risk of human immunodeficiency virus infection. Am J Epidemiol 1992; 135:1.

181. Archibald CP, Schechter MT, Craib KJ, et al. Risk factors for Kaposi's sarcoma in the Vancouver Lymphadenopathy-AIDS Study. J AIDS 1990; 3(suppl 1):S18.

182. Lifson AR, Darrow WW, Hessol NA, et al. Kaposi's sarcoma among homosexual and bisexual men enrolled in the San Francisco City Clinic Cohort Study. J AIDS 1990; 3(suppl 1):S32.

183. Rosenberg H, Orkin FK, Springstead J. Abuse of nitrous oxide. Anesth Analg 1979; 58:104.

184. Nitrous oxide hazards. FDA Drug Bull 1980; 10:15.

185. Aston R. Drug abuse. Its relationship to dental practice. Dent Clin North Am 1984; 28:595.

186. Brillant L. Nitrous oxide as a psychedelic drug. N Engl J Med 1970; 283:1522.

187. DiMaio VJM, Garriott JC. Four deaths resulting from abuse of nitrous oxide. J Forens Sci 1978; 23:169.

188. Schwartz RH, Calihan M. Nitrous oxide: a potentially lethal euphoriant inhalant. Am Fam Phys 1984; 30:171.

189. LiPuma JP, Wellman J, Stern HP. Nitrous oxide abuse: a new cause for pneumomediastinum. Radiology 1982; 145:602.

190. Messina FV, Wynne JW. Homemade nitrous oxide: no laughing matter. Ann Intern Med 1982; 96:333.

191. Layzer R, Fishman R, Schafer J. Neuropathy following abuse of nitrous oxide. Neurology 1976; 28:504.

192. Sahenk Z, Mendell JR, Couri D, Nachtman J. Polyneuropathy from inhalation of N_2O cartridges through a whipped-cream dispenser. Neurology 1978; 28:485.

193. Layzer RB. Myeloneuropathy after prolonged exposure to nitrous oxide. Lancet 1978; 2:1227.

194. Paulson GW. "Recreational" misuse of nitrous oxide. J Am Dent Assoc 1979; 98:410.

195. Gutmann L, Farrell B, Crosby TW, Johnson D. Nitrous oxide–induced myelopathy-neuropathy: potential for chronic misuse by dentists. J Am Dent Assoc 1979; 98:58.

196. Nevins MA. Neuropathy after nitrous oxide abuse. JAMA 1980; 244:2264.

197. Gutmann L, Johnsen D. Nitrous oxide-induced myeloneuropathy: report of cases. J Am Dent Assoc 1981; 103:239.

198. Sterman AB, Coyle PK. Subacute toxic delirium following nitrous oxide abuse. Arch Neurol 1983; 40:446.

199. Blanco G, Peters HA. Myeloneuropathy and macrocytosis associated with nitrous oxide abuse. Arch Neurol 1983; 40:416.
200. Heyer EJ, Simpson DM, Bodis-Wollner I, Diamond SP. Nitrous oxide: clinical and electrophysiologic investigation of neurologic complications. Neurology 1986; 36:1618.
201. Stabler SP, Allen RH, Barrett RE, Savage DG, Lindenbaum J. Cerebrospinal fluid methylmalonic acid levels in normal subjects and patients with cobalamin deficiency. Neurology 1991; 41:1627.
202. Dinn JJ, McCann S, Wilson P, et al. Animal model for subacute combined degeneration. Lancet 1978; 2:1154.
203. van der Westhuyzen J, Fernandes-Costa F, Metz J. Cobalamin inactivation by nitrous oxide produces severe neurological impairment in fruit bats: protection by methionine and aggravation by folate. Life Sci 1982; 31:2001.
204. Amess JAC, Burman JF, Rees GM, et al. Megaloblastic hemopoiesis in patients receiving nitrous oxide. Lancet 1978; 2:1023.
205. Schilling RF. Is nitrous oxide a dangerous anesthetic for vitamin B$_{12}$-deficient subjects? JAMA 1986; 255:1605.
206. Berger JJ, Modell JH, Sypert GW. Megaloblastic anemia and brief exposure to nitrous oxide—a causal relationship? Anesth Analg 1988; 67:197.
207. Holloway KL, Alberico AM. Postoperative myeloneuropathy: a preventable complication in patients with B$_{12}$ deficiency. J Neurosurg 1990; 72:732.
208. Deacon R, Perry J, Lamb M, et al. Selective inactivation of vitamin B$_{12}$ in rats by nitrous oxide. Lancet 1978; 2:1023.
209. Kondo H, Osborne ML, Kolhouse JF, et al. Nitrous oxide has multiple deleterious effects on cobalamin metabolism and causes decreases in activities of both mammalian cobalamin-dependent enzymes in rats. J Clin Invest 1981; 67:1270.
210. Van der Westhuyzen J, Van Tonder S, Gibson JE, et al. Plasma amino acids and tissue methionine levels in fruit bats (Rousettus aegyptiacus) with nitrous oxide–induced vitamin B$_{12}$ deficiency. Br J Nutr 1984; 53:657.
211. Spencer JD, Raasch FO, Trefny FA. Halothane abuse in hospital personnel. JAMA 1976; 235:1034.
212. Kaplan HG, Bakken J, Quadracci L, Schubach W. Hepatitis caused by halothane sniffing. Ann Intern Med 1979; 90:797.
213. Yamashita M, Matsuki A, Oyama T. Illicit use of modern volatile anesthetics. Can Anaesth Soc 1984; 31:76.
214. Beer J, Heer G, Schlup P. Chloroform sniffing: a new variant of substance abuse. Schweiz Med Wochenschr 1984; 114:1538.
215. Edwards JG, Holgate ST. Dependency on salbutamol inhalers. Br J Psychiatry 1979; 134:624.
216. Pratt HF. Abuse of salbutamol inhalers in young people. Clin Allergy 1982; 12:203.
217. Raine JM. Addiction to aerosol treatment. BMJ 1984; 288:241.
218. Brennan PO. Addiction to aerosol treatment. BMJ 1983; 287:1877.
219. Thompson PJ, Dhillan P, Cole P. Addiction to aerosol treatment: the asthmatic alternative to glue sniffing. BMJ 1983; 287:1515.
220. Holmberg PC. Central nervous system defects in children born to mothers exposed to organic solvents during pregnancy. Lancet 1979; 2:177.
221. Goodwin JM, Gail C, Grodner B, Metrick S. Inhalant abuse, pregnancy, and neglected children. Am J Psychiatry 1981; 138:1126.
222. Tourant C, Lippmann S. Fetal solvent syndrome. Lancet 1979; 1:1356.
223. Hersh JH, Podruch PE, Rogers G, Weisskopf B. Toluene embryopathy. J Pediatr 1985; 106:922.
224. Hersh JH. Toluene embryopathy: two new cases. J Med Genet 1989; 26:333.
225. Goodwin TM. Toluene abuse and renal tubular acidosis in pregnancy. Obstet Gynecol 1988; 71:715.
226. Fabro S, Brown NA, Scialli AR. Is there a fetal solvent syndrome? Reprod Toxicol Med Lett 1983; 2:17.
227. Kucera J. Exposure to fat solvents: a possible cause of sacral agenesis in man. J Pediatr 1969; 72:857.
228. Holmberg PC, Nurminen M. Congenital defects of the central nervous system and occupational factors during pregnancy. Am J Ind Med 1980; 1:167.
229. Rantala K, Riala R, Nurminen T. Screening for occupational exposures and congenital malformations. Scand J Work Environ Health 1983; 9:89.
230. Holmberg PC, Hernberg S, Kurppa K, et al. Oral clefts and organic solvent exposure during pregnancy. Int Arch Occup Environ Health 1982; 50:371.
231. Tikkanen J, Heinonen OP. Cardiovascular malformations and organic solvent exposure during pregnancy in Finland. Am J Ind Med 1988; 14:1.
232. Eskenazi B, Gaylord L, Bracken MB, Brown D. In utero exposure to organic solvents and human neurodevelopment. Dev Med Child Neurol 1988; 30:492.
233. Eskenazi B, Bracken MB, Holford TR, Crady J. Exposure to organic solvents and hypertensive disorders of pregnancy. Am J Ind Med 1988; 14:177.
234. Hudak A, Rodics K, Stuber I, et al. The effects of toluene inhalation on pregnant CFY rats and their offspring. Orz Munka-Uzemegeszsegugui Intez Munkavedelm 1977; 23(suppl):25.
235. Hudak A, Ungvary G. Embryotoxic effects of benzene and its methyl derivatives: toluene, xylene. Toxicology 1978; 11:53.
236. Nawrot PS, Staples RE. Embryofetal toxicity and teratogenicity of benzene and toluene in the mouse. Teratology 1979; 19:41A.
237. Mazze RI, Fujinaga M, Baden JM. Reproductive and teratogenic effects of nitrous oxide, fentanyl, and their combination in Sprague-Dawley rats. Br J Anaesth 1987; 59:1291.

238. Kugel G, Letelier C, Atallah H, Zive M. Chronic low level nitrous oxide exposure and infertility. J Dent Res 1989; 68:313.

239. Rowland AS, Baird DD, Weinberg CR, et al. Reduced fertility among women employed as dental assistants exposed to high levels of nitrous oxide. N Engl J Med 1992; 327:993.

240. Hunter AG, Thompson D, Evans JA. Is there a fetal gasoline syndrome? Teratology 1979; 20:75.

241. McSherry TM. Program experiences with the solvent abuser in Philadelphia. In: Crider RA, Rouse BA, eds. Epidemiology of Inhalant Abuse: An Update. Rockville, MD: NIDA Research Monograph 85, DHHS, 1988:106.

Chapter 9
Phencyclidine

"Amoeba," "Angel Dust," "Busy Bee,"
"Cadillac," "Crystal Joints," "CJ,"
"Cyclones," "Devil's Dust," "DOA,"
"Dog," "Elephant Tranquilizer,"
"Embalming Fluid," "Goon," "Gorilla
Tab," "Hog," "Horse Tranquilizer,"
"Mr. Lovely," "Monkey Dust," "Peace Pill,"
"Pig Killer," "Rocket Fuel," "Scuffle,"
"Soma Surfer," "Superweed," "Whack,"
"Window Pane," "Wobble Weed," "Worm,"
"Zombie."
— *Street names for phencyclidine*

Arylcyclohexylamine compounds, which include phencyclidine (1-(1-phenylcyclohexyl)piperidine, or PCP), have central nervous system (CNS) stimulant, depressant, hallucinogenic, and analgesic properties (Figure 9–1). Termed *dissociative anesthetics* because of a tendency of patients during anesthesia to keep their eyes open and seem "disconnected" from the environment, these agents appear to be categorically separable from other psychotomimetic drugs, including hallucinogens.[1]

Pharmacology and Animal Studies

In mice and rats PCP elicits amphetamine-like behavior: With low doses there is increased locomotion and with higher doses stereotypic movements—repetitive head weaving, sniffing, rearing, and circling. In contrast to amphetamine, however, higher doses cause marked ataxia.[2–4] In monkeys low doses produce mild ataxia and calming. With higher doses there is nystagmus and catalepsy: The eyes remain open, and there is no respiratory depression, but the animal is immobile and unresponsive to the environment. Pigeons receiving PCP are also rendered cataleptic.

PCP is a competitive inhibitor of dopamine, norepinephrine, and serotonin uptake,[5] and PCP-induced stereotypic behavior is blocked by neuroleptic drugs and by hydroxydopamine lesions of the nucleus accumbens.[6] PCP also has antimuscarinic actions[7] and in rats suppresses opioid withdrawal signs.[8] Its major actions, however, involve N-methyl-D-aspartate (NMDA) receptors and sigma receptors.

The effects of the excitatory amino acids glutamate and aspartate are mediated through at least five receptor subtypes, including those selective for the agonists kainate, quisqualate, and NMDA. Like the gamma-aminobutyric acid (GABA) receptor, the NMDA receptor is part of a macromolecular complex. The ion channel is permeable to sodium, potassium, and calcium ions, and there are specific receptors for NMDA, glycine, magnesium, zinc, polyamines, and PCP. The PCP binding site—termed the *PCP receptor*—lies within the ion channel and is both voltage dependent and "use dependent"; that is, it requires NMDA agonists to open the channel and provide access to the receptor. PCP then blocks ion flux, either through conformational changes or by plugging the channel. Acting at its own receptor, PCP inhibits NMDA agonists noncompetitively. (Competitive antagonists, which act at the NMDA receptor itself, include 2-amino-5-phosphonopentanoate [AP5] and 2-amino-7-phosphonoheptanoate [AP7].) NMDA receptors are most numerous in hippocampus, amygdala, thalamus,

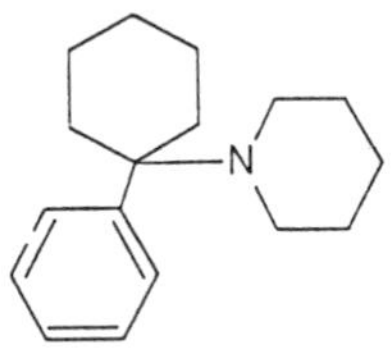

Figure 9–1. Phencyclidine.

caudate, entorhinal cortex, and layers I and II of the somatosensory and motor cortex.[4,9–12]

PCP also binds to so-called sigma receptors, which were originally considered an opioid receptor subtype.[13] Sigma receptor ligands include the benzomorphan class of opioid mixed agonist-antagonists, such as cyclazocine, pentazocine, and N-allynormetazocine (NANM), psychotomimetic effects of which are not blocked by naloxone. Sigma binding sites are most dense in the hippocampus, hypothalamus, limbic forebrain, midbrain, cerebellum, and brain stem. PCP has much greater affinity for PCP receptors than sigma receptors, and different agents have varying degrees of affinity for the two receptor types. A drug with high affinity for PCP receptors, dizocilpine (MK-801), binds hardly at all to sigma receptors. A drug with high affinity for sigma receptors, haloperidol, does not bind to PCP receptors.[14]

The function of sigma receptors is unknown, and the diversity of agents that bind to them implies receptor subtypes.[13,15] It is also unclear to what degree the behavioral effects of PCP are mediated by either sigma receptors or PCP receptors. Biological and behavioral effects have more readily correlated with PCP receptor binding[16,17] than with sigma receptor binding, and in human volunteers the analgesic potency of PCP analogs similarly correlates with PCP receptor affinity.[18] MK-801 in rats, pigeons, and monkeys produces PCP-like behavior[19] yet in human volunteers is not psychotomimetic.[20,21] In animals PCP-like behavior is produced by the competitive NMDA antagonists AP5 and AP7.[3]

Also correlating with their affinities for PCP receptors are the anticonvulsant properties of these agents.[22] MK-801, ketamine, NANM, and PCP suppress seizures induced by electroshock, pentylenetetrazol (PTZ), sound (in audiogenic seizure-prone rodents), and light (in photosensitive baboons).[23,24] Anticonvulsant effects of these noncompetitive NMDA antagonists occur only at doses that produce motor disturbances. By contrast, low doses of competitive NMDA antagonists and some noncompetitive antagonists—for example, 1-phenyl-cyclopentylamine (PPA) and 1-(3-fluorophenyl)-cyclohexylamine (3-F-PCA)—are anticonvulsant without producing other behavioral change.[25] Interestingly,

neonatal rats given PCP or MK-801 are *more* susceptible to audiogenic seizures as adults.[26]

In monkeys, cats, and rats, PCP and related agents impair learning at doses too low to cause gross motor disruption.[27] Such an effect might be related to inhibition of NMDA receptor-dependent long-term potentiation in the hippocampus.[10]

In drug discrimination studies, MK-801, NANM, and ketamine substitute for PCP.[23] Substitution is not always consistent, however, and competitive NMDA antagonists substitute for PCP even less consistently, indicating that NMDA antagonism per se is insufficient to account for PCP discrimination.[28,29] Substitution of potent sigma ligands for PCP is also inconsistent; animals trained to discriminate pentazocine generalize completely to NANM but only partially to PCP,[30] and although haloperidol blocks NANM discrimination, animals trained to discriminate NANM do not generalize to the potent sigma agonist (+)-3-(3-hydroxyphenyl)-N-(1-propyl) piperidine (3-PPP).[31] Animals trained to discriminate PCP do not generalize to dopaminergic, serotonergic, cholinergic, GABAergic, or opioid drugs.[4]

Rats, dogs, monkeys, and baboons self-administer PCP, ketamine, and other PCP receptor ligands.[2,32–35] In studies using long interval schedules, monkeys responded up to 157 times per minute for an hour to receive a single dose.[36] Ketamine is less reinforcing,[35] and neither drug is as reinforcing as cocaine.[37] The reinforcing properties of MK-801 are complex: It is self-administered by monkeys that have recently self-administered PCP or ketamine but, in contrast to PCP, not by monkeys that have recently self-administered cocaine.[38] MK-801 does facilitate intracranial self-stimulation,[39] and PCP receptor ligands—but not sigma receptor ligands—increase punished responding (reward seeking in the face of aversive stimuli).[40] Competitive NMDA antagonists are much less consistently self-administered by animals.[27]

Animals develop tolerance to PCP's behavioral effects. As with a number of other addicting drugs—for example, amphetamine, cocaine, tetrahydrocannabinol, caffeine, and nicotine—signs of physical dependence are less readily identified.[41,42] Rats given PCP for 7 days developed twofold tolerance and on abrupt withdrawal had piloerection, increased susceptibility to audiogenic seizures, transient weight loss, and reduced exploratory activity and rotorod performance.[43] Monkeys receiving large daily intravenous doses of PCP for several weeks developed an abstinence syndrome consisting of tremor, diarrhea, motor and oculomotor hyperactivity, bruxism, priapism, and, in some, convulsions.

Naloxone failed to precipitate these signs, which seemed to require blood levels higher than can be achieved in humans on a long-term basis.[41,44] Monkeys and rats withdrawing from smaller doses demonstrated disruption of food-maintained operant performance without other behavioral abnormalities.[45]

The presence of PCP-binding sites has led to a search for endogenous PCP receptor ligands. A peptide isolated from porcine brain, termed *alpha-endopsychosin*, inhibited PCP binding but not haloperidol binding; its distribution paralleled PCP receptors, with highest concentration in the hippocampus.[46] An endogenous ligand for the sigma receptor (beta-endopsychosin) has also been reported.[3] The significance of these findings remains to be seen.[21]

The pharmacological and behavioral effects of PCP have obvious clinical implications beyond its abuse liability. Resemblance of PCP psychosis to schizophrenia has led to an intensive search for possible abnormalities of PCP or sigma receptors in schizophrenic patients and for antipsychotic drugs acting outside dopamine systems. The association of excitatory amino acids with delayed neuronal death has produced speculation that PCP-like agents such as MK-801 might prevent brain damage associated with seizures, hypoglycemia, ischemia, and even Huntington's and Alzheimer's disease.[47–49]

Historical Background and Epidemiology

Phencyclidine was developed as an anesthetic agent in the 1950s (Sernyl), but postoperative delirium and psychosis prevented its use except in animals (Sernylan).[50] It was first used as a drug of abuse during the 1960s in California, where it became known as *PeaCe Pill*.[51] By the mid-1970s, perhaps related to restricted heroin supplies, its use had spread epidemically across the United States.[52] Sernylan was withdrawn from the market in 1978, and although there is no accepted medical use for PCP, it is currently classified as a schedule II drug.[35]

PCP is easily manufactured by kitchen chemists, and in 1979, 15% of Americans aged 18 to 25, 4% of children aged 12 to 17, and 13% of high school seniors had tried it at least once.[53] During the 1980s, use declined among high school students, perhaps because of the drug's bad reputation as well as increasing availability of cocaine. In a 1987 survey of middle-class and upper-middle-class adolescents in a drug rehabilitation program, 56% had tried PCP, 21% used it once a month to once a week, 16% used

it several times a week, and 8% considered PCP their "best drug experience."[54] In a study of 74 adolescent marijuana users, 24% had PCP in their urine, and it appeared that most of them had taken PCP without knowing it.[55]

Reports from the Drug Abuse Warning Network (DAWN) reflect a shift in the demographics of PCP use, which varies widely among DAWN's 27 metropolitan areas.[56] In 1987, PCP-related emergency room encounters in Washington, D.C. totaled 4235, with 103 deaths—41% of all American PCP-related deaths reported that year. Los Angeles was a distant second with 1589 encounters; New York City reported only 523. In 1976–1977, 51% of PCP encounters involved adolescents, and 24% were black. In 1987 only 15% were adolescent, and 60% were black.

PCP can be eaten, snorted, or injected, and it has been taken rectally and in eye drops. It is most often smoked, sprinkled on tobacco, parsley, or marijuana, and is commonly substituted for or mixed with what is sold as lysergic acid diethylamide (LSD), mescaline, cannabis, amphetamine, or other drugs.[52,57] Street products include powders, pastes, capsules, tablets, and "leaf mixtures" containing mint, oregano, parsley, or, for added hallucinogenic effect, catnip.[51,58,59]

A number of PCP analogs have also appeared as street drugs, including phenylcyclohexylpyrrolidine (PHP), phenylcyclohexylethylamine (PCE), piperidinocyclohexanecarbonitrile (PCC), and thienylcyclohexylpiperidine (TCP).[51,60–64] The structurally related anesthetic, ketamine—"green," "jet," "K," "superacid," "supergrass" (if used with marijuana)—is sold as capsules, tablets, crystals, powder, or in solution and taken intramuscularly, intravenously, intranasally, or by smoking.[59,65,66]

Most PCP users take it about once a week, often in social groups, but some engage in amphetamine-like "runs" lasting 2 to 3 days. A cigarette containing PCP delivers 1 to 100 mg; chronic users may take 1 g daily. Nearly all PCP users take other drugs as well, especially marijuana ("whack," "whacky weed"), ethanol, amphetamine, and hallucinogens.[51] PCP is sometimes smoked with alkaloidal cocaine ("spacebase").[67]

Acute Effects

The effects of PCP are highly variable, and attempts to separate symptoms and signs according to dose oversimplify (Table 9–1).[57,59,68–71] In general, low doses (1 to 5 mg) cause euphoria or dysphoria, emo-

Table 9–1. Phencyclidine Poisoning: Approximate Order of Symptoms with Increasing Dose

Relaxation, euphoria
Anxiety, emotional lability, dysphoria, paranoia
Subjective time-slowing
Decreased sensory perception
Altered body image, sensory illusions
Amnesia
Agitation, bizarre or violent behavior
Analgesia
Synesthesias
Nystagmus
Miosis
Tachycardia, hypertension
Hyperpnea
Fever
Hypersalivation, sweating
Dysarthria, ataxia, vertigo
Psychosis: paranoid or catatonic
Hallucinations
Dystonia, opisthotonus
Myoclonus
Rhabdomyolysis
Seizures
Stupor or coma with blank stare
Extensor posturing
Respiratory depression
Hypotension

tional lability, a sense of time-slowing, and a feeling of numbness. Desired subjective states include mood elevation, heightened sensitivity to stimuli, increased sociability, relaxation, and "hallucinations," although, in contrast to LSD, PCP is more likely to cause sensory distortions and altered body image than a true visual hallucination. Some subjects at the same low dose experience anxiety, hyperirritability, paranoia, disorientation, confusion, and amnesia. At 5 to 15 mg, confusion and agitation, bizarre behavior (for which there is often amnesia), body distortion, synesthesias, decreased sensory perception, and analgesia occur. Higher doses produce frank psychosis mimicking stuporous or excited catatonia or paranoid schizophrenia with persecutory auditory hallucinations. The electroencephalogram shows slowing, sometimes with paroxysmal sharp waves.[72]

Tachycardia, hypertension, fever, hyperpnea, flushing, sweating, miosis, hypersalivation, vertigo, ataxia (including grimacing, torticollis, and tortipelvis), myoclonus, and burst-like horizontal, vertical, or rotatory nystagmus also occur, and anesthetic doses (1 mg/kg or more) produce seizures (including status epilepticus), coma with extensor posturing yet open staring eyes, respiratory depression, and hypotension.[73–76] Fever as high as 42.2°C has been

recorded, sometimes rising hours after admission;[77] malignant hyperthermia causes liver necrosis.[78] Myoglobinuria, possibly from muscle overactivity, causes renal failure,[68,78,79] and there may be hyperkalemia and metabolic acidosis. Uric acid nephropathy also occurs.[81] Abdominal cramps and hematemesis have been attributed to contaminants. Death may be directly from overdose or the result of violence, including homicide, suicide, and accidents.[44,73–75,82–86] A special feature of PCP poisoning is painless self-injury.[84] During recovery, which can take days, any stimulus may provoke agitation or psychotic behavior. Nystagmus often outlasts behavioral abnormalities.

PCP-intoxicated infants and small children are less likely than adults to display agitation or aggression; a report of seven such patients described decreased response to tactile and verbal stimuli and "stupor associated with a blank expressionless stare." Nystagmus was present in only 57%.[87] Small children have been poisoned by PCP after accidental ingestion, inhalation of smoke in an automobile, or following deliberate exposure by siblings or babysitters.[88]

The biological half-life of PCP for most people is around 21 hours but ranges from 11 to 51 hours. About 10% of the drug is excreted unchanged, and the rest is converted in the liver to hydroxyl and glucuronide metabolites. Renal excretion is increased by urinary acidification. Cerebrospinal fluid levels are several times higher than blood levels, and this "trapping" of the drug by the CNS accounts for prolonged duration of action and positive blood and urine toxicology for days or even weeks in chronic users.[64,89,90] In fact, blood levels may continue to rise for several days after large overdoses.[91]

Treatment of PCP intoxication begins with a calm environment (Table 9–2). Delirium and psychosis may be present from the outset or emerge as the patient awakens from coma. "Talking down" is ineffectual in such a setting and may aggravate symptoms. Violent patients must be safely restrained—self-injury is the most common cause of morbidity and mortality.[89]

Because of gastroenteric recirculation, continuous gastric suctioning can shorten PCP's half-life but is difficult in delirious patients, and fluid and electrolyte alterations must then be closely monitored.[1,92,93] Repeated doses of activated charcoal (1 g/kg every 2 to 4 hours) and forced diuresis with furosemide hasten nonrenal and renal clearance. Acidification of the urine—recommended by some[94,95]—is either useless or dangerous. Because only 10% of PCP is excreted unchanged by the kid-

Table 9–2. Treatment of Phencyclidine Poisoning

Calm environment; do not try to "talk the patient down"

Safe restraints for violent patients

Consider continuous gastric suctioning

Activated charcoal (1 g/kg every 2–4 h)

Forced diuresis; do not acidify urine

Tracheal suctioning

Cooling

Antihypertensives

Anticonvulsants

Diazepam intravenously or lorazepam intramuscularly, titered

Consider haloperidol, 2–5 mg, for frank psychosis

Close monitoring of cardiorespiratory status, fluid and electrolyte balance, and renal function (myoglobinuria)

neys, the increased drug clearance is clinically insignificant, and the frequent presence of myoglobinuria sets the stage for renal shutdown.[89] PCP's large volume of distribution, protein binding, and lipid solubility limit the benefit of hemoperfusion or hemodialysis.[89]

Hypersalivation requires frequent suctioning, and there may be need for cooling blankets and ice baths, antihypertensive therapy, or ventilatory support.[75,92,96] Extremely high fever may require gastric or rectal ice water lavage or paralysis with pancuronium.[77] Seizures, which are infrequent, can be treated with diazepam or phenytoin. Treating agitation or psychosis is controversial. The unreliable absorption of intramuscular diazepam or chlordiazepoxide and the difficulty giving intravenous drugs to a violent patient make these agents frequently unsuitable. Moreover, diazepam prolongs PCP's half-life, and sedatives aggravate PCP's depressant actions, including respiratory.[57] Neuroleptics also carry potential problems. Phenothiazines and haloperidol are epileptogenic and can potentiate hypotension or cause a malignant neuroleptic syndrome with exacerbation of myoglobinuria. If neuroleptics are used, haloperidol (starting at 2 to 5 mg) is preferable to phenothiazines, anticholinergic effects of which can aggravate delirium or psychosis.[69] Goldfrank et al.[89] suggest using diazepam for simple agitation and haloperidol for frank psychosis, with intravenous diazepam preferred in doubtful cases. A possible alternative is lorazepam, which is more reliably absorbed intramuscularly.

Anecdotally verapamil has been recommended for PCP intoxication.[97,98] In rats, however, verapamil, nimodipine, and diltiazem potentiate PCP's behavioral effects.[99,100]

PCP's duration of action is dose-related, and symptoms are aggravated by concurrent use of other drugs, such as ethanol and marijuana.[101] In some patients, psychosis requiring neuroleptics (or resistant to them) can last several weeks.[102]

Tolerance develops to PCP's effects in humans.[35] Although craving occurs with abstinence, withdrawal symptoms are usually limited to nervousness, "cold sweats," upset stomach, and tremor.[44,70] Of 37 adult men who had used PCP at least weekly (38% daily) for an average of 7 years, none developed withdrawal symptoms with abstinence.[103] (Only 11% remained abstinent for a year, however.)

Withdrawal signs are frequently encountered in neonates exposed in utero to PCP. Irritability, jitteriness, poor cry, hypertonicity, vomiting, and diarrhea begin within 24 hours of delivery and can be treated with benzodiazepines, barbiturates, or paregoric.[104]

Considerable attention has focused on the resemblance of PCP psychosis to schizophrenia. Amphetamine induces "positive" schizophrenic symptoms—hostility, agitation, paranoia, and delusions—but not "negative"—loss of ego boundaries, concreteness, and loose or bizarre associations. PCP, by contrast, induces a full schizophrenic syndrome, with alterations in body image, apathy, negativism, and disorganized thinking.[105] Volunteers receiving subanesthetic doses of PCP (0.05 to 0.1 mg/kg intravenously) display negativism, withdrawal, and autism, and some develop catatonic posturing, concrete or bizarre responses to proverb interpretation and projective testing, and impoverished speech and thinking. Neuropsychological testing reveals impaired attention, perception, and symbolic thinking similar to what is encountered in schizophrenics. Schizophrenics often have elevated thresholds for pain perception, a striking feature of PCP intoxication. Moreover, CNS abnormalities found in schizophrenics—decreased frontal lobe metabolism and impaired event-related evoked potentials—are induced by PCP but not amphetamine.[106–109] Increased binding of the radiolabeled PCP receptor ligand 1-[1-(2 thienyl)cyclohexyl]piperidine (TCP) was reported in schizophrenic brains.[110]

Chronic schizophrenics are often hyporesponsive to amphetamine or even show symptomatic improvement. PCP exacerbates schizophrenic symptoms, including abnormal affect, disturbed body image, and disordered thinking.[105] (Schizophrenics with prefrontal lobotomies are relatively resistant to PCP exacerbation.[111])

Psychotic symptoms—paranoia, thought disorder, delusions, hallucinations, and catatonia—can last days or weeks after single doses of PCP, and many chronic users demonstrate persistent behavioral and cognitive abnormalities.[52,69,70,102,112–114] As with other drugs, causality is difficult to establish; systematic studies of PCP use and long-term cognitive or psychiatric disturbance have not been conducted.[114a] Preexisting schizophrenia is overrepresented among users with persistent psychosis, but the majority have no history of earlier psychiatric problems.[102]

Of obvious relevance to cognitive or psychiatric disturbance is the observation that PCP and related drugs cause pathological changes in the CNS. Two hours after receiving single doses of PCP, MK801, TCP, or ketamine, rats demonstrated cytoplasmic vacuolization in neurons of the posterior cingulate and retrosplenial cortex. Within 24 hours the reaction subsided, and repeated low doses did not produce a cumulative effect.[106] Higher doses, however, caused irreversible neuronal necrosis.[115,116] The order of potency in producing these changes paralleled binding affinity to the PCP receptor: MK-801 > PCP > TCP > ketamine. The competitive NMDA inhibitor AP5 was also neurotoxic. The mechanism of injury is uncertain, as is its relevance to medial prefrontal hypometabolism in schizophrenia; it is possibly significant that cingulate neurons mediate affective responses to pain.[117] PCP-induced injury is potentiated by pretreatment with the cholinergic agonist pilocarpine and prevented by coadministration of scopolamine. Diazepam provides partial protection, and barbiturates completely protect. The nonbarbiturate anesthetic halothane is not protective.[118] As noted, benzodiazepines reduce psychotomimetic symptoms induced by PCP; anesthetists use diazepam to dampen emergence psychosis in patients receiving ketamine.[119]

The duration of PCP-induced hypertension parallels the mental changes, lasting hours or days.[51,68,74,96] Although hypertension might be related to enhanced catecholamine or serotonin action,[120] contractile responses to PCP of isolated basilar and middle cerebral arteries were not prevented by methysergide, phentolamine, atropine, diphenhydramine, or indomethacin, suggesting the presence of PCP receptors on cerebral vessels.[121] The nature of such receptors is unclear; NMDA receptor agonists *constrict* rat pial arterioles.[122]

Hypertensive encephalopathy followed PCP ingestion in a young woman with systemic lupus erythematosus and a history of migraine.[123] A 13-year-old boy became comatose after taking PCP; blood pressure was normal on admission, and he became alert but 3 days later deteriorated with a blood pressure of 230/130 mm Hg. At autopsy there was intracerebral hemorrhage.[96] Urine contained PCP in

a 6-year-old with seizures and right hemiparesis. Computed tomography demonstrated parieto-occipital lucency and vessel enhancement, suggesting a vascular malformation. He recovered, and cerebral angiography was not done.[124] Subarachnoid hemorrhage has followed PCP use on at least three occasions.[125–127] Two involved adolescents,[125,126] in one of whom autopsy revealed perforation of the ventral surface of the basilar artery without aneurysm or vasculitis.[125] The third was a 33-year-old woman with an anterior communicating artery aneurysm.[127] Cerebral infarction followed PCP smoking in a 56-year-old man with atrial fibrillation; it was suspected that PCP cardiac stimulation caused dislodgment of clot from the heart.[127] Single-photon emission computed tomographic (SPECT) studies on several PCP users revealed asymmetric perfusion abnormalities in the cerebral cortex; each subject also used other drugs, however, including cocaine and ethanol.[128]

PCP specifically binds to lymphocytes and depresses both humoral and cellular immune responses.[129] The lymphocyte receptors are sigma in type and also bind several steroids, including progesterone, testosterone, and deoxycorticosterone.[130] It is uncertain if PCP lymphocyte binding is clinically important or if sigma receptors contribute to steroid-induced mental changes or immunosuppression.

Effects on Pregnancy

In addition to withdrawal signs, infants exposed in utero to PCP have had abnormal behavior; irregular ventilatory patterns during sleep; hydrocephalus; microcephaly; and anomalies of the heart, lungs, urinary or musculoskeletal systems, cerebellum, cerebral commissures, and optic chiasm.[131–136] These anomalies could, of course, be the result of other drugs or poor prenatal care. In a study of 12 infants exposed in utero to PCP, there was no increase in congenital defects, but two-thirds had serious neonatal medical problems, usually respiratory; several infants were still irritable at 6 months of age and at 18 months had mild to severe abnormalities of language, behavior, and fine motor coordination.[104] In another report nine infants exposed to PCP throughout pregnancy had normal psychomotor development at 2 years of age.[137]

References

1. Domino EF. Neurobiology of phencyclidine: an update. In: Petersen RC, Stillman RC, eds. Phencyclidine

(PCP) Abuse: An Appraisal. Washington, DC: NIDA Research Monograph 21, DHEW, 1978:18.

2. Balster RL, Chait LD. The behavioral effects of phencyclidine in animals. In: Petersen RL, Stillman RC, eds. Phencyclidine (PCP) Abuse: An Appraisal. Washington, DC: NIDA Research Monograph 21, DHEW, 1978:53.

3. Contreras PC, Monahan JB, Lanthorn TH, et al. Phencyclidine. Physiological actions, interactions with excitatory amino acids, and endogenous ligands. Mol Neurobiol 1987; 1:191.

4. Johnson KM, Jones SM. Neuropharmacology of phencyclidine: basic mechanisms and therapeutic potential. Annu Rev Pharmacol Toxicol 1990; 30:707.

5. Bowyer JF, Spuhler KP, Weiner N. Effects of phencyclidine, amphetamine, and related compounds on dopamine release from uptake into striatal synaptosomes. J Pharmacol Exp Ther 1984; 229:671.

6. French ED, Dilapil C, Quiron R. Phencyclidine binding sites in the nucleus accumbens and phencyclidine-induced hyperactivity are decreased following lesions of the mesolimbic dopamine system. Eur J Pharmacol 1985; 116:1.

7. Vargas HM, Pechnick RN. Binding affinity and antimuscarinic activity of sigma and phencyclidine receptor ligands. Eur J Pharmacol 1991; 195:151.

8. Rasmussen K, Fuller RW, Stockton ME, et al. NMDA receptor antagonists suppress behaviors but not norepinephrine turnover or locus coeruleus unit activity induced by opiate withdrawal. Eur J Pharmacol 1991; 197:9.

9. Zukin SR, Javitt DC. Mechanisms of phencyclidine (PCP)-n-methyl-d-aspartate (NMDA) receptor interaction: implications for drug abuse research. In: Harris LS, ed. Problems of Drug Dependence 1989. Rockville, MD: NIDA Research Monograph 95, DHHS, 1990:247.

10. Lodge D, Johnson KM. Noncompetitive excitatory amino acid receptor antagonists. Trends Pharmacol Sci 1990; 11:81.

11. Reynolds IJ, Miller RJ. Allosteric modulation of N-methyl-D-aspartate receptors. Adv Pharmacol 1990; 21:101.

12. MacDonald JF, Bartlett MC, Mody I, et al. The PCP site of the NMDA receptor complex. In: Ben Ari Y, ed. Excitatory Amino Acids and Neuronal Plasticity. New York: Plenum Press, 1990:27.

13. Su TP. Sigma receptors. Putative links between nervous, endocrine and immune systems. Eur J Biochem 1991; 200:633.

14. Quiron R, Clicheportiche R, Contreras PC, et al. Classification and nomenclature of phencyclidine and sigma receptor sites. Trends Neurosci 1987; 10:444.

15. Itzhak Y, Stein I, Zhang SH, et al. Binding of sigma-ligands to C57BL/6 mouse brain membranes: effects of monoamine oxidase inhibitors and subcellular distribution studies suggest the existence of sigma-receptor subtypes. J Pharmacol Exp Ther 1991; 257:141.

16. Connick J, Fox P, Nicholson D. Psychotomimetic effects and sigma ligands. Trends Pharmacol Sci 1990; 11:274.

17. Boyce S, Rupniak NM, Steventon MJ, et al. Psychomotor activity and cognitive disruption attributable to NMDA, but not sigma, interactions in primates. Behav Brain Res 1991; 42:115.

18. Klepstad P, Maurset A, Moberg ER, Oye I. Evidence of a role for NMDA receptors in pain perception. Eur J Pharmacol 1990; 187:513.

19. Koek W, Woods JH, Winger GD. MK-801, a proposed noncompetitive antagonist of excitatory amino acid neurotransmission, produces phencyclidine-like behavioral effects in pigeons, rats, and rhesus monkeys. J Pharmacol Exp Ther 1988; 245:969.

20. Troupin AS, Mendius JR, Cheng F, Risinger MW. MK801. In: Meldrum BS, Porter RS, eds. Current Problems in Epilepsy. 4. New Anticonvulsant Drugs. London: John Libby, 1986:191.

21. Sonders MS, Keana JFW, Weber E. Phencyclidine and psychomimetic sigma opiates: recent insights into their biochemical and physiological sites of action. Trends Neurosci 1988; 11:37.

22. Church J, Lodge D. Anticonvulsant actions of phencyclidine receptor ligands: correlation with N-methyl-aspartate antagonism in vivo. Gen Pharmacol 1990; 21:165.

23. Tricklebank MD, Singh L, Oles RJ, et al. The behavioral effects of MK801: a comparison with antagonists acting non-competitively and competitively at the NMDA receptor. Eur J Pharmacol 1989; 167:127.

24. Wood PL, Rao TS, Iyengar S, et al. A review of the in vitro and in vivo neurochemical characterization of the NMDA/PCP/glycine/ion channel receptor macrocomplex. Biochem Res 1990; 15:217.

25. Blake PA, Yamaguchi S, Therkauf A, Rogawski MA. Anticonvulsant 1-phenylcycloalkylamines: two analogues with low motor toxicity when orally administered. Epilepsia 1992; 33:188.

26. Pierson M, Swann J. Sensitization to noise-mediated induction of seizure susceptibility by MK801 and phencyclidine. Brain Res 1991; 560:229.

27. Willetts J, Balster RL, Leander JD. The behavioral pharmacology of NMDA receptor antagonists. Trends Pharmacol Sci 1990; 11:423.

28. Mansbach RS, Balster RL. Pharmacological specificity of the phencyclidine discriminative stimulus in rats. Pharmacol Biochem Behav 1991; 39:971.

29. France CP, Moerschbaecher JM, Woods JH. MK801 and related compounds in monkeys: discriminative stimulus effects on a conditional discrimination. J Pharmacol Exp Ther 1991; 257:727.

30. Steinfels GF, Alberici CP, Tam SW, Cook L. Biochemical, behavioral, and electrophysiologic actions of the selective sigma receptor ligand (+)pentazocine. Neuropsychopharmacology 1988; 1:321.

31. Balster RL. Substitution and antagonism in rats trained to discriminate (+)-N-allylnormetazocine from saline. J Pharmacol Exp Ther 1989; 249:749.

32. Moreton JE, Meisch RA, Stark L, Thompson T. Ketamine self-administration by the rhesus monkey. J Pharmacol Exp Ther 1977; 203:303.

33. Risner ME. Intravenous self-administration of phencyclidine and related compounds in the dog. J Pharmacol Exp Ther 1982; 221:637.
34. Lukas SE, Griffiths RR, Brady JV, Wurster RM. Phencyclidine-analogue self-injection by the baboon. Psychopharmacology 1984; 83:316.
35. Carroll ME. PCP and hallucinogens. Adv Alcohol Subst Abuse 1990; 9:167.
36. Carroll ME. Performance maintained by orally delivered phencyclidine under second-order, tandem, and fixed interval schedules in food satiated and food deprived rhesus monkeys. J Pharmacol Exp Ther 1985; 232:351.
37. Marquis KL, Moreton JE. Animal models of intravenous phencyclidine self-administration. Pharmacol Biochem Behav 1987; 27:385.
38. Beardsley PM, Hayes BA, Balster RL. The self-administration of MK801 can depend on drug-reinforcement history, and its discriminative stimulus properties are phencyclidine-like in rhesus monkeys. J Pharmacol Exp Ther 1990; 252:953.
39. Corbett D. Possible abuse potential of the NMDA antagonist MK801. Behav Brain Res 1989; 34:239.
40. McMillan DE, Hardwick WC, deCosta BR, Rice KC. Effects of drugs that bind to PCP and sigma receptors on punished responding. J Pharmacol Exp Ther 1991; 258:1015.
41. Balster RL. Disruption of schedule-controlled behavior during abstinence from phencyclidine and tetrahydrocannabinol. In: Harris LS, ed. Problems of Drug Dependence 1989. Rockville, MD: NIDA Research Monograph 95, DHHS, 1990:124.
42. Wessinger WD, Owens SM. Phencyclidine dependence: the relationship of dose and serum concentrations to operant behavioral effects. J Pharmacol Exp Ther 1991; 258:207.
43. Spain JW, Klingman GI. Continuous intravenous infusion of phencyclidine in unrestrained rats results in the rapid induction of tolerance and physical dependence. J Pharmacol Exp Ther 1985; 234:415.
44. Pradhan SN. Phencyclidine (PCP): some human studies. Neurosci Biobehav Rev 1984; 8:493.
45. Beardsley PM, Balster RL. Behavioral dependence upon phencyclidine and ketamine in the rat. J Pharmacol Exp Ther 1987; 242:203.
46. DiMaggio DA, Contreras PC, Quirion R, O'Donohue TL. Isolation and identification of an endogenous ligand for the phencyclidine receptor. In: Clouet DH, ed. Phencyclidine: An Update. Rockville, MD: NIDA Research Monograph 64, DHHS, 1986:24.
47. Winger G. PCP-NMDA connection provides hope in cerebral ischemia but new directions for antipsychotics. Trends Pharmacol Sci 1987; 8:323.
48. Rothman SM, Olney JW. Excitotoxicity and the NMDA receptor. Trends Neurosci 1987; 10:299.
49. Zivin J, Choi DW. Stroke therapy. Sci Am 1991; 256:56.
50. Luby ED, Cohen BD, Rosenbaum C, et al. Study of a new schizophrenomimetic drug—Sernyl. Arch Neurol 1959; 81:363.
51. Lerner SE, Burns RS. Phencyclidine use among youth: history, epidemiology, and acute and chronic intoxication. In: Petersen RL, Stillman RC, eds. Phencyclidine (PCP) Abuse: An Appraisal. Washington, DC: NIDA Research Monograph 21, DHEW, 1978:66.
52. Young I, Lawson GW, Gacono CB. Clinical aspects of phencyclidine (PCP). Int J Addict 1987; 22:1.
53. Fishburne PM, Abelson HI, Cisin I. National Survey on Drug Abuse: Main Findings: 1979. Washington, DC: DHHS Publication No (ADM) 80-976, 1980.
54. Schwartz RH, Hoffman NG, Smith D, et al. Use of phencyclidine among adolescents attending a suburban drug treatment facility. J Pediatr 1987; 110:322.
55. Silber TJ, Josefsohn M, Hicks JM, et al. Prevalence of PCP use among adolescent marijuana users. J Pediatr 1988; 112:827.
56. Thombs DL. A review of PCP abuse. Trends and perceptions. Publ Health Rep 1989; 104:325.
57. Khantzian EJ, McKenna GJ. Acute toxic and withdrawal reactions associated with drug use and abuse. Ann Intern Med 1979; 90:361.
58. Lundberg GD, Gupta RL, Montgomery SH. Phencyclidine patterns seen in street drug analysis. Clin Toxicol 1976; 9:503.
59. Siegel RK. Phencyclidine and ketamine intoxication: a study of four populations of recreational users. In: Petersen RC, Stillman RC, eds. Phencyclidine (PCP) Abuse: An Appraisal. Washington, DC: NIDA Research Monograph 21, DHEW, 1978:119.
60. Shulgin AT, MacLean D. Illicit synthesis of phencyclidine (PCP) and several of its analogs. Clin Toxicol 1976; 9:553.
61. Budd RD. PHP, a new drug of abuse. N Engl J Med 1980; 303:588.
62. Gianini AJ, Price WA, Losielle RH, Malone DW. Treatment of phenylcyclohexylpyrrolidine (PHP) psychosis with haloperidol. J Toxicol Clin Toxicol 1985; 23:185.
63. Smialek J, Monforte J, Gault R, Spitz W. Cyclohexamine ("rocket fuel")—phencyclidine's potent analog. J Anal Toxicol 1979; 3:209.
64. Jerrard DA. "Designer drugs"—a current perspective. J Emerg Med 1990; 8:733.
65. Ketamine abuse. FDA Drug Bull 1979; 9:24.
66. Ahmed SN, Petchkovsky L. Abuse of ketamine. Br J Psychiatry 1980; 137:303.
67. Giannini AJ, Loiselle RH, Giannini MC. Space-base abstinence: alleviation of withdrawal symptoms in combinative cocaine-phencyclidine abuse. J Toxicol Clin Toxicol 1987; 25:493.
68. McCarron MM, Schultze BW, Thompson GA, et al. Acute phencyclidine intoxication: incidence of clinical findings in 1000 cases. Ann Emerg Med 1981; 10:237.
69. Allen RM, Young SJ. Phencyclidine-induced psychosis. Am J Psychiatry 1978; 135:1081.
70. Fauman MA, Fauman BJ. The psychiatric aspects of chronic phencyclidine use: a study of chronic PCP users. In: Petersen RC, Stillman RC, eds. Phencyclidine (PCP) Abuse: An Appraisal. Washington, DC: NIDA Research Monograph 21, DHEW, 1978:18.

71. McCarron MM, Schulze BW, Thompson GA, et al. Acute phencyclidine intoxication: clinical patterns, complications, and treatment. Ann Emerg Med 1981; 10:290.

72. Stockard JJ, Werner SS, Albers JA, Chiappa KH. Electroencephalographic findings in phencyclidine intoxication. Arch Neurol 1976; 33:200.

73. Kessler GF, Demers LM, Brennan RW. Phencyclidine and fatal status epilepticus. N Engl J Med 1974; 291:979.

74. Burns RS, Lerner SE. Perspectives: acute phencyclidine intoxication. Clin Toxicol 1976; 9:477.

75. Rappolt RT, Gay GR, Farris RD. Phencyclidine (PCP) intoxication: diagnosis in stages and algorithms of treatment. Clin Toxicol 1980; 16:509.

76. Alldredge BK, Lowenstein DH, Simon RP. Seizures associated with recreational drug abuse. Neurology 1989; 39:1037.

77. Rosenberg J, Pentel P, Pond S, et al. Hyperthermia associated with drug intoxication. Crit Care Med 1986; 14:964.

78. Armen R, Kanel G, Reynolds T. Phencyclidine-induced malignant hyperthermia causing submassive liver necrosis. Am J Med 1984; 77:167.

79. Cogen FC, Rigg G, Simmons JL, Domino EF. Phencyclidine-associated acute rhabdomyolysis. Ann Intern Med 1978; 88:210.

80. Patel R, Das M, Palazzolo M, et al. Myoglobinuric acute renal failure in phencyclidine overdose: report of observations in eight cases. Ann Emerg Med 1980; 9:549.

81. Patel R. Acute uric acid nephropathy: a complication of phencyclidine intoxication. Postgrad Med J 1982; 58:783.

82. Noguchi TT, Nakamura GR. Phencyclidine-related deaths in Los Angeles County, 1976. J Forensic Sci 1978; 23:503.

83. Fauman MA, Fauman BJ. Violence associated with phencyclidine abuse. Am J Psychiatry 1979; 136:1584.

84. Grove VE. Painless self-injury after ingestion of "angel dust." JAMA 1979; 242:655.

85. Lowry PW, Hassig SE, Gunn RA, Mathison JB. Homicide victims in New Orleans: recent trends. Am J Epidemiol 1988; 128:1130.

86. Poklis A, Graham M, Maginn D, et al. Phencyclidine and violent deaths in St. Louis, Missouri: a survey of medical examiners' cases from 1977 through 1986. Am J Drug Alcohol Abuse 1990; 16:265.

87. Schwartz RH, Einhorn A. PCP intoxication in seven young children. Pediatr Emerg Care 1986; 2:238.

88. Schwartz RH. Passive inhalation of marijuana, phencyclidine, and free base cocaine ("crack") by infants. Am J Dis Child 1989; 143:644.

89. Goldfrank LR, Lewin NA, Osborn H. Phencyclidine. In: Goldfrank LR, Flomenbaum NE, Lewin NA, et al, eds. Toxicologic Emergencies, ed. 4. Norwalk, CT: Appleton & Lange, 1990:517.

90. Gorelick DA, Wilkins JN. Inpatient treatment of PCP abusers and users. Am J Drug Alcohol Abuse 1989; 15:1.

91. Jackson JE. Phencyclidine pharmacokinetics after a massive overdose. Ann Intern Med 1989; 111:613.

92. Aronow R, Done A. Phencyclidine overdose: an emergency concept of management. J Am Col Emergency Phys 1978; 7:56.

93. Done AK, Aronow R, Miceli JN. The pharmacokinetics of phencyclidine in overdosage and its treatment. In: Peterson RC, Stillman RC, eds. Phencyclidine (PCP) Abuse: An Appraisal. Washington, DC: NIDA Research Monograph 21, DHEW, 1978:210.

94. Robinson B, Yates A. Angel dust: medical and psychiatric aspects of phencyclidine intoxication. Arizona Med 1984; 41:808.

95. Giannini AJ, Loiselle RH, DiMarzio LR, Giannini MC. Augmentation of haloperidol by ascorbic acid in phencyclidine intoxication. Am J Psychiatry 1987; 144:1207.

96. Eastman JW, Cohen SN. Hypertensive crisis and death associated with phencyclidine poisoning. JAMA 1975; 231:1270.

97. Montgomery PT, Mueller ME. Treatment of PCP intoxication with verapamil. Am J Psychiatry 1985; 142:882.

98. Price WA, Giannini AJ. Management of acute PCP intoxication with verapamil. Clin Toxicol 1986; 24:85.

99. McCann DJ, Winter JC. Effects of phencyclidine, N-alkyl-N-normetazocine (SKF 10047), and verapamil on performance in a radial maze. Pharmacol Biochem Behav 1986; 24:187.

100. Popoli P, Bendedetti M, Scotti-de-Carolis A. Influence of nimodipine and diltiazem, alone and in combination, on phencyclidine-induced effects in rats: an EEG and behavioral study. Eur J Pharmacol 1990; 191:141.

101. Godley PJ, Moore ES, Woodworth JR, Fineg J. Effects of ethanol and delta-9-tetrahydrocannabinol on phencyclidine disposition in dogs. Biopharm Drugs Dispos 1991; 12:189.

102. Luisada PV. The phencyclidine psychosis. In: Petersen RC, Stillman RC, eds. Phencyclidine (PCP) Abuse: An Appraisal. Washington, DC: NIDA Research Monograph 21, DHEW, 1978:241.

103. Gorelick DA, Wilkins JN, Wong C. Outpatient treatment of PCP abusers. Am J Drug Alcohol Abuse 1989; 15:367.

104. Howard J, Kropenske V, Tyler R. The long-term effects on neurodevelopment in infants exposed prenatally to PCP. In: Clouet DH, ed. Phencyclidine: An Update. Washington, DC: NIDA Research Monograph 64, DHHS, 1986:237.

105. Javitt DC, Zukin SR. Recent advances in the phencyclidine model of schizophrenia. Am J Psychiatry 1991; 148:1301.

106. Olney JW, Labruyere J, Price MT. Pathological changes induced in cerebrocortical neurons by phencyclidine and related drugs. Science 1989; 244:1360.

107. Pfefferbaum A, Ford JM, White PM, Roth WT. P3 in schizophrenia is affected by stimulus modality, response requirements, medication status, and negative symptoms. Arch Gen Psychiatry 1989; 46:1035.

108. Weinberger DR, Berman KF. Speculation on the meaning of metabolic "hypofrontality" in schizophrenia. Schizophr Bull 1988; 14:157.

109. Javitt DC, Schroeder CS, Arezzo JC, Vaughan HG. Selective inhibition of processing-contingent auditory event-related potential components by the PCP-like agent MK801. Electroencephalogr Clin Neurophysiol, 1991; 79:65 P.

110. Simpson MD, Sister P, Royston MC, Deakin JF. Alterations in phencyclidine and sigma binding sites in schizophrenic brains. Effects of disease process and neuroleptic medication. Schizophr Res 1991; 6:41.

111. Itil T, Keskiner A, Kiremitci N, Holden JMC. Effect of phencyclidine in chronic schizophrenics. Can Psychiatr Assoc J 1967; 12:209.

112. Rainey JM, Crowder MK. Prolonged psychosis attributed to phencyclidine: report of three cases. Am J Psychiatry 1975; 132:1076.

113. Fauman B, Aldinger G, Fauman M. Psychiatric sequelae of phencyclidine abuse. Clin Toxicol 1976; 9:529.

114. Stillman R, Petersen RC. The paradox of phencyclidine (PCP) abuse. Ann Intern Med 1979; 90:428.

114a. Weinrieb RM, O'Brien CP. Persistent cognitive deficits attributed to substance abuse. In Brust JCM, ed. Neurologic Complications of Drug and Alcohol Abuse. Neurol Clin 1993, in press.

115. Allen HL, Iversen LL. Phencyclidine, dizocilpine, and cerebrocortical neurons. Science 1990; 247:221.

116. Sharp FR, Jasper P, Hall J, et al. MK801 and ketamine induce heat shock protein HSP72 in injured neurons in posterior cingulate and retrosplenial cortex. Ann Neurol 1991; 30:801.

117. Olney JW, Labruyere J, Price MT. Pathological changes induced in cerebrocortical neurons by phencyclidine and related drugs. Science 1989; 244:1360.

118. Olney JW, Labruyere J, Wang G, et al. NMDA antagonist neurotoxicity: mechanism and prevention. Science 1991; 254:1515.

119. Reich D, Silvay G. Ketamine: an update on the first twenty-five years of clinical experience. Can J Anaesth 1989; 36:186.

120. Illett KF, Jarott B, O'Donnell SR, Watstall JC. Mechanism of cardiovascular actions of 1-(phenyl-cyclohexyl)-piperidine hydrochloride (phencylidine). Br J Pharmacol Chemother 1966; 28:73.

121. Altura B, Altura BM. Phencyclidine, lysergic acid diethylamide, and mescaline: cerebral artery spasm and hallucinogenic activity. Science 1981; 212:1051.

122. Altura BM, Huang Q-F, Gebrewold A, et al. Evidence for involvement of the N-methyl-D-aspartate receptor complex in regulation of pial microvasculature. Stroke 1992; 23:153.

123. Burns RS, Lerner SE. The effects of phencyclidine in man: a review. In: Domino EF, ed. PCP (Phencyclidine): Historical and Current Perspectives. Ann Arbor, MI: NPP Books, 1981:449.

124. Crosley CJ, Binet EP. Cerebrovascular complications in phencyclidine intoxication. J Pediatr 1979; 94:316.

125. Boyko OB, Burger PC, Heinz ER. Pathological and radiological correlation of subarachnoid hemorrhage in phencyclidine abuse. Case report. J Neurosurg 1987; 67:446.

126. Besson HA. Intracranial hemorrhage associated with phencyclidine abuse. JAMA 1982; 248:585.

127. Sloan MA, Kittner SJ, Rigamonti D, Price TR. Occurrence of stroke associated with use/abuse of drugs. Neurology 1991; 41:1358.

128. Hertzman M, Reba RC, Kotlyarov EV. Single photon emission computed tomography in phencyclidine and related drug abuse. Am J Psychiatry 1990; 147:255.

129. Khansari N, Whitten HD, Fudenberg HH. Phencyclidine-induced immunodepression. Science 1984; 225:76.

130. Su T-P, London ED, Jaffe JH. Steroid binding at sigma receptors suggests a link between endocrine, nervous, and immune systems. Science 1988; 240:219.

131. Golden NL, Sokol RJ, Rubin IL. Angel dust: possible effects on the fetus. Pediatrics 1980; 65:18.

132. Strauss AA, Modaniou HD, Bosu SK. Neonatal manifestations of maternal phencyclidine (PCP) abuse. Pediatrics 1981; 68:550.

133. Michaud J, Mizrahi EM, Urich H. Agenesis of the vermis with fusion of the cerebellar hemispheres, septo-optic dysplasia, and associated anomalies. Report of a case. Acta Neuropathol 1982; 56:161.

134. Ward SL, Schuetz S, Kirshna V, et al. Abnormal sleeping ventilatory pattern in infants of substance abusing mothers. Am J Dis Child 1986; 140:1015.

135. Golden NL, Kuhnert BR, Sokol RJ, et al. Neonatal manifestations of maternal phencyclidine exposure. J Perinat Med 1987; 15:185.

136. Wachsman L, Schuetz S, Chan LS, Wingert WA. What happens to babies exposed to phencyclidine (PCP) in utero? Am J Drug Alcohol Abuse 1989; 15:31.

137. Chasnoff IJ, Burns KA, Burns WJ, Scholl SH. Prenatal drug exposure: effects on neonatal and infant growth and development. Neurobehav Toxicol Teratol 1986; 8:357.

Chapter 10
Anticholinergics

Your cup with numbing drops of night
and evil, stilled of all remorse,
she will infuse to charm your sight.
—*Homer,* The Odyssey

Upon my secure hour thy uncle stole
With juice of cursed hebona in a vial,
And in the pouches of my ears did pour
The leprous distillment, whose effect
Holds such an enmity with blood of man.
—*William Shakespeare,* Hamlet

A number of plants of the Solanaceae nightshade family contain the belladonna alkaloids atropine (hyoscyamine) and scopolamine (hyoscine), most concentrated in seeds and roots (Table 10–1, Figure 10–1).[1,2] One of these, *Datura stramonium*, grows throughout the United States and is widely used recreationally.

Pharmacology

Atropine and scopolamine are competitive inhibitors of cholinergic muscarinic receptors, located on tissues innervated by postganglionic cholinergic nerves. Except in extremely high doses they are ineffective at autonomic ganglia or the neuromuscular junction. Central nervous system (CNS) cholinergic transmission is mainly nicotinic in the spinal cord and both muscarinic and nicotinic in the brain.[3]

Selective antagonists have defined at least three muscarinic receptor subtypes. M_1 is predominant in cerebral cortex and sympathetic ganglia, M_2 in cardiac muscle, and M_3 in smooth muscle and glands. Moreover, cDNA cloning has revealed at least five structural variants. Muscarinic receptors appear to interact with G proteins.[4,5]

In doses used clinically, atropine has little CNS action, and its peripheral effects are dose related. Toxic doses cause CNS excitation, with restlessness, delir-

ium, or hallucinations, followed by coma, respiratory failure, and circulatory collapse. By contrast, low doses of scopolamine—probably because it more readily crosses the blood–brain barrier—cause euphoria, drowsiness, amnesia, and non–rapid eye movement sleep. Higher doses (or sometimes low doses in the presence of pain) produce excitation.[3]

Historical Background and Epidemiology

Medicinal use of belladonna preparations dates back to ancient Hindu physicians. The ability of anticholinergic plants to induce hallucinations was recognized by the Egyptians and Greeks, who used them to foretell the future. In 38 AD, Marc Antony's troops ate *Datura* as they retreated from Parthia, resulting in delirium, stupor, and fatalities.[1] During the Middle Ages, anticholinergic plants were used by satanic cults to communicate with demons; participating "witches" used brooms as vaginal applicators.[6] The popularity of nightshade as a poison led Linnaeus to name the plant *Atropa belladonna*, after Atropos, the Fate who cuts the thread of life.[3]

In 1676, bizarre behavior in the Jamestown colony was traced to ingestion of *Datura stramonium*, since then known as Jamestown or jimson weed. Thoreau described its use, and it has been suggested that Arthur Dimmesdale's symptoms in *The Scarlet*

Table 10–1. Plants Containing Belladonna Alkaloids

Latin Name	Common Name	Toxin
Atropa belladonna	Belladonna, deadly nightshade	Atropine
Hyoscyamus niger	Henbane, black henbane	Atropine, scopolamine
Mandragora officinarum	Mandrake, Satan's apple	Atropine, scopolamine
Lycium halimifolium	Matrimony vine	Atropine
Lobelia inflata	Lobelia	Atropine, scopolamine, lobeline
Datura stramonium	Jimson weed, sacred Datura, devil's weed, devil's apple, stinkapple, loco weed, thorn apple, malpitte, green dragon	Atropine, scopolamine
Datura sauveolens	Angel's trumpet	Atropine, scopolamine

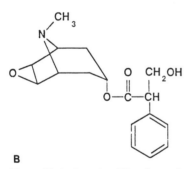

A

B

Figure 10–1. Atropine (A) and scopolamine (B).

Letter were the result of atropine poisoning inflicted by Roger Chillingworth (a physician).[7] Today *Datura* species are used ritualistically by Amazonian natives in a beverage called *yage*, and they have been implicated in the creation of Haitian "zombies" rendered amnestic and submissive and used as slaves.[8] In South America (and sometimes in the United States) scopolamine and extracts from *Datura* or *Brugmansia* species have been employed for less flamboyant criminal purposes; victims unwittingly ingest proffered candy or beverage, become docile, and are robbed with no later recollection of the circumstances.[9,10]

In the United States *Datura* became a popular agent of abuse among adolescents during the 1960s, and widespread use has continued since then.[11–18] In the fall the plant's white trumpet-shaped flower becomes a thorny capsule filled with dark seeds, which weigh approximately 10 mg and contain 4% belladonna alkaloid.[1] Most often seeds are ingested; sometimes flowers are eaten, dried leaves are smoked, roots are chewed, or teas are drunk. Seeds, powders, teas, capsules, and "herbal cigarettes" are also available in "health food" stores, as is "Asthmador," an inhalant preparation cynically promoted as an asthma medication.[19,20] (In France antiasthmatic *Datura* cigarettes are marketed.[21,22]) Also abused in midwestern and southeastern states is *Datura sauveolens* (angel's trumpet),[23] which caused intoxication in a 76-year-old man who ingested "moon flower" wine made from it.[24] Different *Datura* species are popular in other countries;[25,26] henbane abuse has been reported in Germany and Turkey.[27,28]

Belladonna alkaloids are sometimes added to other street drugs or products.[29] Atropine poisoning affected two women who drank a commercial preparation of "burdock root tea"; burdocks do not themselves contain anticholinergic compounds.[30–32]

Less often abused are antiparkinsonian anticholinergics.[33–38] Of 21 trihexyphenidyl abusers from New Zealand, most were young and used ad-

Table 10–2. Dose-Related Effects of Atropine

Dose (mg)	Effects
0.5	Slight bradycardia; dryness of mouth; decreased sweating
1.0	Thirst; tachycardia; mild pupillary dilation
2.0	Tachycardia, palpitations; marked dryness of mouth; dilated pupils; blurring of near vision
5.0	All symptoms above marked; dysarthria; dysphagia; restlessness; fatigue; headache; dry, hot skin; difficulty with micturition; decreased intestinal peristalsis
10.0 or more	Above symptoms more marked; rapid, weak pulse; extreme mydriasis; very blurred vision; skin flushed, hot, dry; ataxia; delirium, hallucinations; coma

(Modified from Brown JH. Atropine, scopolamine, and related antimuscarinic drugs. In: Gilman AG, Rall TW, Nies AS, Taylor P, eds. The Pharmacologic Basis of Therapeutics, ed. 8. New York: Pergamon Press, 1990:150, with permission of the publisher.)

ditional drugs recreationally, but abuse is also well-recognized among prisoners and among schizophrenics receiving anticholinergics for extrapyramidal symptoms, who sometimes escalate dosage when they discover the drug's euphorigenic properties.[36]

To what degree amitriptyline abuse is related to its anticholinergic properties—it also has dopaminergic actions—is uncertain, but amitriptyline overdose produces prominent anticholinergic symptoms and signs.[39,40] Many H$_1$-antihistamines have anticholinergic activity, and recreational use occurs.[41] Tripelennamine is abused parenterally in combination with pentazocine ("T's and blues") (see Chapter 2). Although phenothiazine neuroleptics have anticholinergic actions, they are not abused as street drugs. Scopolamine patches (Transderm) for motion sickness have caused disorientation, memory loss, restlessness, and hallucinations, but deliberate abuse of this product has not been reported.[42] Abuse of cyclopentolate eye drops ("Cyclogel")—instilled topically with absorption likely in the nasal mucosa—has been described in several patients.[43,44]

Acute Effects and Treatment

Datura contains more atropine than scopolamine, and so although scopolamine is chiefly responsible for the mental effects, systemic anticholinergic toxicity is a predictable accompaniment (Table 10–2).[45,46] Within 2 to 6 hours of seed ingestion there is euphoria and then, with sufficient dosage, excitement, delirium, or psychosis with hallucinations that are usually visual and often terrifying—for example, monsters, devils, or "buildings melting and pulsating";[23,47] insight as to their reality is often lost. (Although hallucinations are often a desired effect,

they do not—in contrast to lysergic acid diethylamide (LSD) hallucinations—occur in the absence of excitement or delirium.) Vision is blurred; pupils are dilated and unreactive; and there is dysphagia, urinary retention, dry flushed skin, high fever, hypertension, tachypnea, and tachycardia.[9,47–50] Agitation may alternate with relative calm. The most prominent signs have been summarized as, "hot as a hare, red as a beet, dry as a bone, blind as a bat, and mad as a hatter."

Sometimes seen are nystagmus, hyperreflexia, Babinski signs, extensor posturing, myoclonus, major motor seizures, coma, circulatory collapse, respiratory failure, and death.[48] Delusions and hallucinations can lead to fatal accidents.[47] In a report of 10 cases of "angel's trumpet psychosis," flaccid paralysis was reported in subjects ingesting more than six flowers—enough to deliver at least 1.2 mg of atropine and 3.9 mg of scopolamine; in one case death was attributed to drowning after falling paralyzed into a puddle 3 inches deep.[23] The electroencephalogram shows diffuse slowing and paroxysmal sharp forms.[49] Hallucinations may be most prominent during recovery. Symptoms last hours to days, and survivors are unlikely to have neurological residua, although pupillary dilation can outlast other symptoms by days.[14,17,47,48]

Anticholinergic poisoning is seldom directly fatal, but lethality varies markedly among individuals. Survival has followed 500 mg of scopolamine and 1000 mg of atropine, yet children have died after less than 10 mg of either drug. Alarming idiosyncratic reactions are more common with scopolamine.[3]

The diagnosis of anticholinergic poisoning can be confirmed by giving an intramuscular injection of 1.0 mg physostigmine; a patient intoxicated by anticholinergics fails to develop salivation, sweating, or intestinal hyperactivity, and symptoms may improve

Table 10–3. Treatment of Anticholinergic Poisoning

Ipecac or gastric lavage
Activated charcoal, magnesium sulfate
Physostigmine, 0.5–3 mg intravenously every 30 min to
  2 h as needed
Aspirin, cooling blanket, ice bags, alcohol sponges, or
  bypass cooling
Bladder catheterization
Cardiac, respiratory, and blood pressure monitoring
Diazepam and phenytoin for seizures
Avoid neuroleptics

within minutes.[3] Treatment then follows (Table 10–3): Ipecac or gastric lavage are employed even if ingestion occurred hours earlier—anticholinergics slow gastrointestinal motility. Activated charcoal and magnesium sulfate are then given. Physostigmine, 0.5 to 3 mg, is given intravenously over 2 minutes and repeated as needed every 30 minutes to 2 hours; it is metabolized much more rapidly than atropine or scopolamine. Fever may require aspirin, a cooling blanket, ice bags, alcohol sponges, or bypass cooling. The bladder is catheterized, and fluids are given. Seizures are treated as necessary with diazepam and phenytoin.[1,51–53] Phenothiazines, because of their anticholinergic activity, are contraindicated, and sedatives should be used cautiously.[47,48]

Long-Term Effects

Few anticholinergic abusers take the drug on a daily basis. When they do, they develop tolerance to anticholinergic effects (including euphoria and sedation) and signs of physical dependence. A schizophrenic man who had formerly abused trihexyphenidyl began taking diphenhydramine (in over-the-counter Sominex) and gradually escalated the dose to 1600 mg daily; with abstinence he developed irritability, increased blinking, increased defecation, and craving.[41] A woman who abused cyclopentolate eye drops had withdrawal nausea, vomiting, weakness, and tremor.[44]

Chronic scopolamine administration increases the number of muscarinic receptors in the hippocampus of rats.[54] Animals fed *Datura stramonium* for several weeks had weight loss, decreased serum albumin and calcium levels, and increased blood urea nitrogen and alkaline phosphatase levels.[55] *Datura stramonium* also contains gamma-L-glutamyl-L-aspartate, which inhibits glutamate binding in mouse hippocampus and impairs learning.[56] Rats chronically given *Datura* seeds also have decreased brain content of protein, DNA, and RNA.[57] The

relevance of these observations to human use is unknown.

References

1. Goldfrank LR, Lampe KF. Plants. In: Goldfrank LR, Flomenbaum NE, Lewis NA, et al, eds. Toxicologic Emergencies, ed. 4. Norwalk, CT: Appleton & Lange, 1990:597.
2. Lewin NA, Howland MA, Goldfrank LR. Herbal preparations. In: Goldfrank LR, Flomenbaum NE, Lewin NA, et al, eds. Toxicologic Emergencies, ed. 4. Norwalk, CT: Appleton & Lange, 1990:587.
3. Brown JH. Atropine, scopolamine, and related antimuscarinic drugs. In: Gilman AG, Rall TW, Neis AS, Taylor P, eds. The Pharmacological Basis of Therapeutics, ed. 8. New York: Pergamon Press, 1990:150.
4. Bonner TI, Buckley NJ, Young AC, Brann MR. Identification of a family of muscarinic acetylcholine receptor genes. Science 1987; 237:527.
5. Levine RR, Birdsall MJM, North RA, et al, eds. Symposium: Subtypes of muscarinic receptors, III. Trends Pharmacol Sci 1988(suppl):1.
6. Siegel RK. The natural history of hallucinogens. In: Jacobs BL, ed. Hallucinogens: Neurochemical, Behavioral, and Clinical Perspectives. New York: Raven Press, 1984:1.
7. Khan, JA. Atropine poisoning in Hawthorne's *The Scarlet Letter*. N Engl J Med 1984; 311:414.
8. Davis W. Passage to the Darkness. The Ethnobiology of the Haitian Zombie. Chapel Hill, NC: University of North Carolina Press, 1988.
9. Brizer DA, Manning DW. Delirium induced by poisoning with anticholinergic agents. Am J Psychiatry 1982; 139:1343.
10. Ardila A, Moreno C. Scopolamine intoxication as a model of transient global amnesia. Brain Cogn 1991; 15:236.
11. Keeler MH, Kane FJ. The use of hyoscyamine as a hallucinogen and intoxicant. Am J Psychiatry 1967; 124:852.
12. Muller DJ. Unpublicized hallucinogens. JAMA 1967; 202:650.
13. Gabel MC. Purposeful ingestion of belladonna for hallucinatory effects. J Pediatr 1968; 72:864.
14. Cummins BM, Obetz SW, Wilson MR. Belladonna poisoning as a facet of psychedelia. JAMA 1968; 204:1011.
15. Teitelbaum DT. Stramonium poisoning in "teenyboppers." Ann Intern Med 1968; 68:174.
16. DeYoung C, Cross EG. Stramonium psychedelia. Can Anaesth Soc J 1969; 16:429.
17. Levy R. Jimson seed poisoning: a new hallucinogen on the horizon. J Am Col Emergency Physic 1977; 6:58.
18. Mahler DA. The jimson-weed high. JAMA 1975; 231:138.

19. Siegel RK. Herbal intoxication. Psychoactive effects from herbal cigarettes, tea, and capsules. JAMA 1976; 236:473.

20. Jacobs KW. Asthmador: a legal hallucinogen. Int J Addict 1974; 9:503.

21. Ballantyne A, Lippiett D, Park J. Herbal cigarettes for kicks. BMJ 1976; 2:1539.

22. Larcan A. Conduites toxicomaniaques utilisant des cigarettes antiasthmatiques a base de datura. Bull Acad Natl Med 1984; 168:455.

23. Hall RCW, Popkin MK, McHenry LE. Angel's trumpet psychosis: a central nervous system anticholinergic syndrome. Am J Psychiatry 1977; 134:312.

24. Smith EA, Meloan CE, Pickell JA, Oehme FW. Scopolamine poisoning from home made "moon flower" wine. J Anal Toxicol 1991; 15:216.

25. Hayman J. Datura poisoning: the Angel's Trumpet. Pathology 1985; 17:465.

26. Strobel M, Chevalier J, DeLavarelle B. Coma febrile avec polynucleose du a une intoxication par Datura Stramonium. Presse Med 1991; 20:2214.

27. Betz P, Janzen J, Roider G, Penning R. Psychopathologische Befunde nach oraler Aufnahme von Inhaltsstoffen heimischer Nachtschattengewachse. Arch Kriminol 1991; 188:175.

28. Tugrul L. Abuse of henbane by children in Turkey. Bull Narc 1985; 37:75.

29. Harrison G. The abuse of anticholinergic drugs by adolescents. Br J Psychiatry 1980; 137:495.

30. Bryson PD, Watanabe AS, Rumack BH, Murphy RC. Burdock root tea poisoning. Case report involving a commercial preparation. JAMA 1978; 239:2157.

31. Bryson PD. Burdock root poisoning. JAMA 1978; 240:1586.

32. Rhoads PM, Tong TG, Banner W, Anderson R. Anticholinergic poisonings associated with commercial burdock. J Toxicol Clin Toxicol 1984–1985; 22:581.

33. Pakes GE. Abuse of trihexyphenidyl. JAMA 1978; 240:2434.

34. Goggin DA, Solomon GF. Trihexyphenidyl abuse for euphorigenic effect. Am J Psychiatry 1979; 136:459.

35. Kaminer Y, Munitz H, Wijsenbeck H. Trihexyphenidyl (Artane) abuse: euphoriant and anxiolytic. Br J Psychiatry 1982; 140:473.

36. McInnis M, Petursson H. Trihexyphenidyl dependence. Acta Psychiatr Scand 1984; 69:538.

37. Crawshaw JA, Mullen PE. A study of benzhexol abuse. Br J Psychiatry 1984; 145:300

38. Wells BG, Marken PA, Rickman LA, et al. Characterizing anticholinergic abuse in community mental health. J Clin Psychopharmacol 1989; 9:431.

39. Cohen MJ, Hanbury R, Stimmell B. Abuse of amitriptyline. JAMA 1978; 240:1372.

40. Callahan M, Kassel D. Epidemiology of fatal tricyclic antidepressant ingestion: implications for management. Ann Emerg Med 1985; 14:1.

41. Feldman MD, Behar M. A case of massive diphenhydramine abuse and withdrawal from use of the drug. JAMA 1986; 225:3119.

42. Johnson P, Hansen D, Matarazzo D, et al. Transderm Scop patches for prevention of motion sickness. N Engl J Med 1984; 311:468.

43. Ostler HB. Cycloplegics and mydriatics: tolerance, habituation, and addiction to topical administration. J Paediatr Child Health 1990; 26:106.

44. Sato EH, deFreitas D, Foster CS. Abuse of cyclopentolate hydrochloride (Cyclogyl) drops. N Engl J Med 1992; 326:1363.

45. Arena JM. Atropine poisoning: a report of two cases from jimson weed. Clin Pediatr 1963; 2:182.

46. Farnsworth NR. Hallucinogenic plants. Science 1968; 162:1086.

47. Gowdy JM. Stramonium intoxication. Review of symptomatology in 112 cases. JAMA 1972; 221:585.

48. Mikolich JR, Paulson GW, Cross CJ. Acute anticholinergic syndrome due to jimson seed ingestion. Ann Intern Med 1975; 83:321.

49. Mikolich JR, Paulson GW, Cross CJ, Calhoun R. Neurologic and electroencephalographic effects of jimsonweed intoxication. Clin Electroencephalogr 1976; 7:49.

50. Klein-Schwartz W, Oderda GM. Jimsonweed intoxication in adolescents and young adults. Am J Dis Child 1984; 138:737.

51. Duvoisin RC, Katz R. Reversal of central anticholinergic syndrome in man by physostigmine. JAMA 1968; 206:1963.

52. Orr R. Reversal of datura stramonium delirium with physostigmine: report of three cases. Anesth Analg 1975; 54:158.

53. Shervette RE, Schydlower M, Lampe RM, Fearnow RG. Jimson "loco" weed abuse in adolescents. Pediatrics 1979; 63:520.

54. Ben-Barak J, Dudai Y. Scopolamine induces an increase in muscarinic receptor level in rat hippocampus. Brain Res 1980; 193:309.

55. Dugan GM, Gumbmann MR, Friedman M. Toxicological evaluation of jimson weed (Datura stromonium) seed. Food Chem Toxicol 1989; 27:501.

56. Ungerer A, Schmitz-Bourgeois M, Melan C, et al. Gamma-L-glutamy-L-aspartate induces specific deficits in long-term memory and inhibits [3H]glutamate binding on hippocampal membranes. Brain Res 1988; 446:205.

57. Hasan SS, Kushwaha AK. Chronic effect of datura (seed) extract on the brain of albino rats. Jpn J Pharmacol 1987; 44:1.

Chapter 11
Ethanol

Drink wine, not tears—the sage has said,
"Wine is the antidote for sorrow's poison."
                    —*The Ruba'iat of Omar Khayyam*

Oh! John Barleycorn is a wizard dopester.
Brain and body, scorched and jangled and poisoned,
return to be tuned up by the very poison that
caused the damage.   —*Jack London*

Tens of thousands of years ago, paleolithic people ingested fermented grain, fruit juice, and honey.[1] Today ethanol abuse is a major public health problem throughout much of the world. In the United States ethanol causes more than 100,000 American deaths annually, amounting to nearly 5% of total mortality, and in 1990, the cost of ethanol-related problems—including illness and lost productivity—was estimated at $136 billion.[2-5] Mortality estimates, from the Centers for Disease Control, are based on the relative risk alcohol carries for diseases such as esophageal cancer, cirrhosis, pancreatitis, and stroke, and for automobile accidents, homicide, and suicide (Tables 11–1 and 11–2). Each death represents, on average, 26 "years of potential life lost."[4]

How many Americans are alcoholics? According to the National Institute on Alcoholism and Alcohol Abuse, the answer is 10.4 million: 7.1 million men and 3.3 million women.[6] Such figures are both logistically and definitionally problematic. Screening questionnaires[7,8] and laboratory tests (Table 11–3)[9-19] tend to underestimate use.[3] Moreover, there is no consensus on what constitutes *alcoholism*.[20-23] The term usually refers to a pattern of drinking, either episodic or continuous, that interferes with health, work, home, or social functioning. The two-thirds of Americans who drink, however, occupy a continuum of severity from infrequent to obsessive, and no point clearly separates alcoholics from nonalcoholics. The term *problem drinker* includes both ethanol addicts—that is, psychologically dependent but not

necessarily physically dependent—and those who, even if abstinent most of the time, get into trouble when they drink (e.g., impaired job performance or arrests). The American Psychiatric Association's Diagnostic and Statistical Manual (DSM-III-R) defines *alcohol abuse* in terms of impaired occupational or social functioning and *alcohol dependence* in terms of such impairment plus evidence of tolerance or withdrawal symptoms (see Chapter 1).[21] It is estimated that 19 million Americans 18 years of age or older—or 7% of American adults and 19% of American adolescents—are problem drinkers.[3] A 1988 survey in Wisconsin revealed that 25% of adults were binge drinkers (five or more drinks at least once during the previous month), 8.6% consumed more than 60 drinks per month, and 6.2% had recently driven while intoxicated.[24] So-called skid row alcoholics constitute fewer than 5% of problem drinkers, the great majority of whom are middle-class blue-collar or white-collar workers or housewives.[25] Estimated lifetime rates of ethanol abuse among American physicians have ranged from 4% to 14%.[26]

At Harlem Hospital Center in New York City, 47% of 118 patients consecutively admitted to the general medical service were deemed alcoholic.[27] At the Johns Hopkins Hospital in Baltimore, alcoholism was diagnosed in 25% of inpatients from the Medicine Service, 30% from Psychiatry, 19% from Neurology, 12.5% from Obstetrics/Gynecology, and 23% from Surgery.[28] Twelve percent of American

Table 11–1. Centers for Disease Control Estimates of Alcohol-Attributable Fractions, Total Estimated Mortality, and Estimated Alcohol-Related Mortality, by Sex and Diagnosis—United States, 1987

Diagnosis	AAFs	Male Deaths	ARM	Female Deaths	ARM
Malignant Neoplasms					
Cancer of the lip/oral cavity/pharynx	0.50	5259	2630	2622	1049
Cancer of the esophagus	0.75	6705	5029	2365	1774
Cancer of the stomach	0.20	8178	1636	5428	1086
Cancer of liver/intrahepatic bile ducts	0.15	4215	632	2831	425
Cancer of the larynx	0.50	2968	1484	690	276
Mental Disorders					
Alcoholic psychoses	1.00	302	302	80	80
Alcohol dependence syndrome	1.00	3353	3353	908	908
Alcohol abuse	1.00	537	537	136	136
Cardiovascular Disease					
Essential hypertension	0.08	1663	126	2368	180
Alcoholic cardiomyopathy	1.00	688	688	109	109
Cerebrovascular disease	0.07	58,302	3790	90,068	5854
Respiratory Diseases					
Respiratory tuberculosis	0.25	911	228	396	99
Pneumonia and influenza	0.05	32,379	1619	34,852	1743
Digestive Diseases					
Diseases of esophagus/stomach/duodenum	0.10	4545	455	4520	452
Alcoholic gastritis	1.00	60	60	13	13
Alcoholic fatty liver	1.00	672	672	242	242
Acute alcoholic hepatitis	1.00	518	518	276	276
Alcoholic cirrhosis of the liver	1.00	5517	5517	1991	1991
Alcoholic liver damage, unspecified	1.00	1514	1514	535	535
Other cirrhosis of the liver	0.50	7508	3754	5097	2549
Acute pancreatitis	0.42	1117	469	1005	422
Chronic pancreatitis	0.60	121	73	74	44
Unintentional Injuries					
Motor vehicle accidents	0.42	33,904	14,240	14,386	6042
Other road vehicle accidents	0.20	159	32	72	14
Water transport accidents	0.20	853	171	95	19
Air/space transport accidents	0.16	1032	165	231	37
Alcohol poisonings	1.00	151	151	37	37
Accidental falls	0.35	6091	2132	5485	1920
Accidents caused by fires	0.45	2863	1288	1847	831
Accidental drownings	0.38	3529	1341	831	316
Other injuries	0.25	4469	1117	1410	353
Intentional Injuries					
Suicide	0.28	24,073	6740	6472	1812
Homicide	0.46	15,007	6903	4792	2204
Metabolic Disorder					
Diabetes mellitus	0.05	15,795	790	21,959	1098
Other Alcohol-Related Diagnoses					
Alcoholic polyneuropathy	1.00	4	4	0	0
Excess blood alcohol level	1.00	9	9	2	2
Total			70,168		34,927

AAFs, Alcohol-attributable fractions; ARM, alcohol-related mortality.

Modified from Alcohol-related mortality and years of potential life lost—United States, 1987. MMWR 1990; 39:173.

Table 11–2. Centers for Disease Control Estimates of Alcohol-Related Mortality and Male to Female Ratio, by Sex and Diagnostic Category—United States, 1987

Diagnostic Category Deaths (%)	Male Deaths (%)		Female Deaths (%)		Total	
Malignant neoplasms	11,410	(16.3)	4609	(13.2)	16,019	(15.2)
Mental disorders	4192	(6.0)	1124	(3.2)	5316	(5.1)
Cardiovascular diseases	4604	(6.6)	6143	(17.6)	10,747	(10.2)
Respiratory diseases	1847	(2.6)	1842	(5.3)	3688	(3.5)
Digestive diseases	13,032	(18.6)	6524	(18.7)	19,556	(18.7)
Unintentional injuries	20,637	(29.4)	9569	(27.4)	30,205	(28.7)
Intentional injuries	13,644	(19.4)	4016	(11.5)	17,660	(16.8)
Other alcohol-related diagnoses	803	(1.1)	1100	(3.1)	1903	(1.8)
Total	70,168	(100.0)	34,927	(100.0)	105,095	(100.0)

Modified from Alcohol-related mortality and years of potential life lost—United States, 1987. MMWR 1990; 39:173.

health care expenditure for adults is for alcohol abuse.[24] (Relevant to such figures is that the great majority of alcoholics are also heavy smokers.[29])

If there are any grounds for optimism among these dreary statistics, it is that they seem to have peaked, at least in the United States and Europe. By 1981, per capita consumption of ethanol for Americans older than 14 years of age had risen to 2.76 gallons; it then declined each year, reaching 2.58 gallons in 1986.[30] During this same period, there were also decreases in ethanol-related traffic fatalities and in mortality from cirrhosis.[3]

Metabolism and Mechanism of Action

Ingested ethanol is metabolized by more than one route.[31] Ninety percent is oxidized in the liver to acetaldehyde by cystosolic alcohol dehydrogenase (ADH).[32,33] The enzymatic cofactor, nicotinamide adenine dinucleotide (NAD), is thereby reduced to NADH (Figure 11–1). ADH ordinarily acts on a variety of substrates, perhaps including steroids and

Table 11–3. Laboratory Tests to Identify Alcoholics

Acetaldehyde binding to erythrocytes[9]
Transferrin carbohydrate content[10]
Platelet monoamine oxidase levels[11]
Plasma dopamine beta-hydroxylase levels[11]
Erythrocyte and skeletal muscle Na,K-ATPase activity[12]
Blood dolichol concentration[13]
Serum beta-hexosaminidase levels[14]
Serum methanol levels[15]
Plasma carnitine levels[16]
Auditory evoked potentials[18]

fatty acids, and is present in small amounts in other tissues, including brain, but its function there is unclear.[34,35] Ethanol is also oxidized by a *microsomal ethanol-oxidizing system* (MEOS), which is induced by sustained ethanol ingestion. A third route of ethanol metabolism, by catalase, is probably insignificant in vivo.[31] Very small amounts of ingested ethanol are excreted unchanged in the urine or through the lungs. ("Alcohol breath" is actually the odor of isoamylacetate, ethyl acetate, and other congeners present in different alcoholic beverages.[36])

Acetaldehyde is oxidized to acetate and then acetyl-CoA by NAD-dependent aldehyde dehydrogenase (ALDH), present in liver mitochondria. Following ingestion of C-14-labeled ethanol, the tracer appears in cholesterol, glycerol, and fatty acids.

These biochemical reactions explain a number of ethanol's effects. *Hydrogen equivalents* produced by ethanol oxidation enter mitochondria and bypass the citric acid cycle;[32] fatty acid oxidation is thereby slowed, and much of the carbon skeleton of ethanol is incorporated into fatty acids via acetyl-CoA. The result is hepatic lipid accumulation and eventual organ damage.[37] Depending on the amount and pattern of drinking, ethanol also affects body weight. One gram of ethanol releases 7 kcal of energy. Light to moderate amounts of ethanol, metabolized by ADH, reduce lipid oxidation and increase fatty acid synthesis, favoring lipid storage and weight gain. Heavy ethanol intake stimulates the MEOS system, which generates only heat with consequent weight loss.[38,39] Other effects of ethanol are a consequence of shifts in the ratio of NAD to NADH. An increased NADH to NAD ratio slows metabolism of phosphoenolpyruvate to dihydroacetate and glucose-6-phosphate and of the latter to glycogen, setting the stage for hypoglycemia (Table 11–4).[32] An elevated

$$\text{CH}_3\text{CHOH} + \text{NAD}^+ \xrightarrow{\substack{\text{alcohol} \\ \text{dehydrogenase}}} \text{CH}_3\text{CHO} + \text{NAD} + \text{H}^+$$

ethanol   acetaldehyde

$$\text{CH}_3\text{CHO} + \text{NAD}^+ + \text{H}_2\text{O} \xrightarrow{\substack{\text{aldehyde} \\ \text{dehydrogenase}}} \text{CH}_3\text{COO}^- + \text{NADH} + 2\text{H}^+$$

acetaldehyde   acetate

Figure 11–1. Metabolism of ethanol.

NADH to NAD ratio also interferes with the conversion of lactate to pyruvate, contributing to metabolic acidosis.[33]

Lowered NAD levels slow the oxidation of acetaldehyde, a more potent toxin than ethanol.[32,33] In addition to interfering with tissue metabolism, including heart, liver, and brain, acetaldehyde might contribute to ethanol tolerance, dependence, and withdrawal. Some rats self-administer acetaldehyde but not ethanol intraventricularly,[40] and mice develop physical dependence to acetaldehyde, with ethanol and acetaldehyde each attenuating the other's withdrawal signs.[41] Although ethanol rarely produces pharmacologically significant blood acetaldehyde levels in naive animals or humans, acetaldehyde accumulates in the brains of chronic drinkers,[33] and higher blood levels are found in alcoholics.[42]

Acetaldehyde might have indirect effects by causing central nervous system (CNS) accumulation of a family of compounds called *tetrahydroisoquinolines* (TIQ). These are of two types. Alkyl-substituted TIQs form by condensation of acetaldehyde with catecholamines such as norepinephrine to form 4,6,7-trihydroxy-TIQ or dopamine to form salsolinol.[43] Benzyl-substituted TIQs form by condensation of catecholamines with certain of their own metabolites, present in abnormally high amounts because of competition by acetaldehyde for ALDH. For example, dopamine condenses with phenacetaldehyde to form tetrahydropapaveroline (THP). Acetaldehyde also condenses with indoles to form beta-carboline adducts. TIQs are precursors to morphine in the poppy, and they bind to opioid receptors in the brain. In animals, direct injection of acetaldehyde, TIQs, or beta-carbolines into brain produces addictive-like preference for ethanol, and this behavior is attenuated by naloxone or naltrexone.[44–46] Such findings are consistent with the hypothesis that despite striking differences between their withdrawal syndromes, opioids and ethanol share basic mechanisms of dependence.

Ethanol acts on many levels of the neuraxis, especially complex polysynaptic systems such as the reticular formation (depressed alertness)[47] and the parietal association cortex (impaired eye-hand coordination).[48] Ethanol's action on single neurons is biphasic, initially increasing electrical excitability and then, with higher concentrations, depressing it.[49,50] Although ethanol affects a number of neurotransmitter systems, most investigators believe that its primary action is disruption of the phospholipid bilayer of cell membranes.[51,52] The result, demonstrable by such techniques as electron paramagnetic resonance, is increased *membrane fluidization* and secondary alteration of proteins and ion channels.[53,54] Such action is shared by general anesthetics, which are cross-tolerant with ethanol. In animals, ethanol tolerance correlates with decreased "fluidizability"—or increased membrane "stiffness"—and physical dependence correlates with persistence of this "stiffness" following abstinence.[33,52,55] The increased "stiffness" with chronic ethanol intake is probably the result of increased cholesterol and fatty acid content, which in turn reduces the ability of ethanol to enter the membrane.[52]

A crucial question is whether these changes in physical properties are sufficient to account for ethanol's diverse effects—presumably secondary to conformational changes—on neurotransmitters and ion channels (Table 11–5).[56–93] Most excitatory receptors, including the N-methyl-D-aspartate (NMDA) and kainate subtypes of glutamate receptors and voltage-sensitive calcium channels, are inhibited by

Table 11–4. Contributions to Alcoholic Hypoglycemia

Starvation
Depletion of liver glycogen
Reduced NAD/NADH ratio, limiting gluconeogenesis
Reduced breakdown of fatty acids to acetyl-CoA, further limiting gluconeogenesis
Blunted response to growth hormone

Source: Lieber CS. Metabolism of ethanol. In: Lieber CS, ed. Metabolic Aspects of Alcoholism. Baltimore: University Park Press, 1977:1.

Table 11–5. Neurochemical Effects of Ethanol

Na+/K+ ATPase. Acutely inhibited by ethanol, with development of tolerance and rebound increase during withdrawal[56,57]

Adenylyl cyclase/cyclic AMP. Reports of increased, decreased, or unchanged activity after ethanol.[56] Also reports of ethanol effects on G proteins[58]

Norepinephrine. Increased brain turnover as ethanol blood levels rise and decreased turnover as levels fall. Adrenal catecholamines released dose dependently. Conflicting reports attempting to correlate signs of intoxication or withdrawal with norepinephrine changes[56,59,60]

Dopamine. Increased brain turnover following acute ethanol, most evident in mesolimbic structures.[61] Increased firing of ventral tegmental area neurons and increased extracellular concentrations of dopamine in the nucleus accumbens following acute ethanol[5]

Serotonin. Conflicting reports of increased, decreased, or unaltered brain turnover after acute or chronic ethanol.[56] Depending on animal strain and receptor subtype, serotonin precursors, agonists, and reuptake blockers reported to decrease ethanol preference[62]

Acetylcholine (ACh). Depressed cholinergic transmission, decreased ACh release, and increased ACh levels after acute ethanol; increased ACh synthesis, release, and receptor number after chronic ethanol use.[56] Conflicting reports of acute effects on nicotinic ACh receptors: either enhancement[5] or inhibition with compensatory up-regulation of receptor numbers.[63] Compared with controls, reduced changes in mood and pulse in alcoholics following physostigmine[64]

GABA. Stimulation by ethanol of GABAergic neurotransmission with rapid adaptation of GABA receptors to agonists.[65–67] No effect on GABA synthesis, release, reuptake, brain levels, or turnover; on binding of GABA or benzodiazepines to receptor sites; or on barbiturate-induced modulation of $GABA_A$ receptor binding.[65] Increased number or sensitivity of $GABA_A$ receptors after acute ethanol intake and compensatory reduction in binding with chronic ethanol intake.[68] Ethanol activation of $GABA_A$–gated chloride flux in the absence of GABA and ethanol facilitation of non–GABA-related chloride conductance, suggesting a direct effect on chloride channels.[69] Tolerance to effects on GABA-induced chloride flux, not to direct effects on chloride channels.[70,71] Ethanol enhancement of GABA action dependent on 8 amino acid sequence of GABA receptor's gamma subunit[72]

Calcium. In neuronal cell cultures, brain slices, and living rats, acute inhibition by ethanol of inward calcium currents, neuronal excitability, and calcium-magnesium-ATPase.[81,82] Compensatory up-regulation of L-type calcium channels with chronic ethanol[83]

Adenosine. Stimulation by acute ethanol of adenosine A-2 receptor-dependent cyclic AMP production; compensatory reduction with chronic ethanol use[86]

Endorphins. Increased synthesis of beta-endorphin in the hypothalamus, decreased synthesis of beta-endorphin in the pituitary, and decreased brain met-enkephalin levels following ethanol use.[87,88] Delta-receptor binding acutely decreased, mu-receptor binding increased, and kappa receptors unaffected.[56,89] Much variation with species, brain region, and duration of exposure[90]

Glutamate. Acute inhibition of NMDA-activated ion current in hippocampal neurons.[91] Up-regulation of NMDA receptors in mice receiving chronic ethanol. Reduction of NMDA excitotoxicity in cultured cerebral cortical neurons[92]

---

ethanol. Most inhibitory systems, including gamma-aminobutyric acid (GABA) receptors, are augmented. Exceptions are enhancement of excitatory nicotinic acetylcholine receptors and serotonergic 5-HT_3 receptors.[5]

Some of these effects have obvious clinical implications. Depending on the strain, ethanol ingestion in rats is suppressed by serotonin (5-HT) precursor loading, 5-HT releasers, 5HT uptake blockers, agonists at 5-HT_{1A} receptors, mixed agonists at 5-HT_{1B}/5-HT_{1C} or 5-HT_{1C}/5-HT_2 receptors, and antagonists at 5-HT_3 receptors.[5] Possibly related observations include a reduced density of 5-HT brain stem raphe nucleus fibers innervating limbic structures in strains of ethanol-preferring rats (see later); reduced levels of cerebrospinal fluid (CSF) serotonin and 5-hydroxyindoleacetic acid in many alcoholics; and similar CSF changes in patients with bulimia, obsessive-compulsive disorder, and violent behavior.[62]

Ethanol-induced CNS depression is facilitated by GABA agonists and inhibited by GABA antagonists, and drugs that elevate GABA brain levels suppress ethanol withdrawal signs.[73] Such effects are incomplete, however.[65] For example, in rats the $GABA_A$ agonist muscimol suppresses withdrawal seizures but not forelimb tremors.[74]

In cultured neurons ethanol increases the number of binding sites for benzodiazepine inverse agonists, and the weak benzodiazepine inverse agonist, R015-4513 (an imidazobenzodiazepine), inhibits ethanol-stimulated chloride flux.[70] In rats R015-4513 blocks mild ethanol intoxication without affecting behavioral changes induced by pentobarbital.[75] Whether this effect represents specific antagonism or an intrinsic action is controversial.[76,77] R015-4513 induces seizures in animals recently withdrawn from ethanol but does not itself cause seizures or withdrawal-like signs, and it reverses ethanol's anticonvulsant effects at subconvulsant doses.[78-80] It does not reverse severe ethanol intoxication (i.e., coma).[69]

Up-regulation of L-type calcium channels in animals parallels ethanol tolerance and withdrawal hyperexcitability. Cerebral cortical L-type channels, however, are not increased in the brains of human alcoholics.[84] In animals calcium channel blockers reduce the severity of ethanol withdrawal.[85]

In mice ethanol withdrawal seizures are exacerbated by NMDA and decreased by the NMDA receptor antagonist MK-801.[93]

Bulk membrane fluidization might not explain all of ethanol's actions. There is evidence, for example, that ethanol affects adenylyl cyclase by directly interacting with G proteins; its effects on beta-adrenergic transmission may depend on specific dissociation of G protein subunits or destabilization of the beta-agonist receptor–G protein complex.[94] Others have reported poor correlation between membrane disordering and inhibition of calcium flux.[95] Moreover, cell membranes of aging mice and rats become increasingly stiff and resistant to fluidization, yet such animals are more sensitive to ethanol-induced ataxia and sedation.[96] Some drugs as well as fever increase membrane fluidity without producing intoxication.[53] In mouse brain, membrane fluidization did not correlate with ethanol enhancement of GABA-dependent chloride flux.[97] In an attempt to deal with observations such as these, a modification of the bulk membrane hypothesis proposes that ethanol (and other anesthetics) interacts with particular membrane domains—patches of lipids that differ in chemical composition and fluidity.[53]

Genetic Aspects

The relative risk of ethanol dependence is less than that of addiction to other drugs such as opioids or cocaine.[22] One-third of adult Americans drink occasionally and another third at least weekly, yet alcoholism develops in only a minority. In fact, half the ethanol drunk in America is consumed by 10% of the population.[98] Patterns of ethanol use show striking ethnic and cultural differences. Probably genetic is the much lower incidence of alcoholism among Mongoloid Asians than whites or blacks. Probably nongenetic is the greater prevalence of abstention

Table 11–6. Proposed Genetic Subtypes of Alcoholism[78,107,108]

Type I
High harm avoidance and reward dependence, low novelty seeking
Loss of control when not abstinent
Alcoholism onset in late adulthood
Men and women both affected (*milieu limited*)

Type II
High novelty seeking, low harm avoidance and reward dependence
Inability to abstain
Alcoholism onset in adolescence or early adulthood, with antisocial behavior
Male predominance (*male-limited*)

among American black women compared with white, yet the greater likelihood of black women who drink becoming alcoholic.[3]

ADH, which is the rate-limiting enzyme of ethanol metabolism, consists of multiple isoenzymes, the result of five structural genes encoding five different polypeptide subunits. These isoenzymes differ in their reactivity toward ethanol and contribute to different rates of ethanol metabolism. Peak blood ethanol concentrations (BEC) thus can be very different after equivalent amounts of ethanol, even among individuals of similar age, weight, and prior drinking experience.[99,100]

ALDH is also genetically polymorphous, and its different forms account for striking ethnic differences in response to ethanol.[99,100] Compared with whites, a greater percentage of Mongoloid Asians have acute adverse reactions to ethanol, consisting of facial flushing, tachycardia, abdominal warmth, and dysphoria. The cause is genetic deficiency of an isoenzyme of ALDH, leading to elevated tissue levels of acetaldehyde, which is more vasodilatory and sympathomimetic than ethanol.[101,102] Among the 40% of Chinese, Japanese, and South American Indians who have this isoenzyme deficiency, alcoholism is much less prevalent than among those who do not.

Whites and blacks do not lack this isoenzyme, yet genetic influences contribute to alcoholism in these groups as well.[103,104] There is a twofold higher concordance for alcoholism in identical than in fraternal twins, and adopted-away children of alcoholics have an increased risk of alcoholism even when raised by nonalcoholic adoptive parents.[105,106] On the basis of such studies, Cloninger has postulated two major genetic subtypes of alcoholism (Table 11–6).[1,98,107] Type I alcoholics display the psychological characteristics of passive-dependent or anxious personalities: (1) high harm avoidance ("cautious, apprehensive, pessimistic, inhibited, shy, and susceptible to fatigue"), (2) high reward dependence ("eager to help others, emotionally dependent, warmly sympathetic, sentimental, sensitive to social cues, and persistent"), and (3) low novelty seeking ("rigid, reflective, loyal, orderly, and attentive to details"). By contrast, type II alcoholics have antisocial personalities: (1) low harm avoidance ("confident, relaxed, optimistic, uninhibited, carefree, and energetic"), (2) low reward dependence ("socially detached, emotionally cool, practical, tough-minded, and independently self-willed"), and (3) high novelty seeking ("impulsive, exploratory, excitable, disorderly, distractable"). The drinking pattern of type I alcoholics is one of "loss of control"—they can abstain from ethanol for long periods, but once they begin drinking they cannot stop. Their problems usually begin in late adulthood after many years of exposure to socially encouraged heavy drinking, and they are fearful and guilty about their drinking. Men and women are both affected. Both hereditary and environmental factors are necessary for alcoholism to develop in type I individuals (*milieu limited*). The drinking pattern of type II alcoholics is "inability to abstain entirely"; it is largely limited to men, begins in adolescence or early adulthood with antisocial behavior, and is relatively independent of environmental influences (*male-limited*). They also have high incidence of depression and suicidal ideation.[98,108]

Not every study supports the existence of Cloninger's alcoholism subtypes.[109] Of 456 boys followed to age 47, 116 became alcoholic, 18% before age 20 and 45% after age 31; there was no correlation between age of onset and alcoholic parentage.[110] In a twin study, a strong genetic influence was evident for men with early-onset alcoholism but not for men with late-onset alcoholism or for women with onset at any age.[111] One possibility is that type II alcoholism is simply one manifestation of a broader psychiatric diagnosis—*antisocial personality disorder*—rather than a form of primary alcoholism.[112] Another is that alcoholism is a heterogeneous group of disorders variably dependent on genetic and environmental factors.[106]

Most animals dislike ethanol, and ingenious strategies (such as vaporized cages) have been employed to produce intoxication. Strains of mice and rats have been bred, however, which not only prefer ethanol to water but also seek it out and develop tolerance and physical dependence.[113] Other rodent strains show different physiological responses to ethanol. For example, *long-sleep* (LS) mice are sensitive to ethanol's disruption of the righting reflex, depression of body temperature, elevation of plasma corti

costerone, and inhibition of cerebellar Purkinje cell firing; *short-sleep* (SS) mice are more resistant to these effects and exhibit greater preference for drinking ethanol.[114] In oocytes injected with mRNA from LS mice, ethanol facilitated GABA responses, whereas in oocytes injected with mRNA from SS mice, ethanol was inhibitory.[115] These actions signify different biophysical properties of GABA receptors in LS and SS mice.[116] Such speculation is supported by observations in other mouse strains that a point mutation in the gene for the alpha-6 subunit of the $GABA_A$ receptor, specific to cerebellar granule cells, rendered the animals intolerant to both ethanol and benzodiazepines.[851] Neuronal and erythrocyte membranes from LS mice are more easily "fluidized" by ethanol.[117]

Analogous to human type II alcoholics, other strains of ethanol-seeking mice demonstrate exploratory behavior with little fear; compared with ethanol-avoiding mice they have low basal levels of brain dopamine and increased dopamine turnover.[98] As noted earlier, some strains differ in their responses to serotonin manipulation.[62] The P strain of alcohol-preferring rats has depressed levels of serotonin in several brain areas, including the nucleus accumbens;[118] ethanol consumption increases nucleus accumbens levels of serotonin, and serotonin uptake inhibitors such as fluoxetine block ethanol preference.[119] Ethanol reinforcement in this strain might involve facilitation of serotonergic neurons in the dorsal raphe nucleus. By contrast, the AA strain of ethanol-preferring rats has elevated levels of brain serotonin, and destruction of the dorsal raphe nucleus has no effect on ethanol preference.[120]

Other strains of ethanol-preferring rats have higher densities of GABA-containing nerve terminals in the nucleus accumbens,[5] and ethanol differentially alters brain levels of $GABA_A$ receptor subunit mRNAs in withdrawal seizure-prone compared with withdrawal seizure-resistant mice.[121] Some strains of rodents demonstrate differences in brain levels of [Met]-enkephalin or beta-endorphin.[122,123]

Primary alcoholics (those without other underlying psychiatric illness) and their nonalcoholic children have been studied for possible genetic markers or predictors of disease.[17] Compared with sons of nonalcoholics, sons of alcoholics were less intoxicated (as measured by body sway and psychomotor performance) at equivalent blood ethanol concentrations.[105] Decreased reaction to ethanol could presumably make it harder for someone to learn when to stop drinking. (In the same subjects diazepam did not produce different responses, suggesting ethanol specificity.[124]) Compared with controls, alcoholics and their preadolescent sons have dampened amplitudes of the P300 event-related potential, less electroencephalographic (EEG) alpha activity before ethanol consumption, and a greater amount of EEG alpha activity after ethanol consumption.[105,125,126] Low platelet monoamine oxidase B activity has been observed in alcoholics (especially type I), persisting with abstinence; it is unclear if such changes occur in nonalcoholic offspring.[17,127] Diminished platelet adenylyl cyclase response to stimulants persists in abstinent alcoholics, and diminished lymphocyte adenylyl cyclase response to adenosine persists after the cells are cultured for several generations in ethanol-free media.[128,129] Some children of alcoholics have low levels of platelet adenylyl cyclase even if they are not themselves drinkers.[5] Nonalcoholics at high or low risk have different pituitary beta-endorphin and adrenal cortisol responses to ethanol,[130] and high-risk nonalcoholics have lower plasma GABA-like activity.[131] Compared with controls, sons of familial alcoholics have higher peak serum thyrotropin levels after receiving thyrotropin-releasing hormone.[132]

There have been claims of linkage between a genetic determinant of alcoholism and the genes for the MNS blood groups (chromosome 4) or for esterase-D (chromosome 13).[133,134] In 1990, it was reported that a particular (A1) allele of the dopamine D2 receptor gene, on chromosome 11, was present in 69% of alcoholics compared with 20% of nonalcoholics, apparently conferring "susceptibility to at least one form of alcoholism."[135] Two subsequent studies found no significant difference in the prevalence of the A1 allele between alcoholics and nonalcoholics and no linkage within families of the A1 allele to alcoholism.[136,137] In another report, although the A1 allele did not segregate with alcoholism per se within individual families, it was associated with alcoholism and severe medical complications.[138] In a further study the A1 allele was significantly increased not only in patients with alcoholism (42.3% versus 14.5% for nonalcoholic controls) but also in patients with Tourette's syndrome (44.9%), attention deficit disorder (46.2%), and autism (54.5%) but not schizophrenia.[139] A possible explanation for the association of the A1 allele with alcoholism in the absence of tight linkage is that it is a *modifying gene,* itself neither necessary nor sufficient to cause the disease but affecting its severity.[140] How it modifies whatever other genes are involved in alcoholism is unknown, but it is probably relevant that individuals who carry the A1 allele have reduced striatal binding of the dopamine agonist spiperone com-

Table 11–7. Correlation of Symptoms with Blood Ethanol Concentration

Blood Ethanol Concentration (mg/dL)	Symptoms
50–150	Euphoria or dysphoria, shyness or expansiveness, friendliness or argumentativeness
	Impaired concentration, judgment, and sexual inhibitions
150–250	Slurred speech and ataxic gait, diplopia, nausea, tachycardia, drowsiness, or labile mood with sudden bursts of anger or antisocial acts
300	Stupor alternating with combativeness or incoherent speech, heavy breathing, vomiting
400	Coma
500	Respiratory paralysis, death

pared with individuals who do not.[141] Perhaps such individuals compensate for decreased dopamine activity in the "reward circuit" by drinking ethanol.

Ethanol Intoxication

Ethanol intoxication is so common that physicians tend to forget that it can be fatal, especially when additional drugs have been taken (Table 11–7). Rapidly absorbed from the gastrointestinal tract, ethanol is distributed throughout body water.[142] About 50 g (roughly 2 oz) of 100% ethanol—corresponding to approximately 4 oz of 90-proof spirits, 14 oz of wine, or 48 oz of beer—would produce a mildly intoxicating BEC of 100 mg/dL in a 70-kg man. In nontolerant individuals, ethanol is metabolized at 70 to 150 mg/kg body weight/hour with a fall in BEC of 10 to 25 mg/dL/hour (average 16 mg/dL/hour). Most adults therefore require 6 hours to metabolize a 50-g dose. Drinking only an additional 8 g per hour maintains the BEC at 100 mg/dL; drinking more rapidly raises it. In women, lower activity of gastric ADH leads to higher BECs compared with men.[143,144]

Early saturation of ADH accounts for the constant rate (zero-order kinetics) of ethanol metabolism. Induction of the MEOS by ethanol (and also by other drugs, such as barbiturates) accounts in part for ethanol tolerance, most of which, however, is pharmacodynamic (see Chapter 1).[145] (Zero-order kinetics breaks down at very high ethanol concentration—that is, elimination becomes more dependent on concentration; the mechanism is unclear but does not appear to involve MEOS.[146]) Food in the stomach delays ethanol absorption, and alcoholics learn to enhance intoxication by not eating. Aspirin, cimetidine, and ranitidine reduce gastric ADH activity and when taken with ethanol produce substantially higher blood levels.[147]

Clinically ethanol is a CNS depressant; euphoria and hyperactivity associated with intoxication are the result of cerebral disinhibition, not direct stimulation. At any BEC, intoxication is greater when the level is rising than when it is falling, when the level is reached rapidly, and when the level has been recently achieved.[2] These factors as well as an individual's degree of tolerance mean that a single BEC determination is an unreliable indicator of drunkenness; Table 11–7 offers broad generalizations.[148] (The National Council on Alcoholism defines tolerance as either a blood ethanol level greater than 150 mg without gross evidence of intoxication or daily consumption of at least one-fifth of a gallon of liquor—or equivalent wine or beer—in a 180-lb individual.[149]) Coma, respiratory depression, and death would occur in 50% of subjects at a BEC of 500 mg/dL, but levels of less than 400 mg/dL have been fatal, and levels above 800 mg/dL have been documented in alert patients.[150–153] Most states define legal intoxication as a BEC of at least 100 mg/dL. Driving skills, however, are impaired at levels as low as 50 mg/dL.[154]

Slow saccadic eye movements and interrupted, jerky smooth pursuit, sometimes impairing visual acuity, accompany low to moderate BECs. At these levels, there is increased EEG beta activity ("beta buzz"). Higher concentrations cause nystagmus, esophoria or exophoria, and diplopia, with EEG slowing.[155,156] Ethanol suppresses the rapid eye movement (REM) stage of sleep, followed, as levels fall, by REM "rebound" (and sometimes vivid dreaming). Chronic drinkers have marked disruption of sleep organization, with frequent awakenings and reduction of deep non-REM sleep.[157] Nighttime hypoxemia is common in alcoholics, who may be at increased risk for sleep apnea.[158] Both low and high BECs cause hypothermia; when, as is not unusual, drinkers are exposed to low environmental temperature, hypothermia can be marked—it averaged 84.5°F in a report of 31 patients—with a danger of cardiac arrhythmia.[159,160]

Two forms of ethanol intoxication merit separate categorization. Pathological intoxication, also called idiosyncratic intoxication or acute alcoholic paranoid state, consists of sudden extreme excitement, sometimes with delusions, hallucinations, and violent behavior, even homicide. After minutes to hours, there is sleep and amnesia for the episode. Some cases of pathologic intoxication may represent psychological dissociative reactions; others may be the result of paradoxical excitation, such as occurs with barbiturates. Alcoholic "blackouts" consist of periods of drinking for which the subject has no recollection even though at the time alertness was preserved and behavior appeared normal. Although they are usually associated with frank alcoholism, blackouts also occur in moderate drinkers.[161] The amnesia of pathological intoxication and blackouts is a direct effect of ethanol; BECs as low as 40 mg/dL cause memory impairment, which progresses as the BEC rises. Experimental studies have shown that the effect is on encoding, not consolidation or retrieval. In fact, if ethanol is taken after an event has been encoded, consolidation is enhanced.[162,163] An association of blackouts and low plasma tryptophan levels suggests that alcoholic derangement of serotonin activity might be contributory.[164]

Ethanol can precipitate cardiac arrhythmia, including atrial fibrillation and ventricular tachycardia, in the absence of alcoholic cardiomyopathy or other cardiac disease (holiday heart syndrome). Ethanol releases catecholamines from the adrenal medulla and also directly affects cardiac conduction. A careful drinking history should be obtained in any patient with unexplained palpitations or "lone" atrial fibrillation.[165]

Ethanol intoxication frequently accompanies other serious illness and can intensify depressed consciousness from any cause. Stupor in someone with "alcoholic breath" and signs of vasodilation (flushing, tachycardia, hypotension, and hypothermia) obviously suggests ethanol overdose; such signs, however, can mask the presence of subdural hematoma, meningitis, hepatic encephalopathy, hypoglycemia, ketoacidosis, or other drug poisoning.

For every 100 mg/dL BEC, serum osmolarity rises about 22 mOsm/L. This hyperosmolarity does not cause symptoms because ethanol freely crosses cell membranes without causing shifts of water, but comatose patients whose serum osmolarity is higher than that predicted by serum sodium, glucose, and urea should be suspected of ethanol poisoning.[166] Ethanol suppresses antidiuretic hormone and with high water intake can cause symptomatic hyponatremia ("beer potomania").[167]

The treatment of severe ethanol poisoning is similar to that of other depressant drugs (Table 11–8). Death is from respiratory depression, and so patients require artificial ventilation in an intensive care unit. Hypovolemia, acid–base or electrolyte imbalance, hypoglycemia, and abnormal temperature are often present; if the blood level glucose is not known, 50%

Table 11–8. Treatment of Acute Ethanol Intoxication

For Obstreperous or Violent Patients
Isolation, calming environment, reassurance—avoid sedatives
Close observation

For Stuporous or Comatose Patients
If hypoventilation, artificial respiration in an intensive care unit
If serum glucose in doubt, intravenous 50% glucose
Thiamine, 100 mg, and multivitamins, intramuscularly or intravenously
Careful monitoring of blood pressure; correction of hypovolemia or acid–base imbalance
Consider hemodialysis if patient severely acidotic, deeply comatose, or apneic
Avoid emetics or gastric lavage
Avoid analeptics
Do not forget other possible causes of coma in an alcoholic, as well as concomitant drug use

dextrose is given intravenously with parenteral thiamine. Ethanol's rapid gastrointestinal absorption means that gastric lavage is useful only if other drugs have been ingested. Sedatives or neuroleptics in obstreperous or violent patients can push them into coma and respiratory depression. A familiar feature of ethanol intoxication is a patient's tendency to appear awake during examination only to lapse into stupor and respiratory depression when left alone.

A BEC of 400 mg/dL in a nonhabitual drinker can take 20 hours to become 0. Ethanol metabolism is increased by fructose, which, however, causes gastrointestinal upset, lactic acidosis, hyperuricemia, and osmotic diuresis.[150,161] Hemodialysis or peritoneal dialysis hastens ethanol elimination and should be considered in patients with very high BECs, severe acidosis, or additional drug ingestion (including methanol or ethylene glycol) and in severely intoxicated children. Analeptics, such as ethamivan, caffeine, or amphetamine, are of no value and can precipitate seizures or cardiac arrhythmia.

Numerous other drugs have been studied in ethanol poisoning. In mice low doses of propranolol reduced ethanol-induced depression, but higher doses augmented it, and in humans, propranolol increased ethanol inebriation ratings.[168] L-Dopa, aminophylline, and ephedrine reportedly reduced human ethanol intoxication, perhaps through norepinephrine pathways;[169] the dopamine agonist apomorphine, however, aggravated symptoms.[170] By unclear mechanisms naloxone seems to reverse ethanol-induced coma in a small subset of patients; responders are

not identifiable before treatment, however, and they tend to relapse after only minutes.[171–176]

Not commercially available is the experimental—and controversial—imidazobenzodiazepine drug, R015-4513, which in animals reverses symptoms of mild intoxication but not stupor or respiratory depression.[75]

Ethanol is often ingested with other drugs, either recreationally or in suicide attempts. Although ethanol and barbiturates are cross-tolerant, together the intoxicating or lethal dose for each may be strikingly lowered. Death from apnea followed a secobarbital blood level of 50 μg/mL and a BEC of 100 mg/dL.[177] Ethanol combined with chloral hydrate ("Mickey Finn") has a particularly notorious reputation.[178]

Such additive or synergistic effects also occur when ethanol is taken with sedating antihistamines; neuroleptics; and other sedatives or tranquilizers, such as methaqualone (now a schedule 1 drug), meprobamate, or benzodiazepines (Table 11–9).[179,180] In one survey, 17% of alcoholics also took benzodiazepines daily, often obtained from a nonmedical source.[181] Diazepam and flurazepam have blood half-lives of more than 24 hours and contribute to intoxication when ethanol is taken the next day. Opioids and ethanol also aggravate each other's effects, and many heroin or methadone users are also alcoholic. Death has followed ethanol taken with propoxyphene. Tricyclic antidepressants have reportedly either antagonized or aggravated ethanol's effects. Ethanol's cross-tolerance with general anesthetics such as diethyl ether, chloroform, or fluorinated agents slows sleep induction, but synergistic interaction then increases the depth and length of the anesthetic stage reached. The balance between cross-tolerance and synergistic effects is complex and unpredictable, however, and this uncertainty, coupled with decreased adrenocortical response to stress, impending withdrawal, and associated disease (especially cardiomyopathy), makes alcoholics high anesthetic and surgical risks.[182]

Ethanol interacts in different ways with many drugs (see Table 11–7).[183] For example, it initially retards and then accelerates phenytoin metabolism, producing either drug toxicity or inadequate seizure control.[184] Ethanol inhibits warfarin metabolism. In patients taking antihypertensives, it aggravates postural hypotension. When ethanol is taken with sulfonylurea hypoglycemics, procarbazine, sulfonamides, chloramphenicol, griseofulvin, quinacrine, or metronidazole, a disulfiram-like reaction results (see later). When ethanol is taken with disulfiram itself, the reaction can be fatal.[184]

Table 11–9. Some Ethanol-Drug Interactions[179–184]

Additive or Supraadditive Sedation (in some cases despite cross-tolerance)
General anesthetics
Barbiturates
Benzodiazepines
Nonbenzodiazepine, nonbarbiturate sedatives (e.g., chloral hydrate, glutethimide, meprobamate)
Antihistamines
Tricyclic antidepressants
Neuroleptics
Opioids

Metabolic Effects
Phenytoin (acute ethanol decreases phenytoin metabolism; chronic ethanol increases it)
Warfarin (acute ethanol decreases warfarin metabolism; chronic ethanol increases it)
Aspirin, cimetidine, ranitidine (reduction of gastric alcohol dehydrogenase activity, producing higher blood ethanol levels)

Other Additive Effects
Antihypertensives (postural hypotension)
Insulin and oral hypoglycemics (hypoglycemia)
Neuroleptics (lowered seizure threshold, liver damage)
Chloral hydrate (vasodilation)

Disulfiram-like Reactions
Sulfonylurea hypoglycemics
Chloramphenicol
Griseofulvin
Isoniazid
Metronidazole
Quinacrine

Interactions with Congeners
Monoamine oxidase inhibitors and tyramine in certain wines—e.g., Chianti—produce acute hypertensive crisis
Cobalt in beer produces cardiomyopathy—additive to direct ethanol cardiotoxicity?

Ethanol Withdrawal

"Hangover," consisting of headache, malaise, nausea, sweating, and tremulousness, does not require chronic drinking. It is not an entirely harmless condition, however; studies of motor coordination (e.g., pilots tested in a flight simulator) have shown impairment.[185] More severe or prolonged symptoms indicate physical dependence. Ethanol withdrawal has traditionally been divided into early and late syndromes (Table 11–10).[155,186]

The most common symptom of early ethanol withdrawal is gross tremor, which requires at least several days of heavy drinking and is promptly relieved by ethanol. With continued abstinence, it be-

Table 11–10. Ethanol Withdrawal Syndromes

Early
Tremulousness
Hallucinosis
Seizures

Late
Delirium tremens

comes more intense and is accompanied by easy startling, anxiety, insomnia, nystagmus, flushing, sweating, anorexia, nausea, vomiting, weakness, tachypnea, tachycardia, and systolic hypertension. Except for agitation and inattentiveness, mentation remains intact during early withdrawal; altered mentation suggests the presence of other disturbances, such as seizures, Wernicke-Korsakoff syndrome, meningitis, or subdural hematoma. Tremor is distal, coarse, irregular, rapid, and worse with movement, interfering with eating or even standing. Without treatment it usually subsides over several days, although some patients feel "shaky inside" for a few weeks.[186,187]

Perceptual disturbances occur in about one-fourth of these patients and include vivid dreams, nightmares, illusions, and hallucinations, which can be auditory, visual, tactile, olfactory, or a combination (*alcoholic hallucinosis*). Visual hallucinations are most common, with imagery of insects, animals, people, or disembodied heads. Sometimes occurring only with eye closure, they are mostly fragmentary and tend to last minutes at a time over several days. Insight varies, and there are often paranoid delusions.[186,188] Hallucinations sometimes occur during active drinking or after more than a week of abstinence.[189] A Harlem Hospital patient, blind from bilateral eye injury, during ethanol withdrawal developed not only formed visual hallucinations, which he recognized as such (e.g., little orange people walking through walls), but also Anton's syndrome—he believed his vision had returned and confabulated descriptions.[190] Withdrawal hallucinations have been restricted to the right visual hemifield in patients with left hemineglect, consistent with "inner representation" hypotheses of the neglect syndrome.[191]

Of 70 patients with alcoholic hallucinosis (auditory, visual, or both) 24 had no other symptoms, and the rest had varying combinations of tremor, seizures, and delusions; 4 later developed delirium tremens. Consistent with other reports,[189] eight continued to have hallucinations for months or years, sometimes with ideas of reference, loose associations, and flat affect. Ethanol or its withdrawal might have precipitated schizophrenia in some of these patients, but in none was that diagnosis apparent before the first bout of hallucinosis.[188] Another study, using controls, found no increased incidence of schizophrenia either among patients before their hallucinosis or among their relatives.[192]

Transient parkinsonism and transient chorea have each occurred during ethanol withdrawal.[187,193] Parkinsonism affects patients older than 50 years of age, beginning within a few days of the last drink or sometimes during drinking.[194] It tends to clear over days or weeks without treatment, and patients have been followed for years without developing Parkinson's disease.[195] Oral-lingual choreiform dyskinesias, sometimes spreading to neck or arm muscles, typically affect younger patients during the second week of abstinence.[196] Acutely ethanol decreases striatal dopamine release, perhaps accounting for parkinsonism. Chorea might be secondary to dopamine receptor supersensitivity.[187,197] Neuroleptic-induced tardive dyskinesia is more common among drinkers than nondrinkers.[198]

Panic disorder is unexpectedly prevalent among alcoholics, especially in those with repeated episodes of withdrawal.[199] Ethanol can precipitate seizures in known epileptics, but the amount required is uncertain.[200–202] In nondrinking epileptics, "social" amounts of vodka (10 to 30 g of ethanol) twice weekly for 16 weeks had no effect on seizure frequency, anticonvulsant blood levels, or EEG.[203] How much a nonalcoholic epileptic can safely drink is unknown.

By contrast, ethanol causes seizures in alcoholics whether or not they are epileptic.[203a] The most widely cited study of ethanol-related seizures is by Victor and Brausch,[204] who reviewed 241 patients seen over 15 years with both alcoholism and seizures, either prevalent or incident. This and subsequent studies reinforced the concept that otherwise unexplained seizures in alcoholics ("alcohol seizures," "rum fits") are the result of withdrawal.[205] Either a single major motor seizure or a cluster occurring over several hours typically begins between 6 and 48 hours after cessation of chronic drinking. Status epilepticus occurs in fewer than 10%, but in communities with high alcoholism prevalence, ethanol accounts for a substantial proportion of status epilepticus cases.[206–208] Focal features, not always attributable to previous head injury or other brain lesions, are seen in up to 25%.[204,206] Alcohol seizures sometimes occur in otherwise asymptomatic patients and sometimes accompany tremor or hallucinosis.

How much ethanol is required to provoke alcohol seizures? In a classic review, Victor and Adams[186]

stated that such seizures "tend to affect alcoholics only after many years of excessive drinking." Isbell et al,[155] studying 10 opioid-dependent volunteers, observed seizures in two made abruptly abstinent after several weeks of continuous drinking; both had been alcoholic in the past, however, and one may have had previous ethanol-related seizures. A seizure prevalence of 20% during ethanol withdrawal, moreover, is unusually high; in one study of 1024 alcoholics detoxified without psychoactive drugs, only 1% had seizures during withdrawal.[209] In a case-control study of incident seizures at Harlem Hospital Center, chronic daily ingestion of 50 g ethanol raised the odds ratio above 1, and at 200 g daily it was 20, but the minimal duration of drinking that conferred increased risk of seizures could not be determined.[210] In that study statistical analysis failed to demonstrate a clear-cut temporal relationship between seizures and early abstinence; many seizures occurred either during active drinking or more than a week after stopping, and those who had recently increased their ethanol consumption tended to have seizures sooner after the last drink than those who had decreased their consumption.

Both animal and human studies have led to a general acceptance of the concept of *alcohol withdrawal seizures.*[205,211] *Relative* and *protracted* withdrawal have been invoked to explain seizures occurring outside the period of early abstinence. An alternative possibility is that ethanol causes seizures by more than one mechanism.[212] In the past, the diagnosis of alcohol withdrawal seizures has been made by exclusion in heavy drinkers. The Harlem Hospital study, suggesting that some seizures considered withdrawal are not necessarily so, is consistent with a trend in the literature: As diagnostic accuracy has improved, fewer seizures in drinkers have been presumptively attributed to withdrawal, from 88% in 1967[204] to 59% in 1976[206] and 31% in 1980.[213] Further studies are necessary to determine if ethanol is a risk factor for seizures independently of withdrawal, associated illness such as head injury, or other drugs.[214,215] Animal studies indicate that seizures during ethanol withdrawal are of more than one type, with different time courses, phenomenology, and presumed neuronal mechanisms.[216]

Ethanol-related seizures often occur in patients with previous brain injury, and periodic lateralizing epileptiform discharges (PLEDS) are sometimes observed during ethanol withdrawal.[217,218] Some studies found the risk of seizures to increase with repeated ethanol detoxification, compatible with a kindling phenomenon.[219–221] This observation led to speculation that repeated severe withdrawal symptoms, including seizures, could result in permanent synaptic alteration and the development of nonwithdrawal *alcoholic epilepsy*.[65,201]

The diagnosis of alcohol seizures requires exclusion of other lesions. Even though the yield is low in the absence of focal neurological signs,[222] computed tomography (CT) scan or magnetic resonance imaging (MRI) is indicated when seizures are of new onset, and a spinal tap is necessary if meningitis or subarachnoid hemorrhage is suspected. Previous alcohol seizures do not exclude the possibility that a recurrent seizure has a more ominous cause. The EEG in patients with alcohol seizures is usually normal; a report[204] that photomyoclonic or photoconvulsive responses were common during early withdrawal—with or without seizures—was not borne out by subsequent studies,[221,223] including a prospective analysis of 49 untreated patients from Harlem Hospital Center in whom photomyoclonic response occurred in only two (4%) and photoconvulsive response in none.[224]

In contrast to tremor, hallucinosis, and seizures, *delirium tremens* typically begins 48 to 72 hours after the last drink. Because of the popular misconception that any alcoholic with tremor and hallucinations has delirium tremens, it is overdiagnosed. In fact, delirium tremens consists of not only tremor and disordered sensory perception (illusions or hallucinations) but also delirium (defined as extreme inattentiveness and apparent nonawareness of the environment, usually with agitation and sometimes with depressed alertness), autonomic overactivity, and frequently a fatal outcome. In one series the syndrome was present in fewer than 5% of hospitalized patients with symptomatic ethanol withdrawal.[186] About one-third of patients with early alcohol seizures develop delirium tremens, but seizures during delirium tremens are unusual and suggest an additional diagnosis such as meningitis.

Delirium tremens tends to begin and end abruptly, lasting hours to a few days. Inattentiveness and confusion may rapidly alternate with lucidity, or symptoms may subside gradually. Concurrent disease such as liver failure, pneumonia, or pancreatitis increases the severity of delirium tremens, and relapses can occur for up to several weeks.[217,225,226] Elderly patients have more severe symptoms.[227] A typical patient is agitated and grossly tremulous, with fever, tachycardia, and profuse sweating. Tremor may be so widespread as to involve the face, tongue, and pharynx.[187] The patient picks at the bedclothes or stares wildly about, shouting at hallucinated objects or trying to fend them off. Fluid loss can be marked, and heat stroke or myoglobinuria are occasional

features.[226] Less readily diagnosed are patients with *quiet delirium* or those with a single predominant symptom such as confusion, hallucinations, or delusions. Patients otherwise calm may have striking misperceptions, believing that they are drinking in a bar or, with extreme suggestibility, claiming to see objects described by the examiner but not actually present. In contrast to patients with early hallucinosis, who later can describe their illusions or hallucinations, those with full-blown delirium tremens seldom recall the episode.

The level of severity that separates the early and late ethanol withdrawal syndromes is not easy to define. A patient with early tremor, hallucinations, and otherwise clear sensorium is easily distinguished from one with full-blown delirium tremens, but some patients seem to fall between these extremes. Ethanol withdrawal might be viewed as a continuum of severity, determined not only by the amount of recent drinking but, again analogous to kindling, by the total duration of drinking and the number of previous withdrawal episodes. Moreover, chronic alcoholics have at least a brief withdrawal period every day. Even in drinkers without previous overt withdrawal symptoms, a kindling model might explain the observation that delirium tremens occurs most often after at least 10 years of alcoholism.[228]

Reported mortality for delirium tremens is as high as 15%, mostly attributable to associated disease such as pneumonia or sepsis; patients with delirium tremens have often been hospitalized for a different problem. Sometimes death follows unexplained shock or occurs suddenly without apparent cause. Fatalities have been variably attributed to cardiac arrhythmia, fat emboli, and heat stroke.

An added hazard of ethanol withdrawal is altered drug pharmacokinetics. For example, plasma protein binding of warfarin decreases, leading to a 20% increase in the free fraction.

Treatment of Ethanol Withdrawal

Dozens of drugs have been studied in patients withdrawing from ethanol; unfortunately, most of the literature on treatment is useless. Controls are lacking, and it is seldom stated what in fact was the aim of therapy, for example, relief of tremor, prevention of delirium tremens, or management of delirium tremens.[150,229] Some workers believe that early treatment of ethanol withdrawal can prevent delirium tremens;[230] others doubt that such intervention can either prevent it or reduce its mortality.[161]

Table 11–11. Treatment of Ethanol Withdrawal

Prevention or Reduction of Early Symptoms

Diazepam, 10–40 mg orally or IV, repeated hourly until sedation or mild intoxication. If successive daily doses required, taper by about one-fourth of preceding day's dose with resumption of higher dose if withdrawal symptoms recur. (Consider short-acting benzodiazepines in patients with abnormal liver function)

Alternatively, pentobarbital, 200 mg, orally, IM, or IV, and then 100 mg hourly as needed. Maintenance dose and duration determined by symptoms. Subsequent tapering at about 100 mg/day

Alternatively, paraldehyde, 5–15 mg, orally or PR, repeated hourly as needed. Maintenance and tapering titrated with symptoms

Thiamine, 100 mg, and multivitamins, IM or IV

Magnesium, potassium, and calcium replacement as needed

Delirium tremens

Diazepam, 10 mg IV, then 5 mg or more (up to 40 mg) IV or IM every 5 min until calming. Maintenance diazepam, 5 mg or more IV or IM, every 1–4 h as needed

Careful attention to fluid and electrolyte balance; several liters of saline per day, or even pressors, may be needed

Cooling blanket or alcohol sponges for high fever

Prevent or correct hypoglycemia

Thiamine and multivitamins

Consider coexisting illness, e.g., liver failure, pancreatitis, sepsis, meningitis, or subdural hematoma

IV, Intravenously; IM intramuscularly; PR, per rectum.

Some recommend that mildly symptomatic patients be managed nonpharmacologically with reassurance, reduced sensory stimuli, rest, hydration, and nutrition.[217,231,232] In addition to avoiding unnecessary medication, such patients might experience negatively reinforcing symptoms that would decrease the likelihood of later relapse.[217] Others recommend sedatives either to prevent or to relieve early mild withdrawal symptoms (Table 11–11).[233] Such is the usual practice at Harlem Hospital Center, an acute care–oriented and frequently understaffed institution with frequent admissions for ethanol-related illness. Obviously sedatives must be used cautiously in patients with liver disease, head injury, or chronic obstructive pulmonary disease; indeed, respiratory depression following sedation can cause hypoxic mental changes that are misdiagnosed as worsening withdrawal symptoms.[217]

Cross-tolerance with ethanol favors agents such as paraldehyde, barbiturates, or benzodiazepines, and the latter are currently the drugs of choice.[234] Whatever sedative is used, it should be given in a loading dose sufficient to produce symptoms of mild intoxication (calming, dysarthria, ataxia, fine nystagmus); subsequent doses are adjusted to avoid both intoxication and withdrawal tremor. After a few days, dosage is gradually tapered, with reinstitution of intoxicating doses should withdrawal symptoms appear. For benzodiazepines, an initial dose might consist of 10 to 40 mg diazepam repeated at intervals of 1 to a few hours and titrated against symptoms; up to 400 mg may be needed the first day. It can be given orally or parenterally, but intramuscular absorption is unpredictable. Because of long biological half-life, diazepam accumulation causes delayed toxicity (including precipitation of hepatic encephalopathy), and so after initial loading, subsequent doses are tapered by 25% each day unless increasing withdrawal symptoms dictate otherwise. If symptoms are mild, patients who have received a loading dose of diazepam may require no further medication.[235] An alternative choice is a benzodiazepine with a short half-life such as oxazepam or triazolam. Older patients and heavy smokers may require unusually high doses of benzodiazepines.[227]

Many patients with mild to moderate withdrawal symptoms can be effectively treated as outpatients, with substantially reduced cost. Such an approach is of course impractical in some communities; in one study more inpatients (95%) than outpatients (72%) completed detoxification.[236]

Reports have been conflicting on the efficacy of neuroleptics in early hallucinosis. They are not cross-tolerant with ethanol; they lower seizure threshold; and they cause hypotension, liver damage, acute dystonia, skin rash, bone marrow suppression, and impaired thermoregulation. Several studies found an increased frequency of seizures, delirium tremens, and death in patients receiving phenothiazines compared with those given placebo,[237–242] and recommendations that haloperidol be added to a benzodiazepine for control of hallucinations have lacked evidence of efficacy.[231,243] Neuroleptics are appropriately considered in patients whose only symptoms are hallucinations (especially when accompanied by delusions) or in whom hallucinations have outlasted other withdrawal symptoms.[189]

Blood and urinary catecholamines and their metabolites are increased during ethanol withdrawal and probably contribute to symptoms.[244] Propranolol decreases tremor and cardiac arrhythmia[245,246] but is no more effective than benzodiazepines and in one study exacerbated hallucinations.[247] Some workers have reported favorable results with clonidine,[234,244,248] atenolol,[249–251] or lofexidine.[244,252,253] One study of clonidine, however, found high frequencies of hallucinations, seizures, orthostatic hypotension, and drowsiness.[254] Consistent with ethanol's effects on membrane calcium flux, preliminary studies of both animals and humans suggest that calcium channel blockers might be useful in the treatment of ethanol withdrawal.[255–257] In animals GABA-ergic drugs relieve withdrawal symptoms selectively. For example, muscimol, a $GABA_A$ agonist, suppresses seizures but not tremor in rats, whereas progabide, which is both a $GABA_A$ and a $GABA_B$ agonist, suppresses both seizures and tremor.[65] In mice, the NMDA receptor blocker MK-801 decreased the occurrence and severity of withdrawal seizures.[258]

A seemingly logical approach to therapy would be ethanol itself, the treatment nonhospitalized patients choose for themselves. Parenteral ethanol, however, has a low therapeutic index and is potentially hazardous. Moreover, ethanol has direct organ toxicity (e.g., liver and possibly CNS). Even though most patients resume drinking on discharge, ethanol has no role in the prevention or treatment of withdrawal symptoms.

Because most ethanol-related seizures occur singly or in brief clusters, once they have occurred, anticonvulsants are unnecessary unless the diagnosis is doubtful. In animals and humans, phenytoin failed to prevent alcohol seizures.[226,259] In rats, valproate and carbamazepine prevented withdrawal seizures.[260] In abstinent humans carbamazepine prevented seizures, tremor, sweating, gastrointestinal symptoms, irritability, and insomnia.[261]

The treatment of status epilepticus during ethanol withdrawal is conventional. Intravenous diazepam and phenobarbital have the advantage, compared with phenytoin, of preventing or reducing other withdrawal symptoms.

Long-term anticonvulsants are generally not indicated in patients with alcohol seizures. Abstainers do not need them, and drinkers do not take them. Of agents that can be taken once daily, phenytoin is probably ineffective and phenobarbital can cause synergistic CNS depression. Of safer agents with demonstrable efficacy, valproate and carbamazepine require thrice-daily dosage, virtually ensuring noncompliance.

Respiratory alkalosis and hypomagnesemia occur during early ethanol withdrawal and return to normal before the appearance of delirium tremens.[262] Hyperventilation may recur during delirium tremens, but hypomagnesemia does not.[156] Intracellular shift and body loss probably each contribute to hypomagnesemia.[263] Attempts to correlate hypomagnesemia with alcohol seizures failed to produce convincing evidence of cause and effect, but it could be contributory, and so magnesium sulfate is given to hypomagnesemic patients in early withdrawal.[262] Hypokalemia and hypocalcemia may also be present, and the latter sometimes responds to treatment only after hypomagnesemia is corrected.[264]

Thiamine and multivitamins are indicated even if there are no clinical signs of their depletion, for glucose can precipitate Wernicke's disease in patients with borderline thiamine deficiency. There is often impaired gastrointestinal absorption of thiamine, which is therefore given parenterally.

In contrast to early ethanol withdrawal—or to withdrawal from other drugs such as opioids—delirium tremens once present cannot be abruptly reversed by any agent, including sedatives crosstolerant with ethanol (see Table 11–11). The treatment of delirium tremens is an emergency, and its cornerstone is sedation. In a prospective study comparing parenteral diazepam and rectal paraldehyde in patients with "characteristic advanced delirium tremens," diazepam produced more rapid calming, less respiratory depression, and lower mortality.[265] Initial diazepam doses (10 mg intravenously followed by 5 mg intramuscularly every 5 minutes as needed) ranged from 15 to 215 mg. Once quieted, patients were maintained with 5 to 10 mg intramuscularly every 1 to 4 hours. In view of the unpredictable absorption of intramuscular diazepam, its efficacy is surprising, and intravenous maintenance doses should be considered in patients with poor responses. Moreover, patients vary greatly in the dosage of diazepam necessary for effective sedation; huge amounts are often required—sometimes more than 1000 mg in the first 24 hours. The major hazard of this treatment is hepatic encephalopathy; not only does liver disease decrease the metabolism of diazepam, but also brains of patients with liver failure are hypersensitive to sedatives. The result can be coma lasting days.

The treatment of delirium tremens calls for an intensive care unit. Patients should be prone or in lat-

Table 11–12. Major Nutritional Disturbances in Alcoholics

Disorder	Clinical Features	Deficiency
Wernicke syndrome	Dementia, with lethargy, inattentiveness, apathy, and amnesia Ophthalmoparesis Gait ataxia	Thiamine
Korsakoff syndrome	Dementia, mainly amnesia, with or without confabulation	Thiamine
Cerebellar degeneration	Gait ataxia; limb coordination relatively preserved	?
Polyneuropathy	Distal limb sensory loss and weakness; less often autonomic dysfunction	?
Amblyopia	Optic atrophy, decreased visual acuity, central scotomas; total blindness rare	?
Pellagra	Skin rash, vomiting and diarrhea, delirium or dementia	Nicotinic acid

eral decubitus position and restrained as needed. Oral medications are avoided. Most patients are dehydrated, some severely so, and many require up to 10 L of intravenous saline daily.[161] Patients with liver disease, however, retain sodium and water. Hyponatremia must be treated cautiously to avoid central pontine myelinolysis, and hypokalemia can cause cardiac arrhythmia. Fever, with or without infection, is often marked, requiring alcohol sponges, a cooling blanket, or parenteral cooling. Hypoglycemia may be unrecognized, and possible coexisting illnesses include liver failure, pancreatitis, sepsis, meningitis, and subdural hematoma.

Indirect Effects of Ethanol: Nutritional

Wernicke-Korsakoff Syndrome

History and Definition

In 1881 Carl Wernicke described altered mentation, abnormal eye movements, and ataxic gait in three patients; two were alcoholic, and one had persistent vomiting. All died, and at autopsy there were hemorrhagic lesions adjacent to the third and fourth ventricles and the aqueduct of Sylvius.[266] A few years later, S. S. Korsakoff described mental disturbance and polyneuropathy in alcoholics and noted a particular vulnerability of recent memory.[267] It has since become apparent that Wernicke's and Korsakoff's diseases share the same pathology and are caused by thiamine deficiency. In 1971, the clinical and pathologic spectra of 245 patients with Wernicke-Korsakoff syndrome were the subject of a classic monograph by Victor et al.[268]

Although pathologically similar, Wernicke's and Korsakoff's syndromes are clinically distinct. Full-blown Wernicke's syndrome consists of abnormal mentation, eye movements, and gait. Korsakoff's syndrome is a qualitatively different mental disturbance (Table 11–12).

Wernicke's Syndrome

In acute Wernicke's syndrome mental symptoms evolve over days or weeks to a "global confusional state,"[268] with varying degrees of lethargy, inattentiveness, abulia, decreased spontaneous speech, and impaired memory.[269] Disordered perception is common; a patient might identify the hospital room as his or her apartment or a bar. In fewer than 10% is mentation normal. Stupor and coma were unusual in Victor's series but were the main findings in patients reported from Norway[270] and New Zealand.[271] In fact, in the Norwegian series, only one of 22 cases of autopsy-verified Wernicke's disease had been diagnosed clinically. Similarly, in Perth, Australia, Wernicke's disease was present at 2.8% of autopsies but had been diagnosed clinically only one-fifth of the time.[272]

Abnormal eye movements include nystagmus (horizontal and less often vertical or rotatory), lateral rectus palsy (bilateral but usually asymmetric), and conjugate gaze palsy (horizontal with or without vertical, usually upward). Progression leads to complete ophthalmoplegia. Sluggish pupillary reflexes and mild anisocoria are common, but unreactivity to light and ptosis are rare. *Pretectal syndrome*—pupillary light-near dissociation, limited upgaze, and convergence-retraction nystagmus—has been observed.[273] So have internuclear ophthalmoplegia and ocular bobbing.[274]

More than 80% of patients have truncal ataxia, sometimes of a severity that prevents standing or walking. Limb ataxia is infrequent, especially in the arms. So is dysarthria. Peripheral neuropathy is present in the great majority.[268] Abnormal caloric vestibular testing was found in 17 consecutive patients with acute Wernicke's syndrome, gradually improving over several months.[275]

Patients with Wernicke's syndrome frequently have signs of nutritional deficiency, such as skin changes, red tongue, and cheilosis. They also often have jaundice, ascites, or spider angiomas. Although beri-beri heart disease is rare, tachycardia, dyspnea on exertion, and postural hypotension (unexplained by hypovolemia) are common, and sudden circulatory collapse can follow mild exertion.[276] Hypothermia and thermolability are not unusual.[277] Fever usually indicates infection.

The EEG during acute Wernicke's syndrome may show diffuse slowing or be normal.[268] Cerebral blood flow and cerebral oxygen and glucose consumption are "strikingly reduced" independently of the level of alertness or the EEG.[278] CSF is normal except for occasional mild protein elevation. Elevated blood pyruvate, falling with treatment, is nonspecific. Decreased blood transketolase activity (which requires thiamine pyrophosphate as a cofactor) more reliably indicates thiamine deficiency and in experimental animals falls after only 2 days of restriction.[268] CT scanning sometimes shows diencephalic periventricular low-density abnormalities.[279–281] MRI shows abnormal signals in the periaqueductal area, medial thalamus, and, less often, splenium of the corpus callosum as well as mammillary body atrophy, sometimes evolving after treatment has been given.[282,283]

Korsakoff's Syndrome

In the great majority of cases the more purely amnesic syndrome of Korsakoff emerges as other mental symptoms of Wernicke's syndrome respond to treatment. How often Korsakoff's syndrome arises without preceding Wernicke's syndrome and how often the mental abnormality is restricted to memory are important questions in the current controversy over alcoholic dementia (see later). The amnesia of such patients is both anterograde, with inability to retain new information, and retrograde, with lost recall for events months or years old. Alertness, attentiveness, and behavior are relatively preserved, but there tends to be a lack of spontaneous speech or activity. Confabulation is not invariable and if initially present tends gradually to disappear. Insight is usually impaired, and there may be flagrant anosognosia for the mental disturbance.

In patients with pathologically verified Korsakoff's syndrome psychological testing reveals cognitive impairment not explained by pure memory loss,[268] and different investigators have considered the fundamental defect either a disorder of temporal sequencing, an inability to adopt a new "mental set" to a changing situation, or separable perceptual and mnemonic disturbances.[284] Some have found remote memory to be as impaired as recent,[285] whereas others have observed steep temporal gradients in the retrograde amnesia.[286,287] Many patients are as likely

to scramble past information as to forget it, for example, producing a year and a president that do not match. Such temporal confusion may influence the content of confabulation, with the information proffered signifying temporal displacement rather than complete fabrication. In any event the combination of anterograde and retrograde disturbance indicates abnormalities of both memorization and retrieval. In contrast to patients with Alzheimer's disease, Korsakoff patients tend to have normal *primary or working memory* (retention over 30 seconds, e.g., digit span) and *semantic memory* (memory for facts, concepts, or language); their impairment is one of *episodic memory*—specific verbal and visuo-spacial learning and retrieval. Similar to patients with Alzheimer's disease, Korsakoff patients have normal *procedural memory* (skill learning).[288]

Pathology of Wernicke-Korsakoff Syndrome

The histopathological lesions of Wernicke-Korsakoff syndrome consist of variable degrees of neuronal, axonal, and myelin loss; prominent blood vessels (secondary to endothelial and adventitial thickening); reactive microglia, macrophages, and astrocytes; and, infrequently, small hemorrhages.[268] (Large brain stem and thalamic hemorrhages were found at autopsy in two patients who had Wernicke's disease plus liver and kidney failure.[289]) Nerve cells may be relatively preserved in the presence of extensive myelin destruction and gliosis, and chronically astrocytosis predominates. Patients with "active" (acute and subacute) disease are more likely than patients with "inactive" (chronic) disease to have swollen capillary endothelium, macrophage response, and reactive astrocytes and less likely to have spongy tissue, gliosis, and hemosiderin-filled old macrophages.[290] Lesions affect the thalamus (especially the dorsomedial nucleus and the medial pulvinar), the hypothalamus (especially, and perhaps invariably, the mammillary bodies), the midbrain (especially the periaqueductal areas), and the pons and medulla (especially the abducens and medial vestibular nuclei). In the cerebellum severe Purkinje cell loss with Bergmann astrocytosis accompanies lesser degrees of neuronal loss and gliosis in the molecular and granular layers. Such changes are usually limited to the anterior-superior vermis.[268]

Clinical-Pathological Correlation

Attempts to correlate the anatomical lesions with symptoms and signs have been controversial. Blaming the memory loss of Korsakoff's syndrome on mammillary body damage is tempting in view of that structure's extensive connections with the hippocampus. There are, however, examples of severe mammillary body damage without memory impairment, and amnesia correlates better with lesions of the dorsomedial thalamic nuclei.[268] The combination of severely impaired anterograde verbal and visuospacial learning and retrieval with preserved primary working memory, semantic memory, and procedural memory is compatible with cholinergic impairment, in fact, more so than the broader amnestic constellation of Alzheimer's disease. Indeed, thiamine depletion inhibits acetylcholine synthesis[291] and cholinergic neurons in the basal forebrain are depleted in Korsakoff's syndrome.[292] The global confusion of Wernicke's syndrome, on the other hand, has occurred without visible thalamic lesions and may be related to cerebral thiamine depletion.[268] Patients with either Korsakoff's or Alzheimer's disease have a more temporally extensive retrograde amnesia than is usually found with traumatic amnesia, hippocampal ischemia, or transient global amnesia, and the extent of retrograde amnesia parallels psychometric frontal lobe dysfunction. These findings suggest that although diencephalic lesions may account for anterograde amnesia, additional cortical pathology is responsible for retrograde amnesia as well as non-mnestic cognitive abnormalities.[293-295]

Periaqueductal and oculomotor or abducens nucleus lesions are often found in patients whose eye movements became normal before death.[268] Both cerebellar and vestibular lesions probably contribute to ataxia; avian thiamine deficiency causes peripheral labyrinthine degeneration.[296]

Thiamine and Wernicke-Korsakoff Syndrome

Experimental and clinical evidence supports the specific role of thiamine in the Wernicke-Korsakoff syndrome. Thiamine is a cofactor for several enzymes involved in glucose metabolism, including transketolase, alpha-ketoglutarate dehydrogenase, pyruvate dehydrogenase, and branched-chain alpha-ketoacid dehydrogenase.[2] It may have direct actions on axonal conduction and synaptic transmission,[297] and brain contains thiamine triphosphate, the function of which is obscure. Thiamine deficiency rapidly leads to decreased cerebral glucose utilization, and increased lactate production precedes visible lesions in vulnerable brain areas, probably reflecting a shift from aerobic metabolism to anaerobic glycolysis.[298,299]

After an observation period, patients with acute Wernicke's syndrome were given different vitamins,

and improvement occurred only after thiamine.[300] Thiamine-deficient foxes, cats, pigeons, rats, and monkeys develop lesions similar to those of Wernicke-Korsakoff syndrome.[296,301] Thiamine deficiency in Rhesus monkeys caused anorexia, apathy, lethargy, and lower extremity weakness, promptly relieved by thiamine; during subsequent episodes of thiamine deprivation, symptoms were more severe and included ataxia and abnormal eye movements; pair fed controls remained asymptomatic.[302] Oscillations of thiamine levels, comparable to what occurs in alcoholic patients, may be worse than chronic low levels.[302]

Wernicke-Korsakoff syndrome occurs in only a small minority of alcoholic or otherwise malnourished people and seems particularly to affect whites, suggesting genetic influence. At Harlem Hospital Center, where nearly half of medical admissions are ethanol-related, 12 cases of Wernicke-Korsakoff syndrome were seen during 1975 through 1979; by contrast, 90 cases were seen at the Boston City Hospital during 1950 through 1951 and 129 cases at the Massachusetts General Hospital during 1952 through 1961.[268] Particular strains of pigeons have a hereditary predisposition to the neurological effects of thiamine deficiency,[303] and in a preliminary study genetically determined transketolase deficiency was found in four patients with Wernicke-Korsakoff syndrome.[304] Perhaps Wernicke-Korsakoff syndrome, similar to other inborn errors of metabolism (e.g., glucose-6-phosphate-dehydrogenase deficiency) is the result of a genetic fault that causes symptoms only in the presence of a particular environmental stress.

Course and Treatment

Untreated acute Wernicke-Korsakofff syndrome is fatal.[305] Mortality was 10% among Victor et al.'s treated patients, and the presence of liver failure, infection, and delirium tremens often made the cause of death unclear.[268] Postural hypotension and tachycardia call for strict bed rest; associated medical problems may require intensive care. Thiamine, 50 to 100 mg, is given daily until a normal diet can be taken. The intravenous route is preferred because gastrointestinal absorption of thiamine is impaired in chronic alcoholics;[306] acute Wernicke's encephalopathy followed 12 days of intramuscular thiamine.[307] Alternatively, fat-soluble allithiamines (e.g., thiamine propyl disulfide or thiamine tetrahydrofurfuryl disulfide) are well-absorbed in alcoholic patients.[308] Particularly at need for high, efficiently delivered thiamine doses are a subgroup of patients with so-called low-affinity transketolase variant.[309] Hypomagnesemia, which can retard the response to thiamine, requires early correction, along with other vitamins.[310–312] Protein intake may have to be titrated against the patient's liver status. Animal studies suggest that thiamine deficiency causes excitatory neurotransmitter neuronal toxicity and that NMDA receptor antagonists (e.g., MK-801) are of therapeutic benefit.[313] Such work is not yet clinically applicable.

Following thiamine treatment, ocular abnormalities, especially abducens and gaze palsies, begin to improve within a few hours and usually resolve within a week; horizontal nystagmus often persists indefinitely. Mentation begins to improve within hours or days, and most patients are alert and attentive within a month; amnesia is then present in more than 80% and eventually clears in fewer than a quarter of cases. Improvement in ataxia begins within a few days but is complete in less than half, and nearly a third show no improvement at all.[164]

Improvement in memory was reported in patients with Korsakoff's syndrome who received the serotonin uptake inhibitor fluvoxamine.[314] The role of serotonin pathways in mnemonic performance is complex, and the efficacy of such agents requires confirmation. Clonidine (but not L-dopa or ephedrine) reportedly improved anterograde but not retrograde amnesia in patients with Korsakoff's syndrome;[315] such benefit was not found by others, however.[316]

The best approach to Wernicke's disease is preventive. Any alcoholic patient should receive thiamine, as should any patient receiving glucose for unexplained seizures or coma. Wernicke's disease too often appears in patients hospitalized a few days earlier for some other problem.

On the assumption that 1200 patients with Korsakoff's syndrome require institutionalization annually in the United States, with long-term stay in one-third, it has been proposed that fortification of alcoholic beverages with thiamine would be cost-effective.[317]

Alcoholic Cerebellar Degeneration

Definition and Clinical Picture

A "restricted form of cerebellar cortical degeneration" occurs in nutritionally deficient alcoholics without other signs of Wernicke-Korsakoff syndrome (see Table 11–12).[318,319] Truncal instability is the major symptom, often with incoordination of individual leg movements. Arm ataxia is much less

prominent, and nystagmus, dysarthria, hypotonia, and independent head tremor are rare. Symptoms evolve over years, weeks, or days and eventually stabilize, sometimes even with continued drinking and poor nutrition. Ataxia unassociated with Wernicke's disease is less likely to appear abruptly or to improve.[268] Stabilization does not occur at the same level of severity in all patients, and in some, years of unchanging ataxia are interrupted by further progression.

Pathology and Pathogenesis

Pathologically the superior vermis is invariably involved, with nerve cell loss and gliosis in the molecular, granular, and especially Purkinje cell layers. There may be secondary degeneration of the olives and the fastigial, emboliform, globose, and vestibular nuclei.[319,320] Involvement of the cerebellar hemispheric cortex is exceptional and limited to the anterior lobes. Pathological evidence of Wernicke's disease may coexist even though unsuspected clinically. CT and autopsies, moreover, have revealed cerebellar atrophy in alcoholics not clinically ataxic.[321–323] In ataxic patients, positron-emission tomography reveals superior vermal hypometabolism, which correlates with symptoms better than does CT atrophy.[324]

Although ethanol acutely inhibits Purkinje cell firing,[325] perhaps contributing to the ataxia of inebriation,[326] alcoholic cerebellar degeneration is probably nutritional in origin. Identical lesions were observed in a nonalcoholic man with intestinal obstruction and "protracted nutritional depletion,"[327] and ataxia can begin in malnourished alcoholics after days or weeks of abstinence.[319] The clinical and pathological similarity of alcoholic cerebellar degeneration to the cerebellar component of Wernicke's syndrome suggests shared mechanisms.[268] Unexplained, however, is why the majority of patients with alcoholic cerebellar degeneration do not have pathological evidence of Wernicke's disease. At Harlem Hospital Center Wernicke's syndrome is unusual, yet alcoholic cerebellar degeneration occurs often, clinically and pathologically. Perhaps genetic factors play a role, or perhaps deficiencies other than thiamine are operative. Some workers have demonstrated direct toxicity by ethanol or acetaldehyde.[328,329] In rats, cerebellar neuronal loss followed rapid correction of hyponatremia,[330] and ethanol ingestion caused Purkinje cell dendritic abnormalities not found in pair-fed controls.[331]

Alcoholic Polyneuropathy

Definition and Clinical Picture

Alcoholic polyneuropathy refers to progressive sensorimotor peripheral neuropathy, probably of nutritional origin, which stabilizes or improves with abstinence and an adequate diet (see Table 11–12). Alcoholic polyneuropathy is present in most patients with Wernicke-Korsakoff syndrome but more often occurs alone. It tends to be underdiagnosed. Fewer than 10% of alcoholics in one series were said to have peripheral neuropathy (usually in association with Wernicke-Korsakoff syndrome),[186] yet clinical evidence of polyneuropathy was found in one-third of alcoholic patients at Harlem Hospital Center.[332] A careful neurological examination often elicits sensory loss, and nerve conduction and electromyographic abnormalities (especially of the H-reflex) occur in alcoholics without symptoms or signs.[333–336] In several series of patients with alcoholic polyneuropathy, women were over-represented.[186,337]

Paresthesias are usually the first symptom, progressing over days or weeks to numbness. Burning or lancinating pain and exquisite tenderness of the calves or soles resemble reflex sympathetic dystrophy, and paravertebral sympathetic block sometimes provides temporary relief. Mildly to moderately impaired vibratory sense is the earliest sign of neuropathy in the great majority of patients; proprioception is usually preserved until other sensory loss has become substantial.

Loss of ankle tendon reflexes is another early sign; eventually there is diffuse hyporeflexia or areflexia. Weakness appears at any time and can become severe after only a few days, resembling Guillain-Barré neuropathy.[338] The distal legs are affected first, although in some patients proximal weakness is greater than distal.[339] Radiologically demonstrable neuropathic arthropathy of the feet is common, as is skin thinning, glossiness, reddening, cyanosis, and hyperhidrosis.[332] Peripheral autonomic involvement, although usually less prominent than in diabetic neuropathy, causes urinary and fecal incontinence, hypotension, hypothermia, cardiac arrhythmia, dysphagia, dysphonia,[339] impaired esophageal peristalsis,[340] altered sweat patterns, and abnormal Valsalva ratio.[341,342] Pupillary parasympathetic denervation is rare.[343] Autonomic signs are associated with increased mortality.[344] The CSF in alcoholic polyneuropathy is normal except for occasional mild elevation of protein.

Pathology and Pathogenesis

Pathologically there is degeneration of both myelin and axons, and controversy exists over which occurs first.[333,337,345–347] Electron microscopic evidence suggests that the earliest changes occur in Schwann cells.[348] Nerve root involvement causes secondary degeneration of the dorsal columns. Damage to the vagus nerves and the sympathetic trunks occurs in both humans and animals.[339,349]

The basis of alcoholic polyneuropathy has been debated for years. Severe weight loss is common, improvement occurs with nutritional supplements despite continued drinking, and abstinent alcoholics receiving a vitamin B–free diet have progressive neuropathic symptoms.[350,351] Moreover, heavy ethanol consumption for 4 weeks, with adequate diet, failed to produce electromyographic evidence of peripheral nerve damage in three volunteers.[352] Deficiency of more than thiamine may be operative, for although thiamine alone corrects neuropathy in vitamin-deficient pigeons,[353] polyneuropathy is not a feature of experimental thiamine deprivation in mice,[354] cats,[355] pigs,[356] or monkeys,[357] and thiamine deficiency for months produced only mild symptoms and signs of peripheral neuropathy in human volunteers.[358] Polyneuropathy follows deficiency of pantothenic acid,[359,360] pyridoxine,[359,361] and riboflavin[362] in animals and humans. By contrast, mildly slowed nerve conduction velocities, markedly reduced sensory amplitudes, and histologic axonal degeneration were observed in alcoholics with polyneuropathy, whereas patients malnourished following gastrectomy had electromyographic and histologic abnormalities more consistent with segmental demyelination.[337] The alcoholic patients, moreover, had normal blood thiamine levels, and only a minority had clinical evidence of malnutrition, which did not correlate with severity of neuropathy. That study suggests ethanol is toxic to peripheral nerves. Ethanol does directly impair fast axonal transport.[363] Such a view does not exclude the possibility that nutritional deficiency is contributory, and in any event thiamine and multivitamins should be given to any alcoholic.

Amblyopia

Optic atrophy is common in alcoholics, with progressive visual loss, central or centrocecal scotomas, and temporal disc pallor (see Table 11–12).[364] Red-green color blindness occurs.[365] Demyelination affects the optic nerves, chiasm, and tracts, with predilection for the maculopapular bundle; electrophysiologic and MRI studies favor the retina as the primary site of pathology.[366,367] The condition used to be called *tobacco-alcohol amblyopia* and was thought to represent direct toxicity. Amblyopia improved, however, in 25 patients who received dietary supplements but continued to drink ethanol and to smoke. In five of these, the only supplement was thiamine.[368] Amblyopia, moreover, was common among prisoners-of-war during World War II. Nutritional amblyopia rarely progresses to total blindness, and improvement, albeit incomplete, nearly always follows nutritional replacement.[366]

Pellagra

Nicotinic acid deficiency in alcoholics produces clinical pellagra, with skin, gastrointestinal, and mental abnormalities.[161,186,369–371] Stomatitis and enteritis can be severe, with nausea, vomiting, and diarrhea. CNS symptoms include headache, irritability, and insomnia progressing to impaired memory, delusions, hallucinations, dementia, or delirium. In a review of 22 cases, signs progressed over hours, days, or weeks before or during hospitalization; death in several instances followed administration of thiamine and pyridoxine.[370] Frequent were fluctuating "confusion" and "clouding of consciousness," marked oppositional hypertonus (*gegenhalten*), and startle myoclonus. Pathologically there was neuronal chromatolysis, prominent in the brain stem (especially the pontine nuclei) and the cerebellar dentate nuclei. Several patients also had clinical signs of peripheral neuropathy and pathological evidence of Wernicke-Korsakoff or Marchiafava-Bignami disease.

Treatment of pellagra is with nicotinic acid or nicotinamide, orally at a dose of 50 mg up to 10 times daily or intravenously 25 mg twice or three times daily; thiamine and multivitamins are also given. Response is usually rapid; delirium may clear within hours. As with Wernicke's disease, prevention is preferable to treatment.

Nutritional Deficiency Anemia

Anemia in alcoholics may be microcytic owing to iron deficiency, sideroblastic owing to malnutrition, or megaloblastic owing to folate deficiency.[372] The latter can mask true vitamin B_{12} deficiency secondary to ethanol-induced malabsorption.[373]

Indirect Effects of Ethanol: Nonnutritional

Hepatic Encephalopathy

Cirrhosis of the liver, encountered most often in alcoholics, is the ninth leading cause of death in the United States and the third leading cause of death among 25- to 64-year-olds living in urban areas such as New York City.[374] Alcoholic liver disease causes neurological symptoms and signs—hepatic encephalopathy—that can be masked by simultaneous intoxication, withdrawal, Wernicke-Korsakoff disease, meningitis, subdural hematoma, hypoglycemia, or other ethanol-related diseases. The mechanisms underlying both alcoholic liver disease and hepatic encephalopathy are incompletely understood.

Alcoholic liver disease—steatosis, steatonecrosis (alcoholic hepatitis), and cirrhosis—is mainly the result of direct toxicity, not nutritional deficiency.[38,375] By replacing fatty acids as mitochondrial fuel, ethanol decreases lipid oxidation and increases lipid synthesis. MEOS oxidation of ethanol generates only heat and thus induces hypermetabolism, increased oxygen demand, local hypoxia, and perivenular (centrolobular) necrosis. MEOS induction also increases the production of acetaldehyde, which forms adducts with proteins, thereby altering microtubules (*Mallory bodies*), stimulating antibodies, inactivating enzymes, decreasing DNA repair, damaging mitochondria, depleting glutathione, increasing free radical toxicity, and stimulating collagen synthesis. In addition, MEOS induction activates the metabolism of exogenous hepatotoxins, including carbon tetrachloride, halothane, isoniazid, phenylbutazone, acetaminophen, and cocaine; alcoholics are susceptible to liver disease from these agents. They are also at risk for hepatic cancer. Nutritional deficiency, especially protein, aggravates liver damage.

Several features of alcoholic liver disease remain unexplained by these mechanisms. First, alcoholic hepatitis, considered the precursor of cirrhosis, has never been produced in an animal model. Second, most heavy drinkers do not develop serious liver disease; in a study of alcoholics who had consumed an average of 160 g ethanol daily for more than 10 years, 40% to 50% had no histologic evidence of hepatic necrosis or fibrosis. Third, women are more vulnerable than men to alcoholic liver disease, which in most men requires more than 80 g ethanol daily compared with only 20 g ethanol daily in women.[376,377] Attempts to identify a genetic basis for these differences in susceptibility (e.g., collagen synthesis or histocompatibility antigens) have been

Table 11–13. Hepatic Encephalopathy—Symptoms and Signs

Systemic
  Jaundice
  Ascites
  Spider angiomata
  Fever
  Hyperventilation
  Fetor hepaticus

Neurological
  Altered mentation
    Behavioral change (psychosis)
    Inattentiveness (delirium)
    Decreased alertness (coma)
  Asterixis
  Dysarthria
  Hyperreflexia
  Extensor posturing
  Grimacing
  Downward eye deviation

Table 11–14. Precipitators of Hepatic Encephalopathy

  Infection
  Surgery
  Sedatives
  Analgesics
  Tranquilizers
  Phenothiazines
  Ethanol
  Azotemia
  Diuretics
  Gastrointestinal hemorrhage
  Hypokalemia
  Metabolic encephalopathy
  Protein intoxication
  Constipation

conflicting.[378] Lower gastric metabolism of ethanol in women delivers larger amounts of ethanol to the liver after oral consumption.[379]

The clinical manifestations of alcoholic liver disease correlate poorly with hepatic histopathology and range from asymptomatic hepatomegaly to anorexia, malaise, fever, jaundice, ascites, variceal bleeding, and encephalopathy (Table 11–13). Neurological symptoms and signs comprise a characteristic (although nonspecific) syndrome. Altered mentation includes behavioral change progressing to psychosis, inattentiveness progressing to delirium, and lethargy progressing to coma. Symptoms emerge abruptly or gradually, often accompanied by hyperventilation and fever.[380,381] Asterixis—a fleeting, repetitive loss of voluntary posture holding—is most easily demonstrated in extended wrists and fingers but also occurs in dorsiflexed ankles, closed eyelids, lips, and tongue; in comatose patients it is sometimes elicited by pressing on the fingertips to cause dorsiflexion of the hand. In contrast to myoclonus, asterixis is the result of electrical lapses in contracted muscles. (Without electromyography, myoclonus is diagnosed by observing muscle jerks against gravity.) Myoclonus is rarely if ever the result of liver failure, and its presence should suggest alternate diagnoses such as uremia. Seizures are also an infrequent feature of hepatic encephalopathy; their occurrence probably reflects ethanol withdrawal.[380] Liver failure does cause tremor (fine, rapid, and distal), gegenhalten, dysarthria, hyperactive tendon reflexes, extensor (*decerebrate*) posturing,[382] grimacing, and sucking.

Abnormal eye movements include tonic downward deviation, skew, and ocular bobbing.[383] Focal neurological signs such as hemiparesis suggest structural brain lesions. Many patients have a sweetish, musty odor on the breath, so-called *fetor hepaticus*.[380]

The diagnosis of hepatic encephalopathy is usually easy in patients with known liver disease or jaundice; it can be difficult if there are extrahepatic shunting and only mildly abnormal liver function tests. Encephalopathy is precipitated by a variety of insults (Table 11–14), and coma can then occur abruptly, often in previously stable patients hospitalized for other reasons. Precipitants act in different ways. For example, acetazolamide increases renal venous ammonia levels and decreases renal perfusion, causing azotemia. Metabolic alkalosis favors the formation of nonionized ammonia, which more easily enters the brain. Why sedatives such as barbiturates precipitate hepatic encephalopathy is less clear. The brain in such patients seems to be particularly vulnerable, for elevated serum drug levels secondary to decreased liver metabolism are often insufficient to explain the severity of symptoms. Hepatic coma frequently complicates the treatment of ethanol withdrawal.

Most—but not all—patients with hepatic encephalopathy have hyperammonemia. Tourniquets produce artificial elevations of venous ammonia, and so arterial samples are preferred.[381] Liver enzymes (aspartate aminotransferase and alanine aminotransferase) are usually elevated, but only modestly, and the degree of elevation correlates poorly with the severity of symptoms. CSF pressure and protein in hepatic encephalopathy are usually normal; xanthochromia is present when serum bilirubin reaches 6 mg/dL. Elevated levels of CSF glutamine are found in

Table 11–15. Hepatic Encephalopathy—
Candidate Toxins

Ammonia
Glutamine, alpha-ketoglutaramate
Short-chain fatty acids
Mercaptans
False neurotransmitters (octopamine,
    beta-phenylethanolamine)
Tryptophan, quinolinic acid
Gamma-aminobutyric acid
Benzodiazepine

nearly all patients, and increased brain concentrations of glutamine have been detected in vivo using proton magnetic resonance spectroscopy.[384] The EEG characteristically shows synchronous, symmetric, high-voltage slow waves, especially frontally, at first intermixed with preserved alpha activity but eventually replacing it; such a pattern is nonspecific.[380] Also frequently abnormal are evoked-response potentials.[385] Respiratory alkalosis reflects primary neurogenic drive. Severe hypoglycemia, common in alcoholics with liver disease, can be masked by hepatic encephalopathy, with catastrophic results. Conversely, high blood levels of ammonia stimulate glucagon secretion, and increased hepatic gluconeogenesis from amino acids leads to further ammonia production. Stimulation of insulin then causes increased muscle uptake and metabolism of branched-chain amino acids, resulting in decreased serum levels of valine, leucine, and isoleucine. Blood levels of other amino acids are elevated.[381] Serum vitamin A levels are often decreased, reflecting reduced concentrations in the liver.[386]

Pathology and Pathogenesis

The most striking neuropathological alterations in hepatic encephalopathy are swollen astrocytes in cerebral cortex and other gray structures, including thalamus, basal ganglia, pontine nuclei, and deep cerebellar nuclei. Neuronal damage is far less conspicuous.[380,387] Cerebral edema is a feature of acute fulminating hepatic failure but not of encephalopathy associated with chronic liver disease.[388] Theories of pathogenesis focus on a number of possible circulating toxins (Table 11–15).[389]

In liver failure the synthesis of urea from ammonia decreases and the latter accumulates. The most venerable explanations of hepatic encephalopathy have implicated ammonia, acting either directly as a neurotoxin; synergistically with fatty acids and mercaptans; or indirectly through accumulation of glutamine and alpha-ketoglutaramate or depletion of glutamate, aspartate, and branched-chain amino acids. Ammonia is directly neurotoxic; it interferes with neuronal chloride extrusion and causes both stupor and astrocytic hyperplasia experimentally.[390,391] In animals with portocaval shunts, cerebral blood flow increases without alteration of cerebral oxygen metabolism; ammonium acetate challenge then produces a fall in both, reflecting the sensitivity of a chronically hyperammonemic brain to additional ammonia.[390,392]

The inconsistent presence of elevated serum and CSF ammonia levels in hepatic encephalopathy[393] as well as the observation that treatment with charcoal hemoperfusion reduces symptoms but not serum ammonia levels[394] suggests that ammonia poisoning is insufficient to account for the neurological abnormalities or that its toxic effects are indirect. Short-chain fatty acids and mercaptans accumulate in liver failure and cause coma in experimental animals. Mercaptans, which probably account for fetor hepaticus, enhance the toxicity of ammonia and fatty acids, and blood levels of ammonia, fatty acids, or mercaptans sufficient to cause coma in animals are much less when any two are given together. Phenols have also been implicated in such synergism.[395]

In the liver ammonia is detoxified by the urea cycle. In the brain, however, ammonia combines with glutamate to form glutamine, which is further metabolized to alpha-ketoglutaramate.[396] The presence of glutamine synthetase in glia is possibly related to astrocytic hypertrophy in hepatic encephalopathy.[397] Inhibition of glutamine synthetase (with methionine sulfoximine) protects mice against ammonia intoxication even though brain ammonia is further elevated.[398] Perfusion of alpha-ketoglutaramate into the ventricles of rats produced neurological signs, including myoclonus; a possible explanation is that alpha-ketoglutaramate competes for glutamate receptors in brain. Alternatively, diversion by ammonia of glutamate to glutamine would deplete both glutamate and aspartate; these excitatory neurotransmitters reportedly produce arousal in patients with hepatic encephalopathy.[396,399]

In contrast to hypotheses implicating ammonia, a "false neurotransmitter" hypothesis proposes that amines such as octopamine or beta-phenylethanolamine, absorbed from the gut and bypassing the liver, enter peripheral and central catecholamine nerve terminals and, in effect, inhibit them.[381,400] Possible precursors of such inhibitory false neurotransmitters are aromatic amino acids, increased brain uptake of which would be secondary to depressed blood levels of branched-chain amino acids.[401] Elevation of brain octopamine in experimental animals, however, failed to reproduce signs of hepatic encephalopathy.[402] Serum levels of tryptophan are elevated in hepatic encephalopathy, and ammonia facilitates the transport of tryptophan across the blood–brain barrier.[403] Raised levels of brain tryptophan lead to increases in brain and CSF quinolinic acid, a potentially toxic excitatory neurotransmitter.[404] Rats with portacaval shunts, but not normal rats, develop neuronal degeneration and astrocytic hypertrophy after tryptophan loading.[405]

An alternative hypothesis proposes that the crucial neurotoxin is either GABA or an endogenous benzodiazepine acting at the GABA receptor complex. GABA produced by enteric bacteria is believed to cross an abnormally permeable blood–brain barrier, producing neuronal inhibition. In support of this mechanism are increased serum levels of GABA and increased densities of GABA receptors preceding overt encephalopathy in experimental animals. Additionally, an abnormal visual-evoked potential pattern in hepatic encephalopathy is identical to that associated with coma secondary to barbiturates, benzodiazepines, or GABA agonists and unlike that associated with coma secondary to ammonia or mercaptans.[406–409] GABA antagonists such as bicuculline and chloride channel blockers such as isopropylbicyclophosphate reverse the clinical and electrophysiologic signs of hepatic encephalopathy in rabbits.[410] On the other hand, blood GABA levels correlate poorly with the encephalopathy, and normal brain levels of GABA have been reported in encephalopathic animals and humans. It is claimed, moreover, that even increased blood–brain barrier permeability would not allow increased penetration of GABA, which would be metabolized at the barrier by GABA-transaminase.[411]

Increased *GABA-ergic tone* could be the basis of hepatic encephalopathy without GABA itself accumulating. Possibilities include a toxin acting agonistically at benzodiazepine receptors on the GABA receptor complex.[412,413] Behavioral and electrophysiologic abnormalities in rats with liver failure are reversed by the benzodiazepine antagonist flumazenil.[414] Urine, blood, and CSF benzodiazepine receptor-binding activity was much higher in patients with hepatic encephalopathy than in controls (including uremic patients),[415] and the elevated levels of benzodiazepines—identified by mass spectroscopy as diazepam and N-desmethyldiazepam—were found in the brains of patients dying with hepatic encephalopathy.[416] Flumazenil improves the clinical and electrophysiologic signs of hepatic encephalopathy in the majority of patients.[417]

Table 11–16. Treatment of Hepatic Encephalopathy

Identify and treat precipitating factor(s)
Adequate calories (with protein restriction): provide at least 1600 calories per day from carbohydrate, orally or intravenously
Eliminate protein initially and then after a few days increase by 10 to 20 g per day every few days, depending on symptoms
Bowel cleansing: enemas, colonic lavage. Colonic exclusion in severe, chronic cases
Lactulose, 50–150 mg orally daily in divided doses, or as enema, 300 mL in 700 mL water
Alternatively: neomycin, 2–4 g orally daily, or as enema, 1% solution once or twice daily
Benzodiazepine antagonists
Attention to accompanying medical problems: acid–base disturbance, hypertension or hypotension, coagulation abnormalities, gastrointestinal bleeding, acute pancreatitis, sepsis. Ethanol withdrawal, meningitis, hypoglycemia, or intracranial hematoma or abscess may be masked

If a benzodiazepine agonist is indeed the encephalopathic toxin, its source is obscure.[415] Attempts to identify an endogenous benzodiazepine receptor ligand (e.g., beta-carboline, diazepam-binding inhibitor, or desmethyldiazepam) have produced conflicting results (see Chapter 5). It is possible that in hepatic encephalopathy the source of such a ligand is enteric bacteria or food.

Increased GABA-ergic tone would explain better than ammonia toxicity some features of hepatic encephalopathy. Ammonia is proconvulsant, whereas GABA is anticonvulsant, and myoclonus and seizures are not features of hepatic encephalopathy. Increased GABA-ergic tone would also explain the marked sensitivity of such patients to barbiturates and benzodiazepines.[418]

Treatment

Much of the treatment of hepatic encephalopathy is directed toward decreasing ammonia levels in blood and brain (Table 11–16). Dietary protein restriction is an obviously two-edged sword in malnourished patients. Bowel cleansing and surgical colonic exclusion eliminate urease-producing bacteria. So does neomycin, which can be given orally, 2 to 4 g daily, or by enema as a 1% solution once or twice daily.[419] Absorbed oral or rectal neomycin causes nephrotoxicity and ototoxicity, however, and in most patients the preferred agent is lactulose. This synthetic dissaccharide is metabolized by colonic bacteria to lactic, acetic, and formic acids, producing a gradient that converts ammonia to ammonium ion, which is then trapped in the gut and not absorbed. Lactulose causes diarrhea, which can be a problem in dehydrated or hypotensive patients. The oral dose is therefore titrated to cause two or three soft stools per day with acidic pH.

A controlled study demonstrated that lactulose and neomycin were equally effective in hepatic encephalopathy.[420] Although the two treatments should be mutually exclusive (because neomycin eliminates the bacteria that allow lactulose to work), additive benefits were found in one report, suggesting lactulose acts by mechanisms not yet understood.[421]

The false transmitter hypothesis led to trials with L-dopa or bromocriptine in hepatic encephalopathy.[381] Early studies were promising,[422] but subsequent observations, both anecdotal and controlled, were disappointing.[423] Improved mentation was also claimed following treatment with keto-analogs of amino acids[424] or with infusions high in branched-chain and low in aromatic amino acids.[425] Controlled trials failed to show benefit, however.

Reports of improvement in encephalopathic animals following GABA or benzodiazepine antagonists led to trials in humans. GABA and chloride channel antagonists are too epileptogenic to be practical, but as already noted, benzodiazepine antagonists have shown considerable promise.[417] Moreover, oral flumazenil successfully relieved symptoms, including episodic coma, in a patient with chronic intractable portal systemic encephalopathy.[426] Serious side effects have not been observed.[427] Unfortunately, flumazenil is rapidly metabolized, and its duration of action in most people lasts for only minutes to a few hours.[427] Longer acting agents will likely be developed.

More aggressive therapeutic approaches to hepatic encephalopathy include surgical colonic exclusion, cross-circulation with primates or irreversibly comatose donors, charcoal hemoperfusion, and liver transplantation.[381]

General medical management in hepatic encephalopathy can be complex. Patients are often very ill with acid–base disturbances, hyponatremia, hypernatremia, hypokalemia, edema, hypotension, renal failure, coagulation abnormalities, gastrointestinal bleeding, acute pancreatitis, or sepsis.[428,429] Ethanol withdrawal, meningitis, hypoglycemia, and subdural hematoma may be masked. Moreover, in one study, liver biopsy revealed a nonalcohol-related cause in 20% of alcoholics with liver disease.[430]

Chronic Hepatic Encephalopathy

In some cirrhotics neurological symptoms become chronic, and in alcoholics the clinical picture can be quite confusing. A group of patients with portacaval anastomoses developed progressive neuropsychiatric symptoms unlike those of acute hepatic encephalopathy.[431] They were usually noisy and hyperactive, and some appeared to be schizophrenic or hypomanic. In addition, they had variable combinations of slowly progressive paraparesis and spastic bladder, cerebellar ataxia, parkinsonism, seizures, myoclonus, and focal cortical signs. In one of the paraparetic patients, and in others subsequently reported,[432] autopsy revealed "widespread demyelination" in the spinal cord, not resembling multiple sclerosis. EEG slowing and elevated serum ammonia concentrations were usually present, yet only a few had had previous episodes of acute hepatic encephalopathy. Symptomatic improvement after dietary restriction, neomycin, or colonic exclusion was infrequent. A controlled study suggested favorable response to L-dopa;[433] trials with bromocriptine claimed [434] and denied [435] benefit.

Similar to such patients are those with *acquired chronic hepatocerebral degeneration*, a characteristic syndrome of dementia, dysarthria, ataxia, intention tremor, and choreoathetosis affecting especially cranial muscles. Muscle rigidity, grasp reflexes, mild pyramidal signs, nystagmus, and asterixis are common. The EEG is diffusely abnormal. Pathologically, astrocytosis and neuronal degeneration in the cerebrum, cerebellum, and diencephalon progress to laminar or pseudolaminar necrosis at corticomedullary junctions and microcavitation in the putamen. In the original description of this syndrome, 23 of 27 patients had had previous bouts of hepatic coma, and although all had either elevated serum ammonia levels or abnormal responses to ammonium citrate challenge, lowering of serum ammonia produced no improvement.[436]

Such stereotypic chronic hepatic encephalopathy is infrequently encountered at Harlem Hospital Center, but the question is often raised whether the mental changes of some chronically demented alcoholics without obvious motor disturbance could be on the basis of liver disease. Certainly the nature of *alcoholic cerebral atrophy* is far from clear (see later). In any event, a spectrum of hepatic encephalopathic disease seems to exist, and it is possible that symptomatic irreversibility depends on the degree of structural change.[419]

Table 11–17. Hypoglycemic Symptoms in 125 Consecutive Patients at Harlem Hospital Center (Alcoholism, Alone or Associated with Diabetes or Sepsis, in 60)

Depressed sensorium	
Coma	39
Stupor	16
Obtundation	10
Behavior change	
Confusion	24
Bizarre behavior	14
Dizziness, tremor	10
Seizures	9
Sudden hemiparesis	3

Source: Malouf R, Brust JCM. Hypoglycemia: causes, neurological manifestations, and outcome. Ann Neurol 1985; 17: 421.

Hypoglycemia

Impaired insulin response and glucose intolerance are frequent in alcoholics.[437] More serious is episodic hypoglycemia (Table 11–17), which tends to occur after 6 to 36 hours of moderate to heavy drinking, albeit infrequently; a blood glucose level below 50 mg/dL was found in only one of 131 intoxicated subjects.[438]

During a 12-month prospective survey of the Harlem Hospital emergency room, there were 125 visits for symptomatic hypoglycemia (Table 11–17).[439] In 60, ethanol played a role, either alone or in association with diabetes mellitus or sepsis. Symptoms included dizziness and tremor, abnormal behavior, depressed sensorium, and seizures. Hemiparesis was common on recovery from seizures or coma and in three instances was the presenting symptom in otherwise alert patients. Blood glucose levels tended to be lowest in comatose patients, but there was considerable overlap between groups, and overall there was little correlation between cause, glucose levels, and symptoms. Hypothermia was especially common among alcoholics. Eight patients relapsed after either admission or discharge from the emergency room, demonstrating that treated hypoglycemic patients should not be prematurely sent home but should be admitted, preferably to an intensive care unit. Relapse is especially likely when sepsis or diabetes is present. Overall mortality was 11%, yet only one death was attributable to hypoglycemia per se, and only four survivors had focal neurological residua.

Consistent with other reports, these patients demonstrated that hypoglycemic coma is less dangerous than equivalent degrees of anoxic/ischemic coma. Pathological changes are also different. Although anoxia/ischemia usually damages vascular border zones and end zones of the cerebrum, diencephalon, and cerebellum,[440] hypoglycemia affects the cerebrum and basal ganglia more diffusely and tends to spare the cerebellum. In hypoglycemia, cerebral oxygen consumption does not fall to the same extent as cerebral glucose metabolism, implying as yet unidentified energy sources. Nonetheless, symptomatic hypoglycemia is a medical emergency, for neurological residua do occur, and subtle cognitive changes are undoubtedly underdetected.[441,442] (They would be particularly difficult to demonstrate in alcoholics.) Any patient, alcoholic or not, with unexplained behavioral change, seizures, or depressed alertness should receive glucose and thiamine; those with status epilepticus or coma should be treated intravenously.

Nonalcoholics are vulnerable to ethanol-induced hypoglycemia by a different mechanism. Ethanol stimulates intestinal secretin, which in turn increases the insulin response to glucose. The result can be severe reactive hypoglycemia after a few drinks and a small meal.[443] Coma and seizures occurred in a 3-year-old who became severely hypoglycemic after drinking brandy,[179] and at Harlem Hospital Center ethanol-induced reactive hypoglycemia accounts for more pediatric admissions than does uncomplicated stupor following accidental ethanol ingestion.

Other Endocrinologic Effects

Ethanol's effects on sexual activity have long been recognized; it " ... provokes the desire but takes away the performance."[444] In men chronic ethanol decreases testosterone production and causes testicular atrophy, impotence, and gynecomastia.[445] Increased estrogen levels associated with liver disease contribute to feminization. Alcoholic women develop hyperprolactinemia, amenorrhea, and uterine atrophy. They are more likely to be infertile and once pregnant to have spontaneous abortion.[446]

Ethanol inhibits antidiuretic hormone release at the level of the hypothalamus; diuresis occurs when the blood ethanol concentration is rising but not when it is falling.[447]

Ethanol stimulates adrenocorticotropic hormone (ACTH) release from the pituitary.[448] *Pseudo-Cushing's syndrome* consists of characteristic signs, increased cortisol secretion, absent diurnal cortisol rhythm, and inadequate suppression of cortisol by dexamethasone.[449] Ethanol withdrawal also stimulates ACTH release, sometimes for weeks.[450] Cushingoid signs eventually clear with abstinence.

Acutely and chronically ethanol inhibits growth hormone, although in alcoholics with cirrhosis, levels may be elevated.[56]

Hypocalcemia is common in alcoholics. Hypoalbuminemia, poor nutrition, and increased urinary and intestinal loss each contribute; impaired intestinal calcium absorption has been attributed to hypovitaminosis D, hypoparathyroidism, and parathormone resistance secondary to magnesium deficiency.[451] Osteoporosis is a frequent consequence.[452] In normal volunteers, short-term ethanol administration caused transient hypoparathyroidism with hypocalcemia, hypercalciuria, and hypermagnesuria.[453]

Temperature

Through actions on the hypothalamus, ethanol increases skin blood flow and sweating and lowers body temperature.[454] When environmental temperature is low, life-threatening hypothermia can occur. Ethanol increases mortality in hyperthermic mice; conversely, elevated body temperature increases ethanol toxicity.[455]

Alcoholic Ketoacidosis

Acid–base disturbances in alcoholics are often difficult to interpret.[456,457] Respiratory alkalosis accompanies ethanol withdrawal or hepatic encephalopathy; metabolic alkalosis follows vomiting associated with gastritis or pancreatitis; and lactic acidosis results from seizures, infection, and gastrointestinal or traumatic hemorrhage. (By inhibiting lactate metabolism, ethanol prolongs lactic acidosis of any cause.) These conditions of course can coexist.

Alcoholic ketoacidosis refers to ketosis and an increased anion gap resulting from accumulation of acetoacetate and hydroxybutyrate.[456,457] Typical patients are young binge drinkers who stop drinking when overcome by anorexia or vomiting, sometimes owing to gastritis or pancreatitis. Acute starvation for several days is followed by confusion, obtundation, and Kussmaul respirations; depressed consciousness tends to be less than with a similar degree of diabetic ketoacidosis. There may be coexisting lactic acidosis and metabolic or respiratory alkalosis, with complex dissociations of serum pH, ketosis, and anion gap. When beta-hydroxybutyrate predom-

inates over acetoacetate, the nitroprusside test (Acetest) can be negative. Starvation and impaired gluconeogenesis produce hypoglycemia, but more often blood glucose levels are normal or moderately elevated. Decreased renal excretion of urate causes hyperuricemia. Serum insulin levels are often low, and serum levels of growth hormone, epinephrine, glucagon, and cortisol are high, yet glucose intolerance usually clears without insulin and is inapparent on recovery. Ethanol is rarely detectable in the blood. Repeated attacks of alcoholic ketoacidosis are common.

The cause of the ketosis is increased lipolysis and impaired fatty acid oxidation. Starvation is a major factor, and the role of ethanol per se is uncertain. (Normal rat liver slices incubated with ethanol do not display increased ketogenesis; liver slices from rats fed ethanol do.[458]) Treatment begins with attention to coexisting serious illness. Ketosis usually responds promptly to intravenous glucose (given with thiamine). Insulin is unnecessary unless the patient is diabetic; alcoholic ketoacidosis cannot then be distinguished from diabetic ketoacidosis, and insulin is given.[456] Sodium bicarbonate is also seldom needed, but dehydration and potassium depletion require saline and potassium salts (including potassium phosphate). Hypocalcemia in excess of hypoalbuminemia may reflect hypomagnesemia, correctable with magnesium sulfate.

Infection

Alcoholics have vacuolated white blood cells and granulocytopenia, depressed leukocyte migration, suppressed interferon systems, and decreased serum bactericidal activity.[459–461] Cirrhosis, by uncertain mechanisms, further predisposes to infection.[462] Twenty-nine percent of adults with pneumococcal meningitis at Harlem Hospital Center were alcoholic,[463] as were five of eight patients with nontraumatic gram-negative meningitis at the Detroit Medical Center.[464] Similar susceptibility to tuberculosis leads to meningitis, tuberculoma, and Pott's disease, and cure is difficult if alcoholism is not simultaneously treated.[465] Infectious meningitis must always be considered in alcoholics with seizures or altered mentation, even when the clinical picture seems fully explained by intoxication, withdrawal, thiamine deficiency, hepatic encephalopathy, or hypoglycemia. An epidemic of diphtheria occurred among homeless alcoholics in Seattle.[466] Whether alcoholics are at special risk for acquired immunodeficiency syndrome (AIDS) or early CNS involvement in human immunodeficiency virus (HIV) infection is controversial.[467-469]

Gastrointestinal Effects

Ethanol causes esophagitis, esophageal spasm, Mallory-Weiss tear, acute and chronic gastritis, peptic ulcer, alcoholic diarrhea, and acute and chronic pancreatitis. Malabsorption of folic acid, iron, and vitamins, including pyridoxine and cobalamin, compounds dietary insufficiency and produces a variety of neurological symptoms.

Cancer

Alcoholics have increased risk for cancer of the mouth, pharynx, larynx, and esophagus.[470] Ethanol does not cause cancer in experimental animals and in humans may act as a cocarcinogen with tobacco.[471] Whether ethanol increases risk for breast, gastric, pancreatic, or colonic cancer is controversial; studies claiming an association have lacked adequate controls. Hepatoma in alcoholics is closely linked with cirrhosis.

Trauma

Trauma can be an indicator of early ethanol abuse,[472,473] and ethanol intoxication makes serious injury more likely when trauma occurs.[474] Fifty percent to 55% of traffic fatalities involve either a drunk driver or a drunk pedestrian (see Table 11–1).[475] Ethanol also contributes heavily to aviation and boating accidents, falls, drownings, and fires.[476,477] In one-third of suicides the victims have been drinking and suicide among alcoholics ranges from 8% to 21%.[478] Ethanol is also a major contributor to assault and homicide.[475] In one report, half of murderers or their victims had been drinking at the time of the crime.[479]

Alcoholics bleed easily. Thrombocytopenia is both a direct effect of ethanol and a consequence of cirrhosis with hypersplenism.[372] Liver disease also alters clotting factors, and experimentally ethanol enhances blood–brain barrier leakage around areas of cerebral trauma.[480,481] In rats with spinal cord trauma, ethanol exacerbated the release of free fatty acids and excitatory amino acids and the reduction of tissue magnesium levels; mortality and neurological residua were increased in ethanol-treated rats compared to controls.[481a] Close observation is essential after even mild head trauma in intoxicated patients; altered mentation must not be dismissed as drunkenness.

Peripheral Nerve Pressure Palsies

Radial and peroneal nerve palsies are common in alcoholics. Underlying polyneuropathy increases the vulnerability of peripheral nerves to compression injury, and intoxicated subjects tend to sleep deeply in unusual locations and positions. Recovery takes days or weeks; splints during this period can prevent contractures.

Central Pontine Myelinolysis

Central pontine myelinolysis is an underdiagnosed disease characterized by demyelinating lesions in the central part of the basis pontis. It is not restricted to alcoholics and can be asymptomatic. Of the four original autopsy cases, three were chronic alcoholics with malnutrition and dehydration.[482] Two of these developed pseudobulbar palsy and quadriplegia over several days and died 2 to 4 weeks later. A single large symmetric demyelinating lesion occupied much of the basis pontis, affecting all fiber tracts but sparing all but the most central axons, neurons, and vessels. The third patient had similar but smaller lesions without having had apparent symptoms. Since then, there have been more than 200 reports of central pontine myelinolysis, which occurs in roughly 0.25% of autopsied adults. When severe, lesions extend into the pontine tegmentum, causing sensory loss, abnormal eye movements, and coma. Histologically similar lesions also occur in midbrain, cerebellum, diencephalon, and cerebrum.[483,484]

Central pontine myelinolysis most often affects patients with debilitating conditions such as liver disease, burns, amyloidosis, cerebral trauma, diabetes, kidney transplantation, brain tumor, and leukemia. It has coexisted with pellagra and Wernicke-Korsakoff disease[485] and occurs in children.[486] Although MRI has improved diagnostic accuracy,[487] it is still identified more often at autopsy than during life, especially when the underlying disease also causes neurological symptoms and signs. The demyelinating lesions are caused by overvigorous correction of hyponatremia, the basis pontis being particularly vulnerable because of its unique "anatomic grid structure."[483,488,489] Whether speed of correction or overcorrection to hypernatremia is more dangerous is disputed; animal studies suggest that rapid correction of chronic hyponatremia is especially hazardous.[490,491] In any case, central pontine myelinolysis is most often a preventable iatrogenic disease.

No specific treatment exists once central pontine myelinolysis occurs, although neurological signs occasionally remit with supportive therapy.[492–494] Prevention involves treating hyponatremia such that serum sodium levels do not exceed 130 mEq/L; free water restriction and small amounts of hypertonic saline are titrated to raise serum sodium levels no more rapidly than 0.55 mEq/L/hour or 12 mEq/L/day.[2,495–498]

Effects of Ethanol of Uncertain Cause

Myopathy

Alcoholic myopathy was first recognized as recurrent and sometimes fatal myoglobinuria.[499] Subsequent reports described chronic progressive weakness, and today alcoholic myopathy is classified, clinically and pathologically, as subclinical, chronic, or acute.[500–503] The subclinical variety consists of elevated serum creatine phosphokinase (CPK) levels and electromyographic abnormalities, sometimes with intermittent cramps, weakness, or dark urine. Blood lactate may fail to rise after ischemic exercise, suggesting abnormal muscle phosphorylase. Subclinical myopathy is common; electromyographic abnormalities are found in a majority of chronic alcoholics, and histologic changes—fiber vacuolation and degeneration, macrophages, and increased interstitial fat—occur in nearly half.

Chronic myopathy causes progressive proximal weakness, muscle tenderness, and more pronounced pathological alterations. Acute rhabdomyolysis, often exertional, causes sudden severe weakness and muscle pain, sometimes superimposed on chronic weakness during a drinking binge. Only one limb or muscle group may be affected, and sometimes the face or pharynx is involved.[504] Tenderness and swelling suggest thrombophlebitis. Myoglobinuria causes renal shutdown, and potassium release and hyperkalemia predispose to fatal cardiac arrhythmia. The diagnosis of acute alcoholic myoglobinuria is usually easy; in myopathic patients denying heavy ethanol, an ethanol challenge to produce myalgia has been recommended.[505] To be kept in mind are other causes of proximal weakness in alcoholics, such as hypokalemia following diarrhea,[506] pseudo-Cushing's syndrome,[449] and atypical polyneuropathy.

Whether subclinical, chronic, or acute, alcoholic myopathy improves with abstinence. Although subjects are often malnourished, ethanol toxicity is probably more important than nutritional deficiency. Twenty-three of 50 alcoholic men had histologic evidence of myopathy, which correlated better with the amount of ethanol consumed than with nutrition; it occurred only in those who for many years had drunk the equivalent of at least 12 oz of whiskey a day.[506] Nonalcoholic volunteers consuming ethanol with adequate diets developed, by electron microscopy, intracellular edema, lipid and glycogen accumulation, and abnormal mitochondria and sarcoplasmic reticulum.[508,509] Unclear is the relevance of these structural alterations to the acute reversible effects of ethanol on muscle function.[510] For example, both ethanol and acetaldehyde inhibit sodium-potassium-ATPase, mitochondrial fatty acid oxidation, protein synthesis, and calcium binding to troponin.[511] In alcoholic humans nuclear magnetic resonance spectroscopy is consistent with impaired glycolysis.[512]

Hereditary recurrent rhabdomyolysis affected two brothers whose symptoms—muscle pain and myoglobinuria—were provoked by strenuous exercise or ethanol ingestion. Muscle biopsy revealed ragged red fibers with abnormal mitochondria, and polymerase chain reaction detected deletions of mitochondrial DNA. Ethanol sensitivity in these patients might have been related to impaired oxidation of NADH (generated by alcohol dehydrogenase) secondary to defective mitochondrial energy transduction.[513]

Cardiomyopathy

Ethanol also damages cardiac muscle, and alcoholic cardiomyopathy, a low-output state clearly distinguishable from beri-beri heart disease, is possibly "the major cause of cardiomyopathy . . . in the Western World."[510] Nearly 90% of autopsies on chronic alcoholics reveal cardiomegaly with fiber hypertrophy, fibrosis, lipid and glycogen accumulation, swollen mitchondria, and necrosis. Congestive heart failure, pulmonary emboli, conduction defects, and arrhythmias are frequent; heart disease accounts for up to 15% of alcoholic deaths. In symptomatic patients mortality is 80% within 3 years unless abstinence occurs.[514,515]

Atrial and ventricular arrhythmia following acute heavy ethanol consumption, so-called "holiday heart," can cause sudden death in alcoholics.[516] Whether moderate ethanol consumption precipitates cardiac arrhythmia in otherwise healthy people is less certain, as is the contribution of cigarette smoking.[517] Acute congestive heart failure and arrhythmia have accompanied myoglobinuria after heavy drinking,[518] and in normal volunteers, acute ethanol ingestion causes myocardial depression.[519]

Marchiafava-Bignami Disease

Although an autopsy incidence among alcoholics of 6% has been claimed, Marchiafava-Bignami disease is probably much rarer.[520] It is defined by characteristic demyelinating lesions in the corpus callosum; the clinical spectrum is uncertain. Specifically associated with alcoholism, Marchiafava-Bignami disease was originally described in Italian men addicted to red wine[521] but has since been reported in non-Italians drinking beer or whiskey.[522] Rare cases have occurred in nonalcoholics.[523,524] Early symptoms are typically mental and include psychotic mania, depression, paranoia, and dementia. Major motor seizures are common, and there may be fluctuating hemiparesis, aphasia, rigidity, abnormal movements, dysarthria, and astasia-abasia. A callosal disconnection syndrome has infrequently been described.[522,525] There is usually progression to coma and death over a few months, although sometimes the course evolves acutely over days or chronically over years. A patient with apraxia, grasp reflexes, and gait ataxia improved spontaneously; following his death 3 years later from liver failure, autopsy revealed Marchiafava-Bignami disease.[526] The callosal lesions have been detected with MRI, and in a patient with clinical recovery, CT and MRI abnormalities regressed.[527,528]

Histologic changes resemble those of central pontine myelinolysis but are located, with sharp demarcation, in the medial zone of the corpus callosum, sparing the dorsal and ventral rims and spreading rostrocaudally. The anterior and posterior commissures as well as the subcortical white matter, centrum semiovale, and middle cerebellar peduncles (but not the basis pontis) can also be affected, with striking symmetry. The internal capsule is usually spared. In nearly half the cases, there are cortical lesions corresponding to *Morel's laminar sclerosis*.[520,529] These lesions, originally believed to cause dementia in alcoholics, consist of neuronal loss and gliosis in the third cortical layer of the frontal and parietal convexities. They are sometimes found in the absence of callosal damage.[530] Although the histologic similarity of central pontine myelinolysis and Marchiafava-Bignami disease suggests common mechanisms, rarely have the two diseases occurred together.[531]

The cause of Marchiafava-Bignami disease is unknown, and there is no explanation for such severe symptoms with such mild lesions. Similar pathology can be created experimentally with cyanide, apparently by damaging oligodendroglia,[532] but a relation of such toxicity to either ethanol or malnutrition is dubious.

Alcoholic Dementia

The term *alcoholic dementia* refers to progressive mental decline in alcoholics without apparent cause, nutritional or otherwise. It is a controversial concept. Some believe ethanol is directly neurotoxic, causing cerebral atrophy and progressive intellectual impairment qualitatively different from the amnestic syndrome of Korsakoff. Others deny that ethanol exerts clinically significant neurotoxicity and believe dementia in alcoholics can always be explained by indirect causes, such as nutritional deficiency, head trauma, episodic hypoglycemia, or chronic liver failure.

The notion that alcoholic dementia is a distinct disease entity is based on three lines of evidence. First is the clinical observation that alcoholics frequently have cognitive loss more gradual in onset and more "global" than would be expected with Korsakoff's syndrome. Prior episodes of Wernicke's syndrome are not identified, more than memory is affected, and there is neither history nor clinical evidence of nutritional deficiency or other dementing illness, ethanol-related or not.[533,534] Korsakoff's syndrome is infrequent after nonalcoholic Wernicke's syndrome (as with pernicious vomiting, starvation, renal dialysis, cancer, or AIDS),[2,268,535] and some believe alcoholic dementia represents a synergism between subclinical thiamine deficiency and direct ethanol toxicity.[536]

Opposed to this view is Victor, who points out that in fact Korsakoff's syndrome often evolves subacutely or chronically and includes intellectual and behavioral disturbances quite independent of memory.[161,537–540a] In a series of 20 pathologically proved cases of "inactive Wernicke's encephalopathy," two-thirds had exhibited "more or less pronounced global dementia and not a pure Korsakoff syndrome."[290] In none were there cerebral cortical or hippocampal lesions to suggest Alzheimer's disease, anoxia, or liver failure. Victor asserts, moreover, that autopsies on patients with the clinical diagnosis of alcoholic dementia "practically always" show lesions of Wernicke-Korsakoff disease, cerebral trauma, anoxic encephalopathy, acute and chronic hepatic encephalopathy, hydrocephalus, Alzheimer's disease, Marchiafava-Bignami disease, or stroke.[161,540] In an often-cited report, Courville[541] described histologic changes in allegedly atrophic alcoholic brains; these, in Victor's view, were artifacts. More recent reports of neuronal loss in the superior frontal cortex of alcoholics were confounded by coexisting Wernicke's encephalopathy and cirrhosis.[542,543] Similar drawbacks beset reports of reduced neuronal size in the cingulate cortex of alcoholics,[544] of decreased glucose metabolism (by positron-emission tomography) in medial frontal areas,[290,545] and of cholinergic receptor loss in the temporal cortex.[546]

Second are reports of radiographic "cerebral atrophy," first observed at pneumoencephalography[547–549] and later at CT scanning.[550–560] This literature has been conflicting. Some reports emphasize enlarged ventricles and others widened sulci. Some correlate atrophy with dementia, and others do not. For example, 12 alcoholic patients had CT evidence of enlarged ventricles compared with controls, but only 2 had widened sulci, and all were mentally normal.[550] Conversely, in another study, nearly half of demented alcoholics had no CT abnormalities.[551] In a report of 34 demented alcoholics, psychometric abnormalities correlated only modestly with ventricular size and better for the third than the lateral ventricles.[549] Moreover, some reports claim that both cognition and atrophy improve with abstinence.[561–565] Victor[161] stresses that such morphologic reversibility is more consistent with fluid shifts than tissue loss and that the term *atrophy* is therefore inappropriate. MRI studies on alcoholics have shown abnormalities in cerebral gray and white matter consistent with increased intracellular or extracellular water; cognitive impairment correlated better with these changes than with ventricular size.[566,567]

Third are animal studies, which have shown both behavioral and morphologic abnormalities in nutritionally maintained rodents receiving chronic ethanol. Experimental design has involved pair-fed controls and a sufficient period of abstinence to discount the effects of ethanol withdrawal. Such animals demonstrate impaired learning that tends to be subtle and selective, affecting some tasks but not others.[568–569] In mice and rats large doses of ethanol produce loss of dendritic spines, decreased dendritic branching, and cell death in hippocampal neurons.[570–578] Physiological abnormalities include decreased response of dentate granule cells to perforant path input and depressed inhibitory postsynaptic potentials in dentate granule and CA-1

cells.[579,580] In one study rats receiving daily ethanol to maintain the BEC at 80 to 120 mg/dL for 12 months had loss of hippocampal granule and pyramidal cells with preserved numbers of mossy fiber-CA3 synapses, suggesting new synapse formation; at 18 months, synapses were also decreased, suggesting collapse of this plastic response.[581] Loss of dendritic spines and branches has also been observed in cerebellar Purkinje cells of mice and rats.[569,582–584] Although in one study rat cerebral cortical neurons were unchanged after sufficient ethanol to cause apnea, others have reported that chronic ethanol produces pathological changes in cerebral cortex, mammillary bodies, and brain stem.[584,585] Well-nourished rats receiving chronic ethanol had impaired learning, reduced brain choline acetyltransferase levels and choline uptake, and mild neuronal loss in the nucleus basalis of Meynert;[586] transplantation of cholinergic neurons into hippocampus or cerebral cortex corrected both the abnormal memory and the cholinergic deficit.[587] On the other hand, "adolescent" rats given ethanol had *increased* numbers of spines on apical dendrites of pyramidal neurons in the somatosensory cortex, probably reflecting impairment of the naturally occurring elimination of redundant synapses during youth.[588]

The issue of alcoholic dementia is obviously of enormous importance. If ethanol is directly toxic to brain, either alone or synergistically with other risk factors, it becomes imperative to define a safe dose threshold. It could turn out there is none.

Stroke

Low to moderate amounts of ethanol probably decrease the risk of coronary artery disease and myocardial infarction,[589–599] although not all investigators have found such protection.[600–603] Heavy drinking increases the risk of coronary artery disease, but the dose at which protection turns to risk has not been defined.[604–606] Coronary artery disease in heavy drinkers carries an indirect risk for cardioembolic stroke secondary to cardiac wall hypokinesia or arrhythmia. Thromboembolism is also a prominent feature of alcoholic cardiomyopathy.[607]

Does ethanol increase the risk of stroke independent of its cardiac effects or other risk factors? Finnish investigators reported an association between recent heavy ethanol ingestion and both occlusive and hemorrhagic stroke.[608–611] These studies were retrospective and used population prevalence data as controls; other similarly designed analyses either failed to identify such an association[612] or found it only for intracerebral hemorrhage.[613] Chicago investigators reported that an association between ethanol intoxication and stroke disappeared when corrected for cigarette smoking.[614,615]

Numerous case-control and cohort studies have addressed the relationship of stroke to chronic ethanol use.[616–635a] Such studies have differed in end points selected (e.g., total stroke, occlusive stroke, hemorrhagic stroke, or stroke mortality), amount and duration of ethanol consumption, correction for other risk factors (e.g., hypertension and smoking), ethnicity, and socioeconomics. Among cohort studies, the Yugoslavia Cardiovascular Disease Study found increased stroke mortality among drinkers, and although the association was especially strong for hypertensives, it persisted with adjustment for blood pressure.[597,636] A reduced risk was found for modest drinkers. In the Honolulu Heart Study, heavy drinkers had an increased risk of hemorrhagic stroke independent of other risk factors, including hypertension and smoking.[604,637–639] There was no comparable risk for occlusive stroke. Early reports from the Framingham Study found both positive[640] and negative[641–644] associations; a later report described lower than expected stroke incidence among "moderate" drinkers and higher rates in both heavy drinkers and nondrinkers.[645] The Nurses' Health Study, adjusting for smoking and hypertension, found an inverse association between modest drinking and occlusive stroke and an increased risk at higher intake; both modest and heavy drinkers had an increased risk of subarachnoid hemorrhage.[646] In the Lausanne Stroke Registry, severity of internal carotid artery stenosis inversely correlated with "light to moderate" drinking; there were too few patients to assess heavy intake.[647] The Japanese Hisayama Study initially reported positive correlations,[648] but later, after adjusting for other variables, found no independent association between ethanol and occlusive or hemorrhagic stroke.[649] A study of Japanese physicians found a positive association between stroke mortality and ethanol.[650,651] Other Japanese investigators reported variable risk for hemorrhagic or occlusive stroke among drinkers[652,653]

In a review of 62 epidemiologic studies that examined the relation between stroke and "moderate" ethanol consumption (less than two drinks, or 1 oz of ethanol, daily), it was concluded that ethnicity plays a decisive role.[654] Among whites moderate doses of ethanol protected against ischemic stroke, but higher doses increased risk. Among Japanese little association existed between ethanol and ischemic stroke. In both populations all doses of ethanol in-creased the risk of both intracerebral and subarachnoid hemorrhage. Some studies suggested that the risk of hemorrhagic stroke declines with abstinence. There was insufficient evidence to draw an association between stroke and recent intoxication per se.

As with coronary artery disease, several mechanisms might explain the association between drinking and stroke. Ethanol acutely and chronically causes hypertension,[597,604,606,655–658] perhaps by increasing adrenergic activity and raising blood levels of cortisol, renin, aldosterone, and vasopressin.[659] With abstinence blood pressure sometimes returns to normal.[660]

Ethanol lowers blood levels of low-density lipoproteins (LDL) and elevates levels of high-density lipoproteins (HDL).[661,662] Ethanol reportedly protects large vessels from atherosclerosis, perhaps accounting for ethnic differences in patterns of risk.[663] The relationship is uncertain, however, for ethanol may not raise blood levels of the more protective HDL_2-subfraction.[664,665]

Acutely ethanol decreases fibrinolytic activity, raises levels of factor VIII, increases platelet reactivity to adenosine diphosphate (ADP), and shortens bleeding time.[666–669] On the other hand moderate doses of ethanol increase levels of prostacyclin,[670,671] and some studies have found that ethanol decreases platelet function.[672–675] Alcoholics with liver disease have decreased levels of clotting factors, excessive fibrinolysis, and platelet abnormalities.[659] During ethanol withdrawal, "rebound thrombocytosis" and platelet hyperaggregability have been observed.[676,677] So has decreased platelet response to activators, however.[678]

Acute ethanol intoxication causes cerebral vasodilation[679,680] and blood–brain barrier leakage of albumin.[681] Increased cerebral blood flow also occurs during withdrawal, although dehydration during hangover could reduce cerebral perfusion.[682] Chronic drinking is associated with decreased cerebral blood flow, mainly from reduced cerebral metabolism.[683] In vitro, however, ethanol causes constriction of both large and small cerebral vessels, and some investigators have observed decreased cerebral blood flow and impaired cerebrovascular autoregulation during acute intoxication.[684] Ethanol-related hemoconcentration and reduced erythrocyte flexibility may also lower cerebral blood flow.[609,659] Bilateral anterior cerebral artery occlusion occurred in a young alcoholic woman with sickle cell trait; platelets showed hyperaggregation to epinephrine, raising the possibility that ethanol-induced catecholamine release contributed to cerebral thrombosis.[685]

Fetal Alcohol Syndrome

The "gin epidemic" of 18th century England led to speculation that ethanol abuse caused feeble-mindedness in offspring,[686] and during the 19th century high prevalences of stillbirth and infant mortality were reported among children of alcoholic women.[687] In 1968, French workers reported an association of maternal alcoholism with congenital malformations, delayed psychomotor development, and behavioral problems.[688] Shortly thereafter pediatricians in Seattle, noting frequent failure to thrive in offspring of alcoholic mothers, defined the *fetal alcohol syndrome* (Table 11–18).[689,690]

Major clinical features include CNS dysfunction, growth deficiency, and distinctive faces; less often there are abnormalities of the heart, skeleton, urogenital organs, skin, and muscles.[3,691–693] Microphthalmia, malformed retinal vessels, optic atrophy, and blindness are common.[694] Neuropathological abnormalities include absence of corpus callosum, hydrocephalus, cerebellar dysplasia, microcephaly, and abnormal neuronal migration with heterotopic cell clusters. Prospective controlled studies reveal that the fetal alcohol syndrome occurs independently of maternal malnutrition, smoking, caffeine, other drugs, and age.[695] (That is not to say that other drug exposure or the quality of prenatal care are irrelevant.) Binge drinking that produces high ethanol levels at a critical fetal period may be more important than chronic exposure, and early gestation appears to be the most vulnerable period.[691,696] For reasons unclear, beer may carry greater risk than wine or liquor.[694] In the United States, blacks and certain American Indian tribes are at special risk; the degree to which such risk is independent of socioeconomic status is uncertain.[694]

Children of alcoholic mothers are often intellectually borderline or retarded without other features of the fetal alcohol syndrome;[693] fetal effects of ethanol thus cover a broad spectrum. Stillbirths and attention deficit disorder are especially frequent among offspring of heavy drinkers,[689,697] and each anomaly of the fetal alcohol syndrome can occur alone or in combination with others.[698,699] An association between maternal drinking and spasmus nutans has been suggested.[700] The face of a typical patient with the fetal alcohol syndrome is distinctive and, as in Down's syndrome, easily recognized at birth.[701] Irritability, tremulousness, poor suck, and apparent hyperacusis last weeks to months; some symptoms (e.g., seizures) suggest ethanol withdrawal.[702] Eighty-five percent perform more than 2 standard deviations below the mean on psychometric tests, and it is rare for those not grossly retarded to have even average mental ability.[689] In one series the average IQ was 65 with a range of 16 to 105, and the lowest IQs were in those with the most complete phenotype.[703]

Older children are frequently hyperactive and clumsy, with hypotonia or hypertonia. A 10-year follow-up of 10 children with fetal alcohol syndrome revealed that 2 were dead and 8 were still growth deficient and dysmorphic; 4 were of borderline intelligence, and 4 were severely retarded.[704] Several had eustachian tube abnormalities, chronic otitis media, and deafness. Even more dramatically, a 30 year follow-up of 105 French fetal alcohol syndrome victims (77 of whom were patients from the authors' original report) revealed facial dysmorphism (especially a long face and bulky nose and chin), persistent though less marked growth failure, and even more pronounced microcephaly, with mental retardation frequent and abnormal behavior invariable; interestingly, several siblings without evident dysmorphism at birth also demonstrated psychological impairment.[704a]

Ethanol toxicity is the cause of the fetal alcohol syndrome, which has been reproduced in carefully controlled animal models that include chickens, rodents, dogs, pigs, and primates.[705–710] Rats exposed to ethanol in utero exhibit bony changes in the face and limbs and microcephaly.[711] Litter weight, not litter size, is decreased compared with pair-fed controls in rats exposed to ethanol in utero; with surrogate mothers after delivery, there is catch-up in the weight among animals that received low doses of ethanol but not among the high-dose group.[712] Some exposed rats exhibit impaired mental ability without other physical signs.[713] Fetal ethanol exposure in mice produces neurological, ocular, cardiac, and skeletal anomalies, including exencephaly, hydrocephalus, and microphthalmia.[696] Although adult mice receiving chronic ethanol exhibit audiogenic seizures only transiently, prenatal and neonatal exposure causes long-lasting seizures.[714] In dogs high doses of ethanol prevent intrauterine tissue differentiation, moderate doses cause spontaneous abortion, and low doses cause significant increases in stillbirths.[715] In Macaque monkeys exposure comparable to binge drinking causes craniofacial and nervous system abnormalities similar to the human fetal alcohol syndrome.[709,716] In mice a single exposure to ethanol on the seventh day of pregnancy (corresponding to the third week of human pregnancy) also produces typical features of the fetal alcohol syndrome.[717]

Table 11–18. Clinical Features of the Fetal Alcohol Syndrome

Feature	Majority	Minority
CNS	Mental retardation Microcephaly Hypotonia Poor coordination Hyperactivity	
Impaired growth	Prenatal and postnatal for length and weight Diminished adipose tissue	
Abnormal face		
Eyes	Short palpebral fissures	Ptosis Strabismus Epicanthal folds Myopia Microophthalmia Blepharophimosis Cataracts Retinal pigmentary abnormalities
Nose	Short, upturned Hypoplastic philtrum	

Mouth	Thin vermilion lip borders
	
	Retrognathia in infancy
	Micrognathia or prognathia
	  in adolescence
		Prominent lateral
		  palatine ridges
		Cleft lip or palate
		Small teeth with
		  faulty enamel

Maxilla	Hypoplastic	
Ears		Posteriorly rotated Poorly formed concha

Skeletal		Pectus excavatum
		  or carinatum
		Syndactyly,
		  clinodactyly,
		  or camptodactyly
		Limited joint movements
		Nail hypoplasia
		Radiolunar synostosis
		Bifid xiphoid
		Scoliosis
		Klippel-Feil anomaly

Cardiac		Septal defects Great vessel anomalies
Cutaneous		Abnormal palmar creases Hemangiomas Infantile hirsutism
Muscular		Diaphragmatic, inguinal, or umbilical hernias Diastasis recti
Urogenital		Labial hypoplasia Hypospadias Small rotated kidneys Hydronephrosis

Ethanol-exposed rats have endocrine abnormalities that persist into adulthood. Decreased testosterone levels lead to lasting female-like behavior among males, and increased secretion of adrenal corticosteroids leads to male-like behavior among females.[718]

Both paternal and maternal ethanol consumption lead to increased susceptibility to infection in offspring.[719]

The mechanism of ethanol's teratogenicity is unknown. Easily crossing the placenta, ethanol maintains a fetal blood concentration considerably longer than the maternal level.[720] Failure of neuronal and glial migration suggests effects early in pregnancy,[689] but subtle alterations in sleep patterns suggest later effects.[721] Maternal ethanol use during the third trimester, including its use to inhibit premature labor by suppressing oxytocin release, might carry additional hazards. Newborns of alcoholic mothers have low blood levels of somatomedin C and high levels of growth hormone.[722] Neonatal rats continuously ingesting ethanol are less likely to show histologic brain damage than rats receiving smaller overall doses given over short periods (comparable to binge drinking).[723] Ingested ethanol passes through the liver before reaching the systemic circulation, and continuous small doses are fully metabolized. Much of a single large dose, however, passes through the liver and reaches the brain. The special vulnerability of neurons in the CA-1 region of the hippocampus and cerebellar Purkinje cells parallels vulnerability to neonatal asphyxia, lending support to the hypothesis that ethanol's teratogenicity is the result of vasospasm and CNS ischemia.[684,724–726] Consistent with such a mechanism are studies in sheep and monkey fetuses in which ethanol infusion caused metabolic and then mixed acidosis with EEG slowing and eventual isoelectricity.[727–729]

Ethanol withdrawal may itself be specifically damaging to nervous tissue.[730,731] Prevention of withdrawal signs by tapering ethanol dosage did not prevent CNS damage in fetal rats, however.[732]

Injections of acetaldehyde in pregnant mice led to delayed neural tube closure in fetuses.[733] Acetaldehyde could be an additional teratogen in the fetal alcohol syndrome, although in this experiment its teratogenicity could have been the result of metabolism back to ethanol.

Ethanol inhibits nerve growth factor and neuronal process formation; by this mechanism it might selectively damage those neurons most rapidly growing at the time of exposure.[723,734] Ethanol may also be toxic to the placenta, interfering with uptake of essential nutrients.[690,735–737]

Given to female mice at the time of conception, ethanol interferes with chromosomal segregation, and acetaldehyde interferes with mitotic spindle mechanisms and is clastogenic.[738] Isochrome 9q abnormality was reported in a dysmorphic 2-year-old whose mother had drunk heavily during the first several weeks of pregnancy.[739]

Exposure of male animals or humans to ethanol before conception may predispose their offspring to lower birth weight and decreased viability, but the data are tenuous.[740]

Extrapolating from reports that aspirin and other prostaglandin inhibitors antagonize ethanol-induced sleep, hypothermia, and increased activity, investigators pretreated pregnant mice with aspirin before they received ethanol. Signs comparable to fetal alcohol syndrome developed in 25% of fetuses whose mothers received aspirin, compared with 50% of fetuses whose mothers did not.[741]

The teratogenic risk of ethanol is established, but a threshold of safety has not been defined.[742] The incidence of fetal alcohol syndrome may be as high as one to two live births per 1000 with partial expressions of three to five per 1000.[701] It may affect 1% of children whose mothers drink 1 oz of ethanol per day early in pregnancy and over 30% of the offspring of heavy drinkers.[695] In one study, which corrected for confounding variables, including tobacco, reduced infant size correlated with drinking only 100 g of ethanol per week at the time of conception.[743] In another report low birth weight and decreased head circumference and body length correlated with only one drink per day during the first 2 months of the first trimester.[744] In another study dysmorphism in 4-year-olds was assessed without knowledge of maternal drinking patterns; it was found in 20.4% of children whose mothers had drunk at least 1 oz of ethanol daily early in pregnancy compared with 9.3% of those whose mothers had drunk less.[745] "Social drinking" during pregnancy led to EEG abnormalities in offspring, more severe in infants of intermittent drinkers than of frank alcoholics.[746]

In studies from Seattle and Canada ethanol consumption as low as one-tenth of an ounce daily carried risk for subtle neurological and behavioral effects, including slow habituating responses and delayed weak sucking.[747–749] Only 10 g ethanol daily during early pregnancy was associated with low birth weight,[750] and in mice a single exposure to ethanol at a critical time caused craniofacial anomalies.[751]

Considering that ethanol use during pregnancy tends to be underreported,[752] these findings raise the worrisome possibility that very low doses can cause subtle cognitive changes—that in fact there may be no such thing as a safe dose. They also imply that by the time a woman reaches the antenatal clinic, damage has already been done. Some investigators criticize the studies cited, claiming that when other risk factors are properly considered, there is no hazard association with one or two drinks a day.[753-758] The burden of proof, however, is on those who believe that there is a safe dose of what is probably the leading teratogenic cause of mental retardation in the western world.[701]

Ethanol is detectable in breast milk of mothers who drink alcoholic beverages, and their nursing infants display altered feeding and sleeping behavior.[759] Moreover, motor development was mildly delayed at 1 year in infants breast-fed by mothers who drank ethanol.[760] An obvious problem in interpreting these findings is correcting for substandard maternal behavior.[761,762]

Ethanol Substitutes

Methanol

Methanol (methyl alcohol, wood alcohol) is present in industrial solvents, gasohol, carburetor fluid, duplicator fluid, shellac, antifreeze, solid canned fuels, and windshield washing solution.[763,764] Contamination of bootleg spirits has resulted in epidemics of methanol poisoning. In 1951, 323 poisonings—with 41 deaths—followed the distribution of contaminated bootleg whiskey in Atlanta, Georgia.[765] A smaller outbreak involved the ingestion of duplicating fluid by inmates of a Michigan prison.[766]

Although methanol is rapidly absorbed from the gastrointestinal tract, inebriation is not prominent, and symptoms usually appear only after 12 to 36 hours. Methanol's metabolic products are directly toxic to retinal ganglion cells; visual blurring, sometimes with yellow spots or central scotomas, progresses to complete blindness, unreactive pupils, optic disc hyperemia, engorged retinal veins, and later optic atrophy. Other symptoms include headache, dizziness, nausea, vomiting, abdominal pain (often due to pancreatitis), delirium, seizures, and coma. Respirations become slow, shallow, and gasping. Bradycardia signifies a grave prognosis.[763,764,766]

Blindness has followed ingestion of only 15 ml of methanol. It nearly always precedes death, which is usually associated with doses of 70 to 100 ml. There is much individual variation in the lethal dose, however. Death followed ingestion of only 6 ml absolute methanol, and survival has followed ingestion of more than 500 ml.[763]

Methanol is metabolized by ADH to formaldehyde and then to formic acid, which is responsible for severe anion gap metabolic acidosis.[767,768] (If hypotension is present, lactic acid contributes.) Treatment begins with cardiovascular and respiratory support and gastric emptying. Sodium bicarbonate may be required for several days, as acidosis commonly recurs after seemingly successful treatment. Bicarbonate therapy itself causes hypokalemia. Ethanol is given, because the affinity of ethanol for ADH greatly exceeds that of methanol, and ethanol thereby blocks the conversion of methanol to toxic metabolites. The aim is to achieve a blood ethanol concentration of 100 mg/dL. A usual loading dose is 7.6 to 10 mL/kg 10% ethanol in 5% dextrose intravenously (or 0.8 to 1.0 mL/kg 95% ethanol orally); maintenance dosage is then 1.4 mL/kg/hour of 10% ethanol by continuous intravenous drip (or 0.15 mL/kg 95% ethanol orally).[763] Chronic alcoholics and patients receiving hemodialysis require more. Hemodialysis has been recommended for patients with blood methanol levels above 500 mg/dL.[763,764] Folate is also given, as the oxidation of formic acid to carbon dioxide is folate dependent. 4-Methylpyrazole, which inhibits ADH, has been used successfully in animals and recommended for human methanol poisoning but is not yet available for general use in the United States.[769]

Survivors of methanol poisoning sometimes have movement disorders, including parkinsonism and dystonia. CT scans have revealed putaminal destruction.[770-772] Electromyography demonstrates denervation consistent with anterior horn cell damage. Autopsy shows putaminal necrosis and widespread neuronal damage in the cerebrum, cerebellum, brain stem, and spinal cord.[773]

Ethylene Glycol

Found in antifreezes, windshield de-icers, and brake fluids, ethylene glycol is deliberately drunk as an ethanol substitute.[763] Within a few hours, inebriation is followed by nausea, vomiting, ataxia, nystagmus, ophthalmoparesis, myoclonus, seizures, hypoactive tendon reflexes, and stupor or coma. There may be hypothermia or mild fever. Metabolic acidosis with a marked anion gap is the result of several ethylene glycol metabolites, the most important of which, oxylate, chelates calcium and causes tetany and cardiac symptoms, including pulmonary edema.[763,764,769,774] Calcium oxylate crystals are often (but not always) seen in the urine within a few hours of ingestion. Their precipitation leads to renal failure several days later. Survivors sometimes have lasting cranial neuropathies—especially facial paralysis—appearing up to 18 days after ethylene glycol ingestion; a possible mechanism is deposition of oxylate crystals.[775]

Treatment begins with gastric emptying and respiratory support. Like methanol, ethylene glycol is metabolized by ADH, and so ethanol is given. Hemodialysis is recommended for ethylene glycol blood levels above 50 mg/dL or when renal failure is present.[763,764,766] Forced diuresis can prevent oxalate crystal precipitation, and thiamine and pyridoxine might help to divert ethylene glycol metabolism to products other than oxalate. 4-Methylpyrazole has been effective in ethylene glycol–poisoned animals and dramatically reversed symptoms in a man who drank 1.5 L of antifreeze in a suicide attempt.[777]

Isopropanol

Isopropanol, contained in rubbing alcohol, household cements, glass cleaners, and windshield deicers, is also an occasional ethanol substitute.[763] Metabolized to acetone, it usually causes ketosis without lactic acidosis.[456] Gastritis, abdominal pain, and vomiting are prominent, followed by ataxia, confusion, or coma. Miosis, decreased tendon reflexes, hypothermia, renal tubular necrosis, myopathy, and hemolytic anemia occur. Hypotension is secondary to direct cardiac depression. Treatment is supportive, beginning with continuous gastric lavage—isopropanol continues to be secreted into the stomach. Hemodialysis is used for hypotensive or comatose patients.[763,778] Because isopropanol itself is the major toxin, ethanol is not given.

Treatment of Chronic Alcoholism

Making the Diagnosis

Despite the fact that 90% of adults seen by primary care physicians report using ethanol and up to 45% report abuse,[7] physicians frequently do not ask patients about drinking or advise them to cut back.[779] Simple screening questionnaires can be an effective starting point. For example, CAGE scores of 1 to 4 (Table 11–19) carry probabilities for ethanol abuse of 7%, 46%, 72%, and 98%.[7]

Table 11–19. The CAGE Score

1. Have you ever felt you should *cut down* on your drinking?
2. Have people *annoyed* you by criticizing your drinking?
3. Have you ever felt bad or *guilty* about your drinking?
4. Have you ever had a drink first thing in the morning to steady your nerves or to get rid of a hangover (*eye-opener*)?

Heterogeneity of Patients and Therapies

In the voluminous literature on the treatment of alcoholism, strong opinions outweigh scientific data. Noteworthy are the diversity of the patients being treated.[780] As discussed earlier, a problem drinker is not necessarily physically dependent; no personality type defines an alcoholic; and genetics, associated psychiatric illness, and social deprivation play varying roles. The vast majority of American alcoholics are employed and live with their families.[110,781] Over the past 2 decades, however, alcoholics have increasingly abused other drugs. In a 1985 study additional drug abuse was found in 45% of male and 11% of female alcoholics,[782] and in a report from the San Diego Veterans Administration Medical Center, 53% of primary alcoholics used marijuana; 23%, psychostimulants; 14%, cocaine; and 11%, sedatives.[783] Coexisting psychiatric illness is also common. In one series 50% of female alcoholics had additional psychiatric diagnoses, including unipolar depression (24%), bipolar depression (4%), anxiety disorders (10%), and psychosis (6%).[784] In another study of alcoholics, 18% of men and 38% of women were depressed, 15% of men and 29% of women had phobias, and 5% of men and 9% of women had panic attacks.[782] Further complicating treatment are attitudinal differences. For example, the U.S. Veterans Administration defines *secondary alcoholism* ("secondary to and a manifestation of an acquired psychiatric disorder") as a disease qualifying for disability. *Primary alcoholism*, on the other hand, is defined as "willful misconduct."[785] Finally, ethanol directly or indirectly causes disturbances of memory and cognition that are bound to interfere with treatment.[786]

Such heterogeneity has led to a variety of treatment approaches: for example, psychotherapy, group psychotherapy, family or "social network" therapy, drug therapy, or behavioral (aversion) therapy. Settings also vary: for example, a general hospital, a halfway house, a vocational rehabilitation clinic, or Alcoholics Anonymous. Taken overall, outcome seems to be independent of the particular treatment

Table 11–20. Chronic Alcoholism—Varieties of Treatment

> Tranquilizers
> Disulfiram
> Lithium
> Serotonin uptake inhibitors
> Dopamine agonists
> Opioids
> Psychotherapy
> Alcoholics Anonymous
> Acupuncture

given.[787,788] That does not mean that for an individual patient one treatment is not preferable to another (Table 11–20).

Tranquilizers

The use of tranquilizing or sedating drugs is especially controversial.[789, 790] Benzodiazepines and barbiturates are cross-tolerant with ethanol and might therefore have the same rationale for treating alcoholism that methadone has in treating opioid addiction. Sedatives carry their own abuse potential, however; in fact, the vast majority of benzodiazepine abusers are also alcoholic.[791] Despite their cross-tolerance, tranquilizers and sedatives can also interact synergistically with ethanol. Their use in chronic alcoholism therefore must be judicious and selective.

For anxious patients a recommended approach is short-term use of a benzodiazepine in dosage high enough to reduce "the underlying predisposing tensions" that lead to ethanol use but without blocking symptoms of ethanol withdrawal.[792] Better retention in treatment programs was reported among patients taking chlordiazepoxide compared with those taking disulfiram, imipramine, phenothiazines, or no medicine.[793]

More selective approaches include use of benzodiazepines in type I but not type II alcoholics; impulsivity in the latter may be aggravated by such treatment. Type I alcoholics without other psychiatric disorder, however, may not benefit from any pharmacotherapy.[790] Those with secondary alcoholism should be treated for the primary mental disorder. Panic attacks respond to monoamine oxidase inhibitors, tricyclic antidepressants, serotonin reuptake blockers, or benzodiazepines, including alprazolam, clonazepam, and lorazepam. Social phobias are more likely to respond to beta-adrenergic blockers and single phobias to behavioral therapy. For general anxiety, with or without depression, some favor imipramine or amitriptyline over benzodiazepines.[794] Buspirone may also be preferable to benzodiazepines in alcoholics.[795,796] Similarly, although alprazolam can be effective in depression,[797] tricyclic antidepressants and serotonin reuptake blockers are probably safer in alcoholics. Nearly half of schizophrenics abuse ethanol or other drugs; pharmacotherapy in such patients is especially daunting.[798]

Disulfiram

By inhibiting ALDH, disulfiram (Antabuse) blocks the oxidation of acetaldehyde and produces a constellation of disagreeable symptoms.[799] Within 5 to 10 minutes of ethanol ingestion there is warmth and flushing of the face and chest, throbbing headache, dyspnea, nausea, vomiting, sweating, thirst, chest pain, palpitations, hypotension, anxiety, confusion, weakness, vertigo, and blurred vision.[800] Severity and duration depend on the amount of ethanol drunk. Small amounts cause mild symptoms followed by drowsiness, sleep, and recovery; severe reactions are potentially fatal and require hospitalization and careful management of hypotension, cardiac ischemia, or arrhythmia. In up to 25% of patients taking more than 500 mg per day, fatigue and confusion progress to toxic psychosis, stupor, or catatonia.[801,802] Disulfiram reactions can occur within a week of the last dose; if there is liver disease, the interval is even longer.[803]

Although 150,000 to 200,000 Americans are currently maintained on disulfiram, evidence of efficacy is limited. Taken in the morning when the urge to drink is least, 250 or 500 mg daily does not alter the taste for ethanol and so helps only those who strongly wish to abstain. Two questions then arise: (1) Is disulfiram of any benefit? (2) If so, is benefit based on true pharmacological aversion, or is it simply psychological? Nearly 100 studies attempting to answer the first question are invalid because of lack of controls or insufficient power.[804,805] In two well-designed trials, male alcoholics were randomized to disulfiram, 250 mg; disulfiram 1 mg (i.e., placebo); or no drug. All groups received counseling.[806,807] In the first study at 6 months there was a small but significant increase in total abstinence among those taking disulfiram in either dosage; this finding suggests the effect was mainly due to the patients' fear. In the second study at 12 months there were no differences in total abstinence, time to first drink, or social stability, but those receiving the full disulfiram dose had fewer drinking days than those receiving placebo or no drug. This difference is consistent with true pharmacological aversion. Disulfiram thus helps to reduce drinking frequency after relapse but is no better than counseling alone in sustaining continuous abstinence. It seems to be most effective in older, employed, socially stable patients and should be viewed as only adjunctive therapy.[808–810]

Side effects of disulfiram—in the absence of ethanol—are dose related and include hypertension, drowsiness, forgetfulness, ataxia, dysarthria, peripheral neuropathy, and seizures.[811] It may be difficult to separate disulfiram's complications from the effects of ethanol itself.[812,813] Such side effects can occur in patients taking only 250 mg daily, and one-fourth of patients taking more than 500 mg daily develop fatigue, confusion, psychosis, or stupor.[801] Acute hepatitis also occurs, and inhibition of microsomal enzymes increases blood levels of warfarin, phenytoin, and isoniazid.[799]

A European study comparing disulfiram implants (unavailable in the United States), placebo implants, and no implants found fewer drinking days in patients with either type of implant, again suggesting a behavioral rather than a pharmacological effect.[814]

Also available in Europe and Canada is calcium carbamide, believed by some to produce a milder aversive reaction than disulfiram.[801] It causes hypothyroidism in patients with already reduced thyroid function, a common occurrence in alcoholics. In contrast to disulfiram, calcium carbamide does not inhibit dopamine-beta-hydroxylase and is less likely to cause or exacerbate depression or psychosis.[815]

As noted earlier, a number of other drugs produce disulfiram-like reactions after ethanol, but the effects are usually mild, and such agents are of no use in treating alcoholics. Patients taking disulfiram have had aversive reactions when exposed to occupational solvents (e.g., paint or ceramics)[816] or to other medications containing ethanol (e.g., asthma elixirs).[803,817] Symptoms suggestive of disulfiram reactions can occur in patients who take ethanol with chloral hydrate or who take monoamine oxidase inhibitors with tyramine-containing alcoholic beverages, such as Chianti wine.[803]

Lithium

The frequent mood swings of alcoholics led to a controlled trial with lithium, which demonstrated decreased need for hospitalization among treated subjects.[818] Rats receiving lithium also had reduced ethanol preference.[819] Subsequent human controlled trials, however, failed to demonstrate benefit in either depressed or nondepressed alcoholics.[820,821] Lithium would still be appropriate for patients with bipolar disorder and secondary alcoholism. As with disulfiram, compliance is a problem, and ethanol lowers the threshold for lithium toxicity.

Serotonin Uptake Inhibitors

To cross the blood–brain barrier, tryptophan competes with other amino acids, and relatively low blood levels of tryptophan are found in early-onset alcoholics with depressive or aggressive tendencies.[822] The idea that altered serotonergic neurotransmission might contribute to ethanol-seeking behavior led to trials of serotonin uptake inhibitors in animals and humans.[823,824] Such agents attenuate ethanol intake in rats. In nondepressed humans with "early-stage problem drinking" (about 54 g ethanol daily), zimelidine, citalopram, viqualine, and fluoxetine decreased drinking by 20% to 30%.[825–827] Unfortunately these studies did not identify patient traits that would predict response. Zimelidine was subsequently withdrawn from further trials because of hepatotoxicity and Guillain-Barré syndrome. Fluoxetine is comercially available as an antidepressant.

Dopaminergic Compounds

The dopamine agonists apomorphine and bromocriptine reduce ethanol ingestion by rats. Paradoxically, so does the dopamine release suppressor dihydroergotoxine combined with the dopamine blocker thioridazine. Such drugs await trials in humans.[828]

Opioids

In rats ethanol consumption is suppressed by morphine, methadone, levorphanol, and enkephalinase inhibition, and these effects are blocked by naloxone.[829] In the 19th century alcoholics were frequently treated with opioids, and a number of studies have suggested that opioids reduce craving for ethanol.[830] Although alcoholism is common among patients receiving methadone maintenance treatment, methadone per se is more likely to reduce craving for ethanol than to increase it.[831] On the other hand, naltrexone reduces ethanol drinking by monkeys[832] and in a placebo-controlled trial in humans reduced ethanol consumption.[833]

Alcoholics Anonymous

Benjamin Rush was one of the first to propose that alcoholism is a disease and that alcoholics are unable by themselves to stop drinking.[834] This concept of "powerlessness in the face of alcohol" is the basic ideology of Alcoholics Anonymous (AA), which, since its founding by "Bill W" and "Dr. Bob" in Akron, Ohio in 1935, has grown to more than 700,000 members in the United States and a million and a half worldwide.[835] The "success rate" of AA is difficult to estimate because many drop out early and medical records are not kept.[836,837] Abstinence at 1 year is probably between 26% and 50%.[805] Of 100 alcoholics who first received inpatient counseling and then attended AA meetings, 8-year follow-up revealed that 29% had achieved at least 3 years of stable abstinence, 24% had intermittent drinking, and 47% had continuing serious alcoholism.[110] Ancillary self-help organizations are Al-Anon for families of alcoholics and Alateen for teenage children of alcoholics.

Acupuncture

In a randomized prospective trial severe recidivist alcoholics received acupuncture using either specific or nonspecific insertion points. "Treated" patients were more likely to complete the course of therapy.[838] This study has been criticized for faulty design; moreover, the specificity of acupuncture insertion points in any condition is doubtful.[839,840]

Conclusion

Although the need for hospitalization has been questioned,[841,842] "current standard treatment" of alcoholism consists of detoxification followed by several weeks of inpatient rehabilitation, including psychotherapy and behavior modification.[781,805] Referral is then made to an outpatient facility, often AA. Pharmacotherapy is given cautiously for associated psychiatric problems. In 1984, more than 540,000 Americans were in treatment programs for alcoholism or combined alcohol and other drug dependency. Eight percent were inpatients, 10% were in residential facilities, and 82% were active outpatients.[805]

Especially controversial is whether an alcoholic can ever safely resume "social drinking." Some believe that with "successful life adjustment" alcoholics can drink again.[843] Needless to say, many disagree, and there is considerable evidence that stable moderate drinking is rarely accomplished in physically dependent alcoholics.[110,844–846] What is generally recognized is that treatment must be individualized for each patient and that trial and error must be anticipated. For psychotherapy and drug

treatment, evidence of benefit is sparse; for more unorthodox measures, which include not only acupuncture, but also such radical interventions as stereotactic cingulotomy[847] or hypothalamotomy,[848] meaningful data are nonexistent.

Relevant but beyond the bounds of this discussion are preventive measures, including taxation and price manipulation, advertising restrictions and counteradvertising, depiction in the public media, education programs, establishment of legal drinking ages, and laws on drunken driving. As with other drugs, workplace screening programs raise serious ethical questions.[849] The failure of Prohibition does not exonerate society's role in establishing responsible public policies related to ethanol abuse. During 1987 there were more than five times as many American alcoholics as cocaine or crack users and 30 times as many as heroin users; two-thirds of Americans seeking treatment in substance abuse programs report alcoholism as their primary problem. Yet in 1990 100% of a proposed $100 million increase for federal block-grant funding of state substance abuse programs was mandated for users of illegal drugs.[850]

References

1. Devor EJ, Cloninger CR. Genetics of alcoholism. Ann Rev Genet 1989; 23:19.
2. Charness ME, Simon RP, Greenberg DA. Ethanol and the nervous system. N Engl J Med 1989; 321:442.
3. Seventh Special Report to the US Congress on Alcohol and Health. Rockville, MD: DHHS, Publication No (ADM)-281-88-0002NIAAA, 1990.
4. Alcohol-related mortality and years of potential life lost—United States, 1987. MMWR 1990; 39:173.
5. Samson HH, Harris RA. Neurobiology of alcohol abuse. Trends Pharmacol Sci 1992; 13:206.
6. Williams GD, Stinson FS, Parker DA, et al. Demographic trends, alcohol abuse and alcoholism, 1985–1995. Alcohol Health Res World 1987; 11:80.
7. Buchsbaum DG, Buchanan RG, Centor RM, et al. Screening for alcohol abuse using CAGE scores and likelihood ratios. Ann Intern Med 1991; 115:774.
8. Yersin B, Trisconi Y, Paccaud F, et al. Accuracy of the Michigan Alcoholism Screening Test for screening of alcoholism in patients of a medical department. Arch Intern Med 1989; 149:2071.
9. Hernandez-Munoz R, Baraona E, Blackberg I, Lieber CS. Characterization of the increased binding of acetaldehyde to red blood cells in alcoholics. Alcoholism 1989; 13:654.
10. Schellenberg F, Benard JY, Le Goff AM, et al. Evaluation of carbohydrate-deficient transferrin compared with TF index and other markers of alcohol use. Alcoholism 1989; 13:605.
11. Lykouras E, Markianos M, Moussas G. Platelet monoamine oxidase, plasma dopamine beta hydroxy-

lase activity, dementia and family history of alcoholism in chronic alcoholics. Acta Psychiatr Scand 1989; 80:487.

12. Johnson JH, Crider BP. Increase in Na,K-ATPase activity of erythrocytes and skeletal muscle after chronic ethanol consumption: evidence for reduced efficiency of the enzyme. Proc Natl Acad Sci USA 1989; 86:7857.

13. Roine RP, Nykanen I, Ylikahri R, et al. Effects of alcohol on blood dolichol concentration. Alcoholism 1989; 13:519.

14. Karkkainen P, Poikolainen K, Salaspuro M. Serum beta-hexosaminidase as a marker of heavy drinking. Alcoholism 1990; 14:187.

15. Roine RP, Eriksson CJ, Ylikahri R, et al. Methanol as a marker of alcohol abuse. Alcoholism 1989; 13:172.

16. Glass IB, Chalmers R, Bartlett B, Littleton J. Increased plasma carnitine in severe alcohol dependence. Br J Addict 1989; 84:689.

17. Crabb DW. Biological markers for increased risk of alcoholism and for quantitation of alcohol consumption. J Clin Invest 1990; 85:311.

18. Diaz F, Cadaveira F, Grau C. Short- and middle-latency auditory-evoked potentials in abstinent chronic alcoholics: preliminary findings. Electroencephalogr Clin Neurophysiol 1990; 77:145.

19. Tabakoff B, Hoffman PL, Lee JM, et al. Differences in platelet enzyme activity between alcoholics and nonalcoholics. N Engl J Med 1988; 318:134.

20. Mendelson JH, Mello NK. Diagnostic criteria for alcoholism and alcohol abuse. In: Mendelson JH, Mello NK. The Diagnosis of Alcoholism. New York: McGraw-Hill, 1979:1.

21. American Psychiatric Association, Committee on Nomenclature and Statistics: Diagnostic and Statistical Manual of Mental Disorders, 3rd Edition, Revised (DSM-3R). Washington, DC: American Psychiatric Association, 1987.

22. Criteria Committee, National Council on Alcoholism: Criteria for the diagnosis of alcoholism. Ann Intern Med 1972; 77:249.

23. Miller W, Mombour W, Mettelhammer J. A systematic evaluation of the DSM-III-R criteria for alcohol dependence. Compr Psychiatry 1989; 30:403.

24. Alcohol-related disease impact—Wisconsin 1988. MMWR 1990; 39:178.

25. Ashley MJ, Olin JS, LeRiche WH. Skid row alcoholism: a distinct sociomedical entity. Arch Intern Med 1976; 136:272.

26. Hughes PH, Brandenburg N, Baldwin DC, et al. Prevalence of substance use among US physicians. JAMA 1992; 267:2333.

27. McClusker J, Cherubin CE, Zimberg S. Prevalence of alcoholism in general municipal hospital population. NY State J Med 1971; 71:751.

28. Moore RD, Bone LR, Geller G, et al. Prevalence, detection, and treatment of alcoholism in hospitalized patients. JAMA 1989; 261:403.

29. DiFranza JR, Guerrera MP. Alcoholism and smoking. J Stud Alcohol 1990; 51:130.

30. Apparent per capita ethanol consumption—United States, 1977–1986. MMWR 1989; 38:800.

31. Mezey E. Ethanol metabolism and ethanol-drug interactions. Biochem Pharmacol 1976; 25:869.

32. Lieber CS. Metabolism of ethanol. In: Lieber CS, ed. Metabolic Aspects of Alcoholism. Baltimore: University Park Press, 1977:1.

33. Cavey CV. Alcoholism—a biological approach. Trends Neurosci 1979; 2:23.

34. Raskin NH, Sokoloff L. Brain alcohol dehydrogenase. Science 1968; 162:131.

35. Mendelson JH, Mello NK. Behavioral and biochemical interrelations in alcoholism. Annu Rev Med 1976; 27:321.

36. Griezerstein HB. Tolerance to ethanol: effect of congeners present in bourbon. Psychopharmacology 1977; 53:201.

37. Lieber CS, DiCarli LM. Metabolic effects of alcohol on the liver. In: Lieber CS, ed. Metabolic Aspects of Alcoholism. Baltimore: University Park Press, 1977:31.

38. Lieber CS. Biochemical and molecular basis of alcohol-induced injury to liver and other tissues. N Engl J Med 1988; 319:1639.

39. Suter PM, Schutz Y, Jequier E. The effect of ethanol on fat storage in healthy subjects. N Engl J Med 1992; 326:983.

40. Brown ZW, Amit Z, Rockman GE. Intraventricular self-administration of acetaldehyde, but not ethanol, in naive laboratory rats. Psychopharmacology 1979; 64:271–276.

41. Ortiz A, Griffiths PJ, Littleton JM. A comparison of the effects of chronic administration of ethanol and acetaldehyde to mice: evidence for a role of acetaldehyde in ethanol dependence. J Pharm Pharmacol 1974; 26:249.

42. Korsten MA, Matsuzaki S, Feinman L, et al. High blood acetaldehyde levels after ethanol administration. Differences between alcoholic and non-alcoholic subjects. N Engl J Med 1975; 292:386.

43. Rahwan RG. Toxic effects of ethanol: possible role of acetaldehyde, tetrahydroisoquinolines, and tetrahydro-beta-carbolines. Toxicol Appl Pharmacol 1975; 34:3.

44. Myers RD. Isoquinolines, beta-carbolines and alcohol drinking: involvement of opioid and dopminergic mechanisms. Experientia 1989; 45:436.

45. Tuomisto L, Airaksinen MM, Peura P, Eriksson CJP. Alcohol drinking in the rat: increases following intracerebroventricular treatment with tetrahydro-beta-carbolines. Pharmacol Biochem Behav 1982; 17:831.

46. Myers RD, Melchior CL. Alcohol drinking: abnormal intake caused by tetrahydropapaveroline in the brain. Science 1977; 196:554.

47. Kalant H. Direct effects of ethanol on the nervous system. Fed Proc 1975; 34:1930.

48. Hyvarinen J, Laakso M, Roine R, et al. Effect of ethanol on neuronal activity in the parietal association cortex of alert monkeys. Brain 1978; 101:701.

49. Kalant H, Woo N. Electrophysiological effects of ethanol on the nervous system. Pharmacol Ther 1981; 14:431.

50. Pohorecky LA. Biphasic action of alcohol. Biol Behav Res 1978; 1:231.

51. Chin JH, Goldstein DB. Drug tolerance in biomembranes. A spin label study of the effects of ethanol. Science 1977; 196:684.

52. Goldstein DB. Effect of alcohol on cellular membranes. Ann Emerg Med 1986; 15:1013.

53. Wood WG, Schroeder F. Membrane effects of ethanol: bulk lipid versus lipid domains. Life Sci 1988; 43:467.

54. Alling C. The effects of alcohol on lipids in neuronal membranes. In: Porter RJ, Mattson RH, Cramer JA, et al., eds. Alcohol and Seizures. Basic Mechanisms and Clinical Concepts. Philadelphia: FA Davis, 1990:44.

55. Harris RA, Baxter DM, Mitchell MA, et al. Physical properties and lipid composition of brain membranes from ethanol tolerant-dependent mice. Mol Pharmacol 1984; 25:401.

56. Pohorecky LA, Brick J. Pharmacology of ethanol. Pharmacol Ther 1988; 36:335.

57. Rangaraj N, Kalant H, Beauge F. Alpha-1-adrenergic receptor involvement in norepinephrine-ethanol inhibition of rat brain Na-K-ATPase and in ethanol tolerance. Can J Physiol Pharmacol 1985; 63:1075.

58. Hoffman PL, Tabakoff B. Ethanol and guanine nucleotide binding proteins: a selective interaction. FASEB J 1990; 4:2612.

59. Adams MA, Hirst M. The ethanol withdrawal syndrome in the rat: effect of drug treatment on adrenal gland and urinary catecholamines. Subst Alc Actions Misuse 1982; 3:287.

60. Holman RB, Snape BM. Effects of ethanol in vitro and in vivo on the release of endogenous catecholamines from specific regions of rat brain. J Neurochem 1985; 44:357.

61. Imperato A, DiChiara G. Preferential stimulation of dopamine release in the nucleus accumbens of freely moving rats by ethanol. J Pharmacol Exp Ther 1986; 239:219.

62. Sellers EM, Higgins GA, Sobell MB. 5HT and alcohol abuse. Trend Pharmacol Sci 1992; 13:69.

63. Collins AC. Interactions of ethanol and nicotine at the receptor level. Rec Dev Alc 1989; 7:221.

64. Janowsky DS, Risch SC, Irwin M, Schuckit MA. Behavioral hyporeactivity to physostigmine in detoxified primary alcoholics. Am J Psychiatry 1989; 146:538.

65. Frye GD. Gamma-aminobutyric acid (GABA) changes in alcohol withdrawal. In: Porter RJ, Mattson RH, Cramer JA, et al, eds. Alcohol and Seizures. Basic Mechanisms and Clinical Concepts. Philadelphia: FA Davis, 1990:87.

66. Suzdak P, Schwartz R, Skolnick P, Paul SM. Alcohols stimulate gamma-aminobutyric acid receptor-mediated chloride uptake in brain vesicles. Correlation with intoxication potency. Brain Res 1988; 444:340.

67. Mehta G, Ticku MK. Ethanol potentiation of GABAergic transmission in cultured spinal cord neurons involves gamma-aminobutyric acid-gated chloride channels. J Pharmacol Exp Ther 1988; 246:558.

68. Ticku M, Kulkarni S. Molecular interations of ethanol with GABAergic system and potential of RO15-4513 as an ethanol antagonist. Pharmacol Biochem Behav 1988; 30:501.

69. Morrow AL, Suzdak PD, Paul SM. Ethanol and the GABA/benzodiazepine receptor complex. In: Porter RJ, Mattson RH, Cramer JA, et al, eds. Alcohol and Seizures. Basic Mechanisms and Clinical Concepts. Philadelphia: FA Davis, 1990:102.

70. Mhatre M, Ticku MK. Chronic ethanol treatment selectively increases the binding of inverse agonists for benzodiazepine binding sites in cultured spinal cord neurons. J Pharmacol Exp Ther 1989; 251:164.

71. Morrow A, Suzdak PD, Karanian JW, Paul SM. Chronic ethanol administration alters gamma-aminobutyric acid, pentobarbital and ethanol-mediated 36-Cl uptake in cerebrocortical synaptoneurosomes. J Pharmacol Exp Ther 1988; 246:158.

72. Wafford KA, Burnett DM, Leidenheimer NJ, et al. Ethanol sensitivity of the GABA-A receptor expressed in Xenopus oocytes requires 8 amino acids contained in the gamma 2L subunit. Neuron 1991; 7:27.

73. Liljequist S, Engel J. Effects of GABAergic agonists and antagonists on various ethanol-induced behavioral changes. Psychopharmacology 1982; 78:71.

74. Frye GD, McCown TJ, Breese GR. Differential sensitivity of ethanol withdrawal signs in the rat to gamma-aminobutyric acid (GABA) mimetics: blockade of audiogenic seizures but not forelimb tremors. J Pharmacol Exp Ther 1983; 226:720.

75. Suzdak PD, Glowa JR, Crawley JN, et al. A selective imidazobenzodiazepine antagonist of ethanol in the rat. Science 1986; 234:1243.

76. Lister RG, Nutt DJ. Is RO15-4513 a specific alcohol antagonist? Trends Neurosci 1987; 10:223.

77. Britton KT, Ehlers CL, Koob GF. Is ethanol antagonist RO15-4513 selective for ethanol? Science 1988; 239:648.

78. Liste RG, Karanian JW. RO15-4513 induces seizures in DBA/2 mice undergoing ethanol withdrawal. Alcohol 1987; 4:409.

79. Lister RG, Nutt DJ. Interactions of the imidazobenzodiazepine RO15-4513 with convulsants. Br J Pharmacol 1988; 93:210.

80. Nutt DJ, Lister RG. The effect of the imidazobenzodiazepine RO15-4513 on the anticonvulsant effect of diazepam, sodium pentobarbital and ethanol. Brain Res 1987; 413:193.

81. Carlen P, Rougier-Naquet I, Reynolds JN. Alterations of neuronal calcium and potassium currents during alcohol administration and withdrawal. In: Porter RJ, Mattson RH, Cramer JA, et al, eds. Alcohol and Seizures. Basic Mechanisms and Clinical Concepts. Philadelphia: FA Davis, 1990:68.

82. Gandhi CR, Ross DH. Influence of ethanol on calcium, inositol phospholipids and intracellular signaling mechanisms. Experientia 1989; 45:407.

83. Greenberg DA, Messing RO, Marks SS, Carpenter CL. Calcium channel changes during alcohol withdrawal.

In: Porter RJ, Mattson RH, Cramer JA, et al, eds. Alcohol and Seizures. Basic Mechanisms and Clinical Concepts. Philadelphia: FA Davis, 1990:60.

84. Kril JJ, Gundlach AL, Dodd PR, et al. Cortical dihydropyridine binding sites are unaltered in human alcoholic brain. Ann Neurol 1989; 26:395.

85. Little HJ, Dolin SJ, Halsey MJ. Calcium channel antagonists decrease the ethanol withdrawal syndrome. Life Sci 1986; 39:2059.

86. Diamond I, Mochley-Rosen D, Gordon AS. Reduced adenosine receptor activation in alcoholism. Implications for alcohol withdrawal seizures. In: Porter RJ, Mattson RH, Cramer JA, et al, eds. Alcohol and Seizures. Basic Mechanisms and Clinical Concepts. Philadelphia: FA Davis, 1990:79.

87. Seizinger BR, Bovermann K, Hollt V, Herz A. Enhanced activity of the beta-endorphinergic system in the anterior and neurointermediate lobe of the rat pituitary after chronic treatment with ethanol liquid diet. J Pharmacol Exp Ther 1984; 230:455.

88. Seizinger BR, Bovermann K, Maysinga D, et al. Differential effects of acute and chronic ethanol treatment on particular opioid peptide systems in discrete regions of rat brain and pituitary. Pharmacol Biochem Behav 1983; 18(suppl 1):361.

89. Charness ME. Ethanol and opioid receptor signaling. Experientia 1989; 45:418.

90. Gianoulakis C. The effect of ethanol on the biosynthesis and regulation of opioid peptides. Experientia 1989; 45:428.

91. Lovinger DM, White G, Weight FF. NMDA receptor-mediated synaptic excitation selectively inhibited by ethanol in hippocampal slice from adult rat. J Neurosci 1990; 10:1372.

92. Lustig HS, Chan J, Greenberg DA. Ethanol inhibits excitotoxicity in cerebral cortical cultures. Neurosci Lett 1992; 135:259.

93. Goodwin FK, Gause EM. From the Alcohol, Drug Abuse, and Mental Health Administration. JAMA 1990; 263:352.

94. Valverius P, Hoffman PL, Tabakoff B. Effect of ethanol on mouse cerebral cortical beta-adrenergic receptors. Mol Pharmacol 1987; 32:217.

95. Harris RA, Bruno P. Membrane disordering by anesthetic drugs: relationship to synaptosomal sodium and calcium fluxes. J Neurochem 1985; 44:1274.

96. Armbrecht HJ, Wood WG, Wise RW, et al. Ethanol-induced disordering of membranes from different age groups of C57BL/CNNIA mice. J Pharmacol Exp Ther 1983; 226:387.

97. Huidobro-Toro P, Bleck V, Allan AM, Harris RA. Neurochemical actions of anesthetic drugs on the gamma-aminobutyric acid receptor-chloride channel complex. J Pharmacol Exp Ther 1987; 242:963.

98. Cloninger CR. Neurogenetic adaptive mechanisms in alcoholism. Science 1987; 236:410.

99. Li T-K, Bosron WF. Genetic variability of enzymes of alcohol metabolism in human beings. Ann Emerg Med 1986; 15:997.

100. Bosron WF, Lumeng L, Li TK. Genetic polymorphism of enzymes of alcohol metabolism and susceptibility to alcoholic liver disease. Mol Aspects Med 1988; 10:147.

101. Agarwal DP, Goedde HW. Human aldehyde dehydrogenases: their role in alcoholism. Alcohol 1989; 6:517.

102. Goedde HW, Agarwal DP. Pharmacogenetics of aldehyde dehydrogenase (ALDH). Pharmacol Ther 1990; 45:345.

103. Mullan M. Alcoholism and the "new genetics." Br J Addict 1989; 84:1433.

104. Wallace J. The new disease model of alcoholism. West J Med 1990; 152:502.

105. Schukit M. Genetic aspects of alcoholism. Ann Emerg Med 1986; 15:991.

106. Pickens RW, Svikis DS, McGue M, et al. Heterogeneity in the inheritance of alcoholism. Arch Gen Psychiatry 1991; 48:19.

107. Cloninger CR. Genetic and environmental factors in the development of alcoholism. J Psychiatric Treat Eval 1983; 5:487.

108. Buydens-Branchey L, Branchey MH, Noumair D. Age of alcoholism onset. 1. Relationship to psychopathology. Arch Gen Psychiatry 1989; 46:225.

109. Schukit MA, Irwin M. An analysis of the clinical relevance of type 1 and type 2 alcoholics. Br J Addict 1989; 84:869.

110. Vaillant GE. The Natural History of Alcoholism. Cambridge, MA: Harvard University Press, 1983.

111. McGue M, Pickens RW, Svikis DS. Sex and age effects on the inheritance of alcohol problems: a twin study. J Abnorm Psychol 1992; 101:3.

112. Irwin M, Schukit M, Smith TL. Clinical importance of age of onset in type 1 and type 2 primary alcoholics. Arch Gen Psychiatry 1990; 47:320.

113. Li TK, Lumeng L, McBride WJ, et al. Rodent lines selected for factors affecting alcohol consumption. Alcohol 1987; (suppl 1):91.

114. Phillips TJ, Feller DJ, Crabbe JC. Selected mouse lines, alcohol and behavior. Experientia 1989; 45:805.

115. Wafford KA, Burnett DM, Dunwiddie TV, Harris RA. Genetic differences in the ethanol sensitivity of GABA-A receptors expressed in xenopus oocytes. Science 1990; 249:291.

116. McIntyre TD, Trullas R, Skonick P. Differences in biophysical properties of the benzodiazepine/gamma-aminobutyric acid receptor chloride channel complex in the long-sleep and short-sleep mouse lines. J Neurochem 1988; 51:642.

117. Goldstein DB, Chin JH, Lyon RC. Ethanol disordering of spin-labelled mouse brain membranes: correlation with genetically determined ethanol sensitivity of mice. Proc Natl Acad Sci USA 1982; 79:4231.

118. Wong DT, Threlkeld PG, Lumeng L, Li T-K. Higher density of serotonin-1A receptors in the hippocampus and cerebral cortex of alcohol-preferring rats. Life Sci 1990; 46:231.

119. McBride WJ, Murphy JM, Lumeng L, Li T-K. Serotonin and ethanol preference. Rec Dev Alcohol 1989; 7:187.

120. Sinclair JD, Le AD, Kiianmaa K. The AA and ANA rat lines, selected for differences in voluntary alcohol consumption. Experientia 1989; 45:798.

121. Buck KJ, Hahner L, Sikela J, Harris RA. Chronic ethanol treatment alters brain levels of gamma-aminobutyric acid-A receptor subunit in RNAs: relationship to genetic differences in ethanol withdrawal seizure severity. J Neurochem 1991; 57:1452.

122. Blum K, Briggs AH, Wallace JE, et al. Regional brain [Met]-enkephalin in alcohol-preferring and non-alcohol preferring inbred strains of mice. Experentia 1986; 43:408.

123. Gianoulakis C, Gupta A. Inbred strains of mice with variable sensitivity to ethanol exhibit differences in the content and processing of beta-endorphin. Life Sci 1986; 39:2315.

124. Holden C. Probing the complex genetics of alcoholism. Science 1991; 251:163.

125. Hill SY, Steinhauer S, Park J, Zubin J. Event-related potential characteristics in children of alcoholics from high density families. Alcoholism 1990; 14:6.

126. Ehlers CL, Schukit MA. EEG fast frequency activity in the sons of alcoholics. Biol Psychiatry 1990; 27:631.

127. Sullivan JL, Baenziger JC, Wagner DL, Rauscher FP. Platelet MAO in subtypes of alcoholism. Biol Psychiatry 1990; 27:911.

128. Gordis E, Tabakokff B, Goldman D, Berg K. Finding the gene(s) for alcoholism. JAMA 1990; 263:2094.

129. Tabakoff B, Hoffman PL, Lee JM, et al. Differences in platelet enzyme activity between alcoholics and non-alcoholics. N Engl J Med 1988; 318:134.

130. Gianoulakis C, Beliveau D, Angelogianni P, et al. Different pituitary beta-endorphin and adrenal cortical response to ethanol in individuals with high and low risk for future development of alcoholism. Life Sci 1989; 45:1097.

131. Moss HB, Yao J, Burns M, et al. Plasma GABA-like activity in response to ethanol challenge in men at high risk for alcoholism. Biol Psychiatry 1990; 27:617.

132. Moss HB, Guthrie S, Linnoila M. Enhanced thyrotropin response to thyrotropin releasing hormone in boys at risk for development of alcoholism. Arch Gen Psychiatry 1986; 43:1137.

133. Hill SY, Aston C, Rabin B. Suggestive evidence of genetic linkage between alcoholism and MNS blood group. Alcoholism 1988; 12:811.

134. Tanna VL, Wilson AF, Winokur G, Elston RC. Possible linkage between alcoholism and esterase-D. J Stud Alcohol 1988; 49:472.

135. Blum K, Noble EP, Sheridan PJ, et al. Allelic association of human dopamine D-2 receptor gene in alcoholism. JAMA 1990; 263:2055.

136. Bolos AM, Dean M, Lucas-Derse S, et al. Population and pedigree studies reveal a lack of association between the dopamine D-2 receptor gene and alcoholism. JAMA 1990; 264:3156.

137. Gelernter J, O'Malley S, Risch N, et al. No association between an allele at the D2 dopamine receptor gene (DRD2) and alcoholism. JAMA 1991; 266: 1801.

138. Parsian A, Todd RD, Devor EJ, et al. Alcoholism and alleles of the human dopamine D2 receptor locus: studies of association and linkage. Arch Gen Psychiatry 1991; 48:655.

139. Comings DE, Comings BG, Muhleman D, et al. The dopamine D2 receptor locus as a modifying gene in neuropsychiatric disorders. JAMA 1991; 266:1793.

140. Cloninger CR. D2 dopamine receptor gene is associated but not linked with alcoholism. JAMA 1991; 266:1833.

141. Noble EP, Blum K, Ritchie T, et al. Allelic association of the D2 dopamine receptor gene with receptor binding characteristics in alcoholism. Arch Gen Psychiatry 1991; 48:648.

142. Rall TW. Hypnotics and sedatives; ethanol. In: Gilman AG, Rall TW, Nies As, Taylor P, eds. The Pharmacological Basics of Therapeutics, ed 8. New York: Pergamon Press, 1990:345.

143. Frezza M, diPadova C, Pozzato G, et al. High blood alcohol levels in women. The role of decreased alcohol dehydrogenase activity and first-pass metabolism. N Engl J Med 1990; 322:95.

144. Schenker S, Speeg KV. The risk of alcohol intake in men and women. N Engl J Med 1990; 322:127.

145. Tabakoff B, Cornell N, Hoffman PL. Alcohol tolerance. Ann Emerg Med 1986; 15:1005.

146. Holford NHG. Clinical pharmacokinetics of ethanol. Clin Pharmacokinetics 1987; 13:273.

147. Roine R, Gentry T, Hernandez-Munoz R, et al. Aspirin increases blood alcohol concentrations in humans after ingestion of ethanol. JAMA 1990; 264:2406.

148. Minion GE, Slovis CM, Boutiette L. Severe alcohol intoxication: a study of 204 consecutive patients. J Toxicol Clin Toxicol 1989; 27:375.

149. Behnke RH. Recognition and management of alcohol withdrawal syndrome. Hosp Pract 1976; 11:79.

150. Sellers EM, Kalant HL. Alcohol intoxication and withdrawal. N Engl J Med 1976; 294:757.

151. Davis AR, Lipson AH. Central nervous system depression and high blood ethanol levels. Lancet 1986; 1:566.

152. Redmond AD. Central nervous system depression and high blood ethanol levels. Lancet 1986; 1:805.

153. Johnson RA, Noll EC, Rodney WM. Survival after a serum ethanol concentration of 1 1/2%. Lancet 1982; 2:1394.

154. AMA Council on Scientific Affairs: Alcohol and the driver. JAMA 1986; 255:522.

155. Isbell H, Fraser HF, Wikler A. An experimental study of the etiology of "rum fits" and delirium tremens. QJ Stud Alcohol 1955; 16:1.

156. Kalant H. Direct effects of ethanol on the nervous system. Fed Proc 1975; 34:1930.

157. Roth T, Roehrs T, Zorick F, Conway W. Pharmacological effects of sedative-hypnotics, narcotic analgesics, and alcohol during sleep. Med Clin North Am 1985; 69:1281.

158. Vitiello MV, Prinz PN, Personius JP, et al. Relationship of alcohol abuse history to nighttime hypoxemia in abstaining chronic alcoholic men. J Stud Alcohol 1990; 51:29.

159. Woodhouse P, Keatings WP, Coleshaw SR. Factors associated with hypothermia in patients admitted to a group of inner hospitals. Lancet 1989; 2:1201.

160. Weyman AE, Greenbaum DM, Grace WJ. Accidental hypothermia in an alcoholic population. Am J Med 1974; 56:13.

161. Victor M. Neurologic disorders due to alcoholism and malnutrition. In: Joynt RJ, ed. Clinical Neurology. Philadelphia: JB Lippincott, Ch 61, 1986:1.

162. Sweeney DF. Alcoholic blackouts: legal implications. J Subst Abuse Treatment 1990; 7:155.

163. Parker ES. Alcohol and cognition. Psychopharmacol Bull 1984; 20:494.

164. Martin PR, Adinoff B, Eckardt MJ, et al. Effective pharmacotherapy of alcoholic amnestic disorder with fluvoxamine. Arch Gen Psychiatry 1989; 46:617.

165. Editorial. Alcohol and atrial fibrillation. Lancet 1985; 1:1374.

166. Loeb JN. The hyperosmolar state. N Engl J Med 1974; 290:1184.

167. Harrow AS. Beer potomania syndrome in an alcoholic. Va Med 1989; 116:270.

168. Alkana RL, Parker ES, Cohen HB, et al. Reversal of ethanol intoxication in humans: an assessment of the efficacy of propranolol. Psychopharmacology 1976; 51:29.

169. Alkana RL, Parker ES, Cohen HB, et al. Reversal of ethanol intoxication in humans: an assessment of the efficacy of L-DOPA, aminophylline, and ephedrine. Psychopharmacology 1977; 55:203.

170. Alkana RL, Willingham TA, Cohen HB, et al. Apomorphine and amantadine: interaction with ethanol in humans. Fed Proc 1976; 36:331.

171. Guerin JM, Friedberg G. Naloxone and ethanol intoxication. Ann Intern Med 1982; 97:932.

172. Lyon LJ, Antony J. Reversal of alcohol coma by naloxone. Ann Intern Med 1982; 96:464.

173. Jefferys DB, Flanagan RF, Volans GN. Reversal of ethanol induced coma with naloxone. Lancet 1980; 1:308.

174. Mattila MJ, Nuotto E, Seppala T. Naloxone is not an effective antagonist of ethanol. Lancet 1981; 1:775.

175. Ducobu J. Naloxone and alcohol intoxication. Ann Intern Med 1984; 100:617.

176. Lignian H, Fontaine J, Askenasi R. Naloxone and alcoholic intoxication. Ann Intern Med 1982; 97:455.

177. Gupta RC, Kofoed J. Toxicological statistics for barbiturates, other sedatives, and tranquilizers in Ontario: a 10-year survey. Can Med Assoc J 1966; 94:863.

178. Gessner PK. Effect of trichloroethanol and of chloral hydrate on the in vivo disappearance of ethanol in mice. Arch Int Pharmacodyn Ther 1973; 202:392.

179. Alcohol-drug interactions. FDA Drug Bull 1979; 9:10.

180. Rada RT, Kellner R, Buchanan JG. Chlordiazepoxide and alcohol: a fatal overdose. J Forens Sci 1975; 20:544.

181. Busto U, Simpkins J, Sellers EM, et al. Objective determination of benzodiazepine use and abuse in alcoholics. Br J Addict 1983; 78:429.

182. Edwards R. Anesthesia and alcohol. BMJ 1985; 291:423.

183. Seixas FA. Alcohol and its drug interactions. Ann Intern Med 1975; 83:86.

184. Interaction of alcohol with drugs. Med Lett 1977; 19:47.

185. Yesavage JA, Leirer VO. Hangover effects on aircraft pilots 14 hours after alcohol ingestion: a preliminary report. Am J Psychiatry 1986; 143:1546.

186. Victor M, Adams RD. The effect of alcohol on the nervous system. Res Publ Assoc Res Nerv Ment Dis 1953; 32:526.

187. Neiman J, Lang AE, Fornazarri L, Carlen PL. Movement disorders in alcoholism. A review. Neurology 1990; 40:741.

188. Victor M, Hope JM. The phenomenon of auditory hallucinations in chronic alcoholism. J Nerv Ment Dis 1958; 126:451.

189. Surawicz FG. Alcoholic hallucinosis: a missed diagnosis. Can J Psychiatry 1980; 25:57.

190. Schwarz BE, Brust JCM. Anton's syndrome accompanying withdrawal hallucinosis in a blind alcoholic. Neurology 1984; 34:969.

191. Chamorro AA, Sacco RL, Ciecierski K, et al. Visual hemineglect and hemihallucinations in a patient with a subcortical infarction. Neurology 1990; 40:1463.

192. Schukit MA, Winokur G. Alcoholic hallucinosis and schizophrenia. A negative study. Br J Psychiatry 1971; 119:549.

193. Shen WW. Extrapyramidal symptoms associated with alcohol withdrawal. Biol Psychiatry 1984; 19:1037.

194. Shandling M, Carlen PL, Lang AE. Parkinsonism in alcohol withdrawal: a follow-up study. Movement Disord 1990; 5:36.

195. Carlen PL, Lee MA, Jacob MA, Livshits O. Parkinsonism provoked by alcoholism. Ann Neurol 1981; 9:84.

196. Fornazarri L, Carlen PL. Transient chorieform dyskinesias during alcohol withdrawal. Can J Neurol Sci 1982; 9:89.

197. Balldin J, Alling C, Gottfries CG, et al. Changes in dopamine receptor sensitivity in humans after heavy alcohol intake. Psychopharmacology 1985; 86:142.

198. Olivera AA, Kiefer MW, Manley NK. Tardive dyskinesia in psychiatric patients with substance use disorders. Am J Drug Alcohol Abuse 1990; 16:57.

199. George DT, Nutt DJ, Dwyer BA, Linnoila M. Alcoholism and panic disorder: is the comorbidity more than coincidence? Acta Psychiatr Scand 1990; 81:97.

200. Heckmatt J, Shaikh AA, Swash M, Scott DF. Seizure induction by alcohol in patients with epilepsy; experience in two hospital clinics. J R Soc Med 1990; 83:6.

201. Chan AWK. Alcoholism and epilepsy. Epilepsia 1985; 26:223.

202. Simon RP. Alcohol and siezures. N Engl J Med 1988; 319:715.

203. Hoppener RJ, Kuyer A, van der Lugt PJM. Epilepsy and alcohol: the influence of social alcohol intake on seizures and treatment in epilepsy. Epilepsia 1983; 24:459.

203a. Earnest MP. Seizures. In Brust JCM ed: Neurologic Complications of Drug and Alcohol Abuse. Neurol Clin 1993, in press.

204. Victor M, Brausch CC. The role of abstinence in the genesis of alcoholic epilepsy. Epilepsia 1967; 8:1.

205. Earnest MP, Feldman H, Marx JA, et al. Alcohol-related first seizures: the role of abstinence. Neurology 1989; 39(suppl):147.

206. Earnest MP, Yarnell PR. Seizure admissions to a city hospital: the role of alcohol. Epilepsia 1976; 17:387.

207. Pilke A, Partinen M, Kovanen J. Status epilepticus and alcohol abuse: analysis of 82 status epilepticus admissions. Acta Neurol Scand 1984; 70:443.

208. Lowenstein DH, Alldredge BK. Status epilepticus at an urban public hospital in the 1980s. Neurology 1993; 43:483.

209. Whitfield CL, Thompson G, Lamb A, et al. Detoxification of 1024 alcoholic patients without psychoactive drugs. JAMA 1978; 239:1409.

210. Ng SKC, Hauser WA, Brust JCM, Susser M. Alcohol consumption and withdrawal in new-onset seizures. N Engl J Med 1988; 319:666.

211. Goldstein DB. The alcohol withdrawal syndrome. A view from the laboratory. Rec Dev Alcohol 1986; 4:213.

212. Hauser WA, Ng SKC, Brust JCM. Alcohol, seizures, and epilepsy. Epilepsia 1988; 29(suppl 2):S66.

213. Hillbom ME. Occurrence of cerebral seizures provoked by alcohol abuse. Epilepsia 1980; 21:459.

214. Ng SKC, Hauser WA, Brust JCM, Susser M. Alcohol consumption and withdrawal in new onset seizures. N Engl J Med 1989; 320:597.

215. Meyer-Wahl JG, Braun J. Epileptic seizures and cerebral atrophy in alcoholics. J Neurol 1982; 228:17.

216. Gonzalez LP, Czachura JF, Brewer KW. Spontaneous versus elicited seizures following ethanol withdrawal: differential time course. Alcohol 1989; 6:481.

217. Gorelick DA, Wilkins JN. Special aspects of human alcohol withdrawal. Rec Dev Alcohol 1986; 4:283.

218. Chu N-S. Periodic lateralized epileptiform discharges with pre-existing focal brain lesion. Role of alcohol withdrawal and anoxic encephalopathy. Arch Neurol 1980; 37:551.

219. Maier DM, Pohorecky LA. The effect of repeated withdrawal episodes on subsequent withdrawal severity in ethanol treated rats. Drug Alcohol Depend 1989; 23:103.

220. Brown ME, Anton RF, Malcolm R, Ballenger JC. Alcohol detoxification and withdrawal seizures: clinical support for a kindling hypothesis. Biol Psychiatry 1988; 23:507.

221. Lechtenberg R, Worner TM. Seizure risk with recurrent alcohol detoxification. Arch Neurol 1990; 47:535.

222. Feussner JR, Linfors EW, Blessing CL, Starmer CF. Computed tomography brain scanning in alcohol withdrawal seizures. Ann Intern Med 1981; 94:519.

223. Vossler DG, Browne TR. Rarity of EEG photoparoxysmal and photomyogenic responses following treated alcohol-related seizures. Neurology 1990; 40:723.

224. Fisch BJ, Hauser WA, Brust JCM, et al. The EEG response to diffuse and patterned photic stimulation during acute untreated alcohol withdrawal. Neurology 1989; 39:434.

225. Tavel ME, Davidson W, Baterton TD. A critical analysis of mortality associated with delirium tremens. Am J Med 1961; 242:18.

226. Thompson WL. Management of alcohol withdrawal syndromes. Arch Intern Med 1978; 138:278.

227. Liskow BI, Rinck C, Campbell J, DeSouza C. Alcohol withdrawal in the elderly. J Stud Alcohol 1989; 50:414.

228. Ballenger JC, Post RM. Kindling as a model for alcohol withdrawal syndromes. Br J Psychiatry 1978; 133:1.

229. Moskowitz G, Chalmers TC, Sacks HS, et al. Deficiencies of clinical trials of alcohol withdrawal. Alcoholism 1983; 7:42.

230. Majumdar SK. Chlormethiazole: current status in the treatment of acute ethanol withdrawal syndrome. Drug Alcohol Depend 1991; 27:201.

231. Naranjo CA, Sellers EM. Clinical assessment and pharmacotherapy of the alcohol withdrawal syndrome. Rec Dev Alcohol 1986; 4:265.

232. Whitfield EL, Thompson G, Lamb A, et al. Detoxification of 1024 alcoholic patients without psychoactive drugs. JAMA 1978; 293:1409.

233. Devenyi P, Harrison ML. Prevention of alcohol withdrawal seizures with oral diazepam loading. Can Med Assoc J 1985; 132:798.

234. Guthrie SK. The treatment of alcohol withdrawal. Pharmacotherapy 1989; 9:131.

235. Sellers EM, Naranjo CA, Harrison M, et al. Oral diazepam loading: simplified treatment of alcohol withdrawal. Clin Pharmacol Ther 1983; 34:822.

236. Hayashida M, Alterman AI, McLellan AT, et al. Comparative effectiveness and costs of inpatient and outpatient detoxification of patients with mild-

to-moderate alcohol withdrawal syndrome. N Engl J Med 1989; 320:358.

237. Thomas DW, Freedman DX. Treatment of the alcohol withdrawal syndrome; comparison of promazine and paraldehyde. JAMA 1964; 188:316.

238. Muller DJ. A comparison of three approaches to alcohol withdrawal states. South Med J 1969; 62:495.

239. Sereny G, Kalant H. Comparative clinical evaluation of chlordiazepoxide and promazine in treatment of alcohol withdrawal syndrome. BMJ 1965; 1:92.

240. Goldbert TM, Sanz CJ, Rose HE, et al. Comparative evaluation of treatments of alcohol withdrawal syndromes. JAMA 1967; 201:99.

241. Kaim SC, Kett CJ, Rothfeld B. Treatment of the acute alcohol withdrawal state: a comparison of four drugs. Am J Psychiatry 1969; 125:1640.

242. Kaim SC, Klett CJ. Treatment of delirium tremens: a comparison of four drugs. Q J Stud Alcohol 1972; 33:1065.

243. Sellers EM, Kalant H. Alcohol withdrawal and delirium tremens. In: Pattison EM, Kaufman E, eds. Encyclopedic Handbook of Alcoholism. New York: Gardner Press, 1982:147.

244. Linnoila M, Mefford I, Nutt D, Adinoff B. Alcohol withdrawal and noradrenergic function. Ann Intern Med 1987; 107:875.

245. Zilm DH, Sellers EM, MacLeod SM, et al. Propranolol effect on tremor in alcohol withdrawal. Ann Intern Med 1975; 83:234.

246. Zilm DH, Jacob MS, MacLeod SM, et al. Propranolol and chlordiazepoxide effects on cardiac arrhythmias during alcohol withdrawal. Alcoholism Clin Exp Res 1980; 4:400.

247. Jacob MS, Zilm DH, MacLeod SM, et al. Propranolol-associated confused states during alcohol withdrawal. J Clin Psychopharmacol 1983; 3:185.

248. Wilkins AJ, Jenkins WJ, Steiner JA. Efficacy of clonidine in treatment of alcohol withdrawal state. Psychopharmacology 1983; 81:78.

249. Kraus ML, Gottlieb LD, Horwitz RI, Anscher M. Randomized clinical trial of atenolol in patients with alcohol withdrawal. N Engl J Med 1985; 313:905.

250. Horwitz RI, Gottlieb LD, Kraus ML. The efficacy of atenolol in the outpatient management of the alcohol withdrawal syndrome. Results of a randomized clinical trial. Arch Intern Med 1989; 149:1089.

251. Lerner WD, Fallon HJ. The alcohol withdrawal syndrome. N Engl J Med 1985; 313:951.

252. Cushman P, Sowers JP. Alcohol withdrawal syndrome: clinical and hormonal responses to alpha-2-adrenergic agonist treatment. Alcoholism 1989; 13:361.

253. Cushman P, Forbes R, Lerner W, Stewart M. Alcohol withdrawal syndromes: clinical management with lofexidine. Alcoholism 1985; 9:103.

254. Robinson BJ, Robinson GM, Maling TJ, Johnson RH. Is clonidine useful in the treatment of alcohol withdrawal? Alcoholism 1989; 13:95.

255. Greenburg DA, Carpenter FL, Messing RO. Ethanol-induced component of 45-Ca-2+ uptake in PC 12 cells is sensitive to Ca-2+ channel modulating drugs. Brain Res 1987; 410:143.

256. Little HJ, Dolin SJ, Halsley MJ. Calcium channel antagonists decrease the ethanol withdrawal syndrome. Life Sci 1986; 39:2059.

257. Koppi S, Eberhardt G, Haller R, Koig P. Calcium channel-blocking agent in the treatment of acute alcohol withdrawal—caroverine versus meprobamate in a randomized double-blind study. Neuropsychobiology 1987; 17:49.

258. Grant KA, Valverius P, Hudspith M, Tabakoff B. Ethanol withdrawal seizures and the NMDA receptor complex. Eur J Pharmacol 1990; 176:289.

259. Alldredge BK, Lowenstein DH, Simon RP. A placebo-controlled trial of intravenous diphenylhydantoin for the short-term treatment of alcohol withdrawal seizures. Am J Med 1989; 87:645.

260. Stornebring B. Treatment of alcohol withdrawal seizures with carbamazepine and valproate. In: Porter RJ, Mattson RH, Cramer JA, et al, eds. Alcohol and Seizures. Basic Mechanisms and Clinical Concepts. Philadelphia: FA Davis, 1990:315.

261. Bjorkqvist SE, Isohanni M, Makela P, et al. Ambulant treatment of alcohol withdrawal symptoms with cabamazepine: a formal multicentre double-blind comparison with placebo. Acta Psychiatr Scand 1976; 53:333.

262. Victor M. The role of hypomagnesemia and respiratory alkalosis in the genesis of alcohol-withdrawal symptoms. Ann NY Acad Sci 1973; 215:235.

263. Flink EB. Magnesium deficiency in alcoholism. Alcoholism 1986; 10:590.

264. Meyer JG, Urban K. Electrolyte changes and acid-base balance after alcohol withdrawal, with special reference to rum fits and magnesium deficiency. J Neurol 1977; 215:135.

265. Thompson WL, Johnson AD, Maddrey WL, et al. Diazepam and paraldehyde for treatment of severe delirium tremens. A controlled trial. Ann Intern Med 1975; 82:175.

266. Wernicke C. Lehrbuch der Gehirnkrankheiten fur Aertze und Studierende, Vol 2. Kassel: Theodore Fischer, 1881:229.

267. Victor M, Yakovlev PL. SS Korsakoff's psychic disorder in conjunction with peripheral neuritis. A translation of Korsakoff's original article with brief comments on the author and his contribution to clinical medicine. Neurology 1955; 5:394.

268. Victor M, Adams RD, Collins GH. The Wernicke-Korsakoff Syndrome, ed 2. Philadelphia: FA Davis, 1989.

269. Reuler JB, Girard DE, Cooney TG. Wernicke's encephalopathy. N Engl J Med 1985; 312:1035.

270. Torvik A, Lindboe CF, Rodge S. Brain lesions in alcoholics. A neuropathological study with clinical correlations. J Neurol Sci 1982; 56:233.

271. Wallis WE, Willoughby E, Baker P. Coma in the Wernicke-Korsakoff syndrome. Lancet 1978; 2:400.

272. Harper C. The incidence of Wernicke's encephalopathy in Australia—a neuropathological study of 131 cases. J Neurol Neurosurg Psychiatry 1983; 46:593.

273. Keane JR. The pretectal syndrome. 206 patients. Neurology 1990; 40:684.

274. Luda E. Le signe du bobbing oculaire dans l'encephalopathie de Wernicke. Rev Otoneuroophtalmol 1980; 52:123.

275. Ghez C. Vestibular paresis: a clinical feature of Wernicke's disease. J Neurol Neurosurg Psychiatry 1969; 32:134.

276. Birchfield RL. Postural hypotension in Wernicke's disease. A manifestation of autonomic nervous system involvement. Am J Med 1964; 36:404.

277. Lipton JM, Payne H, Garza HR, Rosenberg RN. Thermolability in Wernicke's encephalopathy. Arch Neurol 1978; 35:750.

278. Shimojyo S, Scheinberg P, Reinmuth O. Cerebral blood flow and metabolism in the Wernicke-Korsakoff syndrome. J Clin Invest 1967; 46:849.

279. McDowell JR, LeBlanc HJ. Computed tomographic findings in Wernicke-Korsakoff syndrome. Arch Neurol 1984; 41:453.

280. Mensing JW, Hoogland PH, Sloof JL. Computed tomography in the diagnosis of Wernicke's encephalopathy: a radiological-neuropathological correlation. Ann Neurol 1984; 16:363.

281. Jacobson RR, Lishman WA. Cortical and diencephalic lesions in Korsakoff's syndrome: a clinical and CT scan study. Psychol Med 1990; 20:63.

282. Charness ME, DeLaPaz RL. Mamillary body atrophy in Wernicke's encephalopathy: antemortem identification using magnetic resonance imaging. Ann Neurol 1987; 22:595.

283. Park SH, Na DL, Lee SB, Myung HJ. MRI findings in Wernicke's encephalopathy: in the acute phase and follow-up. Neurology 1992; 42(suppl 3):278.

284. Victor M, Talland G, Adams RD. Psychological studies of Korsakoff's psychosis. I. General intellectual functions. J Nerv Ment Dis 1959; 128:528.

285. Sanders HI, Warrington EK. Memory for remote events in amnestic patients. Brain 1971; 94:661.

286. Albert MS, Butters N, Levin J. Temporal gradients in the retrograde amnesia of patients with alcoholic Korsakoff's disease. Arch Neurol 1979; 36:211.

287. Sacks O. The Man Who Mistook His Wife for a Hat and Other Clinical Tales. New York: Summit Books, 1985:22.

288. Kopelman MD, Corn TH. Cholinergic "blockade" as a model for cholinergic depletion. A comparison of the memory deficits with those of Alzheimer-type dementia and the alcoholic Korsakoff syndrome. Brain 1988; 111:1079.

289. Rosenblum WI, Feigen I. The hemorrhagic component of Wernicke's encephalopathy. Arch Neurol 1965; 13:627.

290. Torvik A, Lindboe CF, Rogde S. Brain lesions in alcoholics. A neuropathological study with clinical correlations. J Neurol Sci 1982; 56:233.

291. Witt ED. Neuroanatomical consequences of thiamine deficiency: a comparative analysis. Alcohol Alcoholism 1985; 20:201.

292. Arendt T, Bigl V, Arendt A, Tennstedt A. Loss of neurons in the nucleus basalis of Meynert in Alzheimer's disease, paralysis agitans and Korsakoff's disease. Acta Neuropathol (Berlin) 1983; 61:101.

293. Kopelman MD. Remote and autobiographical memory, temporal context memory, and frontal atrophy in Korsakoff and Alzheimer patients. Neuropsychologia 1989; 27:437.

294. Kopelman MD. Frontal dysfunction and memory deficits in the alcoholic Korsakoff syndrome and Alzheimer-type dementia. Brain 1991; 114:117.

295. Becker JT, Furman JMR, Panisset M, Smith C. Characteristics of the memory loss of a patient with Wernicke-Korsakoff's syndrome without alcoholism. Neuropsychologia 1990; 28:171.

296. Swank RL, Prados M. Avian thiamine deficiency. II. Pathologic changes in the brain and cranial nerves (especially the vestibular) and their relation to the clinical behavior. Arch Neurol Psychiat 1942; 47:97.

297. Iwata H. Possible role of thiamine in the nervous system. Trends Pharmacol Sci 1982; 3:171.

298. Hakim AM, Pappius HM. Sequence of metabolic, clinical, and histological events in experimental thiamine deficiency. Ann Neurol 1983; 13:365.

299. Hakim AM. The induction and reversibility of cerebral acidosis in thiamine deficiency. Ann Neurol 1984; 16:673.

300. Phillips GB, Victor M, Adams RD, et al. A study of the nutritional defect in Wernicke's syndrome: the effect of a purified diet, thiamine, and other vitamins on the clinical manifestations. J Clin Invest 1952; 31:859.

301. Dreyfus PM, Victor M. Effects of thiamine deficiency on the central nervous system. Am J Clin Nutrition 1961; 9:414.

302. Mesulam M-M, Van Hoesen GW, Butters N. Clinical manifestations of chronic thiamine deficiency in the rhesus monkey. Neurology 1977; 27:239.

303. Lofland HB, Goodman HO, Clarkson TB, et al. Enzyme studies in thiamine deficient pigeons. J Nutrition 1963; 79:188.

304. Blass JP, Gibson GE. Abnormality of a thiamine-requiring enzyme in patients with Wernicke-Korsakoff syndrome. N Engl J Med 1977; 297:1367.

305. Rosenbaum M, Merritt HH. Korsakoff's syndrome. Clinical study of the alcoholic form, with special regard to prognosis. Arch Neurol Psychiatry 1939; 41:978.

306. Thompson A, Baker H, Leevy CM. Thiamine absorption in alcoholism. Am J Clin Nutrition 1968; 21:537.

307. Harper CG, Giles M, Finlay-Jones R. Clinical signs in the Wernicke-Korsakoff complex: a retrospective analysis of 131 cases diagnosed at necropsy. J Neurol Neurosurg Psychiatry 1986; 49:341.

308. Thompson A, Frank O, Baker H, et al. Thiamine propyl disulfide: absorption and utilization. Ann Intern Med 1971; 74:529.

309. Jeyasingham MD, Pratt OE, Burns A, et al. The activation of red blood cell transketolase in groups of patients especially at risk from thiamine deficiency. Psychol Med 1987; 17:311.

310. Ross J, Birmingham CL. Wernicke's encephalopathy. N Engl J Med 1985; 313:637.

311. Traviesa DC. Magnesium deficiency: a possible cause of thiamine refractoriness in Wernicke-Korsakoff encephalopathy. J Neurol Neurosurg Psychiatry 1974; 37:959.

312. Flink EB. Role of magnesium depletion in Wernicke-Korsakoff syndrome. N Engl J Med 1978; 298:743.

313. Langlais PJ, Mair RG, McEntee WJ. Acute thiamine deficiency in the rat: brain lesions, amino acid changes, and MK-801 pretreatment. Soc Neurosci 1988; 14:774.

314. McEntee WJ, Mair RG. Memory improvement in Korsakoff's disease with fluvoxamine. Arch Gen Psychiatry 1990; 47:978.

315. Mair RG, McEntee WJ. Cognitive enhancement in Korsakoff's psychosis by clonidine: a comparison with L-DOPA and ephedrine. Psychopharmacology 1986; 88:374.

316. Martin PR, Ebert MH, Gordon EK, et al. Catecholamine metabolism during clonidine withdrawal. Psychopharmacology 1984; 84:58.

317. Centerwall BS, Criqui MH. Prevention of the Wernicke-Korsakoff syndrome: a cost-benefit analysis. N Engl J Med 1978; 299:285.

318. Romano J, Michael M, Merritt HH. Alcoholic cerebellar degeneration. Arch Neurol Psychiatry 1940; 44:1230.

319. Victor M, Adams RD, Mancall EL. A restricted form of cerebellar cortical degeneration occurring in alcoholic patients. Arch Neurol 1959; 71:579.

320. Phillips SC, Harper CG, Kril J. A quantitative histological study of the cerebellar vermis in alcoholic patients. Brain 1987; 110:301.

321. Hillbom M, Muuronen A, Holm L, Lindmarsh T. The clinical versus radiological diagnosis of alcoholic cerebellar degeneration. J Neurol Sci 1986; 73:45.

322. Dano P, Le Guyade J. Atrophie cerebrale et alcoolisme chronique. Rev Neurol 1988; 144:202.

323. Melgaard B, Ahlgren P. Ataxia and cerebellar atrophy in chronic alcoholics. J Neurol 1986; 233:13.

324. Gilman S, Adams K, Koeppe RA, et al. Cerebellar and frontal hypometabolism in alcoholic cerebellar degeneration studied with position emission tomography. Ann Neurol 1990; 28:775.

325. Eidelberg E, Bond ML, Kelter A. Effects of alcohol on cerebellar and vestibular neurons. Arch Int Pharmacodyn Ther 1973; 185:583.

326. Northrup LR. Additive effects of ethanol and Purkinje cell loss in the production of ataxia in mice. Psychopharmacology 1976; 48:189.

327. Mancall EL, McEntee WJ. Alterations of the cerebellar cortex—nutritional encephalopathy. Neurology 1965; 15:303.

328. Tavares MA, Paula-Barbosa MM, Gray EG. A morphometric Golgi analysis of the Purkinje cell dendritic tree after long-term alcohol consumption in the adult rat. J Neurocytol 1983; 12:939.

329. Phillips SC. Qualitative and quantitative changes of mouse cerebellar synapses after chronic alcohol consumption and withdrawal. Exp Neurol 1985; 88:748.

330. Kleinschmidt-DeMasters BK, Norenberg MD. Cerebellar degeneration in the rat following rapid correction of hyponatremia. Ann Neurol 1981; 10:561.

331. Pentney RJ, Quackenbush LJ, O'Neill M. Length changes in dendritic networks of cerebellar Purkinje cells of old rats after chronic ethanol treatment. Alcoholism 1989; 13:413.

332. Thornhill HL, Richter RW, Shelton MV, et al. Neuropathic arthropathy (Charcot forefeet) in alcoholics. Orthoped Clin North Am 1973; 4:7.

333. Mawdsley C, Mayer RF. Nerve conduction in alcoholic polyneuropathy. Brain 1965; 88:335.

334. Guiheneuc P, Bathien N. Two patterns of results in polyneuropathies investigated with the H-reflex. J Neurol Sci 1976; 30:83.

335. Willer JC, Dehen H. Le reflexe H du muscle pedieux: etude au cours des neuropathies alcoholiques latentes. Electroencephalogr Clin Neurophysiol 1977; 42:205.

336. Lefebvre D'Amour M, Shahani BT, Young RR, et al. The importance of studying sural nerve conduction and late responses in the evaluation of alcoholic subjects. Neurology 1979; 29:1600.

337. Behse F, Buchthal F. Alcoholic neuropathy: clinical, electrophysiological, and biopsy findings. Ann Neurol 1977; 2:95.

338. Vallet JM, Hugon J, Tabaraud F, et al. Acute or subacute alcoholic polyradiculoneuropathy: clinical, electrophysical, and histological findings in nine cases. Neurology 1988; 38(suppl 1):222.

339. Novak DJ, Victor M. The vagus and sympathetic nerves in alcoholic polyneuropathy. Arch Neurol 1974; 30:273.

340. Winship DH, Caflisch CR, Zboralske FF, et al. Deterioration of esophageal peristalsis in patients with alcoholic neuropathy. Gastroenterology 1968; 55:173.

341. Low PA, Walsh JC, Huang CY, et al. The sympathetic nervous system in alcoholic neuropathy—a clinical and pathological study. Brain 1975; 98:357.

342. Villalta J, Estruch R, Antunes E, et al. Vagal neuropathy in chronic alcoholics: relation to ethanol consumption. Alcohol Alcoholism 1989; 24:421.

343. Myers W, Willis K, Reeves A. Absence of parasympathetic denervation of the iris in alcoholics. J Neurol Neurosurg Psychiatry 1979; 42:1018.

344. Johnson RH, Robinson BJ. Mortality in alcoholics with autonomic neuropathy. J Neurol Neurosurg Psychiatry 1988; 51:476.

345. Walsh JC, McLeod JG. Alcoholic neuropathy. An electro-physical and histological study. J Neurol Sci 1970; 10:457.

346. Tackmann W, Minkenberg R, Strenge H. Correlation of electro-physiological and quantitative histological findings in the sural nerve of man. Studies on alcoholic neuropathy. J Neurol 1977; 216:289.

347. Said G, Landrieu P. Etude quantitative des fibres nerveuses isolee dans les polynevrites alcooliques. J Neurol Sci 1978; 35:317.

348. Juntunen J, Teravainen H, Eriksson K, et al. Experimental alcoholic neuropathy in the rat: histological and electrophysiological study on the myoneural junctions and the peripheral nerves. Acta Neuropathol 1978; 41:131.

349. Rossi MA, Zucoloto S. Effect of alcohol on ganglion cells in the superior cervical ganglion of young rats. Beitr Pathol 976; 157:183.

350. Strauss MB. The etiology of "alcoholic" polyneuritis. Am J Med Sci 1935; 189:378.

351. Graham JR, Woodhouse D, Read FH. Massive thiamine dosage in an alcoholic with cerebellar cortical degeneration. Lancet 1971; 2:107.

352. Mayer RF. Peripheral nerve conduction in alcoholics. Studies of the effects of acute and chronic intoxication. Psychosom Med 1966; 28:475.

353. Swank RL. Avian thiamine deficiency; correlation of pathology and clinical behavior. J Exp Med 1940; 71:683.

354. Dunn TB, Morris HP, Dubnik CS. Lesions of chronic thiamine deficiency in mice. J Nat Cancer Inst 1947; 8:139.

355. Berry C, Neumann C, Hinsey JC. Nerve regeneration in cats on vitamin B1 deficient diets. J Neurophysiol 1945; 8:315.

356. Wintrobe MM, Follis RH, Humphreys S, et al. Absence of nerve degeneration in chronic thiamine deficiency in pigs. J Nutr 1944; 28:283.

357. Rinehart JF, Friedman M, Greenberg LD. Effect of experimental thiamine deficiency on the nervous system of the rhesus monkey. Arch Pathol 1949; 48:129.

358. Williams RD, Mason HL, Power MH, et al. Induced thiamine (vitamin B1) deficiency in man. Arch Intern Med 1943; 71:38.

359. Swank RL, Adams RD. Pyridoxine and pantothenic acid deficiency in swine. J Neuropath Exp Neurol 1948; 7:274.

360. Bean WB, Hodges RE, Daum KE. Pantothenic acid deficiency induced in human beings. J Clin Invest 1955; 34:1073.

361. Vilter RW, Mueller JF, Glazer HS, et al. Effect of vitamin B6 deficiency induced by desoxypyridoxine in human beings. J Lab Clin Med 1953; 42:335.

362. Lane M, Alfrey CP, Mengel CE, et al. The rapid induction of human riboflavin deficiency with galactoflavin. J Clin Invest 1964; 43:357.

363. McLane JA. Decreased axonal transport in rat nerve following acute and chronic ethanol exposure. Alcohol 1987; 4:385.

364. Victor M. Tobacco-alcohol amblyopia. A critique of current concepts of this disorder, with special reference to the role of nutritional deficiency in its causation. Arch Ophthalmol 1963; 70:313.

365. Sivyer G. Evidence of limited repair of brain damage in a patient with alcohol-tobacco amblyopia. Med J Aust 1989; 151:541.

366. Victor M, Dreyfus PM. Tobacco-alcohol amblyopia. Further comments on its pathology. Arch Ophthalmol 1965; 74:649.

367. Kermode AG, Plant GT, Miller DH, et al. Tobacco-alcohol amblyopia: magnetic resonance imaging findings. J Neurol Neurosurg Psychiatry 1989; 52:1447.

368. Carroll FD. The etiology and treatment of tobacco-alcohol amblyopia. Am J Ophthalmol 1944; 27:713.

369. Vannuci H, Moreno FS. Interaction of niacin and zinc metabolism in patients with alcoholic pellagra. Am J Clin Nutr 1989; 50:364.

370. Serdaru M, Hausser-Hauw C, LaPlane D, et al. The clinical spectrum of alcoholic pellagra encephalopathy. Brain 1988; 111:829.

371. Hauw J-J, deBaecque C, Hausser-Hauw C, Serdaru M. Chromatolysis in alcoholic encephalopathies. Pellagra-like changes in 22 cases. Brain 1988; 111:843.

372. Lindenbaum J. Metabolic effects of alcohol on the blood and bone marrow. In: Lieber CS, ed. Metabolic Aspects of Alcoholism. Baltimore: University Park Press, 1977:215.

373. Lindenbaum J, Lieber CS. Alcohol-induced malabsorption of vitamin B12 in man. Nature 1969; 224:806.

374. New York City. Summary of Vital Statistics 1984. New York: Department of Health, Bureau of Health Statistics and Analysis.

375. Diehl AM. Alcoholic liver disease. Med Clin North Am 1989; 73:815.

376. Pares A, Caballeria J, Bruguera M, et al. Histological course of alcoholic hepatitis. Influence of abstinence, sex, and extent of hepatic damage. J Hepatol 1986; 2:33.

377. Sorensen TIA, Orholm M, Bensten KD, et al. Prospective evaluation of alcohol abuse and alcoholic liver disease in men as predictors of development of cirrhosis. Lancet 1984; 1:241.

378. Montiero E, Alves MP, Santos ML, et al. Histocompatibility antigens: markers of susceptibility to and protection from alcoholic liver disease in a Portuguese population. Hepatology 1988; 8:455.

379. Saunders JB, Davis M, Williams R. Do women develop alcoholic liver disease more readily than men? BMJ 1981; 282:1140.

380. Adams RD, Foley JM. The neurological disorder associated with liver disease. Res Publ Assoc Res Nerv Ment Dis 1953; 32:198.

381. Gammal SH, Jones EA. Hepatic encephalopathy. Med Clin North Am 1989; 73:793.
382. Conomy JP, Swash M. Reversible decerebrate and decorticate postures in hepatic coma. N Engl J Med 1968; 278:876.
383. Rai G, Buxton-Thomas M, Scanlon M. Ocular bobbing in hepatic encephalopathy. Br J Clin Pract 1976; 30:202.
384. Kreis R, Farrow N, Ross BD. Diagnosis of hepatic encephalopathy by proton magnetic resonance spectroscopy. Lancet 1990; 336:635.
385. Yang S-S, Chu N-S, Liaw Y-F. Somatosensory evoked potentials in hepatic encephalopathy. Gastroenterology 1985; 89:625.
386. Leo MA, Lieber CS. Hepatic vitamin A depletion in alcoholic liver injury. N Engl J Med 1982; 307:597.
387. Diemer NH. Glial and neuronal changes in experimental hepatic encephalopathy. A quantitative morphological investigation. Acta Neurol Scand 1978; 58(suppl 71):1.
388. Traber PG. Hepatic encephalopathy. N Engl J Med 1986; 314:786.
389. Butterworth RF. Pathogenesis and treatment of portal-systemic encephalopathy. An update. Digest Dis Sci 1992; 37:321.
390. Raabe W, Onsted G. Portacaval shunting changes neuronal tolerance to ammonia. Ann Neurol 1980; 8:106.
391. Cole M, Rutherford RB, Smith FO. Experimental ammonia encephalopathy in the primate. Arch Neurol 1972; 26:130.
392. Gjedde A, Lockwood AH, Duffy TE, et al. Cerebral blood flow and metabolism in chronically hyperammonemic rats: effect of acute ammonia challenge. Ann Neurol 1978; 3:325.
393. Plum F. The CSF in hepatic encephalopathy. Exp Biol Med 1971; 4:34.
394. Gazzard BD, Weston MJ, Murray-Lyon IM, et al. Charcoal haemoperfusion in the treatment of fulminant hepatic failure. Lancet 1974; 1:1301.
395. Zieve L, Brunner G. Encephalopathy due to mercaptans and phenols. In: McCandless DW, ed. Cerebral Energy Metabolism and Metabolic Encephalopathy. New York: Plenum, 1985:179.
396. Duffy TE, Vergara F, Plum F. Alpha-ketoglutaramate in hepatic encephalopathy. Res Publ Assoc Res Nerv Ment Dis 1974; 53:39.
397. Martinez-Hernandez A, Bell KP, Norenberg MD. Glutamine synthetase: glial localization in brain. Science 1977; 195:1356.
398. Warren KS, Schenker S. Effect of an inhibitor of glutamine synthesis (methionine sulfoximine) on ammonia toxicity and metabolism. J Lab Clin Med 1964; 64:442.
399. Lockwood AH, McCandless DW. Hepatic encephalopathy. N Engl J Med 1986; 314:785.
400. Fischer JE, Baldessarini RJ. Neurotransmitter metabolism in hepatic encephalopathy. N Engl J Med 1975; 293:1152.
401. James JH, Ziparo V, Jepsson B, et al. Hyperammonemia, plasma amino acid imbalance, and blood-brain amino acid transport: a unified theory of portal systemic encephalopathy. Lancet 1979; 2:772.
402. False neurotransmitters and liver failure. Lancet 1982; 1:86.
403. Freese A, Swartz KJ, During MJ, Martin JB. Kynurenine metabolites of tryptophan: implications for neurologic diseases. Neurology 1990; 40:691.
404. Moroni F, Lombardi G, Carla V, et al. Increase in the content of quinolinic acid in cerebrospinal fluid and frontal cortex of patients with hepatic failure. J Neurochem 1986; 47:1667.
405. Bucci L, Ioppolo A, Chiavarelli R, Biogotti A. The central nervous system toxicity of long-term oral administration of L-tryptophan to porto-caval shunted rats. Br J Exp Pathol 1982; 63:235.
406. Jones EA, Schafer DF. Hepatic encephalopathy: a neurochemical disorder. Prog Liver Dis 1986; 8:525.
407. Pappas SC. Increased gamma-aminobutyric acid (GABA) receptors in the brain precedes hepatic encephalopathy in fulminant hepatic failure. Hepatology 1984; 4:1051.
408. Ferenci P, Schafer DF, Kleinberger G, et al. Serum levels of gamma-aminobutyric acid-like activity in acute and chronic hepatocellular disease. Lancet 1983; 2:811.
409. Tran VT, Snyder SH, Major LF, et al. GABA receptors are increased in the brains of alcoholics. Ann Neurol 1981; 9:289.
410. Bassett ML, Mullen KD, Skolnick P, et al. Amelioration of hepatic encephalopathy by pharmacologic antagonism of the GABA-A/benzodiazepine receptor complex in a rabbit model of fulminant hepatic failure. Gastroenterology 1987; 93:1069.
411. Cooper AJL, Ehrlich ME, Plum F. Hepatic encephalopathy: GABA or ammonia? Lancet 1984; 2:158.
412. Jones EA, Skolnick P, Gammal SH, et al. The gamma-aminobutyric acid A (GABA-A) receptor complex and hepatic encephalopathy. Some recent advances. Ann Intern Med 1989; 110:532.
413. Basile AS, Jones EA, Skolnick P. The pathogenesis and treatment of hepatic encephalopathy: evidence for the involvement of benzodiazepine ligands. Pharmacol Rev 1991; 43:28.
414. Bosman DK, van den Buijs CA, de Haan JG, et al. The effects of benzodiazepine antagonists and partial inverse agonists on acute hepatic encephalopathy in the rat. Gastroenterology 1991; 101:772.
415. Mullen KD, Szauter KM, Kaminsky-Ross K. "Endogenous" benzodiazepine activity in body fluids of patients with hepatic encephalopathy. Lancet 1990; 336:81.
416. Basile AS, Hughes RD, Harrison PM, et al. Elevated brain concentrations of 1,4-benzodiazepines in fulminant hepatic failure. N Engl J Med 1991; 325:473.
417. Ferenci P, Grimm G. Benzodiazepine antagonist in the treatment of human hepatic encephalopathy. Adv Exp Med Biol 1990; 272:255.

418. Bakti G, Fisch HV, Karlaganis G, et al. Mechanism of the excessive sedative response of cirrhotics to benzodiazepines: model experiments with triazolam. Hepatology 1987; 7:629.

419. Hoyumpa AM, Desmond PV, Avant GR, et al. Hepatic encephalopathy. Gastroenterology 1979; 76:184.

420. Conn HO, Leevy CM, Vlahcevic ZR, et al. Comparison of lactulose and neomycin in the treatment of chronic portal-systemic encephalopathy. Gastroenterology 1977; 72:573.

421. Pirotte J, Guffens JM, Devos J. Comparative study of basal arterial ammonemia and of orally-induced hyperammonemia in chronic portalsystemic encephalopathy, treated with neomycin and lactulose. Digestion 1974; 10:435.

422. Parkes JD, Sharpstone P, Williams R. Levodopa in hepatic coma. Lancet 1970; 2:1341.

423. Michel H, Cauvet G, Grainer PM, et al. Treatment of cirrhotic hepatic encephalopathy by L-DOPA: a double-blind study of 58 patients. Digestion 1977; 15:232.

424. Maddrey WG, Weber FL, Coulter AW, et al. Effects of ketoanalogues of essential amino acids in portal systemic encephalopathy. Gastroenterology 1976; 71:190.

425. Smith AR, Rossi-Fanelli F, Ziparo V, et al. Alterations in plasma and CSF amino acids, amines, and metabolites in hepatic coma. Ann Surg 1978; 187:343.

426. Ferenci P, Grimm G, Meryn S, et al. Successful long-term treatment of portal-systemic encephalopathy by the benzodiazepine antagonist flumazenil. Gastroenterology 1989; 96:240.

427. Jones EA, Skolnick P. Benzodiazepine receptor ligands and the syndrome of hepatic encephalopathy. Prog Liver Dis 1990; 9:345.

428. Warren SE, Mitas JA, Swerdlin A. Hypernatremia in hepatic failure. JAMA 1980; 243:1257.

429. Nelson DC, McGrew WRG, Hoyumpa AM. Hypernatremia and lactulose therapy. JAMA 1983; 249:1295.

430. Levin DM, Baker AL, Rochman H, et al. Nonalcoholic liver disease: overlooked causes of liver injury in patients with heavy alcohol consumption. Am J Med 1979; 66:429.

431. Reade AE, Sherlock S, Laidlaw J, et al. The neuropsychiatric syndromes associated with chronic liver disease and an extensive portal-systemic collateral circulation. Q J Med 1967; 36:135.

432. Gauthier G, Wildi E. L'encephalo-myelopathie portosystemique. Rev Neurol 1975; 131:319.

433. Lunzer M, James IM, Weinman J, et al. Treatment of chronic hepatic encephalopathy with levodopa. Gut 1974; 15:555.

434. Morgan MY, Jacobovits AW, James IM, et al. Bromocriptine in the treatment of chronic portal-systemic encephalopathy. Gut 1978; 19:453.

435. Uribe M, Farca A, Marquez MA, et al. Treatment of chronic portal systemic encephalopathy with bromocriptine. Gastroenterology 1979; 76:1347.

436. Victor M, Adams RD, Cole M. The acquired (non-Wilsonian) type of chronic hepatocerebral degeneration. Medicine 1965; 44:345.

437. Bunout D, Petermann M, Bravo M, et al. Glucose turnover rate and peripheral insulin sensitivity in alcoholic patients without liver damage. Ann Nutr Metab 1989; 33:31.

438. Kallas P, Sellers EM. Blood glucose in intoxicated chronic alcoholics. Can Med Assoc J 1975; 112:590.

439. Malouf R, Brust JCM. Hypoglycemia: causes, neurological manifestations, and outcome. Ann Neurol 1985; 17:421.

440. Kalimo H, Olsson Y. Effects of severe hypoglycemia on the human brain: neuropathological case reports. Acta Neurol Scand 1980; 62:345.

441. Bale RN. Brain damage in diabetes mellitus. Br J Psychiatry 1973; 122:337.

442. Haumont D, Dorchy H, Pele S. EEG abnormalities in diabetic children: influence of hypoglycemia and vascular complications. Clin Pediatr 1979; 18:750.

443. O'Keefe SJD, Marks V. Lunchtime gin and tonic as a cause of reactive hypoglycemia. Lancet 1977; 1:1286.

444. Shakespeare W. Macbeth, Act II, Scene 3.

445. Van Thiel DH, Gavaler JS. Hypothalamic-pituitary-gonadal function in liver disease with particular attention to the endocrine effects of chronic alcohol abuse. Prog Liver Dis 1986; 8:273.

446. Mello NK, Mendelson JH, Teoh SK. Neuroendocrine consequences of alcohol abuse in women. Ann NY Acad Sci 1981; 562:211.

447. Eisenhoffer G, Johnson RH. Effect of ethanol ingestion on plasma vasopressin and water balance in humans. Am J Physiol 1982; 242:R522.

448. Rivier C, Bruhn T, Vale W. Effect of ethanol on the hypothalamic-pituitary-adrenal axis in the rat. Role of corticotropin-releasing factor (CRF). J Pharmacol Exp Ther 1984; 229:127.

449. Lamberts SWJ, Klijn JGM, deJong FH, et al. Hormone secretion in alcohol-induced pseudo-Cushing's syndrome. Differential diagnosis with Cushing's disease. JAMA 1979; 242:1640.

450. Willenbring ML, Morley JE, Niewoehner CB, et al. Adrenocortical hyperactivity in newly admitted alcoholics. Prevalence, course, and associated variables. Psychoneuroendocrinology 1984; 9:415.

451. Bjorneboe GE, Bjorneboe A, Johnson J, et al. Calcium status and calcium-regulating hormones in alcoholics. Alcoholism 1988; 12:229.

452. Spencer H, Rubio N, Rubio E, et al. Chronic alcoholism: frequently overlooked cause of osteoporosis in men. Am J Med 1986; 80:393.

453. Laitinen KK, Lamberg-Allardt C, Tunninen R, et al. Transient hypoparathyroidism during acute alcohol intoxication. N Engl J Med 1991; 324:721.

454. Moore JA, Kakihana R. Ethanol-induced hypothermia in mice: influence of genotype on the development of tolerance. Life Sci 1978; 23:2331.

455. Dinh TKH, Gailis L. Effect of body temperature on acute ethanol toxicity. Life Sci 1979; 25:547.

456. Fulop M. Alcoholism, ketoacidosis, and lactic acidosis. Diabetes Metab Rev 1989; 5:365.
457. Goldfrank LR, Starke CL. Metabolic acidosis in the alcoholic. In: Goldfrank LR, Flomenbaum NE, Lewin NA, et al, eds. Toxicologic Emergencies, ed 4. Norwalk, CT: Appleton & Lange, 1990:465.
458. Lefevre A, Adler H, Lieber CS. Effect of ethanol on ketone metabolism. J Clin Invest 1970; 49:1775.
459. Jerrells TR, Eckardt MJ, Weinberg J. Mechanisms of ethanol-induced immunsuppression. In: Seminara D, Watson RR, Pawlowski A, eds. Alcohol, Immunomodulation, and AIDS. New York: Alan R. Liss, 1990:173.
460. MacGregor RR. Alcohol and immune defense. JAMA 1986; 256:1474.
461. Dunne FJ. Alcohol and the immune system. BMJ 1989; 298:543.
462. Anderson BR. Host factors causing increased susceptibility to infection in patients with Laennec's cirrhosis. Ann NY Acad Sci 1975; 252:348.
463. Richter RW, Brust JCM. Pneumococcal meningitis at Harlem Hospital. NY State J Med 1971; 71:2747.
464. Crane LR, Lerner AM. Non-traumatic gram-negative bacillary meningitis in the Detroit Medical Center, 1964–1974 (with special mention of cases due to Escherichia coli). Medicine 1978; 57:197.
465. Hudolin V. Tuberculosis and alcoholism. Ann NY Acad Sci 1975; 252:353.
466. Harnisch JP, Tronca E, Nolan CM, et al. Diphtheria among alcoholic urban adults. A decade of experience in Seattle. Ann Intern Med 1989; 111:71.
467. Kaslow RA, Blackwelder WC, Ostrow DG, et al. No evidence for a role of alcohol or other psychoactive drugs in accelerating immunodeficiency in HIV-1-positive individuals. A report from the multicenter AIDS Cohort Study. JAMA 1989; 261:3424.
468. Schleifer SJ, Keller SE, Lombardo JM, et al. HIV-1 antibody reactivity in inner-city alcoholics. JAMA 1989; 262:2680.
469. Drexler KPG, Brown GR. Psychoactive drug use and AIDS. JAMA 1990; 263:371.
470. Garro AJ, Lieber CS. Alcohol and cancer. Annu Rev Pharmacol Toxicol 1990; 30:219.
471. McCoy GD, Napier K. Alcohol and tobacco consumption as risk factors for cancer. Alcohol Health Res World 1986; 10:28.
472. Rudzinski M, Stankaitis JA. Recognizing the alcoholic patient. N Engl J Med 1989; 320:125.
473. Skinner HA, Holt S, Schuller R, et al. Identification of alcohol abuse using laboratory tests and a history of trauma. Ann Intern Med 1984; 101:846.
474. Luna GK, Maier RV, Swoder L, et al. The influence of ethanol intoxication on outcome of injured motorcyclists. J Trauma 1984; 24:695.
475. Epidemiology. In: Hurley J, Horowitz J, eds. Alcohol and Health. DHHS. New York: Hemisphere Publishing, 1987:1.
476. Abel EL, Zeidenberg P. Age, alcohol and violent death: a postmortem study. J Stud Alcohol 1985; 46:228.
477. Modell JG, Mountz JM. Drinking and flying—the problem of alcohol use by pilots. N Engl J Med 1990; 323:455.
478. Berglund M. Suicide in alcoholism. Arch Gen Psychiatry 1984; 41:888.
479. Combs-Orme T, Taylor JR, Scott EB, Holmes SJ. Violent deaths among alcoholics: a descriptive study. J Stud Alcohol 1983; 44:938.
480. Rosengren L, Persson L, Johansson B. Enhanced blood-brain barrier leakage to Evans blue-labeled albumin after air embolism in ethanol-intoxicated rats. Acta Neuropathol (Berlin) 1977; 38:149.
481. Flamm ES, Demopoulos HB, Seligman ML, et al. Ethanol potentiation of CNS trauma. J Neurosurg 1977; 46:328.
481a. Halt PS, Swanson RA, Faden AI. Alcohol exacerbates behavioral and neurochemical effects of rat spinal cord trauma. Arch Neurol 1992; 49:1178.
482. Adams RD, Victor M, Mancall EL. Central pontine myelinolysis. A hitherto undescribed disease occurring in alcoholic and malnourished subjects. Arch Neurol Psychiatr 1959; 81:154.
483. Tomlinson BE, Pierides AM, Bradley WG. Central pontine myelinolysis. Two cases with associated electrolyte disturbance. Q J Med 1976; 45:373.
484. Wright DG, Laureno R, Victor M. Pontine and extra-pontine myelinolysis. Brain 1979; 102:361.
485. Cole M, Richardson EP, Segarra JM. Central pontine myelinolysis: further evidence relating the lesion to malnutrition. Neurology 1964; 14:165.
486. Valsamis MP, Peress NE, Wright LD. Central pontine myelinolysis in childhood. Arch Neurol 1971; 25:307.
487. Miller GM, Baker HL, Okasaki H, Whisnant JP. Central pontine myelinolysis and its imitators; MR findings. Radiology 1988; 168:795.
488. Burcar PJ, Norenberg MD, Yarnell PR. Hyponatremia and central pontine myelinolysis. Neurology 1977; 27:223.
489. Messert B, Orrison WW, Hawkins MJ, et al. Central pontine myelinolysis. Considerations on etiology, diagnosis, and treatment. Neurology 1979; 29:147.
490. Norenberg MD, Papendick RE. Chronicity of hyponatremia as a factor in experimental myelinolysis. Ann Neurol 1984; 15:544.
491. Illowsky BP, Laureno R. Encephalopathy and myelinolysis after rapid correction of hyponatremia. Brain 1987; 110:855.
492. Khurana R, Post JC, Kalyanaraman K. Bulbar paralysis in chronic alcoholism with recovery. Dis Nerv Syst 1974; 35:135.
493. Wiederholt WC, Kobayashi RM, Stockard JJ, et al. Central pontine myelinolysis. A clinical reappraisal. Arch Neurol 1977; 34:220.
494. Estol CJ, Caplan LR. Reversible central pontine myelinolysis. Neurology 1990; 40(suppl 1):211.
495. Narins RG. Therapy of hyponatremia: does haste make waste? N Engl J Med 1986; 314:1573.

496. Ayus JC, Krothapalli RK, Arieff AI. Treatment of symptomatic hyponatremia and its relation to brain damage: a prospective study. N Engl J Med 1987; 317:1190.

497. Sterns RH. Severe symptomatic hyponatremia. Treatment and outcome: a study of 64 cases. Ann Intern Med 1987; 107:656.

498. Laureno R, Karp BI. Pontine and extrapontine myelinolysis following rapid correction of hyponatremia. Lancet 1988; 1:1439.

499. Hed R, Larrson H, Fahlgren H. Acute myoglobinuria. Acta Med Scand 1955; 152:459.

500. Perkoff GI, Dioso MM, Bleisch V, et al. A spectrum of myopathy associated with alcoholism. I. Clinical and laboratory features. Ann Intern Med 1967; 67:481.

501. Haller RG, Knochel JP. Skeletal muscle disease in alcoholism. Med Clin North Am 1984; 68:91.

502. Urbano-Marquez A, Estruch R, Grau JM, et al. On alcoholic myopathy. Ann Neurol 1985; 17:418.

503. Diamond I. Alcoholic myopathy and cardiomyopathy. N Engl J Med 1989; 320:458.

504. Weber LD, Nashel DJ, Mellow MH. Pharyngeal dysphagia in alcoholic myopathy. Ann Intern Med 1981; 95:189.

505. Spector R, Choudhury A, Cancilla P, et al. Alcoholic myopathy. Diagnosis by alcohol challenge. JAMA 1979; 242:1648.

506. Rubenstein AE, Wainapel SF. Acute hypokalemic myopathy in alcoholism. Arch Neurol 1977; 34:553.

507. Urbano-Marquez A, Estruch R, Navarro-Lopez F, et al. The effects of alcoholism on skeletal and cardiac muscle. N Engl J Med 1989; 320:409.

508. Song SK, Rubin E. Ethanol produces muscle damage in human volunteers. Science 1972; 175:327.

509. Rubin E, Katz AM, Lieber CS, et al. Muscle damage produced by chronic alcohol consumption. Am J Pathol 1976; 83:499.

510. Rubin E. Alcoholic myopathy in heart and skeletal muscle. N Engl J Med 1979; 301:28.

511. Psuzkin S, Rubin E. Adenosine diphosphate effect on contractility of human actomyosin: inhibition by ethanol and acetaldehyde. Science 1975; 188:1319.

512. Bollaert PE, Robin-Lherbier B, Escayne JM, et al. Phosphorus nuclear magnetic resonance evidence of abnormal skeletal muscle metabolism in chronic alcoholics. Neurology 1989; 39:821.

513. Ohno K, Tanaka M, Sahashi K, et al. Mitochondrial DNA deletions in inherited recurrent myogolobinuria. Ann Neurol 1991; 29:364.

514. Bing RJ, Tillmanns H. The effect of alcohol on the heart. In: Lieber CS, ed. Metabolic Aspects of Alcoholism, Baltimore: University Park Press, 1977:117.

515. Demakis JG, Proskey A, Rahimtoola SH, et al. The natural course of alcoholic cardiomyopathy. Ann Intern Med 1974; 80:293.

516. Greenspon AJ, Schaal SF. The "holiday heart": electrophysiologic studies of alcohol effects in alcoholics. Ann Intern Med 1983; 98:135.

517. Regan TJ. Of beverages, cigarettes, and cardiac arrhythmias. N Engl J Med 1979; 301:1060.

518. Seneviratne BIB. Acute cardiomyopathy with rhabdomyolysis in chronic alcoholism. BMJ 1975; 3:378.

519. Lang RM, Borow KM, Neumann A, Feldman T. Adverse cardiac effects of acute alcohol ingestion in young adults. Ann Intern Med 1985; 103:742.

520. Brion S. Marchiafava-Bignami syndrome. In: Vinken PJ, Bruyn GW, eds. Handbook of Clinical Neurology, Vol 28. Metabolic and Deficiency Diseases of the Nervous System, Part II. Amsterdam: North-Holland Publishing, 1976:317.

521. Marchiafava E, Bignami A. Sopra un alterzione del corpor calloso osservata in soggetti acoolisti. Riv Pat Nerv Ment 1903; 8:544.

522. Ironside R, Bosanquet FD, McMenemey WH. Central demyelination of the corpus callosum (Marchiafava-Bignami disease) with report of a second case in Great Britain. Brain 1961; 84:212.

523. Kosaka K, Aoki M, Kawashaki N, et al. A non-alcoholic Japanese patient with Wernicke's encephalopathy and Marchiafava-Bignami disease. Clin Neuropathol 1984; 3:231.

524. Leong ASY. Marchiafava-Bignami disease in a non-alcoholic Indian male. Pathology 1979; 11:241.

525. Lechevalier B, Andersson JC, Morin P. Hemispheric disconnection syndrome with a "crossed avoiding" reaction in a case of Marchiafava-Bignami disease. J Neurol Neurosurg Psychiatry 1977; 40:483.

526. Leventhal CM, Baringer JR, Arnason BG, et al. A case of Marchiafava-Bignami disease with clinical recovery. Trans Am Neurol Assoc 1965; 90:87.

527. Baron R, Heuser K, Marioth G. Marchiafava-Bignami disease with recovery diagnosed by CT and MRI: demyelination affects several CNS structures. J Neurol 1989; 236:364.

528. Ikeda A, Antoku Y, Abe T, et al. Marchiafava-Bignami disease: consecutive observation at acute stage by magnetic resonance imaging and computerized tomography. Jpn J Med 1989; 28:740.

529. Morel F. Une forme anatomo-clinique particuliere de l'alcoolisme chronique: sclerose corticale laminaire alcoolique. Rev Neurol 1939; 71:280.

530. Naeije R, Franken L, Jacobivitz D, et al. Morel's laminar sclerosis. Eur Neurol 1978; 17:155.

531. Ghatak NR, Hadfield G, Rosenblum WI. Association of central pontine myelinolysis and Marchiafava-Bignami disease. Neurology 1978; 28:1295.

532. Levine S, Stypulkowski W. Experimental cyanide encephalopathy. Arch Pathol 1959; 67:306.

533. Horvath TB. Clinical spectrum and epidemiological features of alcoholic dementia. In: Rankin JG, ed. Alcohol, Drug, and Brain Damage. Toronto: Alcoholism and Drug Addiction Research Foundation of Ontario, 1975:1.

534. Lishman WA. Cerebral disorder in alcoholism: syndrome of impairment. Brain 1981; 104:1.

535. Davtyan DG, Vinters HV. Wernicke's encephalopathy in AIDS patient treated with zidovudine. Lancet 1987; 1:919.

536. Lishman WA. Alcoholic dementia: a hypothesis. Lancet 1986; 1:1184.

537. Bowden SC. Separating cognitive impairment in neurologically asymptomatic alcoholism from Wernicke-Korsakoff syndrome: is the neuropsychological distinction justified? Psychol Bull 1990; 107:355.

538. Jacobson RR, Lishman WA. Selective memory loss and global intellectual deficits in alcoholic Korsakoff's syndrome. Psychol Med 1987; 17:549.

540. Victor M, Adams RD. The alcoholic dementias. In: Frederiks JAM, ed. Handbook of Clinical Neurology, Vol 2 (46): Neuro-behavioral Disorders. Amsterdam: Elsevier Science Publishers, 1985:335.

540a. Victor M: Persistent altered mentation due to ethanol. In Brust JCM, ed. Neurologic Complications of Drug and Alcohol Abuse. Neurol Clin 1993, in press.

541. Courville CB. Effects of Alcohol on the Nervous System of Man. Los Angeles: San Lucas, 1955.

542. Harper C, Kril J. Patterns of neuronal loss in the cerebral cortex in chronic alcoholic patients. J Neurol Sci 1989; 92:81.

543. Harper CJ, Kril J, Daly J. Are we drinking our neurons away? BMJ 1987; 294:534.

544. Krill J, Harper CG. Neuronal counts from four cortical regions of alcoholic brains. Acta Neuropathol 1989; 79:200.

545. Samson Y, Baron J-C, Feline A, et al. Local cerebral glucose utilisation in chronic alcoholics: a positron tomographic study. J Neurol Neurosurg Psychiatry 1986; 49:1165.

546. Freund G, Ballinger WE. Loss of muscarinic cholinergic receptors from the temporal cortex of alcohol abusers. Metab Brain Dis 1989; 4:121.

547. Postel J, Cossa P. L'atrophie cerebrale des alcooliques chroniques, etude pneumoencephalographique. Rev Neurol 1956; 94:604.

548. Brewer C, Perrett L. Brain damage due to alcohol consumption: an air-encephalographic, psychometric, and electroencephalographic study. Br J Addict 1971; 66:170.

549. Carlsson C, Claeson L-E, Karlsson K-I, Petterson L-E. Clinical, psychometric, and radiologic signs of brain damage in chronic alcoholism. Acta Neurol Scand 1979; 60:85.

550. Fox JH, Ramsey RG, Huckman MS, Proske AE. Cerebral ventricular enlargement: chronic alcoholics examined by computerized tomography. JAMA 1976; 236:365.

551. Epstein PS, Pisani VD, Fawcett JA. Alcoholism and cerebral atrophy. Clin Exp Res 1977; 1:61.

552. von Gall M, Becker H, Artmann H, et al. Results of computer tomography on chronic alcoholics. Neuroradiology 1978; 16:329.

553. Cala LA, Jones B, Mastaglia FL, Wiley B. Brain atrophy and intellectual impairment in heavy drinkers—a clinical, psychometric and computerized tomographic study. Aust N Z J Med 1978; 8:147.

554. Lee K, Moller L, Hardt F, et al. Alcohol-induced brain damage and liver damage in young males. Lancet 1979; 2:759.

555. Hill SY, Mikhael MA. Computerized transaxial tomographic and neuropsychological evaluations in chronic alcoholics and heroin abusers. Am J Psychiatry 1979; 136:598.

556. Lusins J, Zimberg S, Smokler H, Gurley K. Alcoholism and cerebral atrophy: a study of 50 patients with CT scan and psychological testing. Alcohol Clin Exp Res 1980; 4:406.

557. Kroll P, Seigel R, O'Neill B, Edwards RP. Cerebral cortical atrophy in alcoholic men. J Clin Psychiatry 1980; 41:417.

558. Sarabia F, Bowden CL. Computerized tomographic evidence of cerebral atrophy in heavy drinkers. South Med J 1980; 73:716.

559. Feusssner JR, Linfors EW, Blessing CL, Starmer F. Computed tomography brain scanning in alcohol withdrawal seizures. Value of the neurological examination. Ann Intern Med 1981; 94:519.

560. Wilkinson DA. Examination of alcoholics by computed tomographic (CT) scans: a critical review. Alcohol Clin Exp Res 1982; 6:31.

561. Carlen PL, Wortzman G, Holgate RC, et al. Reversible cerebral atrophy in recently abstinent chronic alcoholics measured by computed tomography scans. Science 1978; 200:1076.

562. Artmann H, Gall MV, Hacker H, Herrlich J. Reversible enlargement of cerebral spinal fluid spaces in chronic alcoholics. Am J Neuroradiol 1981; 2:23.

563. Ron MA, Acker W, Shaw GK, Lishman WA. Computerized tomography of the brain in chronic alcoholism. A survey and follow-up study. Brain 1982; 105:497.

564. Zipursky RB, Lim KC, Pfefferbaum A. MRI study of brain changes with short-term abstinence from alcohol. Alcoholism 1989; 13:664.

565. Muuronen A, Bergman H, Hindmarsh T, Telakivi T. Influence of improved drinking habits on brain atrophy and cognitive performance in alcoholic patients: a 5-year follow-up study. Alcoholism 1989; 13:137.

566. Chick JD, Smith MA, Englemann HM, et al. Magnetic resonance imaging of the brain in alcoholics: cerebral atrophy, lifetime alcohol consumption, and cognitive deficits. Alcoholism 1989; 13:512.

567. Gallucci M, Amicarelli I, Rossi A, et al. MR imaging of white matter lesions in uncomplicated chronic alcoholism. J Comput Assist Tomogr 1989; 13:395.

568. File SE, Mabbutt PS. Long-lasting effects on habituation and passive avoidance performance of a period of chronic ethanol administration in the rat. Behav Brain Res 1990; 36:171.

569. Walker DW, Hunter BE, Abraham WC. Neuroanatomical and functional deficits subsequent to chronic ethanol administration in animals. Alcohol Clin Exp Res 1981; 5:267.

570. Phillips SC. The threshold concentration of dietary ethanol necessary to produce toxic effects of hippocampal cells and synapses in the mouse. Exp Neurol 1989; 104:68.

571. Durand D, St Cyr JA, Curevich N, Carlen PL. Ethanol-induced dendritic alterations in hippocampal granule cells. Brain Res 1989; 477:373.

572. Lescaudron L, Jafford R, Verns A. Modifications in number and morphology of dendritic spines resulting from chronic ethanol consumption and withdrawal: a Golgi study in the mouse anterior and posterior hippocampus. Exp Neurol 198; 106:156.

573. Alvarez MG, Stoltenburg-Didinger G, Aruffo C. "Ageing" of spine morphology in hippocampal pyramidal cells of rats prenatally exposed to ethanol—a Golgi study. Int Congr Neuropathol 1986; 10:282.

574. Davies DL, Smith DE. A Golgi study of mouse hippocampal CA1 pyramidal neurones folowing perinatal ethanol exposure. Neurosci Lett 1981; 26:49.

575. Walker DW, Barnes DE, Zornetzer SF, et al. Neuronal loss in hippocampus induced by prolonged ethanol consumption in rats. Science 1980; 209:711.

576. West JR, Lind MD, Demut RM, et al. Lesion-induced sprouting in the rat dentate gyrus is inhibited by repeated ethanol administration. Science 1982; 218:808.

577. Riley JN, Walker DW. Morphological alterations in hippocampus after long-term alcohol consumption in mice. Science 1978; 701:646.

578. McMullen PA, St Cyr JA, Carlen PL. Morphological alterations in rat hippocampal pyramidal cell dendrites resulting from chronic ethanol consumption and withdrawal. J Comp Neurol 1984; 225:111.

579. Abraham WC, Rogers CJ, Hunter BE. Chronic ethanol-induced decreases in the response of dentate granule cells to perforant path input in the rat. Exp Brain Res 1984; 54:406.

580. Durand D, Carlen PL. Impariment of long-term potentiation in rat hippocampus following chronic ethanol treatment. Brain Res 1984; 308:325.

581. Cadete-Leite A, Tavares MA, Pacheco MM, et al. Hippocampal mossy fiber CA2 synapses after chronic alcohol consumption and withdrawal. Alcohol 1989; 6:303.

582. Tavares MA, Paula-Barbosa MM. Alcohol-induced granule cell loss in the cerebellar cortex of the adult rat. Exp Neurol 1982; 78:574.

583. Tavares MA, Paula-Barbosa MM, Gray EG, Volk B. Dendritic inclusions in the cerebellar granular layer after long-term alcohol consumption in adult rats. Alcohol Clin Exp Res 1985; 9:45.

584. Goldstein B, Maxwell DS, Ellison G, Hammer RP. Dendritic vacuolation in the central nervous system of rats after long term voluntary consumption of ethanol. J Neuropathol Exp Neurol 1983; 42:579.

585. Lescaudron L, Verna A. Effects of chronic ethanol consumption on pyramidal neurons of the mouse dorsal and ventral hippocampus: a quantitative histological analysis. Exp Brain Res 1985; 58:362.

586. Arendt T, Henning D, Gray JA, Marchbanks R. Loss of neurons in the rat basal forebrain cholinergic projection system after prolonged intake of ethanol. Brain Res Bull; 21:563.

587. Arendt T, Allen Y, Sinden J, et al. Cholinergic-rich brain transplants reverse alcohol-induced memory deficits. Nature 1988; 332:448.

588. Ferrer I, Galofre E, Fabriques I, Lopez-Tejero D. Effects of chronic ethanol consumption beginning at adolescence: increased numbers of dendritic spines on cortical pyramidal cells in adulthood. Acta Neuropathol 1989; 78:528.

589. Yano K, Rhoads GG, Kagan V. Coffee, alcohol, and risk of coronary heart disease among Japanese men living in Hawaii. N Engl J Med 1977; 297:405.

590. Ashley MJ. Alcohol consumption, ischemic heart disease, and cerebrovascular disease. J Stud Alcohol 1982; 43:869.

591. US National Institute on Alcohol Abuse and Alcoholism. Alcohol and Health, Second Special Report to the Congress. Washington, DC: DHEW Publication No (ADM) 75-212, US Government Printing Office, 1975.

592. Dyer AR, Stamler J, Paul O, et al. Alcohol consumption and 17-year mortality in the Chicago Western Electric Company. Prev Med 1980; 9:78.

593. St Leger AS, Cocrane AL, Moore F. Factors associated with cardiac mortality in developed countries with particular reference to the consumption of wine. Lancet 1979; 1:1017.

594. Hennekens CH, Rosner B, Cole DS. Daily alcohol consumption and fatal coronary heart disease. Am J Epidemiol 1978; 107:196.

595. Stason WB, Neff RK, Meittinen OS, Jick H. Alcohol consumption and nonfatal myocardial infarction. Am J Epidemiol 1976; 104:603.

596. Klatsky AJ, Friedman GD, Siegelaub AB. Alcohol consumption before myocardial infarction: results from the Kaiser-Permanente epidemiologic study of myocardial infarction. Ann Intern Med 1974; 81:294.

597. Kozaravic D, McGee D, Vojvodic N, et al. Frequency of alcohol consumption and morbidity and mortality. The Yugoslavia cardiovascular disease study. Lancet 1980; 1:613.

598. Petitti DB, Wingerd J, Pellegrin F, Ramcharan S. Risk of vascular disease in women: smoking, oral contraceptives, noncontraceptive estrogens, and other factors. JAMA 1979; 242:1150.

599. La Porte RE, Cresanta JL, Kuller LH. The relationship of alcohol consumption to atherosclerotic heart disease. Prev Med 1980; 9:32.

600. Morris JN, Kagan A, Pattison DC, et al. Incidence and prediction of ischemic heart disease in London busmen. Lancet 1966; 2:553.

601. Doyle JT, Heslin AS, Hilleboe HE, et al. A prospective study of degenerative cardiovascular disease in Albany: report of three years' experience. 1. Ischemic heart disease. Am J Publ Health 1957; 47:25.

602. Grieg M, Pemberton J, Hay I, MacKensie G. A prospective study of the development of coronary heart disease in a group of 1202 middle-aged men. J Epidemiol Commun Health 1980; 34:23.

603. Friedman GD, Dales LG, Ury HK. Mortality in middle-aged smokers and non-smokers. N Engl J Med 1979; 300:213.
604. Blackwelder WC, Yano K, Rhoads GC, et al. Alcohol and mortality: the Honolulu Heart Study. Am J Med 1980; 68:164.
605. Tibblin G, Wilhelmsen L, Werko L. Risk factors for myocardial infarction and death due to ischemic heart disease and other causes. Am J Cardiol 1975; 35:513.
606. Dyer A, Stamler J, Paul O, et al. Alcohol consumption, cardiovascular risk factors, and mortality in two Chicago epidemiologic studies. Circulation 1977; 56:1067.
607. Caplan LR, Hier DB, DeCruz I. Cerebral embolism in the Michael Reese Stroke Registry. Stroke 1983; 14:530.
608. Hillbom M, Kaste M. Does ethanol intoxication promote brain infarction in young adults? Lancet 1978; 2:1181.
609. Hillbom M, Kaste M. Ethanol intoxication: a risk factor for ischemic brain infarction in adolescents and young adults. Stroke 1981; 12:422.
610. Hillbom M, Kaste M. Ethanol intoxication: a risk factor for ischemic brain infarction. Stroke 1983; 14:694.
611. Syrjanen J, Valtonen VV, Ivananainen M, et al. Association between cerebral infarction and increased serum bacterial antibody levels in young adults. Acta Neurol Scand 1986; 73:273.
612. Hilton-Jones O, Warlow CP. The cause of stroke in the young. J Neurol 1985; 232:137.
613. Moorthy G, Price TR, Thurim S, et al. Relationship between recent alcohol intake and stroke type? The NINDS Stroke Data Bank. Stroke 1986; 17:141.
614. Gorelick PB, Rodin MB, Longenberg P, et al. Is acute alcohol ingestion a risk factor for ischemic stroke? Results of a controlled study in middle-aged and elderly stroke patients at three urban medical centers. Stroke 1987; 18:359.
615. Gorelick PB, Rodin MB, Langenberg P, et al. Weekly alcohol consumption, cigarette smoking, and the risk of ischemic stroke: results of a case-control study at urban medical centers in Chicago, Illinois. Neurology 1989; 39:339.
616. Von Arbin M, Britton M, Du Faire U, Tissell A. Circulatory manifestations and risk factors in patients with acute cerebrovascular disease and in matched controls. Acta Med Scand 1985; 218:373.
617. Boysen G, Nyboe J, Appleyard M, et al. Stroke incidence and risk factors for stroke in Copenhagen, Denmark. Stroke 1988; 19:1345.
618. Taylor JR, Combs-Orme T. Alcohol and strokes in young adults. Am J Psychiatry 1985; 142:116.
619. Cullen K, Stenhouse NS, Wearne KL. Alcohol and mortality in the Busselton Study. Int J Epidemiol 1982; 11:67.
620. Stemmermann GN, Hayashi T, Resch JA, et al. Risk factors related to ischemic and hemorrhage cerebrovascular disease at autopsy: the Honolulu Heart Study. Stroke 1984; 15:23.
621. Gill JS, Zezulka AV, Shipley MJ, et al. Stroke and alcohol consumption. N Engl J Med 1986; 315:1041.
622. Gordon T, Doyle JT. Drinking and mortality: the Albany Study. Am J Epidemiol 1987; 125:263.
623. Semenciw RM, Morrison MI, Mao Y, et al. Major risk factors for cardiovascular disease mortality in adults: results from the Nutrition Canada Survey Study. Int J Epidemiol 1988; 17:317.
624. Herman B, Schmintz PIM, Leyten ACM, et al. Multivariate logistic analysis of risk factors for stroke in Tilborg, the Netherlands. Am J Epidemiol 1983; 118:514.
625. Peacock PB, Riley CP, Lampton TD, et al. The Birmingham Stroke, Epidemiology, and Rehabilitation Study. In: Stewart G, ed. Trends in Epidemiology: Applications to Health Service Research and Training. Springfield, IL: Charles C. Thomas, 1972:231.
626. Khaw AL, Barrett-Conner E. Dietary potassium and stroke-associated mortality: a 12-year prospective study. N Engl J Med 1987; 316:235.
627. Paganini-Hill A, Ross RK, Henderson BE. Postmenapausal oestrogen treatment and stroke: a prospective study. N Engl J Med 1988; 297:519.
628. Oleckno WA. The risk of stroke in young adults: an analysis of the contribution of cigarette smoking and alcohol consumption. Public Health 1988; 102:5.
629. Klatsky AL, Friedman GD, Siegelaub AB. Alcohol and mortality: a ten-year Kaiser-Permanente experience. Ann Intern Med 1981; 95:139.
630. Lieber CS. To drink (moderately) or not to drink. N Engl J Med 1984; 310:846.
631. Henrich JB, Horwitz RI. Evidence against the association between alcohol use and ischemic stroke risk. Arch Intern Med 1989; 149:1413.
632. Editorial. Alcohol and hemorrhagic stroke. Lancet 1986; 2:256.
633. Monforte R, Estruch R, Graus F, et al. High ethanol consumption as risk factor for intracerebral hemorrhage in young and middle-aged people. Stroke 1990; 21:1529.
634. Donahue RB, Abbott RD. Alcohol and hemorrhagic stroke. Lancet 1986; 2:515.
635. Palomaki H, Kaste M. Does light to moderate consumption of alcohol protect against ischemic brain infarction? Stroke 1991; 22:2.
635a. Ben-Shlomo Y, Markowe H, Shipley M, Marmot MG. Stroke risk from alcohol consumption using different control groups. Stroke 1992; 23:1093.
636. Korarevic DJ, Vodvodic N, Gordon T, et al. Drinking habits and death: the Yugoslavia Cardiovascular Disease Study. Int J Epidemiol 1983; 12:145.
637. Donahue RP, Abbott RD, Reed DM, Yano K. Alcohol and hemorrhagic stroke: the Honolulu Heart Study. JAMA 1986; 255:2311.
638. Kagan A, Popper JS, Rhoads GG, Yano K. Dietary and other risk factors for stroke in Hawaiian Japanese men. Stroke 1985; 16:390.

639. Tayeka Y, Popper JS, Shimizu Y, et al. Epidemiologic studies of coronary heart disease and stroke in Japanese men living in Japan, Hawaii, and California: incidence of stroke in Japan and Hawaii. Stroke 1984; 15:15.
640. Wolf PA, Kannel WB, Verter J. Current status of risk factors for stroke. In Barnett HJM, (ed.): Cerebrovascular Disease, Neurologic Clinics Vol 1. Cerebrovascular Disease. Philadelphia, WB Saunders 1983:317.
641. Gordon T, Kannel WB. Drinking habits and cardiovascular disease: the Framingham Study. Am Heart J 1983; 105:667.
642. Kannel WB. Current status of the epidemiology of brain infarction associated with occlusive arterial disease. Stroke 1971; 2:295.
643. Kannel WB, Woosley P. Alcohol and cardiovascular risk. Circulation 1975; 52(suppl 2):200.
644. Kannel WB, Wolf PA, Dawber TR. An evaluation of the epidemiology of atherothrombotic brain infarction. Milbank Memorial Fund Q 1975; 53:405.
645. Wolf PA, D'Agostino RB, Odell P, et al. Alcohol consumption as a risk factor for stroke: the Framingham Study. Ann Neurol 1988; 24:177.
646. Stamfer MJ, Coditz GA, Willett WC, et al. A prospective study of moderate alcohol consumption and the risk of coronary disease and stroke in women. N Engl J Med 1988; 319:267.
647. Bogousslavsky J, Van Melle G, Despland PA, Regli F. Alcohol consumption and carotid atherosclerosis in the Lausanne Stroke Registry. Stroke 1990; 21:715.
648. Katsuki S. Hisayama study. Jpn J Med 1971; 10:167.
649. Ueda K, Hasuo Y, Kiyohara Y, et al. Hisayama: incidence, changing pattern during long-term follow-up, and related factors. Stroke 1988; 19:48.
650. Kono S, Ikeda M, Ogata M, et al. The relationship between alcohol and mortality among Japanese physicians. Int J Epidemiol 1983; 12:437.
651. Kono S, Ikeda M, Tokudome S, et al. Alcohol and mortality. A cohort study of male Japanese physicians. Int J Epidemiol 1986; 15:527.
652. Tanaka H, Ueda Y, Hayashi M, et al. Risk factors for cerebral hemorrhage and cerebral infarction in a Japanese rural community. Stroke 1992; 13:62.
653. Tanaka H, Hayashi M, Date C, et al. Epidemiologic studies of stroke in Shibata, a Japanese provincial city: preliminary report on risk factors for cerebral infarction. Stroke 1985; 16:773.
654. Camargo CA. Moderate alcohol consumption and stroke. The epidemiologic evidence. Stroke 1989; 20:1611.
655. Russel M, Cooper ML, Frone M, et al. Drinking patterns and blood pressure. Am J Epidemiol 1988; 128:917.
656. Klatsky AL, Friedman GD, Seigelaub AB, et al. Alcohol consumption and blood pressure. Kaiser-Permanente Multiphasic Health Examination data. N Engl J Med 1977; 296:1194.
657. MacMahon SW. Alcohol consumption and hypertension. Hypertension 1987; 9:111.
658. MacMahon SW, Norton RN. Alcohol and hypertension: implications for prevention and treatment. Ann Intern Med 1986; 105:124.
659. Gorelick PB. Alcohol and stroke. Stroke 1987; 18:268.
660. Longstreth WT, Koepsell TD, Yerby MS, van Belle G. Risk factors for subarachnoid hemorrhage. Stroke 1985; 16:377.
661. Camargo CA, Williams PT, Vranizan KM, et al. The effect of moderate alcohol intake on serum apolipoproteins A-I and A-II: a controlled study. JAMA 1985; 253:2854.
662. Haskell WJ, Camargo C, Williams PT, et al. The effect of cessation and resumption of moderate alcohol intake on serum high-density lipoprotein subfractions. A controlled study. N Engl J Med 1984; 310:805.
663. Reed DM, Resch JA, Hayashi T, et al. A prospective study of cerebral artery atherosclerosis. Stroke 1988; 19:820.
664. Avogaro P, Cazzolato G, Belussi F, Bittolo Bon G. Altered apoprotein composition of HDL-2 and HDL-3 in chronic alcoholics. Artery 1982; 10:317.
665. Gorelick PB. The status of alcohol as a risk factor for stroke. Stroke 1989; 20:1607.
666. Hillbom M, Kaste M, Rasi V. Can ethanol intoxication affect hemocoagulation to increase the risk of brain infarction in young adults? Neurology 1983; 33:381.
667. Lee K, Neilsen JD, Zeeberg I, Gormasen J. Platelet aggregation and fibrinolytic activity in young alcoholics. Acta Neurol Scand 1980; 621:287.
668. Hillbom M, Kangasaho M, Kaste M, et al. Acute ethanol ingestion increases platelet reactivity. Is there a relationship to stroke? Stroke 1985; 16:19.
669. Lang WE. Ethyl alcohol enhances plasminogen activator secretion by endothelial cells. JAMA 1983; 250:772.
670. Jakubowski JA, Vailloncourt R, Deykin D. Interaction of ethanol, prostacyclin, and aspirin in determining human platelet reactivity in vitro. Arteriosclerosis 1988; 8:436.
671. Landolfi R, Steiner M. Ethanol raises prostacyclin in vivo and in vitro. Blood 1984; 64:679.
672. Fenn CG, Littleton JM. Inhibition of platelet aggregation by ethanol: the role of plasma and platelet membrane lipids. Br J Pharmacol 1981; 73:305P.
673. Haut MJ, Cowan DH. The effect of ethanol on hemostatic properties of human blood platelets. Am J Med 1974; 56:22.
674. Kangasaho M, Hillbom M, Kaste M, Vapaatolo H. Effects of ethanol intoxication and hangover on plasma levels of thromboxane B-2 formation by platelets in man. Thromb Haemostat 1982; 48:232.
675. Mikhailidis DP, Barradas MA, Jeremy JY. The effect of ethanol on platelet function and vascular prostanoids. Alcohol 1990; 7:171.
676. Haselager EM, Vreeken J. Rebound thrombocytosis after alcohol abuse: a possible factor in the pathogenesis of thromboembolic disease. Lancet 1977; 1:774.

677. Hutton RA, Fink FR, Wilson DT, Margot DH. Platelet hyperaggregability during alcohol withdrawal. Clin Lab Haematol 1981; 3:223.

678. Neiman J, Rand ML, Jakowec DM, Packham MA. Platelet responses to platelet-activating factor are inhibited in alcoholics undergoing alcohol withdrawal. Thromb Res 1989; 56:399.

679. McQueen JD, Sklar FK, Posey JB. Autoregulation of cerebral blood flow during alcohol infusion. J Stud Alcohol 1978; 39:1477.

680. Weiss MH, Craig JR. The influence of acute ethanol intoxication on intracranial physical dynamics. Bull Los Angeles Neurol Soc 1978; 43:1.

681. Persson LI, Rosengren LE, Johansson BB, Hansson HA. Blood brain barrier dysfunction to peroxidase after air embolism, aggravated by acute ethanol intoxication. J Neurol Sci 1979; 42:65.

682. Wilkins MR, Kendall MJ. Stroke affecting young men after alcoholic binges. BMJ 1985; 291:1342.

683. Berglund M. Cerebral blood flow in chronic alcoholics. Alcoholism Clin Exp Res 1981; 5:295.

684. Altura BM, Altura BT, Gebrewold A. Alcohol-induced spasms of cerebral blood vessels. Relations to cerebrovascular accidents and sudden death. Science 1983; 220:331.

685. Swanson TH, Zinkel JL, Peterson PL. Bilateral anterior cerebral artery occlusion in an alcohol abuser with sickle-cell trait. Henry Ford Hosp Med J 1987; 35:67.

686. Warner R, Rosett H. The effects of drinking on offspring: an historical survey of the American and British literature. J Stud Alcohol 1975; 36:1395.

687. Sullivan WC. A note on the influence of materal inebriety on offspring. J Ment Sci 1988; 43:489.

688. Lemoine P, Harousseau H, Borteyru JP, et al. Les enfants de parents alcooliques: anomalies observees. Ouest Med 1968; 25:476.

689. Jones K, Smith DW. Recognition of the fetal alcohol syndrome in early infancy. Lancet 1973; 2:999.

690. Colangelo W, Jones DG. The fetal alcohol syndrome: a review and assessment of the syndrome and its neurological sequelae. Prog Neurobiol 1982; 19:271.

691. Hanson JW, Jones KL, Smith DW. Fetal alcohol syndrome. Experience with 41 patients. JAMA 1976; 235:1458.

692. Day NL, Jasperse D, Richardson G, et al. Prenatal exposure to alcohol: effect on infant growth and morphologic characteristics. Pediatrics 1989; 84:536.

693. Streissguth AP. Psychologic handicaps in children with fetal alcohol syndrome. NY Acad Sci 1976; 273:140.

694. Fetal alcohol syndrome. In: Hurley J. Horowitz J. Alcohol and Health. New York: Hemisphere Publishing Corp, 1987:80.

695. Ouelette EM, Rosett HL, Rosman NP, et al. Adverse effects on offspring of maternal alcohol abuse during pregnancy. N Engl J Med 1977; 297:528.

696. Chernoff GF. The fetal alcohol syndrome in mice: an animal model. Teratology 1977; 15:223.

697. Kaminski M, Rumeau-Rouquette C, Schwartz D. Effects of alcohol on the fetus. N Engl J Med 1978; 298:55.

698. Streissguth AP, Martin DC, Barr HM, et al. Intrauterine alcohol and nicotine exposure: attention and reaction time in 4-year-old children. Dev Psychol 1984; 20:533.

699. Streissguth AP, Barr HM, Sampson PD, et al. Attention, distraction, and reaction time at age 7 years and prenatal alcohol exposure. Neurobehav Toxicol Teratol 1986; 8:717.

700. Bray PF. Can maternal alcoholism cause spasmus nutans in offspring? N Engl J Med 1990; 322:554.

701. Clarren SK, Smith DW. The fetal alcohol syndrome. N Engl J Med 1978; 298:1063.

702. Pierog S, Chandavasu O, Wexler I. Withdrawal symptoms in infants with the fetal alcohol syndrome. J Pediatr 1977; 90:630.

703. Streissguth AP, Herman CS, Smith DW. Intelligence, behavior and dysmorphogenesis in the fetal alcohol syndrome: a report on 20 patients. J Pediatr 1978; 92:363.

704. Streissguth AP, Clarren SK, Jones KL. Natural history of the fetal alcohol syndrome: a ten-year follow-up of eleven patients. Lancet 1985; 2:85.

704a. Lemoine P, Lemoine P. Avenir des enfants de meres alcooliques (etude de 105 cas retrouves a l'age adult) et quelques constatations d'interet prophylactique. Ann Pediatr 1992; 29:226.

705. Chernoff GF. The fetal alcohol syndrome in mice: maternal variables. Teratology 1980; 22:71.

706. Mukherjee AB, Hodgen GD. Maternal ethanol exposure induces transient impairment of umbilical circulation and fetal hypoxia in monkeys. Science 1982; 218:700.

707. Ellis FW, Pick JR. An animal model of the fetal alcohol syndrome in beagles. Alcoholism Clin Exp Res 1980; 4:123.

708. Dexter JD, Tumbleson ME, Decker JD, et al. Fetal alcohol syndrome in Sinclair (S-1) miniature swine. Alcoholism Clin Exp Res 1980; 4:146.

709. Clarren SK, Bowden DM. Fetal alcohol syndrome: a new primate model for binge drinking and its relevance to human ethanol teratogenesis. J Pediatr 1982; 101:819.

710. Altshuler HL, Shippenberg TS. A subhuman primate model for fetal alcohol syndrome research. Neurobehav Toxicol Teratol 1981; 3:121.

711. Tze WJ, Lee M. Adverse effects of maternal alcohol consumption on pregnancy and fetal growth in rats. Nature 1975; 257:479.

712. Abel EL, Dintcheff BA. Effect of prenatal alcohol exposure on growth and development in rats. J Pharmacol Exp Ther 1978; 207:916.

713. Riley EP, Lochry EA, Shapiro NR. Lack of response inhibition in rats prenatally exposed to alcohol. Psychopharmacology 1979; 62:47.

714. Yanai J, Ginsburg BE. Audiogenic seizures in mice whose parents drank alcohol. J Stud Alcohol 1976; 37:1564.

715. Ellis RW, Pick JR. Beagle model of the fetal alcohol syndrome. Pharmacologist 1976; 18:190.

716. Clarren SK, Bowden DM. Measures of alcohol damage in utero in the pigtailed Macaque (Macaca nemestrina). In: Porter R, O'Conner M, Whelan J, eds. Mechanisms of Alcohol Damage in Utero. London: Pittman Publishing Ltd, 1984:157.

717. Sulik KK, Lauder JM, Dehart DB. Brain malformations in prenatal mice following acute maternal ethanol administration. Int J Dev Neurosci 1984; 2:203.

718. McGivern RF, Clancy AN, Hill MA, Noble EP. Prenatal alcohol exposure alters adult expression of sexually dimorphic behavior in the rat. Science 1984; 224:896.

719. Abel EL, Hazlett LS, Berk RS, Mutchnick MG. Neuro-immunotoxic effects in offspring of paternal alcohol consumption. In: Seminara D, Watson RR, Pawlowski A, eds. Alcohol, Immunomodulation, and AIDS. New York: Alan R. Liss, 1990:47.

720. Seppala M, Raiha NC, Tamminen V. Ethanol elimination in a mother and her premature twins. Lancet 1971; 2:1188.

721. Sander LW, Snyder PA, Rosett HL, et al. Effects of alcohol intake during pregnancy in newborn state regulation: a progress report. Alcoholism Clin Exp Res 1977; 1:233.

722. Halmesmaki E, Valimaki M, Karonen SL, Ylikorkala O. Low somatomedin C and high growth hormone levels in newborns damaged by maternal alcohol abuse. Obstet Gynecol 1989; 74:366.

723. Bonthuis DJ, West JR. Alcohol-induced neuronal loss in developing rats: increased brain damage with binge exposure. Alcoholism Clin Exp Res 1990; 14:107.

724. Altura BM, Altura BT, Corella A, et al. Alcohol produces spasms of human umbilical vessels: relationship to FAS. Eur J Pharmacol 1982; 86:311.

725. Wisniewski K. A clinical neuropathological study of the fetal alcohol syndrome. Neuropediatrics 1983; 14:197.

726. Mukherjee AB, Hodgen GD. Maternal ethanol exposure induces transient impairment of umbilical circulation and fetal hypoxia in monkeys. Science 1982; 218:700.

727. Mann LI, Bhakthavathsalan A, Liu M, et al. Placental transport of alcohol and its effect on maternal acid-base balance. Am J Obstet Gynecol 1975; 122:837.

728. Mann LT, Bhakkthavathsalan A, Liu M, et al. Effect of alcohol on fetal cerebral function and metabolism. Am J Obstet Gynecol 1975; 122:845.

729. Horiguchi T, Suzuki K, Comas-Urrutia AC. Effect of ethanol upon uterine activity and fetal acid-base state of the rhesus monkey. Am J Obstet Gynecol 1971; 109:910.

730. Phillips SG, Gragg BG. Alcohol withdrawal causes a loss of cerebellar Purkinje cells in mice. J Stud Alcohol 1984; 45:475.

731. Hemmingsen R, Jorgensen OS. Specific brain proteins during severe ethanol intoxication and withdrawal in the rat. Psychiatr Res 1980; 3:1.

732. Samson HA, Grant KA, Coggan S, Sachs VM. Ethanol induced microcephaly in the neonatal rat: occurrence without withdrawal. Neurobehav Toxicol Teratol 1982; 4:115.

733. O'Shea KS, Kaufman MH. The teratogenic effect of acetaldehyde: implications of the study of the fetal alcohol syndrome. J Anat 1979; 128:65.

734. Dow KE, Riopelle RI. Ethanol neurotoxicity: effects on neurite formation and neurotrophic factor production in vitro. Science 1985; 228:591.

735. Fisher SE, Atkinson M, Jacobson M, et al. Selective fetal malnutrition. The effect of in vivo ethanol exposure upon in vitro placental uptake of amino acids in the non-human primate. Pediatr Res 1983; 17:704.

736. Snyder AK, Singh SP, Pullen GL. Ethanol-induced intrauterine growth retardation: correlation with placental glucose transfer. Alcoholism 1986; 10:167.

737. Fisher SE, Duffy L, Atkinson M. Selective fetal malnutrition: effect of acute and chronic ethanol exposure upon rat placental Na,K-ATPase activity. Alcoholism 1986; 10:150.

738. Kaufman MH. Ethanol-induced chromosomal abnormalities at conception. Nature 1983; 302:258.

739. Gardner LI, Mitter N, Coplan J, et al. Isochromosome 9q in an infant exposed to ethanol prenatally. N Engl J Med 1985; 312:1521.

740. Little RE, Sing CF. Association of father's drinking and infant's birth weight. N Engl J Med 1986; 314:1644.

741. Randall CL, Anton RF. Aspirin reduced alcohol-induced prenatal mortality and malformations in mice. Alcoholism Clin Exp Res 1984; 8:513.

742. Ernhart CB, Sokol RJ, Ager JW, et al. Alcohol-related birth defects: assessing the risk. Ann NY Acad Sci 1989; 562:159.

743. Wright JT, Barrison IG, Waterson EJ, et al. Alcohol consumption, pregnancy, and low birthweight. Lancet 1983; 1:663.

744. Day NL, Jasperse D, Richardson G, et al. Prenatal exposure to alcohol: effect on infant growth and morphologic characteristics. Pediatrics 1989; 84:536.

745. Graham JM, Hansen JW, Darby BL, et al. Independent dysmorphology evaluations at birth and 4 years of age for children exposed to varying amounts of alcohol in utero. Pediatrics 1988; 81:772.

746. Ioffe S, Chernick V. Development of the EEG between 30 and 40 weeks gestation in normal and alcohol-exposed infants. Dev Med Child Neurol 1988; 30:797.

747. Streissguth AP, Martin DC, Barr HM. Maternal alcohol use and neonatal habituation assessed with the Brazelton Scale. Child Dev 1983; 54:1109.

748. Ernhart CH, Wolf AW, Linn PL, et al. Alcohol-related birth defects: syndromal anomalies, intrauterine growth retardation, and neonatal behavioral assessment. Alcoholism Clin Exp Res 1985; 9:447.

749. Mills JL, Graubard BI, Harley EE, et al. Maternal alcohol consumption and birthweight: how much drinking during pregnancy is safe? JAMA 1984; 252:1875.

750. Little RE, Asker RL, Sampson PD, et al. Fetal growth and moderate drinking in early pregnancy. Am J Epidemiol 1986; 123:270.

751. Sulik K, Johnston MS, Webb MA. Fetal alcohol syndrome: embryogenesis in a mouse model. Science 1981; 214:936.

752. Morrow-Tlucak M, Ernhart CB, Soko RJ, et al. Underreporting of alcohol use in pregnancy: relationship to alcohol problem history. Alcoholism 1989; 13:399.

753. Marbury MC, Linn S, Monson R, et al. The association of alcohol consumption with outcome of pregnancy. Am J Publ Health 1983; 73:1165.

754. Tennes K, Blackard C. Maternal alcohol consumption, birthweight, and minor physical anomalies. Am J Obstet Gynecol 1980; 138:774.

755. Hingson R, Alpert JJ, Day N, et al. Effects of maternal drinking and marijuana use on fetal growth and development. Pediatrics 1982; 70:539.

756. Grisso JA, Roman E, Inskip H, et al. Alcohol consumption and outcome of pregnancy. J Epidemiol Commun Health 1984; 38:232.

757. Zuckerman B, Frank DA, Hingson R, et al. Effects of maternal marijuana and cocaine use on fetal growth. N Engl J Med 1989; 320:762.

758. Alpert J, Zuckerman B. High blood alcohol levels in women. N Engl J Med 1990; 323:60.

759. Mennella JA, Beauchamp GK. The transfer of alcohol to human milk—effects on flavor and the infant's behavior. N Engl J Med 1991; 325:981.

760. Little RE, Anderson KW, Ervin CH, et al. Maternal alcohol use during breast feeding and infant mental and motor development at one year. N Engl J Med 1989; 321:425.

761. Lindmark B. Maternal use of alcohol and breast-fed infants. N Engl J Med 1990; 322:338.

762. Little RE. Maternal use of alcohol and breast-fed infants. N Engl J Med 1990; 322:339.

763. Litovitz T. The alcohols: ethanol, methanol, isopropanol, ethylene glycol. Pediatr Clin North Am 33; 311:1986.

764. Goldfrank LR, Flomenbaum NE, Lewin NA, Howland MA. Methanol, ethylene glycol, and isopropanol. In: Goldfrank LR, Flomenbaum NE, Lewin NA, et al, eds. Toxicologic Emergencies, ed 4. Norwalk, CT: Appleton & Lange, 1990:481.

765. Bennett IL, Cary FH, Mitchell GL. Acute methyl alcohol poisoning: review based on experiences in outbreak of 323 cases. Medicine 1953; 32:431.

766. Swartz RD, Millman RP, Billi JE, et al. Epidemic methanol poisoning: clinical and biochemical analysis of a recent episode. Medicine 60; 373:1981.

767. Klaassen CD. Nonmetallic environmental toxicants; air pollutants, solvents and vapors, and pesticides. In: Gilman AG, Rall TW, Nies AS, Taylor P, eds. The Pharmacological Basis of Therapeutics, ed 8. New York: Pergamon Press, 1990:1615.

768. Sejeersted OM, Jacobsen D, Ovrebo S, et al. Formate concentrations in plasma from patients poisoned with methanol. Acta Med Scand 213; 105:1983.

769. Jacobsen D, McMartin KE. Methanol and ethylene glycol poisonings: mechanism of toxicity, clinical course, diagnosis, and treatment. Med Toxicol 1986; 1:309.

770. Guggenheim MA, Couch JR, Weinberg W. Motor dysfunction as a permanent complication of methanol ingestion. Arch Neurol 1971; 24:550.

771. Ley CO, Gali FG. Parkinsonian syndrome after methanol intoxication. Eur Neurol 1983; 22:405.

772. LeWitt PA, Martin SD. Dystonia and hypokinesis with putaminal necrosis after methanol intoxication. Clin Neuropharmacol 1988; 11:161.

773. McLean DR, Jacobs H, Mielke BW. Methanol poisoning: a clinical and pathological study. Ann Neurol 1980; 8:161.

774. Gabow PA, Clay K, Sullivan JB, Lepoff R. Organic acids in ethylene glycol intoxication. Ann Intern Med 1986; 105:16.

775. Spillane L, Roberts JR, Meyer AE. Multiple cranial nerve deficits after ethylene glycol poisoning. Ann Emerg Med 1991; 20:208.

776. Peterson CD, Collins AJ, Himes JM, et al. Ethylene glycol poisoning: pharmacokinetics during therapy with ethanol and hemodialysis. N Engl J Med 1981; 304:21.

777. Baud FJ, Galliot M, Astier A, et al. Treatment of ethylene glycol poisoning with intravenous 4-methylpyrazole. N Engl J Med 1988; 319:97.

778. Lacouture PG, Watson S, Abrams A, et al. Acute isopropyl alcohol intoxication: diagnosis and management. Am J Med 1983; 75:680.

779. Hasin DS, Grant BF, Dufour MG, Endicott J. Alcohol problems increase while physician attention declines. 1967 to 1984. Arch Intern Med 1990; 150:397.

780. Pattison EM. The selection of treatment modalities for the alcoholic patient. In: Mendelson JH, Mello NK, eds. The Diagnosis and Treatment of Alcoholism. New York: McGraw-Hill, 1979:125.

781. Klerman GL. Treatment of alcoholism. N Engl J Med 1989; 320:395.

782. Hesselbrock MH, Eyer RE, Keener JJ. Psychopathology in hospitalized alcoholics. Arch Gen Psychiatry 1985; 42:1050.

783. Schukit MA. The clinical implications of primary diagnostic groups among alcoholics. Arch Gen Psychiatry 1985; 42:1043.

784. Halikas JA, Herzog MA, Mirassou MM, Lyttle MD. Psychiatric diagnoses among female alcoholics. In: Galanter M, ed. Currents in Alcoholism, Vol VIII. New York: Grune & Stratton, 1983:283.

785. Holden C. Is alcoholism a disease? Science 1987; 238:1647.

786. Becker JT, Jaffe JH. Impaired memory for treatment-relevant information in in-patient men alcoholics. J Stud Alcohol 1984; 45:339.

787. Schukit MA, Schuei MG, Gold E. Prediction of outcome in inpatient alcoholics. J Stud Alcohol 1986; 47:151.

788. Finney JW, Moss RH. Matching patients with treatments: conceptual and methodological issues. J Stud Alcohol 1986; 47:122.

789. Ciraulo DA, Sands BF, Shader RI. Critical review of liability for benzodiazepine abuse among alcoholics. Am J Psychiatry 1988; 145:1501.

790. Linnoila MI. Benzodiazepines and alcohol. J Psychiatr Res 1990; 24(suppl 2):121.

791. Hollister LE. Interactions between alcohol and benzodiazepines. Rec Dev Alcohol 1989; 7:233.

792. Kissin B. The use of psychoactive drugs in the long-term treatment of chronic alcoholism. Ann NY Acad Sci 1975; 252:385.

793. Rosenberg CM. Drug maintenance in the outpatient treatment of chronic alcoholism. Arch Gen Psychiatry 1974; 30:373.

794. Johnstone EC, Owens DGC, Frith DC, et al. Neurotic illness and its response to anxiolytic and antidepressant treatment. Psychol Med 1980; 10:321.

795. Bruno F. Buspirone in the treatment of alcoholic patients. Psychopathology 1989; 22(suppl 1):49.

796. Kranzler HR, Meyer RE. An open trial of buspirone in alcoholics. J Clin Psychopharmacol 1989; 9:379.

797. Rickels K, Chung HR, Csanalos IB, et al. Alprazolam, diazepam, imipramine, placebo in outpatients with general depression. Arch Gen Psychiatry 1987; 44:862.

798. Barbee JG, Clark PD, Carpanzano MS, et al. Alcohol and substance abuse among schizophrenic patients presenting to an emergency psychiatric service. J Nerv Ment Dis 1989; 177:400.

799. Becker CE. Pharmacotherapy in the treatment of alcoholism. In: Mendelson JH, Mello NK, eds. The Diagnosis and Treatment of Alcoholism. New York: McGraw-Hill, 1979:283.

800. Kitson TM. The disulfiram-ethanol reaction. A review. J Stud Alcohol 1977; 38:96.

801. Wright C, Moore RD. Disulfiram treatment of alcoholism. Am J Med 1990; 88:647.

802. Fisher DM. "Catatonia" due to disulfiram toxicity. Arch Neurol 1989; 46:798.

803. Goldfrank LR, Brensnitz EA, Melinek M, Weisman RS. Disulfiram. In: Goldfrank LR, Fromenbaum NE, Lewin NA, et al, eds. Toxicologic Emergencies, ed 4. Norwalk, CT: Appleton & Lange, 1990:475.

804. Sellers EM, Naranjo CA, Peachey JE. Drugs to decrease alcohol consumption. N Engl J Med 1981; 305:1255.

805. Treatment. In: Hurley J, Horowitz J, eds. Alcohol and Health. New York: Hemisphere Publishing, 1987:120.

806. Fuller RK, Roth HP. Disulfiram for the treatment of alcoholism: an evaluation of 128 men. Ann Intern Med 1979; 90:901.

807. Fuller RK, Branchey L, Brightwell DR, et al. Disulfiram treatment of alcoholism. A Veteran's Administration Cooperative Study. JAMA 1986; 256:1449.

808. Tennant FS. Disulfiram will reduce medical complications but not cure alcoholism. JAMA 1986; 256:1489.

809. Schukit MA. A one-year follow-up of men given disulfiram. J Stud Alcohol 1985; 46:191.

810. American College of Physicians: Disulfiram treatment of alcoholism. Ann Intern Med 1989; 111:943.

811. Palliyath SK, Schwartz BD, Gant L. Peripheral nerve functions in chronic alcoholic patients on disulfiram: a six-month follow-up. J Neurol Neurosurg Psychiatry 1990; 53:227.

812. Hotson JR, Langston JW. Disulfiram-induced encephalopathy. Arch Neurol 1976; 33:141.

813. Sans P, Deneux A, Magne C, et al. Neurologic complications due to disulfiram. Neuropathies, encephalopathies. Concours Med 1975; 97:3773.

814. Wilson A, Davidson WJ, Blanchard R, White J. Disulfiram implantation: trial using placebo implants and two types of controls. J Stud Alcohol 1980; 41:429.

815. Peachey JE, Annis HM, Bornstein ER, et al. Calcium carbimide in alcoholism treatment. Part 2: medical findings of a short-term, placebo-controlled, double-blind clinical trial. Br J Addict 1989; 84:1359.

816. Scott GE, Little FW. Disulfiram reaction to organic solvents other than ethanol. N Engl J Med 1985; 313:790.

817. Barna P. Alcohol in anti-asthma elixers. Lancet 1985; 1:753.

818. Kline NS, Wren JC, Cooper TB, et al. Evaluation of lithium therapy in chronic and periodic alcoholism. Am J Med Sci 1974; 268:15.

819. Ho AK, Tsai CS. Effects of lithium on alcohol preference and withdrawal. Ann NY Acad Sci 1976; 273:371.

820. Dorus W, Ostow DG, Anton R, et al. Lithium treatment of depressed and non-depressed alcoholics. JAMA 1989; 262:1646.

821. de la Fuente J-R, Morse RM, Niven RG, Ilstrup DM. A controlled study of lithium carbonate in the treatment of alcoholism. Mayo Clin Proc 1989; 64:177.

822. Buydens-Branchey L, Branchey MH, Nomair D, Lieber CS. Age of alcoholism onset. 2. Relationship of susceptibility to serotonin precurser availability. Arch Gen Psychiatry 1989; 46:231.

823. Gorelick DA. Serotonin uptake blockers and the treatment of alcoholism. Rec Dev Alcohol 1989; 7:267.

824. Gill K, Amit Z. Serotonin uptake blockers and voluntary alcohol consumption. A review of recent studies. Rec Dev Alcohol 1989; 7:225.

825. Naranjo CA, Sellers EM, Sullivan JT, et al. The serotonin uptake inhibitor citalopram attenuates alcohol intake. Clin Pharmacol Ther 1987; 41:266.

826. Naranjo CA, Sellers EM, Roach CA, et al. Zimelidine-induced variations in alcohol intake by non-depressed heavy drinkers. Clin Pharmacol Ther 1984; 35:374.

827. Naranjo CA, Kadlec KE, Sanhueza P, et al. Fluoxetine differentially alters alcohol intake and other consummatory behaviors in problem drinkers. Clin Pharmacol Ther 1990; 47:490.

828. Fadda F, Franch F, Mosca E, et al. Inhibition of voluntary ethanol intake in rats by a combination of dihydroergotoxine and thioridazine. Alcohol Drug Res 1987; 7;285.

829. Blum K. Suppression of alcohol craving by enkephalinase inhibition: a new opportunity in clinical treatment. Alcohol Drug Res 1987; 7:122.

830. Siegel S. Alcohol and opiate dependence: reevaluation of the Victorian perspective. In: Cappell HD, Glaser FB, Isreal Y, et al, eds. Research Advances in Alcohol and Drug Problems, Vol 9. New York: Plenum Press, 1986:279.

831. Sinclair JD. the feasibility of effective psychopharmacological treatments for alcoholism. Br J Addict 1987; 82:1213.

832. Myers RD, Borg S, Mossberg R. Antagonism by naltrexone of voluntary alcohol selection in the chronically drinking macaque monkey. Alcohol 1986; 3:383.

833. Volpicelli JR, Alterman A, Hayashida M, et al. Naltrexone in the treatment of alcohol dependence: intial findings. In: Reid LB, ed. Opioids, Bulimia, Alcohol, and Alcoholism. New York: Springer-Verlag, 1989:195.

834. Classics of the alcohol literature: the first American medical work on the effects of alcohol: Benjamin Rush's "An inquiry into the effects of ardent spirits upon the human body and mind." (1795). QJ Stud Alcohol 1943; 4:321.

835. Trice HM, Staudenmeier WJ. A sociocultural history of Alcoholics Anonymous. Rec Dev Alcohol 1989; 7:11.

836. Ogborne AC. Some limitations of Alcoholics Anonymous. Rec Dev Alcohol 1989; 7:55.

837. Emrick CD. Alcoholics Anonymous: membership characteristics and effectiveness as treatment. Rec Dev Alcohol 1989; 7:37.

838. Bullock ML, Culliton PD, Olander RT. Controlled trial of acupuncture for severe recidivist alcoholism. Lancet 1989; 1:1435.

839. Editorial. Many points to needle. Lancet 1990; 1:20.

840. Ter Riet G, Kleijnen J, Knipschild P. De effectiviteit van acupunctuur: de meta analyse als reviewmethode. Huisarts Wet 1989; 32:176.

841. Goodwin DW. Inpatient treatment of alcoholism—new life for the Minneapolis plan. N Engl J Med 1991; 325:804.

842. Walsh DC, Hingson RW, Merrigan DM, et al. A randomized trial of treatment options for alcohol-abusing workers. N Engl J Med 1991; 325:775.

843. Sobell MB, Sobell LC. Second year treatment outcome of alcoholics treated by individualized behavior therapy: results. Behav Res Ther 1976; 14:195.

844. Helzer JE, Robins LN, Taylor JR, et al. The extent of long-term moderate drinking among alcoholics discharged from medical and psychiatric treatment facilities. N Engl J Med 1985; 312:1678.

845. Kissin B, Hanson M. Integrations of biological and psychological interventions in the treatment of alcoholism. In: McCrady BS, Noel NE, Nirenberg TD, eds. Future Directions in Alcohol Abuse Treatment and Research. Washington, DC: DHHS Publication No. (ADM) 85-1322, US Government Printing Office, 1988:63.

846. Pendery ML, Maltzman IM, West LJ. Controlled drinking by alcoholics: new findings and a reevaluation of a major affirmative study. Science 1982; 217:169.

847. Kanaka TS, Balasubramaniam V. Sterotactic cingulotomy for drug addiction. Appl Neurophysiol 1978; 41:86.

848. Dieckman G, Schneider H. Influence of stereotactic hypothalamotomy on alcohol and drug addiction. Appl Neurophysiol 1978; 41:93.

849. Schottenfeld RS. Drug and alcohol testing in the workplace—objectives, pitfalls, and guidelines. Am J Drug Alcohol Abuse 1989; 15:413.

850. Isikoff M. The nation's alcohol problem is falling through the crack. Washington Post National Weekly Edition, April 9, 1990:30.

851. Korpi ER, Kleingoor C, Kettenmann H, Seeburg PH. Benzodiazepine-induced motor impairment linked to point mutation in cerebellar GABA-A receptor. Nature 1993; 361:356.

Chapter 12
Tobacco

The use of tobacco is growing greatly and conquers men with a certain secret pleasure, so that those who have become accustomed thereto can later hardly be restrained therefrom.
—Sir Francis Bacon, Historia vitae et mortis (1623)

For thy sake, tobacco, I
Would do anything but die.
—Charles Lamb

Each year, more than 400,000 Americans die as a consequence of cigarette smoking. Put another way, tobacco kills more than 1,000 Americans every day. Or, put another way, tobacco accounts for 20% to 25% of all American mortality (compared with 5% for ethanol and less than 3% for all the other drugs discussed in this book).[1-6] Amidst such carnage, most Americans who smoke claim they would stop if they could. There is no question therefore that tobacco is addicting. It is also evident that the addictive substance in tobacco is nicotine (Figure 12–1).[7-9]

Pharmacology and Animal Studies

Nicotine's pharmacological actions are biphasic: low doses stimulate nicotinic receptors, and higher doses block them. Acting both peripherally and centrally, nicotine produces complex effects. For example, heart rate may be either increased or decreased depending on actions at sympathetic and parasympathetic ganglia, carotid and aortic bodies, medullary centers, and the adrenal as well as on compensatory reflexes.[10] Central nervous system (CNS) stimulation causes tremor or seizures; CNS depression causes respiratory failure. An alerting response in the electroencephalogram may be accompanied by decreased muscle tone and reduced amplitude in the electromyogram.

In rats, dogs, and monkeys, high doses of nicotine depress locomotion, often with ataxia.[11] Low doses increase locomotion, and tolerance develops to the depressant effect of high doses but not to the stimulatory effect of low doses. Thus with chronic administration of high doses, increased locomotion emerges. In monkeys nicotine reduces aggression.[12] Nicotine improves the performance of rodents and primates on tasks involving memory, learning, and sustained attention.[13,14] In novices nicotine causes nausea and vomiting by stimulating vagal afferents and the medullary chemoreceptor trigger zone. It also reduces appetite, mainly for sweet-tasting foods; both decreased caloric intake and increased metabolic rate and energy expenditure contribute to weight loss.[15]

Nicotine acts as a discriminative stimulus in animals, generalizing to nicotinic agonists but not to other drugs of abuse (although partial generalization to amphetamine has been reported).[12,16] Place preference and self-administration studies in rats, dogs, and primates confirm that nicotine is reinforcing, although less so than cocaine.[12,16-20] Perhaps reflecting tolerance to nicotine's depressant effects, self-administration steadily increases during the first week of availability. Nicotine's reinforcing actions are blocked by the nicotinic receptor antagonist mecamylamine.[16] The varying degrees of tolerance to nicotine's effects appear to be more pharmacodynamic than dispositional. Withdrawal following chronic administration in animals produces impaired attention and task performance, slower electroencephalographic frequencies, and decreased heart rate

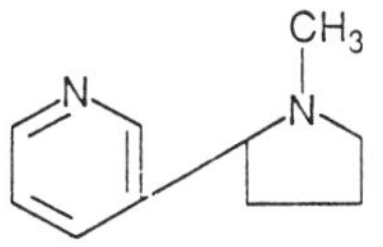

Figure 12–1. Nicotine.

and blood pressure. Monkeys display prominent jaw clenching.[12] However, a predictable prominent abstinence syndrome comparable to what follows opioid or barbiturate withdrawal does not occur.[20]

The pharmacological basis of nicotine's CNS effects—including reinforcement—is unknown.[14,16] Central nicotinic receptors differ from those found peripherally, and subtypes are based on combinations of different alpha and beta subunits.[21] Controversy exists over whether CNS receptors are stimulated or inhibited at smoking doses. Contrary to what would be expected, receptors are up-regulated by chronic exposure to nicotine.[16] Low doses of systemic nicotine release dopamine in the nucleus accumbens, as does direct injection of nicotine into the nucleus accumbens. Lesions of mesolimbic dopaminergic pathways reduce nicotinic receptors in terminal areas, consistent with a presynaptic location.[22] Nicotine injected into the ventral tegmental area (VTA) of rats increases locomotion, and the increased locomotion that follows systemic nicotine, as well as nicotine self-administration itself, is blocked by 6-hydroxydopamine lesions of the nucleus accumbens.[16,23] Dopamine antagonists attenuate nicotine discrimination and place preference.[16]

Nicotine stimulates release of vasopressin—perhaps related to its effects on memory. It also releases beta-endorphin.[24] In rats trained to respond in a fixed schedule of food presentation, nicotine increases responses, and naloxone blocks this effect.[25]

Historical Background and Epidemiology

Columbus and other New World explorers observed tobacco smoking by American Indians and brought the custom back to Europe. The compulsive nature of smoking was quickly recognized, and later world explorers not only carried tobacco with them but also planted it throughout the world. The tobacco plant was named *Nicotiana tabacum* in honor of Jean Nicot, an early importer.[9] Nicotine was isolated from the leaves in 1828, and in the mid-19th century new methods of cultivating and curing tobacco led to the invention of the cigarette.

The obviously addictive nature of tobacco led to early proscriptions. In the 17th century Pope Urban VII issued a bull against tobacco, and its use was banned in Bavaria, Saxony, and Zurich. In Constantinople tobacco smoking was punishable by death. Like other drug prohibitions, such efforts were to no avail.[26]

In the United States, public health campaigns against chewing tobacco (made from alkaline leaves, allowing easy absorption of nicotine through buccal mucosa) coincided with the rising popularity of cigarettes (made from acid leaves, requiring inhalation to accomplish nicotine absorption). In 1900, 4.2 billion cigarettes were produced; by 1970, the figure was 583 billion.[26] During the 1920s, several states banned the sale of cigarettes, but the futility of such laws led to their repeal by the end of the decade. In 1964 the first of a series of reports by the U.S. Surgeon General on the health consequences of smoking ushered in a steady 3-decade decline in the percentage of American adults who smoke: from two-thirds to less than one-third. In 1988, 91 million (52%) of Americans over 18 years of age were ever smokers, and 49 million (28%) were current smokers, including 31% of all men, 26% of all women, 32% of all blacks, and 28% of all whites.[27] Nineteen percent of high school seniors were regular smokers;[7] however, increasing numbers were using "smokeless tobacco"—chewing tobacco or snuff.[28] Smoking prevalence decreases with years of education. As nonsmokers have become a majority, they have succeeded in instituting educational campaigns, restrictions on advertising, warnings on packages, and banning of smoking on airplanes, in public buildings, and in the workplace.

In contrast to other substance abusers, the majority of smokers take their drug continuously or frequently throughout the day, every day, craving a cigarette soon after the last is finished, while quite aware of the health consequences. In 1985 U.S. direct health care costs of smoking were estimated at $16 billion, with indirect costs from lost productivity amounting to $37 billion.[3] The addiction liability of tobacco is aggravated by ready availability of cheap cigarettes, absence of overdose or impaired mental faculties, social acceptability, and the delay—up to decades—before the appearance of such complications as cancer, pulmonary disease, myocardial infarction, and stroke.

In 1993 the U.S. Environmental Protection Agency reported that second-hand tobacco smoke inhalation by non-smokers kills an estimated 3,000 Americans yearly and subjects thousands of children to respiratory disease; 20% of all lung cancers were attributed to indirect environmental tobacco smoke.[29]

Acute Effects

Smoking may be either stimulating or sedating depending on the setting and the subject's methods of titrating dosage. Smoking improves "speed and accuracy of information processing"[24] and long-term memory, reduces tension and anxiety, and increases pain threshold.[30] The usual response is arousal followed by relaxation, and smokers appear to adjust nicotine intake to favor one or the other phase. Overall, they increase or decrease their total smoking as the nicotine content of their cigarettes falls or rises.[31] Smokers do not usually describe alertness, relaxation, or euphoria as the motive for lighting a cigarette; rather the "taste of the cigarette" is perceived as the reason.[6] In fact, many smokers, while claiming inability to quit, report little or no "pleasure" in smoking.[32] On the other hand, nicotine given intravenously to smokers—but not nonsmokers—is euphorigenic, suggesting "reverse tolerance" and perhaps paralleling the locomotor effects seen in animals chronically given nicotine. In fact, among cigarette-smoking drug abusers, intravenous nicotine has been mistaken for cocaine.[19]

Burning tobacco generates more than 4,000 compounds, both gaseous and particulate, including carbon monoxide, nitrogen oxides, ammonia, nitrosamines, hydrogen cyanide, sulfur-containing compounds, hydrocarbons, alcohols, aldehydes, and ketones. Nicotine, a volatile liquid, is suspended in tobacco smoke on minute particles of "tar," consisting largely of aromatic hydrocarbons, some of which are highly carcinogenic.[9] In the lung nicotine is absorbed so quickly that it reaches the brain within 8 seconds; physiologic effects are rapid and brief, increasing reinforcement potential.[9] Similar amounts of nicotine are delivered to the brain by smokeless tobacco. (Tobacco chewers who use 6 wads a day for 30 minutes each are exposed to nicotine and carcinogen concentrations equivalent to two packs of cigarettes.[29]) Most American cigarettes contain about 9 mg of nicotine, of which 1 mg is absorbed during smoking.[33] The half-life of nicotine following inhalation or parenteral administration is about 2 hours; with continuous or frequent smoking, nicotine accumulates and is detectable through the night. Most nicotine is metabolized in the liver. The major metabolite, cotinine, has a half-life of 10 to 27 hours but is not pharmacologically active.[34]

Acute nicotine poisoning is not associated with tobacco smoking or chewing but follows accidental ingestion of tobacco by children (or of certain insecticides by adults). Symptoms appear rapidly and include nausea, vomiting, salivation, lacrimation, abdominal pain, diarrhea, sweating, headache, miosis, agitation, delirium, fasciculations, and weakness.[10,35,36] Tachycardia and hypotension precede seizures, coma, and death from respiratory depression. Treatment consists of gastric lavage, activated charcoal, and ventilatory and blood pressure support. Atropine can be given for parasympathetic overstimulation.[36]

As in animals, tolerance develops variably to nicotine's different effects. Novices but not chronic smokers experience dizziness, nausea, and vomiting; both exhibit tremor and increased blood pressure and pulse rate. Tolerance to some of nicotine's effects seems to develop over the course of a day's smoking. For most smokers the first cigarette of the day produces the greatest subjective response, especially arousal.[9,33]

Chronic smokers experience an abstinence syndrome in which craving is strikingly out of proportion to observable signs. There is irritability, restlessness, anxiety, depression, difficulty concentrating, drowsiness, fatigue, insomnia, and headache. Performance is impaired on tests requiring attentiveness. Infrequently there is sweating, nausea, constipation, or diarrhea. Heart rate, blood pressure, and blood epinephrine levels decrease, and skin temperature and peripheral blood flow increase.[9,36,37] The electroencephalogram, which contains low-voltage fast activity during smoking, shows slower frequencies during abstinence.[37] Craving peaks at 24 to 48 hours and then usually diminishes gradually. In several series irritability, anger, anxiety, and difficulty concentrating occurred in one-half to two-thirds of abstainers; by 6 months these symptoms had largely cleared, yet three-fourths of the subjects still craved cigarettes.[38] Some continue to crave for years. (Similar symptoms follow abstinence from smokeless tobacco or nicotine gum.)

Weight gain occurs in most smokers who quit and is probably secondary both to nicotine's effects on energy expenditure and to increased eating.[39] Women are more likely than men to gain weight, but in either sex major weight gain—more than 13 kg—occurs in only a minority.[40]

Medical and Neurological Complications

In the United States tobacco accounts for 85% of all lung cancer deaths and contributes to cancer of the oropharynx, esophagus, stomach, pancreas, kidney, and bladder. It accounts for 80% of all chronic obstructive pulmonary disease deaths. It is immunosuppressive.[2,41-43] Space does not permit a detailed discussion of the mechanisms of these tobacco-related diseases, which, of course, can produce a myriad of neurological complications. (For example, patients with lung cancer develop brain and spinal cord metastases, paraneoplastic syndromes, CNS infection, and nutritional disturbance.)

A major risk factor for both coronary artery and peripheral vascular disease, tobacco accounts for about 30% of American cardiac mortality.[2,43,44] As regards cerebrovascular disease, although a few reports have been negative or demonstrated only insignificant trends,[45-47] most case control and cohort studies have shown that smoking also increases the risk for both occlusive and hemorrhagic stroke.[7,48-73] In women smokers the risk of occlusive and hemorrhagic stroke is greater in those taking oral contraceptives.[74-78] In a prospective cohort study of middle-aged women, smoking increased stroke risk in a dose-dependent fashion; for those smoking 25 or more cigarettes daily, the relative risk for all stroke was 3.7 and for subarachnoid hemorrhage 9.8 independent of other risk factors, including oral contraceptives, hypertension, and ethanol.[79] In another report, smoking in hypertensive men and women carried a 15-fold risk for subarachnoid hemorrhage and was a greater risk than hypertension itself.[64] In another study the treatment of hypertension reduced stroke incidence in nonsmokers but not in smokers.[80] In the Honolulu Heart Program stroke risk was independent of coronary artery disease.[63] In a French study of women less than 45 years of age, smoking did not confer independent risk of stroke, and migraine conferred marginal risk; when both conditions were present, however, stroke risk was significantly increased.[80a] The Framingham Study found smoking to be a risk factor for subarachnoid hemorrhage and, independent of age and hypertension, for both occlusive and hemorrhagic stroke; this risk was dose dependent and disappeared when smoking ceased.[81,82] Others have confirmed reduction of risk with cessation of smoking.[53,55] One study found that not only was the risk of subarachnoid hemorrhage dose-dependently related to smoking but that it was greatest within three hours of a cigarette.[82a] In the Nurses' Health Study the risk of total and occlusive stroke among former smokers disappeared within 2 to 4 years after cessation,[82b] and in another study of elderly subjects abstention from smoking was followed by improved cerebral perfusion.[82c]

Several possible mechanisms could underlie tobacco's risk for stroke. Smoking aggravates atherosclerosis; in a study of identical twins discordant for smoking,[83] carotid plaques were significantly more prominent in the smokers, and in other reports

smoking correlated in a dose-related fashion with severity of extracranial carotid atherosclerosis.[84-93] The decline of stroke risk with cessation of smoking is against that being the sole mechanism.[82,94,95] In a case-control study, however, an increased risk of cerebral ischemia persisted for at least 10 years in those who had stopped smoking,[70] and others have reported a persistent risk for subarachnoid hemorrhage after more than 5 years abstinence.[95a,95b] In an angiographic study intracranial carotid artery atherosclerosis correlated more with duration of smoking than with hypertension or diabetes mellitus.[96]

Carbon monoxide in cigarette smoke reduces blood's oxygen carrying capacity, and nicotine constricts coronary arteries.[97,98] In animals nicotine damages endothelium, and increased numbers of circulating endothelial cells are found in smokers.[99,100] Smoking acutely raises blood pressure, systole more than diastole; cerebral blood flow is reduced even after such acute effects have worn off.[101,102] Smoking is not a risk factor for chronic hypertension,[103] but it accelerates the progression of chronic hypertension to malignant hypertension.[104] Smokers become tachycardic, and atrial fibrillation has followed nicotine gum chewing.[98] Smoking increases platelet reactivity and inhibits prostacyclin formation.[94,105-108] It also raises blood fibrinogen, a linkage noted in several stroke studies.[44,45,109] Elevated hemoglobin levels in smokers compared with nonsmokers may also be a risk factor.[110] The increased risk of subarachnoid hemorrhage in smokers has been blamed on increased elastolytic activity in the serum.[67]

Progressive multifocal symptoms occurred in four young women who smoked and used oral contraceptives. Cerebral angiography demonstrated moyamoya; abnormal studies included elevated erythrocyte sedimentation rate, positive antinuclear antibodies, and elevated cerebrospinal fluid (CSF) gamma globulin (IgG). Disease progression ceased with discontinuation of oral contraceptives and reduction in smoking.[111]

Many brands of chewing tobacco are flavored with licorice, which contains the hypertensive, sodium-retaining, potassium-depleting glycoside glycyrrhetinic acid.[112] It is not known if this substance is an added risk factor for vascular disease.

Worsening of neurological symptoms or signs has followed tobacco smoking or nicotine ingestion in patients with multiple system atrophy,[113] spinocerebellar degeneration,[114] alcoholic cerebellar degeneration,[115] and multiple sclerosis.[116] Smoking has precipitated myoclonus, ataxia, and weakness in patients with myoclonic epilepsy,[117] an effect blocked with mecamylamine; during nicotine-precipitated quadriparesis in such a patient, the soleus muscle H-reflex increased, an unexpected finding, for smoking depresses the H-reflex in normal humans.[118,119]

In normal subjects, smoking induces a primary-position upbeat nystagmus that is suppressed by fixation.[120] It also impairs horizontal and vertical pursuit movements.[121] Nicotine gum produces similar alterations.[122]

Smokers suffer from diminished smell, and the impairment can last for years after cessation. Anosmia has been attributed to nasal olfactory cell damage by chemicals such as acrolein, acetaldehyde, ammonia, and formaldehyde.[123]

Smoking and depression are linked. Individuals who have experienced major depression are more likely than others to be regular smokers, are less successful at quitting, and are at risk when they do quit of having a recurrence of depressive symptoms.[124,125] Among adolescents, depression appears to contribute to the initiation of cigarette smoking.[126] Uncertain are the relative roles of symptomatic relief and of underlying personality or genetic traits.[127] A prospective cohort study found that first-incidence major depression was significantly higher in subjects with a history of nicotine dependence, whether or not they had smoked during the previous year, and that a history of major depression increased smokers' risk of progressing to nicotine dependence.[127a] A twin study found that when personal smoking history was controlled, family history of smoking predicted risk for major depression and that when personal history of major depression was controlled, family history of major depression predicted smoking.[127b] These findings suggest a genetic but probably non-causal link between smoking and major depression. Smoking undoubtedly contributes to the excess medical mortality associated with major depression.[124,128]

Effects on Pregnancy

Twenty percent to 25% of pregnant American women smoke throughout pregnancy, many heavily.[129] Fetal risks include low birth weight and spontaneous abortion.[130,131] It is estimated that maternal smoking accounts for 21% to 39% of American fetal growth retardation and 4600 perinatal deaths each year, attributable to abruptio placentae, placenta previa, and premature rupture of the membranes.[129] Low Apgar scores are associated with heavy maternal smoking, and some studies found adverse effects on later child development. Children born to smokers have had impaired performance on tests of habit-uation, motor performance, autonomic regulation, reflexes, hearing, and IQ; abnormalities are much more evident at 12 months of age than at 24 months.[131a] As with other drugs, confounders include poor prenatal care, other substance abuse (especially ethanol), socioeconomic class, and education. Low birth weight is also associated with passive smoke inhalation by the mother from smoking by the father.[132] Cardiovascular, gastrointestinal, and urogenital congenital anomalies were reportedly increased among newborns of smoking mothers;[131] other workers do not believe tobacco is teratogenic.[129]

Fetal growth retardation is probably secondary to hypoxia and ischemia caused by nicotine and carbon monoxide. In animals nicotine reduces uterine blood flow,[133] and in pregnant humans two-pack-a-day smoking produces 10% blood carboxyhemoglobin levels, sufficient to cause an equivalent 60% reduction in fetal blood flow.[134] Offspring of rats exposed to tobacco smoke have behavioral abnormalities and altered CNS catecholaminergic and cholinergic neuronal activity;[135,136] acetylcholine possibly exerts trophic influences on developing brain.[136,137] Animal studies suggest that lead, thiocyanate, and cadmium contained in cigarette smoke also harm the fetus.[137a]

Protective Effects: Parkinson's Disease and Alzheimer's Disease

A number of epidemiologic reports suggest that cigarette smoking protects against Parkinson's disease.[138] Cohort and case-control studies have found risk reductions of 20% to 70%.[54,139-146] Possible explanations for the inverse correlation include increased mortality among smokers and a "premorbid personality type" in preparkinsonian patients that makes them less inclined to smoke. In favor of such explanations is the observation that the *amount* of smoking does not correlate with the presence, age of onset, or severity of Parkinson's disease.[147] On the other hand, nicotine does affect dopamine systems and could plausibly prevent the disease or relieve its symptoms. In humans nicotine reduces parkinsonian tremor (but not other tremors).[148] In mice nicotine protects against nigral degeneration induced by 1-methyl-4-phenyl-1,2,3,6-tetrahydropyridine (MPTP),[149,150] and in rats nicotine reduces degeneration of dopamine neurons and terminals following midbrain transection of ascending nigrostriatal fibers.[151] Other workers, unable to verify these findings, believe that whatever risk reduction smoking provides is from other compounds in cigarette smoke.[152,153]

In Alzheimer's disease nicotinic receptor binding is reduced to a greater extent than muscarinic receptor binding.[154] Epidemiologic studies of smoking and Alzheimer's disease, however, have been inconsistent. Anecdotal reports and case-control studies have claimed a decreased risk, [155-159] an increased risk, [160,161] or no correlation in either direction.[162-168] Metaanalysis of eight case-control studies revealed a significant inverse relationship between smoking and Alzheimer's disease.[169] Investigators from Seattle[170] reported a significant reduced risk of Alzheimer's disease among smokers, but with striking modifiers: the greatest benefit occurred among hypertensives with higher education; there was less benefit for those with either hypertension or higher education but not both; and among those with neither hypertension nor higher education smoking actually increased the risk of Alzheimer's disease. Moreover, among all groups those who smoked the least (pack-years) had the greatest risk reduction. These interactions were unexpected and not readily explained. If smoking does in fact reduce the risk of Alzheimer's disease, possible mechanisms include altered cerebral nicotinic receptors or increased release of acetylcholine in the cortex.[171,172] Nicotine reportedly improves attention and information processing in patients with Alzheimer's disease.[158] Potential confounders in epidemiologic studies include smoking-related diseases that select out patients and differences in education and occupation between smokers and nonsmokers.[172,173]

Treatment

No effective treatment of nicotine addiction exists.[32] Mecamylamine, a centrally acting nicotine antagonist, reduced tobacco craving in a small group of volunteers, but smoking rates increased in subjects who were not trying to stop.[174] Both clonidine and the benzodiazepine alprazolam reduced anxiety and irritability during withdrawal; clonidine more effectively reduced craving.[175] In a controlled study clonidine produced higher abstinence rates than diazepam or placebo.[176] In another controlled study clonidine was superior to placebo but only in women.[177] In another controlled study it was not effective at all.[178]

Subcutaneous naloxone reportedly decreased the pleasure of cigarette smoking and helped people trying to stop;[179] another study found it to be without effect.[180] (Heroin, methadone, and buprenorphine increase cigarette smoking, as do ethanol, amphetamine, pentobarbital, and a decrease in accustomed levels of caffeine.[181])

Nicotine-substitution therapy includes nicotine gum, nicotine aerosols, and sustained-release transdermal nicotine.[8] In controlled studies nicotine gum combined with behavioral therapy is more effective than placebo;[182] used alone, nicotine gum is of little value.[183] (Consuming acidic food or beverages—including coffee—before chewing nicotine gum can render it ineffective.[184]) Randomized trials have demonstrated better results with transdermal nicotine patch than with placebo patch,[185,186] although in one widely cited study, in which subjects used a 16-hour patch for 12 weeks and then tapered dosage, only 17% were still abstinent after a year compared with 4% of those receiving placebo.[187] Nicotine gum and patches are used intermittently because of concern that tolerance to nicotine's effects could develop or that sleep could be disrupted. Long-term treatment is avoided for fear of cardiovascular and cerebrovascular complications.[188,189]

Nicotine gum has been used in conjunction with transdermal clonidine patches, clonidine serving to dampen withdrawal symptoms from decreasing doses of nicotine.[190] The efficacy of such an approach has not yet been demonstrated.

Family, twin, and adoption studies have demonstrated genetic influences on tobacco addiction;[191] in one study genetic factors appeared to play a role in light and heavy smokers but not moderate smokers.[192] Whether such heritability will lead to the identification of children at special risk—with preventive measures targeted at them—remains to be seen.

The tobacco industry spends more than $3 billion a year advertising and promoting the single most preventable cause of death in America.[193] Much of the effort is targeted at children.[194,195] Much is devoted to forcing American-made cigarettes into foreign markets, under threat of U.S. governmental trade sanctions toward nations that resist.[196] The consequences of such immorality are staggering. It is estimated that if global cigarette consumption continues to increase at present rates, the *annual* deaths caused by the American tobacco industry will soon exceed the total deaths caused by the Holocaust of Nazi Germany.[197] In China alone, by the year 2025 2 million men will die annually from smoking.[198]

Despite a succession of Surgeon General Reports, the passage of legislation restricting smoking in public places, and, finally in 1992, legal accountability for damages,[199] governmental antismoking efforts have been listless compared with the enthusiastic expenditures of money and energy directed against substances decreed illicit. In 1992, responding to pressures from tobacco lobbyists, the governor of California canceled funding of a highly successful education and research program directed against tobacco addiction.[200,201] Even practicing physicians seem disinclined to do battle with the tobacco industry. Surveys reveal that fewer than half of American smokers seen by a physician during the previous year have been advised to stop.[202] Physicians trained to counsel patients about quitting do make a difference.[203-205] Tobacco's legality should be an incentive, not a deterrent, to such intervention. As elected officials succumb to the pressures of industry lobbyists, physicians should remind themselves that tobacco is the only product legally sold in the United States that causes disease and death when used as intended.[206,207]

References

1. Ravenholt RT. Addiction mortality in the United States 1980: tobacco, alcohol, and other substances. Population Development Rev 1984; 10:697.
2. Schultz JM. Smoking-attributable mortality and years of potential life lost—United States, 1988. MMWR 1991; 40:62.
3. Fielding JE. Smoking health effects and control. N Engl J Med 1985; 313:491, 555.
4. Warner KE. Health and economic implications of a tobacco-free society. JAMA 1987; 258:2080.
5. Nadelman EA. Drug prohibition in the United States: costs, consequences, and alternatives. Science 1989; 245:939.
6. Schelling TC. Addictive drugs: the cigarette experience. Science 1992; 255:430.
7. Department of Health and Human Services. The Health Consequences of Smoking: Nicotine Addiction. A Report of the Surgeon General. Washington, DC: DHHS Publication No (CDC) 88-8406, US Government Printing Office, 1988.
8. Benowitz NL. Pharmacologic aspects of cigarette smoking and nicotine addiction. N Engl J Med 1988; 319:1318.
9. Jaffe J. Drug addiction and drug abuse. In: Gilman AG, Rall TW, Nies AS, Taylor P, eds. The Pharmacological Basis of Therapeutics, ed 8. New York: Pergamon Press, 1990:522.
10. Taylor P. Agents acting at the neuromuscular junction and autonomic ganglia. In: Gilman AG, Rall TW, Nies AS, Taylor P, eds. The Pharmacological Basis of Therapeutics, ed 8. New York: Pergamon Press, 1990:166.
11. Clarke PBS, Kumar R. The effects of nicotine on locomotor activity in non-tolerant and tolerant rats. Br J Pharmacol 1983; 78:329.
12. Clarke PBS. Nicotine and smoking: a perspective from animal studies. Psychopharmacology 1987; 92:135.
13. Warburton DM. Psychopharmacological aspects of nicotine. In: Wonnacott S, Russell MAH, Stolerman IP, eds. Nicotine Psychopharmacology. Molecular, Cellular, and Behavioral Aspects. Oxford: Oxford University Press, 1990:77.
14. Stolerman IP. Behavioral pharmacology of nicotine in animals. In: Wonnacott S, Russell MAH, Stolerman IP, eds. Nicotine Psychopharmacology. Molecular, Cellular, and Behavioral Aspects. Oxford: Oxford University Press, 1990:278.
15. Lupien JR, Bray GA. Nicotine increases thermogenesis in brown adipose tissue in rats. Pharmacol Biochem Behav 1988; 29:33.
16. Stolerman IP, Garcha HS, Pratt JA, Kumar P. Role of training dose in discrimination of nicotine and related compounds by rats. Psychopharmacology 1984; 84:413.
17. Goldberg SR, Spealman RD, Goldberg DM. Persistent high rate behavior maintained by intravenous self-administration of nicotine. Science 1981; 214:573.
18. Cox BM, Goldstein A, Nelson WT. Nicotine self-administration in rats. Br J Pharmacol 1984; 83:49.
19. Henningfield JE, Mijasato K, Jasinski DR. Abuse liability and pharmacodynamic characteristics of intravenous and inhaled nicotine. J Pharmacol Exp Ther 1985; 234:1.
20. Swedberg MDB, Henningfield JE, Goldberg SR. Nicotine dependency: animal studies. In: Wonnacott S, Russell MAH, Stolerman IP, eds. Nicotine Psychopharmacology: Molecular, Cellular, and Behavioral Aspects. Oxford: Oxford University Press, 1990:38.
21. Deneris ES, Connolly J, Rogers SW, Duvoisin R. Pharmacological and functional diversity of neuronal nicotinic acetylcholine receptors. Trends Pharmacol Sci 1991; 12:34.
22. Clarke PBS, Pert A. Autoradiographic evidence for nicotine receptors on nigrostriatal and mesolimbic dopaminergic neurons. Brain Res 1985; 348:355.
23. Clarke PBS, Fu DS, Jakubovic A, Fibiger HC. Evidence that mesolimbic dopaminergic activation underlies the locomotor stimulant action of nicotine in rats. J Pharmacol Exp Ther 1988; 246:701.
24. Pomerleau OF, Pomerleau CS. Neuroregulators and the reinforcement of smoking: towards a behavioral explanation. Neurosci Behav Rev 1984; 8:503.
25. Corrigall WA, Herling S, Coen KM. Evidence for opioid mechanisms in the peripheral effects of nicotine. Psychopharmacology 1988; 96:29.
26. Brecher EM. Licit and Illicit Drugs. Boston: Little, Brown, 1972.
27. Centers for Disease Control. Cigarette smoking among adults—United States 1988. MMWR 1991; 40:757.
28. Marwick C. Increasing use of chewing tobacco, especially among younger persons, alarms surgeon general. JAMA 1993; 269:195.
29. U.S. Environmental Protection Agency. Respiratory Health Effects of Passive Smoking: Lung Cancer and Other Disorders. Washington, DC: U.S. Government Printing Office, 1993.

30. Tripathi J, Martin B, Aceto M. Nicotine-induced antinociception in rats and mice: correlation with nicotine brain levels. J Pharmacol Exp Ther 1982; 221:91.

31. Moss RA, Prue DM. Research on nicotine regulation. Behav Ther 1982; 13:31.

32. Kozlowski LT, Wilkinson A, Skinner W, et al. Comparing tobacco cigarette dependence with other drug dependencies. JAMA 1989; 261:898.

33. Benowitz NL. Clinical pharmacology of inhaled drugs of abuse: implications in understanding nicotine dependence. In: Chiang CN, Hawks RL, eds. Research Findings on Smoking of Abused Substances. Rockville, MD: NIDA Research Monograph 99, DHHS, 1990:12.

34. Wall MA, Johnson J, Jacob P, Benowitz NL. Cotinine in the serum, saliva, and urine of nonsmokers, passive smokers, and active smokers. Am J Publ Health 1988; 78:699.

35. Borys DJ, Setzer SC, Ling LJ. CNS depression in an infant after the ingestion of tobacco: a case report. Vet Hum Toxicol 1988; 30:20.

36. Goldfrank LR, Melinek M, Weisman RS. Nicotine. In: Goldfrank LR, Flomenbaum NE, Lewin NA, et al, eds. Toxicologic Emergencies, ed 4. Norwalk, CT: Appleton & Lange, 1990:613.

37. Gilbert RM, Pope MA. Early effects of quitting smoking. Psychopharmacology 1982; 78:121.

38. Hughes JR, Gust SW, Skoog K, et al. Symptoms of tobacco withdrawal. Arch Gen Psychiatry 1991; 48:52.

39. Perkins KA, Epstein LH, Marks BL, et al. The effect of nicotine on energy expenditure during light physical activity. N Engl J Med 1989; 320:898.

40. Williamson DF, Madans J, Anda RF, et al. Smoking cessation and severity of weight gain in a national cohort. N Engl J Med 1991; 324:739.

41. Berger LR. Cigarette smoking and the acquired immunodeficiency syndrome. Ann Intern Med 1988; 108:638.

42. Henderson BE, Ross RK, Pike MC. Toward the primary prevention of cancer. Science 1991; 254:1131.

43. Smoking and Health. A National Status Report, 2nd Edition. Rockville, MD: DHHS, Publication No (CDC) 87-8396, 1990.

44. Kannel WB, D'Agostino RB, Belanger AL. Fibrinogen, cigarette smoking, and risk of cardiovascular disease: insights from the Framingham Study. Am Heart J 1987; 113:1006.

45. Kannel WB, Dawber TR, Cohen ME, et al. Vascular disease of the brain—epidemiologic aspects. The Framingham Study. Am J Publ Health 1965; 55:1355.

46. Herman B, Leyten ACM, van Luuk JH, et al. An evaluation of risk factors for stroke in a Dutch community. Stroke 1982; 13:334.

47. Davanipour Z, Sobel E, Alter M, et al. Stroke/transient ischemic attack in the Lehigh Valley: evaluation of smoking as a risk factor. Ann Neurol 1988; 24:130.

48. Hammond EC. Smoking in relation to mortality and morbidity: finding in the first 34 months of followup in a prospective study started in 1959. J Natl Cancer Inst 1964; 32:1161.

49. Kahn HA. The Dorn study of smoking and mortality among US veterans: report on 8 1/2 years of observation. Natl Cancer Inst Monogr 1966; 19:1.

50. Paffenbarger RS, Wing A. Characteristics in youth predisposing to fatal stroke in later years. Lancet 1967; 1:753.

51. Kurtzke JF. Epidemiology of Cerebrovascular Disease. New York: Springer-Verlag, 1969.

52. Paffenbarger RS, Williams JL. Chronic disease in former college students. XI. Early precursors of nonfatal stroke. Am J Epidemiol 1971; 94:524.

53. Rogot E. Smoking and General Mortality Among US Veterans, 1954–1969. Bethesda, MD: National Heart and Lung Institute, 1974.

54. Doll R, Peto R. Mortality in relation to smoking: 20 years' observations on male British doctors. BMJ 1976; 2:1525.

55. Koch A, Reuther R, Boos R, et al. Risikofaktoren bei cerebralen Durchblutungsstorungen. Verh Dtsch Ges Inn Med 1977; 83:1977.

56. Abu-Zeid HAH, Choi NW, Maini KK, et al. Relative role of factors associated with cerebral infarction and cerebral hemorrhage: a matched pair case-control study. Stroke 1977; 8:106.

57. Doll R, Gray R, Hafner B, et al. Mortality in relation to smoking: twenty-two years observations on female British doctors. BMJ 1980; 1:967.

58. Salonen JT, Puska P, Tuomilehto J, et al. Relation of blood pressure, serum lipids, and smoking to the risk of cerebral stroke: a longitudinal study in Eastern Finland. Stroke 1982; 13:327.

59. Wolf PA, Kannel WB, Verter J. Current status of risk factors for stroke. Neurol Clin 1983; 1:317.

60. Candelise L, Bianchi F, Galligoni F, et al. Italian multicenter study on cerebral ischemic attacks. III. Influence of age and risk factors on cerebral atherosclerosis. Stroke 1984; 15:379.

61. Herrschaft H. Prophylaxe zerbraler Durchblutungsstorungen. Fortschr Neurol Psychiatr 1985; 53:337.

62. Bloch C, Richard JL. Risk factors for atherosclerotic diseases in the Prospective Parisian Study. I. Comparison with foreign studies. Rev Epidemiol Sante Publ 1985; 33:108.

63. Abbott RD, Reed DM, Yano K. Risk of stroke in male cigarette smokers. N Engl J Med 1986; 315:717.

64. Bonita R. Cigarette smoking, hypertension, and the risk of subarachnoid hemorrhage: a population-based case-control study. Stroke 1986; 17:831.

65. Bonita R, Scragg R, Stewart A, et al. Cigarette smoking and risk of premature stroke in men and women. BMJ 1986; 293:6.

66. Molgaard CA, Bartok A, Peddercord KM, et al. The association between cerebrovascular disease and smoking: a case control study. Neuroepidemiology 1986; 5:88.

67. Fogelholm R. Cigarette smoking and subarachnoid hemorrhage: a population-based case-control study. J Neurol Neurosurg Psychiatry 1987; 50:78.

68. Gorelick PB, Rodin MB, Langenberg P, et al. Weekly alcohol consumption, cigarette smoking, and the risk

of ischemic stroke: results of a case-control study at three urban medical centers in Chicago, Illinois. Neurology 1989; 39:339.

69. Shinton R, Beevers G. Meta-analysis of relation between cigarette smoking and stroke. BMJ 1989; 298:789.

70. Donnan GA, Adena MA, O'Malley HM, et al. Smoking as a risk for cerebral ischemia. Lancet 1989; 2:643.

71. Harmsen P, Rosengren A, Tsipogianni A, Wilhelmsen L. Risk factors for stroke in middle-aged men in Goteborg, Sweden. Stroke 1990; 21:223.

72. Love BB, Biller J, Jones MP, et al. Cigarette smoking. A risk factor for cerebral infarction in young adults. Arch Neurol 1990; 47:693.

73. Tuomilehto J, Bonita R, Stewart A, et al. Hypertension, cigarette smoking, and the decline in stroke incidence in Eastern Finland. Stroke 1991; 22:7.

74. Collaborative Group for the Study of Stroke in Young Women. Oral contraception and increased risk of cerebral ischemia or thrombosis. N Engl J Med 1973; 288:871.

75. Frederiksen H, Ravenholt RT. Thromboembolism, oral contraceptives, and cigarettes. Publ Health Rep 1970; 85:197.

76. Goldbaum GM, Kendrick JS, Hogelin GC, Gentry EM. The relative impact of smoking and oral contraceptive use on women in the United States. JAMA 1987; 258:1339.

77. Pettiti DB, Wingerd J. Use of oral contraceptives; cigarette smoking, and risk of subarachnoid hemorrhage. Lancet 1978; 2:234.

78. Royal College of General Practitioners. Oral Contraceptives and Health. London: Pitman, 1974.

79. Colditz GA, Bonita R, Stampfer MJ, et al. Cigarette smoking and risk of stroke in middle-aged women. N Engl J Med 1988; 318:937.

80. Medical Research Council Working Party. MRC Trial of treatment of mild hypertension: principal results. BMJ 1985; 291:97.

80a. Iglesias S, Visy JM, Hubert JB, et al. Migraine as a risk factor for ischemic stroke. A case-control study. Stroke 1993; 24:171.

81. Sacco RL, Wolf PA, Bharucha NE, et al. Subarachnoid and intracerebral hemorrhage: natural history, prognosis, and precursive factors in the Framingham Study. Neurology 1984; 34:847.

82. Wolf PA, D'Agostino RB, Kannel WB, et al. Cigarette smoking as a risk factor for stroke. The Framingham Study. JAMA 1988; 259:1025.

82a. Longstreth WT, Nelson LM, Koepsell TD, van Belle G. Cigarette smoking, alcohol use, and subarachnoid hemorrhage. Stroke 1992; 23:1242.

82b. Kawachi I, Colditz GA, Stampfer MJ, et al. Smoking cessation and decreased risk of stroke in women. JAMA 1993; 269:232.

82c. Rogers RL, Meyer JS, Judd BW, Mortel KF. Abstention from cigarette smoking improves cerebral perfusion among elderly chronic smokers. JAMA 1985; 253:2970.

83. Haapanen A, Koskenvuo M, Kaprio J, et al. Carotid arteriosclerosis in identical twins discordant for cigarette smoking. Circulation 1989; 80:10.

84. Bogousslavsky J, Van Melle G, Despland PA, Regli F. Alcohol consumption and carotid atherosclerosis in the Lausanne Stroke Registry. Stroke 1990; 21:715.

85. Whisnant JP, Homer D, Ingall TJ, et al. Duration of cigarette smoking is the strongest predictor of severe extracranial carotid atherosclerosis. Stroke 1990; 21:707.

86. Dempsey RJ, Diana AL, Moore RW. Thickness of carotid artery atherosclerotic plaque and ischemic risk. Neurosurgery 1990; 27:343.

87. Crouse JR, Toole JF, McKinney WM, et al. Risk factors for extracranial carotid artery atherosclerosis. Stroke 1987; 18:990.

88. Gostomzyk JG, Heller WD, Gerhardt P, et al. B-scan ultrasound examination of the carotid arteries within a representative population (MONICA Project Augsburg). Klin Wochenschr 1988; 66(suppl XI):58.

89. Salonen R, Seppanen K, Rauramaa R, Salonen JT. Prevalence of carotid atherosclerosis and serum cholesterol levels in Eastern Finland. Arteriosclerosis 1988; 8:788.

90. Lassila R, Seyberth HW, Haapanen A, et al. Vasoactive and atherogenic effects of cigarette smoking: A study of monozygotic twins discordant for smoking. BMJ 1988; 297:955.

91. Tell GS, Howard G, McKinney WM, Toole JF. Cigarette smoking cessation and extracranial carotid atherosclerosis. JAMA 1989; 262:1178.

92. Dempsey RJ, Moore RW. Amount of smoking independently predicts carotid artery atherosclerosis severity. Stroke 1992; 23:693.

93. Dempsey RJ, Moore RW. A causal chain from smoking to stroke. Stroke 1992; 23:A12.

94. Murchison LE, Fyfe T. Effects of cigarette smoking on serum lipids, blood glucose, and platelet adhesiveness. Lancet 1966; 2:182.

95. Rogers RL, Meyer JS, Shaw TG, et al. Cigarette smoking decreases cerebral blood flow suggesting increased risk for stroke. JAMA 1983; 250:2796.

95a. Bell BA, Symon L. Smoking and subarachnoid hemorrhage. BMJ 1979; 1:577.

95b. Taha A, Ball KP, Illingworth RD. Smoking and subarachnoid hemorrhage. J R Soc Med 1982; 75:332.

96. Ingall TJ, Homer D, Baker HL, et al. Predictors of intracranial carotid artery atherosclerosis. Arch Neurol 1991; 48:687.

97. Maouad J, Fernandez F, Barrillon A, et al. Diffuse or segmental narrowing (spasm) of coronary arteries during smoking demonstrated on angiography. Am J Cardiol 1984; 53:354.

98. Benowitz NL. Pharmacologic aspects of cigarette smoking and nicotine addiction. N Engl J Med 1988; 319:1318.

99. Davis JW, Shelton L, Eigenberg DA, et al. Effects of tobacco and non-tobacco cigarette smoking on endothelium and platelets. Clin Pharmacol Ther 1985; 37:529.

100. Zimmerman M, McGreachie J. The effect of nicotine on aortic endothelium: a quantitative ultrastructural study. Atherosclerosis 1987; 63:33.

101. Kubota K, Yamaguchi T, Abe Y. Effects of smoking on regional cerebral blood flow in neurologically normal subjects. Stroke 1983; 14:720.

102. Longstreth WT, Swanson PD. Oral contraceptives and stroke. Stroke 1984; 15:747.

103. Green MS, Jucha E, Luz Y. Blood pressure in smokers and non-smokers: epidemiologic findings. Am Heart J 1986; 111:932.

104. Isles C, Brown JJ, Cumming AM, et al. Excess smoking in malignant phase hypertension. BMJ 1979; 1:579.

105. Seiss W, Lorenz R, Roth P, Weber PC. Plasma catecholamines, platelet aggregation and associated thromboxane formation after physical exercise, smoking, or norepinephrine infusion. Circulation 1982; 66:44.

106. Nadler JL, Velasso JS, Horton R. Cigarette smoking inhibits prostacyclin formation. Lancet 1983; 1:1248.

107. Belch JJ, McArdle BM, Burns P, et al. The effects of acute smoking on platelet behavior, fibrinolysis, and haemorphology in habitual smokers. Thromb Haemost 1984; 51:6.

108. Renaud S, Blache O, Dumont E, et al. Platelet function after cigarette smoking in relation to nicotine and carbon monoxide. Clin Pharmacol Ther 1984; 36:389.

109. Wilhelmsen L, Svardsudd K, Korsan-Bengsten K, et al. Fibrinogen as a risk factor for stroke and myocardial infarction. N Engl J Med 1984; 311:501.

110. Nordenberg D, Yip R, Binkin NJ. The effect of cigarette smoking on hemoglobin levels and anemia screening. JAMA 1990; 264:1556.

111. Levine SR, Fagan SC, Floberg J, et al. Moyamoya, oral contraceptives, and cigarette use. Ann Neurol 1988; 24:155.

112. Morris DJ, Davis E, Latif SA. Licorice, tobacco chewing, and hypertension. N Engl J Med 1990; 322:849.

113. Johnson JA, Miller JT. Tobacco intolerance in multiple system atrophy. Neurology 1986; 36:986.

114. Spillane JD. The effect of nicotine on spinocerebellar ataxia. BMJ 1955; 2:1345.

115. Schmitt J, Seelinger D, Appenzeller O, Orrison W. Nicotine and alcoholic cerebellar degeneration. Neurology 1988; 38(suppl 1):205.

116. Emre M, de Decker C. Nicotine and CNS. Neurology 1987; 37:1887.

117. Yoshimura I, Tabe HK, Fukushima Y, Fuyushi T. The aggravating effect of smoking on myoclonus: a case of Ramsey Hunt syndrome. Neurol Med 1988; 28:636.

118. Yokota T, Kagamihara Y, Hayashi H, et al. Nicotine-sensitive paresis. Neurology 1992; 42:382.

119. Domino EF, Von Baumgarten AM. Tobacco cigarette smoking and patellar reflex depression. Clin Pharmacol Ther 1969; 10:72.

120. Sibony PA, Evinger C, Manning KA. Tobacco-induced primary position upbeat nystagmus. Ann Neurol 1987; 21:53.

121. Sibony PA, Evinger C, Manning KA. The effects of tobacco smoking on smooth pursuit eye movements. Ann Neurol 1988; 23:238.

122. Sibony PA, Evinger C, Manning K, Pellegrini JJ. Nicotine and tobacco-induced nystagmus. Ann Neurol 1990; 28:198.

123. Frye RE, Schwartz BS, Doty RL. Dose-related effects of cigarette smoking on olfactory function. JAMA 1990; 263:1233.

124. Glassman AH, Helzer JE, Covey LS, et al. Smoking, smoking cessation, and major depression. JAMA 1990; 264:1546.

125. Anda RF, Williamson DF, Escobedo LG, et al. Depression and the dynamics of smoking. A national perspective. JAMA 1990; 264:1541.

126. Kandel DB, Davies M. Adult sequelae of adolescent depressive symptoms. Arch Gen Psychiatry 1986; 43:255.

127. Glass RM. Blue mood, blackened lungs. Depression and smoking. JAMA 1990; 264:1584.

127a. Kendler KS, Neale MC, MacLean CJ, et al. Smoking and major depression. A causal analysis. Arch Gen Psychiatry 1993; 50:36.

127b. Breslau N, Kilbey M, Andreski P. Nicotine dependence and major depression. New evidence from a prospective investigation. Arch Gen Psychiatry 1993; 50:31.

128. Bruce ML, Leaf PJ. Psychiatric disorders and 15 month mortality in a community sample of older adults. Am J Publ Health 1989; 79:727.

129. Benowitz NL. Nicotine replacement therapy during pregnancy. JAMA 1990; 266:3174.

130. Cole H. Studying reproductive risks, smoking. JAMA 1986; 255:22.

131. Himmelberger DU, Brown BW, Cohen EN. Cigarette smoking during pregnancy and the occurrence of spontaneous abortion and congenital abnormality. Am J Epidemiol 1978; 108:470.

131a. Chiriboga C. Fetal effects. In Brust JCM, ed. Neurologic Complications of Drug and Alcohol Abuse. Neurol Clin 1993, in press.

132. Rubin DH, Krasilnikoff PA, Leventhal JM, et al. Effect of passive smoking on birth weight. Lancet 1986; 2:415.

133. Resnik R, Brink GW, Wilkes M. Catecholamine mediated reduction in uterine blood flow after nicotine infusion in the pregnant ewe. J Clin Invest 1979; 63:1133.

134. Bureau MA, Monette J, Shapcott D, et al. Carboxyhemoglobin concentration in fetal cord blood and in blood of mothers who smoked during labor. Pediatrics 1982; 69:371.

135. Peters DAV, Taub H, Tang Sk. Postnatal effects of maternal nicotine exposure. Neurobehav Toxicol 1979; 1:221.

136. Navarro HA, Seidler FJ, Whitmore WL, Slotkin TA. Prenatal exposure to nicotine via maternal infusions: effects on development of catecholamine systems. J Pharmacol Exp Ther 1988; 244:940.

137. Navarro HA, Seidler FJ, Eylers JP, et al. Effects of prenatal nicotine exposure on evidence of cholinergic trophic influences in developing brain. J Pharmacol Exp Ther 1989; 251:894.

137a. Kunhert DB. Drug exposure to the fetus. The effect of smoking. In Kilbey MM, Asghar K, eds. Methodological Issues in Controlled Studies on Effects of Prenatal Exposure to Drug Abuse. Rockville, MD: NIDA Research Monograph 114. DHHS, 1991:1.

138. Bharucha NE, Stokes L, Schoenberg BS, et al. A case-control study of twin pairs discordant for Parkinson's disease: a search for environmental risk factors. Neurology 1986; 36:284.

139. Baron JA. Cigarette smoking and Parkinson's disease. Neurology 1986; 36:1490.

140. Nefzger MD, Quadfasel FA, Karl VC. A retrospective study of smoking in Parkinson's disease. Am J Epidemiol 1968; 88:149.

141. Kessler II, Diamond EL. Epidemiologic studies of Parkinson's disease. I. Smoking and Parkinson's disease: a survey and explanatory hypothesis. Am J Epidemiol 1971; 94:16.

142. Marttila RJ, Rinne UK. Smoking and Parkinson's disease. Acta Neurol Scand 1980; 62:322.

143. Haack DG, Baumann RJ, McLean HE, et al. Nicotine exposure and Parkinson's disease. Am J Epidemiol 1981; 114:191.

144. Godwin-Austin RB, Lee PN, Marmot MG, Stern GM. Smoking and Parkinson's disease. J Neurol Neurosurg Psychiatry 1982; 45:577.

145. Kondo K. Epidemiological clues for the etiology of Parkinson's disease. Adv Neurol 1984; 40:345.

146. Rajput AH. Epidemiology of Parkinson's disease. Can J Neurol Sci 1984; 11:156.

147. Golbe LI, Cody RA, Duvoisin RC. Smoking and Parkinson's disease. Search for a dose-response relationship. Arch Neurol 1986; 43:774.

148. Marshall J, Schnieden H. Effect of adrenaline, noradrenaline, atropine, and nicotine on some types of human tremor. J Neurol Neurosurg Psychiatry 1966; 29:214.

149. Reavill C. Action of nicotine on dopamine pathways and implications for Parkinson's disease. In: Wonnacott S, Russell MAH, Stolerman IP, eds. Nicotine Psychopharmology. Molecular, Cellular and Behavioral Aspects. Oxford: Oxford University Press, 1990:307.

150. Janson AM, Fuxe K, Sundstrom E, et al. Chronic nicotine treatment partly protects against the 1-methyl-4-phenyl-1,2,3,6-tetrahydropyridine-induced degeneration of nigrostriatal dopamine neurons in the black mouse. Acta Physiol Scand 1988; 132:589.

151. Janson AM, Fuxe K, Agnati LF, et al. Chronic nicotine treatment counteracts the disappearance of tyrosine hydroxylase-immunoreactive nerve cell bodies, dendrites and terminals in the mesostriatal dopamine system of the male rat after partial hemitransection. Brain Res 1988; 455:332.

152. Fuxe K, Andersson K, Harfstrand A, et al. Effects of nicotine on synaptic transmission in the brain. In:

Wonnacott S, Russell MAH, Stolerman IP, eds. Nicotine Psychopharmacology. Molecular, Cellular, and Behavioral Aspects. Oxford: Oxford University Press, 1990:194.

153. Yong VW, Perry T. Monoamine oxidase B, smoking, and Parkinson's disease. J Neurol Sci 1986; 72:265.

154. Kellar KJ, Wonnacott S. Nicotinic cholinergic receptors in Alzheimer's disease. In: Wonnacott S, Russell MAH, Stolerman IP, eds. Nicotine Psychopharmacology. Molecular, Cellular, and Behavioral Aspects. Oxford: Oxford University Press, 1990:341.

155. Appel SH. Alzheimer's disease. In: Enna SJ, Samorajski T, Beer T, eds. Brain Neurotransmitters and Receptors in Aging and Age-related Disorders. New York: Raven Press, 1981:203.

156. Hofman A, van Duijn CM. Alzheimer's disease, Parkinson's disease, and smoking. Neurobiol Aging 1990; 11:295.

157. Ferini-Strambi L, Smirne S, Garancini P, et al. Clinical and epidemiological aspects of Alzheimer's disease with presenile onset: a case-control study. Neuroepidemiology 1990; 9:39.

158. Grossberg GT, Nakra R, Woodward V, Russell T. Smoking as a risk factor for Alzheimer's disease. J Am Geriatr Soc 1989; 37:822.

159. van Duijn CM, Hofman A. Relation between nicotine intake and Alzheimer's disease. BMJ 1991; 302:1491.

160. Shalat SL, Seltzer B, Pidcock C, Baker EL. Risk factors for Alzheimer's disease: a case-control study. Neurology 1987; 37:1630.

161. Joya CJ, Pardo CA, Londono JL. Risk factors in clinically diagnosed Alzheimer's disease: a case-control study in Colombia (South America). Neurobiol Aging 1990; 11:796.

162. French LR, Schuman LM, Mortimer JA, et al. A case-control study of dementia of the Alzheimer's type. Am J Epidemiol 1985; 121:414.

163. Jones GMM, Reith M, Philpot MP, Sahakian BJ. Smoking and dementia of Alzheimer type. J Neurol Neurosurg Psychiatry 1987; 50:1383.

164. Amaducci LA, Fratiglioni L, Rocca WA, et al. Risk factors for clinically diagnosed Alzheimer's disease: a case-control study of an Italian population. Neurology 1986; 36:922.

165. Chandra V, Philipose V, Bell PA, et al. Case-control study of late onset "probable Alzheimer's disease." Neurology 1987; 37:1295.

166. Broe GA, Henderson AS, Creasey H, et al. A case-control study of Alzheimer's disease in Australia. Neurology 1990; 40:1698.

167. Graves AB, White E, Koepsell T, et al. A case-control study of Alzheimer's disease. Ann Neurol 1990; 28:766.

168. Hebert LE, Scherr PA, Beckett LA, et al. Relation of smoking and alcohol consumption to incident Alzheimer's disease. Am J Epidemiol 1992; 135:347.

169. Graves AB, van Duijn CM, Chandra V. Alcohol and tobacco consumption as risk factors for Alzheimer's disease: a collaborative re-analysis of case-control studies. Int J Epidemiol 1991; 20:548.

170. Brenner DE, Kukull WA, van Belle G, et al. Relationship between cigarette smoking and Alzheimer's disease in a population-based case-control study. Neurology 1993; 43:293.

171. Schwartz RD, Kellar K. In vivo regulation of [3H]acetylcholine recognition sites in brain by nicotinic cholinergic drugs. J Neurochem 1985; 45:427.

172. Rowell PP, Winkler DL. Nicotinic stimulation of [3-H] acetylcholine release from mouse cerebral cortical synaptosomes. J Neurochem 1984; 43:1593.

173. Dartigues JF. Tobacco consumption and risk of cognitive impairment. Results of the Paquid study. Neurology 1992; 42(suppl 3):142.

174. Tennant FS, Tarver AL, Rawson RA. Clinical evaluation of mecamylamine for withdrawal from nicotine dependence. In: Harris LS, ed. Problems of Drug Dependence, 1983. Washington, DC: NIDA Research Monograph 49, DHHS, 1984:239.

175. Glassman AH, Jackson WK, Walsh WK, et al. Cigarette craving, smoking withdrawal, and clonidine. Science 1984; 226:864.

176. Wei H, Young D. Effect of clonidine on cigarette cessation and in the alleviation of withdrawal symptoms. Br J Addict 1988; 83:1221.

177. Glassman AH, Stetner F, Walsh BT, et al. Heavy smokers, smoking cessation, and clonidine: results of a double-blind randomized trial. JAMA 1988; 259:2863.

178. Franks R, Harp J, Bell B. Randomized controlled trial of clonidine for smoking cessation in a primary care setting. JAMA 1989; 262:3011.

179. Karras A, Kane J. Naloxone reduces cigarette smoking. Life Sci 1980; 27:1541.

180. Nemmeth-Coslett R, Griffiths RR. Naloxone does not affect cigarette smoking. Psychopharmacology 1986; 89:261.

181. Mello NK, Lukas SE, Mendelson JH. Buprenorphine effects on cigarette smoking. Psychopharmacology 1985; 86:417.

182. Tonnesen P, Frye V, Hansen M, et al. Effect of nicotine chewing gum in combination with group counselling on the cessation of smoking. N Engl J Med 1988; 318:15.

183. Hughes JR, Gust SW, Keenan RM, et al. Nicotine vs placebo gum in general medical practice. JAMA 1989; 261:1300.

184. Henningfield JE, Radzius A, Cooper TM, Clayton RR. Drinking coffee and carbonated beverages blocks absorption of nicotine from nicotine polacrilex gum. JAMA 1990; 264:1560.

185. Rose J, Levin ED, Behm FM, et al. Transdermal nicotine facilitates smoking cessation. Clin Pharmacol Ther 1900; 47:323.

186. Transdermal Nicotine Study Group. Transdermal nicotine for smoking cessation. JAMA 1991; 266:3134.

187. Tonnesen P, Norregaard J, Simonsen K, Sawe U. A double-blind trial of 16-hour transdermal nicotine patch in smoking cessation. N Engl J Med 1991; 325:311.

188. Benowitz NL. Pharmacodynamics of nicotine: implications for rational treatment of nicotine addiction. Br J Addict 1991; 86:495.

189. Tonnesen P, Norregaard, Simonsen K, Sawe U. Transdermal nicotine patch for smoking cessation. N Engl J Med 1992; 326:344.

190. Sees KL. Cigarette smoking, nicotine dependence, and treatment. West J Med 1990; 152:578.

191. Hughes JR. Genetics of smoking: a brief review. Behav Ther 1986; 17:335.

192. Carmelli D, Swan GE, Robinette D, Fabsitz R. Genetic influences on smoking—a study of male twins. N Engl J Med 1992; 327:829.

193. Jones RT. What have we learned from nicotine, cocaine, and marijuana about addiction? In: O'Brien CP, Jaffe JH, eds. Addictive States. Res Publ Assoc Res Nerv Ment Dis 1992; 70:109

194. DiFranza JR, Richards JW, Paulman PM, et al. RJR Nabisco's cartoon camel promotes Camel cigarettes to children. JAMA 1991; 266:3149.

195. Centers for Disease Control. Comparison of the cigarette brand preferences of adult and teen-aged smokers—United States, 1989, and 10 US communities, 1988 and 1990. MMWR 1992; 41:169.

196. Vateesatokit P. The latest victim of tobacco trade sanctions. JAMA 1990; 264:1522.

197. Foege WH. The growing brown plague. JAMA 1990; 264:1580.

198. Yu SJ, Mattson ME, Boyd GM, et al. A comparison of smoking patterns in the People's Republic of China with the United States. JAMA 1990; 264: 1575.

199. Greenhouse L. Court opens way for damage suits over cigarettes. New York Times, June 25, 1992.

200. Bal DG, Kizer KW, Felten PG, et al. Reducing tobacco consumption in California. Development of a statewide anti-tobacco use campaign. JAMA 1990; 264:1570.

201. Barinaga M. Wilson slashes spending for antismoking effort. Science 1992; 255:1348.

202. Frank E, Winkleby MA, Altman DG, et al. Predictors of physicians' smoking cessation advice. JAMA 1991; 266:3139.

203. Cummings SR, Coates TJ, Richard RJ, et al. Training physicians in counseling about smoking cessation. A randomized trial of the "Quit for Life" Program. Ann Intern Med 1989; 110:640.

204. Cohen SJ, Stookey GK, Katz BP, et al. Encouraging primary care physicians to help smokers quit. A randomized controlled trial. Ann Intern Med 1989; 110:648.

205. Manley M, Epps RP, Husten C, et al. Clinical interventions in tobacco control. A National Cancer Institute training program for physicians. JAMA 1991; 266:3172.

206. Gostin LO, Brandt AM, Cleary PD. Tobacco liability and public health policy. JAMA 1991; 266:3178.

207. Fiore MC. The new vital sign. Assessing and documenting smoking status. JAMA 1991; 266:3184.

Index

Page numbers followed by t and f stand for tables and figures, respectively.